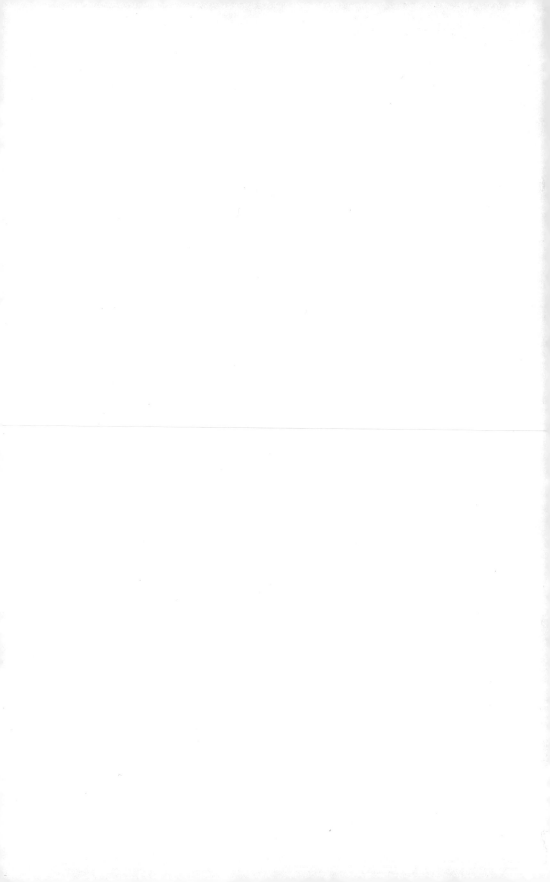

Perinatal Epidemiology

Perinatal Epidemiology

Edited by
MICHAEL B. BRACKEN

New York   Oxford
OXFORD UNIVERSITY PRESS
1984

Copyright © 1984 by Oxford University Press, Inc.

Library of Congress Cataloging in Publication Data
Main entry under title:

Perinatal epidemiology.

Bibliography: p.
Includes index.
1. Pregnancy, Complications of.   2. Infants (Newborn)
—Diseases.   3. Epidemiology.   I. Bracken, Michael B., 1942–
[DNLM: 1. Infant, Newborn, Diseases—Occurrence.
2. Pregnancy complications—Occurrence.   WS 420 P4406]
RG571.P42   1984   618.3′2   83-19350
ISBN 0-19-503389-2

Printing (last digit): 9 8 7 6 5 4 3 2

Printed in the United States of America

Mary Bradley Meyer, 1916–1982: An Appreciation

Epidemiology as a scientific discipline is primarily concerned with studies of population groups. Methods for such investigations have been developed, and an identifiable body of epidemiologic knowledge has emerged. Epidemiologists have increasingly served another role, that of analyzing and synthesizing data and knowledge derived from a variety of scientific disciplines, including the biologic and social sciences. Epidemiologists who are involved in such endeavors clearly must have breadth of knowledge, critical sensitivity, and analytic abilities. A practitioner of this type of epidemiologic activity to a superior degree was Mary Bradley Meyer, whose death occurred while this book was being prepared.

Mary Meyer's initial epidemiologic work was in infectious diseases, and more specifically on mumps. In these studies, she manifested those traits that characterized all of her future work: meticulous care in the collection of original data, insightful analysis, and the ability to make inferences that were both critical and imaginative within the framework of existing biologic knowledge.

While we were completing a study of the putative effects of intrauterine radiation exposure, Mary had the creative insight that this study could be extended to investigate possible radiation effects on the ova of the radiated mother by tracing and following up her children. This study had a ripple effect and stimulated her interest in the prenatal effects of cigarette smoking. She diligently obtained all the existing data sets and analyzed them. She then critically assessed the nature of all the published evidence, reviewed the experimental biologic bases for the epidemiologic data, and finally integrated these into what is the best holistic view of this issue.

Mary had the desire, motivation, and drive to learn the methods and substantive content of those fields that provide biologic insights necessary for interpreting epidemiologic data. Combined with a critical sensitivity and concern for good data, she transmitted these approaches to her colleagues and students. She will be sorely missed by all who had contact with her.

Abraham M. Lilienfeld, M.D., M.P.H., D.Sc.(Hon.)
University Distinguished Service Professor of Epidemiology
The Johns Hopkins University
School of Hygiene and Public Health

Preface

It has long been recognized that events during pregnancy influence the health and well-being of the newborn. This recognition, and the obvious need to provide integrated care to both mother and baby, has led to the establishment of perinatology as the medical specialty that bridges the gap between the obstetrician's concern for the pregnant woman and the care of her newborn by a pediatrician. Only recently have we begun to understand that events occurring long before pregnancy, sometimes inter-generationally, can affect our reproductive capabilities. We also now know that vicissitudes in our own uterine existence may profoundly influence the rest of our lives both physically and behaviorally. Population-based studies of these phenomena fall within the domain of perinatal epidemiology, which has evolved into a major subspecialty of epidemiology and an important component of perinatal medicine.

Illness in pregnancy and the perinatal period continue to be a major disease burden. In less technically developed countries, maternal mortality is fifty times or more greater than that found in Scandinavia and perinatal mortality, though seriously under-reported, is still documented as four or five times greater (World Health Organization, 1982). Areas with relatively high rates of infant mortality persist in the United States; the infant death rate in Washington, D.C. is three times greater than in Wyoming (National Center for Health Statistics, 1983). While the overall improvement in perinatal health over the last fifty years is possibly the single most impressive achievement in public health, the present inter- and intra-national variability in perinatal and maternal morbidity and mortality indicate that significant gains in the health of mothers and newborns continue to be possible. Even though it now appears that the relatively high rate of neonatal mortality in the

United States, compared with Scandinavia, for example, is due to the greater proportion of low birth weight and premature babies born in the United States, the reasons for the higher incidence of these conditions remain elusive and a question of high priority in the next decade.

Not only do pregnancy and the perinatal period incur significant health problems in their own right, but the search for etiologic risk factors for illness in adult life, including cardiovascular disease and cancer, increasingly need to take into account perinatal experiences. The administration of diethylstilbestrol to prevent miscarriage and its association with infertility, poor reproductive outcomes, and cancer in the adult life of the exposed fetus is a perinatal risk factor discussed in several chapters of the present volume. Thus, while the term perinatal has traditionally referred to the immediate period surrounding birth, a broader perspective is becoming increasingly necessary. Birth (or sometimes the inability to give birth) remains the central organizing event for perinatal epidemiology although we now extend our research foci beyond the immediate pre- and post-partum period.

Because mutagenesis is so closely linked to the carcinogenic process, perinatal epidemiology plays an expanding role in the surveillance of potential occupational and environmental health hazards. There is considerable interest in using pregnancy outcomes, especially miscarriage and selected congenital malformations, as early signal indicators for environmental exposures which may increase cancer risks but which might otherwise remain undetected for many years. A chapter in the present book explicitly covers this topic and it is discussed in several others.

Another expanding component of perinatal epidemiology is the evaluation of efficacy and risk attending innovations in perinatal medicine. While innovations often involve high technology (ultrasound, fetal monitoring, and pharmacologic patient management for example), they equally include new approaches to service delivery, e.g. birthing centers, as well as innovations in patient and physician education. Randomized clinical trials are the most elegant method of evaluating innovation but have not yet achieved the widespread acceptance in perinatal medicine that they enjoy in some other medical specialties. Thus, this topic is given some prominence in the book.

All epidemiologists carry a dual obligation. The first is to contribute to knowledge and, we hope, solutions to conditions currently afflicting the public's well-being. The second is to further develop our scientific methodology so that this unique approach to medical research is even better equipped to address the next generation of health problems. Contrary to what we are told by some who would write a requiem for epidemiology (Rothman, 1981), epidemiologists will increasingly be called upon to address the world's major health problems. Identification in the laboratory of "super genes" and powerful toxins will still demand an explanation of how such causal agents operate within the multifactorial complexity of human populations.

The stimulus for the present volume was the need for a contemporary and comprehensive text for students taking my courses in perinatal epidemiology at Yale. This book is in debt to earlier texts (Chipman et al., 1966; Kretchmer and Hasselmyer, 1974; Brent and Harris, 1976) and should be used as a companion to more specialized monographs now available in selected subjects and referred to throughout the volume.

No one is more aware than I of omissions in the topics covered by the volume. Many issues that deserve to have been included in the book were not. Some scientists could not be enticed into the dubious joys of writing a review chapter; others had scheduling difficulties. The epidemiology of respiratory distress syndrome, transplacental carcinogenesis, and some congenital malformations might all have merited a fresh review here but must be sought elsewhere. For other important conditions, such as intra-ventricular hemorrhage, so little is known about their epidemiology that a detailed review was considered premature. The inclusion of some topics admittedly reflect the broad view of perinatal epidemiology adopted by the editor. Thus, hydatidiform mole epidemiology has benefited from recent major advances in our knowledge of the genetics of the disease and provides a rare example of the association between an anomalous pregnancy outcome and subsequent carcinoma.

Unwanted pregnancy and induced abortion exert such profound effects on the epidemiology of many perinatal outcomes, on their etiology as well as on the population groups they most affect, that a review of their own epidemiologies seemed appropriate. Other substantive topics are more obviously central to perinatal epidemiology as well as being active fields of research and of major public health interest. These include the epidemiology of genetic and chromosomal disorders, spontaneous abortion, selected congenital malformations, low birthweight, prematurity, perinatal mortality, sudden infant death syndrome, neurobehavioral disorders, infertility, multiple births, and perinatal viral infections.

The methodological part of the book discusses selected recent advances in techniques for conducting perinatal epidemiologic research. These chapters cover sampling and statistical analysis, the design and conduct of randomized clinical trials, strategies for investigating the drug etiology of congenital malformations, assessments of neurobehavioral dysfunction, evaluation of environmental and occupational exposures, and new techniques for evaluating perinatal mortality.

Perinatal Epidemiology will have served its purpose when it requires complete revision due to research done by those students who are the principal audience for the present volume.

New Haven   M.B.B.
January 1984

REFERENCES

Brent, R.L. and Harris, M.I. (1976). Editors, *Prevention of embryonic, fetal, and perinatal disease.* Bethesda, Md.: National Institutes of Health. Publication No. (NIH) 76-853.

Chipman, S.S., Lilienfeld, A.M., Greenberg, B.G., and Donnelly, J.F. (1966). Editors, *Research methodology and needs in perinatal studies.* Springfield, Ill.: Charles C Thomas.

Kretchmer, N. and Hasselmyer, E.G. (1974). Editors, *Horizons in perinatal research: Implications for clinical care.* New York: John Wiley.

National Center for Health Statistics (1983). Annual Summary of Births, Deaths, Marriages, and Divorce: United States, 1982. *Monthly Vital Statistics Report 31*: No. 13, October 5.

Rothman, K.J. (1981). The rise and fall of epidemiology, 1950–2000 A.D. *New Engl. J. Med. 304*: 600–602.

World Health Organization (1982). *World Health Statistics, Vital Statistics and Causes of Death.* Geneva: World Health Organization.

Acknowledgments

A number of students commented on chapter drafts and offered useful suggestions for changes. These were Carolyn Anderman, Anne Berg, John Collins, Linda Leo, Kristine M. Napier, and Risé K. Phillips. The staff of the Yale Perinatal Epidemiology Unit provided numerous services and I am especially grateful to Carol Bryce-Buchanan, JoAnne Mezger, Lynn Gaylord, Kathleen Pinto, Jean-ellen McSharry, Sue Curtis, Robert Silten, Karen Hellenbrand, Mary Jo Shepard, Bernice Carr, Cheryl Kassow, Michelle Pasternak, Coleen Pendleton, Marsha Silverman, Elaine Scharadin, and Susan Arnold. Jeffrey House, my editor at Oxford University Press, and Managing Editor Ellen B. Fuchs made valued comments and kept the entire project on schedule. The book would never have seen the light of day without the invaluable secretarial, managerial and, occasionally, even diplomatic skills of Ann Wetherbee. Without exception the contributors kept to deadlines (well, almost), were responsive to editorial suggestions, and produced very fine chapters. I am most appreciative of their work and hope they feel the volume is a suitable vehicle for their contributions. As always, the support of my family, Maryann, James, and Sara, proved to be crucial and unwavering.

Contributors*

Eva Alberman, M.D.
Professor of Clinical
Epidemiology
The London Hospital Medical
College
University of London
London, England

Milton Alter, M.D., Ph.D.
Professor and Chairman
Department of Neurology
Temple University
School of Medicine
Philadelphia, Pennsylvania

Gordon Allen, M.D.
Medical Statistician
Division of Biometry and
Epidemiology
National Institute of Mental
Health
U.S. Dept. of Health and
Human Services
Rockville, Maryland

Warren A. Andiman, M.D.
Assistant Professor of
Pediatrics and Epidemiology
School of Medicine
Yale University
New Haven, Connecticut

Leiv S. Bakketeig, M.D.
Professor and Chairman
The University of Trondheim
Faculty of Medicine
Department of Community
Medicine
University Hospital
Trondheim, Norway

Mark A. Belsey, M.D.
Medical Officer
Special Programme of
Research in Human
Reproduction
World Health Organization
Geneva, Switzerland

Michael B. Bracken, Ph.D.,
M.P.H.
Associate Professor of
Research in Epidemiology
and Obstetrics and
Gynecology
Director, Perinatal
Epidemiology Unit
School of Medicine
Yale University
New Haven, Connecticut

* Present affiliations

Willard Cates, Jr., M.D.,
  M.P.H.
Director, Division of Venereal
  Disease Control
Center for Prevention Services
Centers for Disease Control
Atlanta, Georgia

Brenda Eskenazi, Ph.D.
Assistant Professor of
  Epidemiology
  (Environmental Health)
School of Medicine
Yale University
New Haven, Connecticut

Daniel H, Freeman, Jr., Ph.D.
Associate Professor of Public
  Health (Biostatistics)
School of Medicine
Yale University
New Haven, Connecticut

Jane E. Gordon, Ph.D.
National Institute for
  Occupational Safety and
  Health
Robert A. Taft Laboratories
Cincinnati, Ohio

Kenji Hayashi, M.D.
Director, Maternal and Child
  Health Division
Institute of Public Health
Tokyo, Japan

Howard J. Hoffman, M.A.
Chief, Biometry Branch
Epidemiology and Biometry
  Research Program
National Institute of Child
  Health and Human
  Development
National Institutes of Health
Bethesda, Maryland

Theodore R. Holford, Ph.D.
Associate Professor of Public
  Health (Biostatistics)
School of Medicine
Yale University
New Haven, Connecticut

Ernest B. Hook, M.D.
Bureau of Maternal and Child
  Health
Albany, New York

Dorothy M. Horstmann, M.D.,
  Sc.D., Dr. Med. Sci.
John Rodman Paul Professor
  Emeritus of Epidemiology
  and Pediatrics
School of Medicine
Yale University
New Haven, Connecticut

James F. Jekel, M.D., M.P.H.
C.-E.A. Winslow Professor of
  Epidemiology and Public
  Health
School of Medicine
Yale University
New Haven, Connecticut

Lorraine V. Klerman, Dr. P.H.
Professor of Public Health
Heller Graduate School
Brandeis University
Waltham, Massachusetts

Jennie Kline, Ph.D.
Research Scientist
New York State Psychiatric
  Institute and Associate
  Research Scientist
Sergievsky Center
Columbia University
New York, New York

Olav Meirik, M.D.
Associate Professor of
  Obstetrics and Gynecology
University Hospital of Uppsala
Sweden

Ann R. Titmuss Oakley, Ph.D.
National Perinatal
  Epidemiology Unit
Radcliffe Infirmary
Oxford, England

Frank W. Oechsi, Ph.D.
Associate Research
  Demographer
Child Health and Development
  Studies
School of Public Health
University of California,
  Berkeley
Oakland, California

Donald R. Peterson, M.D.,
  M.P.H.
Professor and Chairman
School of Public Health and
  Community Medicine
Department of Epidemiology
University of Washington
Seattle, Washington

David T. Scott, Ph.D.
Assistant Professor of
  Pediatrics
New Born Special Care Unit
School of Medicine
Yale University
New Haven, Connecticut

Zena Stein, M.A., M.B., B. Ch.
Professor of Public Health
  (Epidemiology)
School of Public Health
Columbia University
New York, New York

Bea J. van den Berg, M.D.
Adjunct Professor Biostatistics
Director, Child Health and
  Development Studies
School of Public Health
University of California,
  Berkeley
Oakland, California

Contents

xix

Contents

I
Epidemiology of Perinatal Disorders

1

Human Chromosome Abnormalities*

Ernest B. Hook

TYPES OF CHROMOSOME ABNORMALITIES

Chromosome abnormalities may be distinguished in two independent ways: whether they are of germinal or somatic cell origin and whether they involve numerical or structural abnormality. These distinctions generate four subtypes of abnormality: (1) germinal-numerical (e.g., the 47,+21 pattern of Down syndrome), (2) germinal-structural [e.g., the structural interchange trisomies such as 46,−14, +t(14q,21q), which may also produce Down syndrome], (3) somatic-numerical (e.g., the 45,X/46,XX pattern associated sometimes with Turner syndrome, and (4) somatic-structural (e.g., the various heterogeneous chromosome breaks and rearrangements observed in cultured lymphocytes and other somatic tissues that may occur spontaneously or may be induced by somatic mutagens). There is one outcome, the rare 46,XY/XX pattern resulting in true hermaphroditism, that fits none of these subdivisions but is produced by either dispermy or fusion of two fertilized eggs.

The precise differentiation of individuals whose abnormalities are of germinal cell origin from those whose somatic abnormalities have occurred at an early state of embryogenesis is often impossible, but in

---

* The epidemiology of cytogenetic abnormalities is a vast topic and justice cannot be done to it in a book-length chapter. Moreover, discoveries are being made at a rapid pace. It is likely a good deal of material such as that on maternal age effects for Down's syndrome will not be quickly outdated. But for other topics, such as the associations of fragile chromosomes or chromosome rearrangements with abnormal phenotypes, we are clearly at the beginning of our knowledge. I have not cited all pertinent material but have instead indicated earlier reviews where further citations and discussion can be found. I have tended to cite, in addition to previous reviews, more recent papers that are not listed in the earlier references. Of course, any author is most cognizant of his own work. I have tended to cite my own earlier reviews on some matters because I am familiar with them and believe them to be comprehensive, at least at the time they were written. If I have thereby omitted some papers that should be cited, the reader may find them noted in the earlier references.

the present discussion this will generally not be an issue. This chapter will be confined largely to germinal or somatic abnormalities occurring sufficiently early in gestation to produce abnormal chromosome lines in a significant proportion of the organism's cells.

A distinction should be made between the cytogenetic genotype of an individual and the associated phenotype. For instance, several different genotypes can produce the Down syndrome phenotype: 47,+21 (nonmosaic); 47,+21/46 (i.e., mosaicism); unbalanced Robertsonian translocations involving the long arm of the 21 chromosome [e.g., 46,−14,+(14q,21q), and other rearrangements resulting in a triple dose of 21q22 band]. (For discussion of the latter point, see Summitt, 1981.) The 47,+21 (apparent nonmosaic) occurs in about 92–94% of cases with the phenotype, recognized 47,+21 mosaicism in about 1.5–4.5%, Robertsonian translocation trisomies in about 1.5–4.5%, and other patterns in less than 1%. Occasional instances of Down syndrome phenotype without detectable cytogenetic abnormality have also been reported, perhaps with cryptic mosaicism or structural rearrangement. The ratio of Robertsonian translocation to 47,+21 cases varies with maternal age of the population; the higher the proportion of older mothers, the lower the ratio (see Hook, 1981).

Although numerical chromosome abnormalities have been well described, we are only beginning to learn the extent of structural abnormalities in our species. With diagnostic advances, an increasing number of conditions of hitherto unknown etiology have been associated with subtle structural abnormalities. Chromosome abnormalities have been found even in patients with disorders previously regarded as specific locus mutations. Some of the conditions listed in McKusick's catalog, *Mendelian Inheritance in Man* (1978), that investigators have very recently found to be associated with specific cytogenetic errors are X-linked mental retardation and megalotestes (McKusick No. 30957) with a fragile site at Xq28; Prader-Willi (a possible autosomal recessive—McKusick No. 26400) with deletion of 15q (11–12); aniridia–Wilms' tumor (a possible autosomal recessive—McKusick No. 27780) with an 11p13 deletion; and instances of retinoblastoma (an autosomal dominant—McKusick No. 18020) with a 13q14 deletion (see Hook, 1983a).

PREVALENCE OF CHROMOSOME ABNORMALITIES AT DIFFERENT STAGES OF LIFE

At the time pregnancy is first recognizable clinically, about five weeks after the onset of the last menstrual period, the proportion of recognized human conceptuses with cytogenetic abnormality is about

4

5% (Hook, 1981a, 1983a). Almost all of these abnormalities (4.7%) are clinically significant because in all likelihood they will either cause embryonic or fetal death, or carry a high risk of retardation or congenital defect in conceptuses surviving to livebirth.

Martin et al. (1982) reported that about 9% of human sperm have chromosome abnormalities. These data would imply (assuming that chromosomal composition of gametes does not influence zygote formation and that there is at least as high a proportion of cytogenetically abnormal ova as sperm) that as many as 15% of all zygotes have some chromosome aberration. Assuming this figure, and the 5% estimate at gestational age five weeks, then at least 10% of zygotes are lost in the three weeks after fertilization.

In livebirths studied to date, the proportion with cytogenetic abnormality has dropped to 0.6%, about half of which are clinically significant (Table 1-1). The distribution of types of cytogenetic abnormalities in embryonic and fetal deaths appears in the appropriate section below (p. 14).

These estimates are derived from the pooled results of surveys from Japan, Australia, North America, and Europe done in the late 1960s and 1970s. The precise figures, particularly for trisomics, will vary with the maternal age distribution of the childbearing population. Thus, the livebirth prevalence rate of the 47,+21 genotype is now about 1.0 per 1000 in most European countries and Japan, where the proportion of childbearing women aged 35 and older is about 5–7%, but it has been as high as 1.6–1.8 per 1000 when the proportion of older mothers was 10% or higher (Hook, 1981, 1983c). Environmental factors may affect the maternal age-specific rates to an unknown

Table 1-1. Estimated Prevalence of Chromosome Abnormalities at Various Gestational Stages

Gestational age (weeks)	All abnormalities (%)	Clinically significant abnormalities[a] (%)
5	5.0	4.7
8	4.2	3.8
12	2.4	2.1
16	1.1	0.8
20	0.8	0.5
28	0.7	0.4
Livebirth (mode = 40 weeks)	0.6	0.3

[a] Proportion is 0.1% less if XXXs and XYYx are excluded.
Source: Hook (1981b, 1982).

extent, although evidence for any sizeable contribution to overall frequency or cytogenetic defect is still lacking.

After birth the higher mortality due to congenital defects and other associated disorders results in a progressive decrease in the proportion of those with unbalanced chromosomal genotypes in the population. For Down syndrome, for example, mortality in a group born in the late 1950s and early 1960s had reached nearly 65% by age ten years (Fabia and Drolette, 1970); comparable figures are probably lower now because of more frequent therapeutic intervention for congenital heart defects and infectious disorders (see below). The XXX, XXY, and XYY conditions are apparent exceptions. They are not associated with any demonstrated increase in mortality.

BIOLOGIC AND DEMOGRAPHIC FACTORS

Maternal Age

Advanced maternal age is the only factor (aside from transmissible parental chromosome abnormality) that exhibits an unequivocal association with chromosomal disorders. Trisomies 21, 18, 13, and conditions with extra X chromosomes all demonstrate a maternal age association. The effect is best documented for the $47,+21$ genotype. (See references and discussion in Hook, 1981, 1983c; Carothers et al., 1978.) There is also strong evidence that many of the nonviable trisomies have an association with advanced maternal age, including trisomy 7, 15, 16, 20, and 22 (Stein et al., 1980). It is likely that this association exists for other lethal trisomies as well, but relatively small numbers have been studied. In contrast, monosomy X (45,X) is associated with lower maternal age (Warburton et al., 1980). The reasons for this association are unknown. Penrose suggested that there are maternal age independent and dependent classes of Down syndrome (Penrose and Smith, 1966); that is, there are "background" factors independent of age that may result in Down syndrome, and superimposed upon these are age-related factors. Depending on the maternal age structure of the entire liveborn population, the proportion of putative age-independent cases occurring in all newborns may vary considerably from, say, under 50% when there is a high proportion of older mothers, to over 60% as the number of older mothers declines (Hook, 1981, 1983a).

There are many possible ways of modeling the change in rate of Down syndrome to maternal age (Lamson and Hook, 1981). One that fits the observed data well between maternal ages 20 and 49, and is consistent with the suggestion of Penrose, may be obtained by

6

postulating the combination of a first-order exponential increase with age and a flat background maternal age-independent component (Lamson and Hook, 1980). Thus the equation for the rate y may be given as: $a + \exp(b + cx)$ where a, b, and c are constants (about 6×10^{-4}, -17, and 0.3, respectively, and x is mother's age in years. (The parameter for the maternal age-independent class is a, and the rest of the equation describes the superimposed component that changes with age.) At maternal age 20 the bulk of cases are maternal age independent in this formulation; at about age 30 approximately half are age dependent and half are age independent; and by the 40s the vast majority of cases are age dependent. Data from a recent Swedish study by Lindsjo support this model (Lamson and Hook, 1981).

Under maternal age 20 there may be a slight increase in rate of Down syndrome with decreasing age in at least some populations. (See discussion and references in Hook, 1981, 1983c.)

There are not many analyses correlating age with other chromosome abnormalities. The rate of occurrence of the $47,+18$ genotype appears to increase with age with the same slope that $47,+21$ does. The occurrence rate of $47,XXX$ also increases with maternal age and may, at ages 45 and over, exhibit an even more pronounced correlation than Down syndrome (Hook, 1981b; Carothers et al., 1978). Regression analysis of data gathered at amniocentesis suggests that the maternal age effect for $47,+13$ is not as strong as that for $47,+21$, and that the rate of increase of $47,XXX$ with age at higher ages may not be as pronounced as originally suspected (Schreinemachers et al., 1982).

Ayme and Lippman-Hand (1982) suggest that the maternal age effect for liveborn trisomies is in part attributable to a lower rate of spontaneous abortion of trisomic fetuses in older mothers. There is little evidence for such effect after the usual time of amniocentesis, judging by maternal ages of chromosomally abnormal fetuses that survive to livebirth or are spontaneously aborted (Hook, 1983b). Moreover, this hypothesis is also inconsistent with the observation that there is little if any maternal age effect for translocation trisomies.

Paternal Age

Even though the extra chromosome is of paternal origin in those zygotes with the XYY genotype, in 20–25% of those with the $47,+21$ genotype, in 60% of those with XXY genotype, and probably a large number of other abnormalities (see Hook, 1981, for reference), no firm proof of a strong paternal age effect (independent of a maternal age effect) has been demonstrated. This applies also for those cases with the 45,X genotype, in 75% of whom the missing X chromosome is of paternal origin. For some disorders (e.g., the XYY genotype), the *lack* of increase with paternal age appears well established; in fact, there may even be a negative association (Carothers et al., 1978). For the 47,+21 genotype there is conflicting evidence with some positive and some negative studies. (For citation of studies see Hook, 1983b; Hook and Cross, 1982.) Perhaps this is best explained by evidence of a small increase of the order of 1% per year with paternal age (Hook et al., 1980; Hook and Cross, 1982a). Stene et al. (1981) reported a strong association of paternal age with Down syndrome diagnosed prenatally, in a German study. Although the analysis of Stene et al. appears statistically acceptable, the results were not replicated in a larger data set from New York State (Hook and Cross, 1982b). Statistical fluctuation (despite the reported p values), temporal or geographic variation, or other factors could explain the differences. The extent of inconsistency in the available data renders improbable the consideration of advanced paternal age as a strong ubiquitous risk factor for the occurrence of Down syndrome.

Birth Order

The association of parental age with Down syndrome has been found to be independent of birth order in the majority of studies. Nevertheless, after appropriate age adjustment, there is evidence suggesting a slight positive association of the Down syndrome phenotype with firstborn status (Hook, 1981). There is no evidence for any birth order effect for the sex chromosome abnormalities (see Hook, 1981; Carothers et al., 1978).

Family Clustering

Individuals with a structural chromosome abnormality, even if putatively normal phenotypically because they have only a balanced rearrangement, are at high risk to have children with significant unbalanced rearrangements. Such rearrangements are associated with retardation and congenital anomalies because of the inheritance of translocations in an "unbalanced" state by the offspring (Hamerton, 1971). Even balanced (reciprocal but not Robertsonian) translocations, if de novo mutants, are associated with higher risk for mental retardation (Jacobs, 1974).

The major clinical interest, however, concerns clustering within nuclear families of numerical abnormalities such as the 47,+21 genotype. In liveborns there is good evidence that 47,+21 tends to recur in

8

families. The estimated relative risk for a Down syndrome livebirth is perhaps 10- to 20-fold higher for a younger mother who has already borne an affected child (Hook and Cross, 1982a). (This, moreover, excludes known mosaic parents.) An increased recurrence risk for other types of trisomy has been suggested but not documented in livebirths. For trisomies of all types resulting in spontaneous embryonic and fetal deaths, the studies of Jacobs (1979) indicate that the relative odds of recurrence of a trisomy, not necessarily the same one, if another fetal death occurs, is about 14. Recurrence of the same trisomy (homoaneuploid, as defined by Hecht, 1977) may be attributable to cryptic parental mosaicism. Clustering of different trisomies in families (heteroaneuploidy) may be associated with genetic and environmental factors predisposing to nondisjunction in general; however, such causal factors remain speculative in humans, although they are established in drosophila. (See further discussion and references in Hook, 1981; Hook and Cross, 1982a.)

Temporal and Spatial Clustering Including Seasonality

Considerable literature exists on the purported seasonality of the Down syndrome phenotype, but the data are quite inconsistent. Moreover, it is difficult to find any unifying explanation for the different trends reported, except, perhaps, statistical fluctuation. (See references and discussion in Lilienfeld, 1969; Hook, 1981.) There have also been occasional reports of clusters of 47, +18; but, again, no episodes that conclusively exclude statistical fluctuation as an explanation.

With regard to secular changes in crude livebirth prevalence rates, the diminished relative fertility of older women compared to younger women has resulted in declines in the rates of 47, +21 and other viable abnormalities associated with increased parental age (Hook, 1981; Huether and Gummere, 1982). Amniocentesis and selective induced abortion have also had an effect on rates since 1975, but much less than the demographic changes—at least in New York State through 1981.

Some evidence for an increase in the maternal age-specific rates of Down syndrome livebirths in women 35 years of age and older has been reported, as has an increase in the translocation Down syndrome in 1973. (See discussion and references in Hook and Cross, 1982a.) The explanation for these changes remains unknown, but both may be due to statistical fluctuation. (Very recent analysis based on rates at amniocentesis suggests, however, that this apparent increase has subsided if, in fact, it was real—Schreinemachers et al., 1982.)

9

Ethnic and Racial Factors

Although data are sparse, the clearest trend appears to be a lower rate of the XYY genotype in black than in white livebirths. In six studies to date, five summarized by Hook (1974) and one later study (Hara et al., 1976), there were *no* XYYs among 3732 black male livebirths but 18 XYYs among 19,515 white male livebirths (0.9 per 1000) in the same studies. All were done in the United States during the 1960s and 1970s. The difference is significant at the .04 level (Fisher's exact test, two-tailed). For the XXY genotype there is a suggestive but not significant trend in the other direction: 1.60 per 1000 in blacks versus 1.13 per 1000 in whites. The XXY genotype is associated with increased maternal age, and the mean age of black parents is younger than that of white parents. Thus, if precise data on parental age were available in those studied, adjustment for this factor would enhance the difference between the races in the livebirth prevalence of the XXY genotype.

With regard to Down syndrome, one study reported higher maternal age-specific rates in whites than in blacks at more advanced ages (Stark and White, 1977), whereas data of another study are consistent with lower rates in whites at more advanced ages (Sever et al., 1970). Data from one study in Israel suggest higher maternal age-specific rates of Down syndrome in livebirths to Jews of Asian and African origin than those of European or American origin (Hook and Harlap, 1979). Thus, with the possible exception of Asian or African Jews, there are apparently no grounds for adjusting maternal age-specific risks for ethnic and racial factors in genetic counseling for Down syndrome. (For further discussion and references see Hook and Porter, 1977.)

Socioeconomic Factors

Only one study of Down syndrome has found any association with socioeconomic status (Harlap, 1973). This report from Israel, however (which found higher rates in those of lower status), may have confounded ethnic with socioeconomic factors, because maternal age-specific rates, as noted previously, are higher in the Asian and African Jews in this study—who are of lower average socioeconomic status. Cohen et al. (1977) reported no difference between parents of Down syndrome cases and controls in occupation or education. Warburton et al. (1980a, 1980c), in studies of chromosome abnormalities detected in spontaneous embryonic and fetal deaths, found a higher rate of abnormality in dead fetuses of "private" than those of "public" patients at fetal age 16–28 gestational weeks, but not under 16 weeks. The total rate of abnormality was 39.9% in the private group and 29.5% in the public group. Half of the excess was attributable to triploidy, which represented the only significant difference among the chromosome abnormality categories. The only category higher in the public (10.2%) rather than private (6.9%) group was that involving "other" aberrations, mostly instances in which there were double trisomies or other multiple anomalies. The study population, however, is quite heterogeneous, racially and ethnically, and it is possible that these population characteristics—rather than socioeconomic status—are responsible for the observed differences.

Inbreeding and Consanguinity

There is only one study on human populations, from Kuwait (Alfi et al., 1980), that suggests any association of inbreeding—and, by inference, of autosomal recessive genes—with the livebirth prevalence of Down syndrome. Possibly such genes may be restricted to only a few populations. (For further discussion and references see Hook, 1981, 1983c.)

PUTATIVE ENVIRONMENTAL FACTORS

Radiation

It has long been known that ionizing radiation induces nondisjunction in drosophila (Mavor, 1922). Nevertheless, despite extensive investigation, the evidence to date in humans is inconclusive. Down syndrome has been the most extensively investigated abnormality. There are both positive (e.g., Alberman et al., 1972; Uchida, 1977) and negative studies (Schull and Neel, 1962; Cohen et al., 1977), the results of which are difficult to reconcile. No inferences are yet possible regarding the possible effects of radiation on Down syndrome in livebirths. (See other references and further discussion in Hook and Porter, 1977.) Regarding other abnormalities, data have become available from the studies of Awa on children of parents exposed to the atomic blasts at Hiroshima and Nagasaki. These data are presented in detail here because of their importance and because, to my knowledge, they have yet to be published anywhere, although they were presented at the 1981 International Congress of Human Genetics. The results (Awa, 1981) pertain to 5762 individuals born to exposed parents and 5058 born to control parents between May 1946 and 1958, and subsequently studied at about age 13. Because the children survived to this age, it is unlikely that many phenotypically severe aberrations, such as autosomal trisomies or unbalanced translocations, would be found. Nevertheless, results on sex chromosome abnormalities and balanced translocations are available, and these appear in Table 1-2. There is no evidence for any association of

Table 1-2. Chromosome Abnormality Prevalence in Individuals Born to Parents Exposed to Radiation at Hiroshima–Nagasaki and to Controls[a]

| Abnormalities | Radiation exposed | | | | |
	Father only	Mother only	Mother and Father	Either parent	Controls
Sex chromosome abnormalities[b]					
XYY	3.0	0.6	0	1.1	1.3
XXY	1.5	2.5	2.4	2.3	2.6
Other male sex chromosomal abnormalities	0	0.6	0	0.4	0
XXX	2.6	0.5	2.2	1.3	0.7
45,X	0	0	0	0	0
Other female sex chromosomal abnormalities	0	0.5	2.2	0.6	0.7
Subtotal (all sexes)	3.5	2.3	3.4	2.8	2.6
Autosomal trisomy	0	0	0	0	0
Autosomal structural rearrangement					
Balanced Robertsonian (Dq/Dq)	0.7	0.9	0	0.7	0.2
(Dq/Gq)	0	0.6	0	0.3	0
(Gq/Gq)	0	0	0	0	0
Reciprocal	0.7	0.3	2.3	0.7	1.6
Inversion	0	0.3	0	0.2	0.4
Other	0	0	0	0	0
Subtotal (autosomal structural)	1.4	2.1	2.3	1.9	2.2
Unbalanced autosomal supernumerary	0.7	0	0	0.2	0.2
Other autosomal	0	0.6	0	0.3	0
Subtotal (all autosomal)	2.1	2.7	2.3	2.4	2.4
Grand total	5.6	5.0	5.7	5.2	4.9
Number of cases					
Males	667	1585	410	2662	2267
Females	775	1861	464	3100	2791
Both	1442	3446	874	5762	5058

[a] Rates per 1000 individuals.

[b] Rates of sex chromosome abnormalities are sex specific (e.g., rates of XYYs are in males only). Rates in subtotal are those in both sexes.

Source: Personal communication from A. Awa, September 27, 1981 on data collected through July 17, 1981.

significance, but in view of the low prevalence rates, the numbers analyzed are still relatively few. Further data are being accumulated.

Brewen et al. (1975), in a controversial investigation on prisoners, showed that high doses of radiation induce germinal chromosome structural rearrangements. These observations, however, are not directly pertinent to the question of effects of low-dose irradiation.

Viruses

The association of Down syndrome at livebirth with hepatitis in the mother, suggested some years ago, has not stood up to statistical reexamination. It does appear, however, that individuals with Down syndrome are more likely to develop hepatitis (Blumberg, 1978). The possible implication in the etiology of Down syndrome of a slow virus, that may act by inducing nondisjunction seems a viable possibility. The reported association of Alzheimer disease, leukemia, and Down syndrome within families (Heston, 1977) is consistent with this. In addition, for reasons that are not as yet understood, it appears that most if not all Down syndrome individuals who survive beyond the age of 50 will develop clinical and pathologic findings similar to if not identical to those of Alzheimer disease. A slow virus that induces nondisjunction and then is incorporated into the cellular genome of the individual formed by the affected gamete might account for these observations.

Oral Contraceptives

There is a considerable body of literature on the topic of oral contraceptives and their possible association with chromosomal abnormalities in offspring. Most studies have revealed no significant effect, but Lejeune and Prieur (1979) have claimed a marked association with Down syndrome in a large series from France. (See Hook, 1981, for earlier references.)

Other Agents

A suggestive association of spermicides with tetraploidy in abortuses (Warburton et al., 1980b) and Down syndrome (Jick et al., 1981; Rothman, 1982) has been reported. Three recent studies, however, have failed to find a significant association of Down syndrome with spermicide use (Huggins et al., 1982; Polednak et al., 1982; Bracken and Vita, 1983).

With this possible exception—in addition to the report cited above of Brewen et al. (1975) on radiation-induced structural germinal cell abnormalities in prisoners—there is no direct evidence for association of gonadal chromosome abnormality with environmental factors. Nonetheless, it appears likely that agents that are known to cause germinal specific locus mutations in experimental mammals may well induce germinal *structural* chromosome rearrangements in humans, as has been found for radiation (Brewen et al., 1975). Little is known, however, concerning the gonadal effects of the numerous agents (aside from radiation) that have been observed to induce somatic chromosome *breakage* in vitro or even in vivo. With regard to *numerical* chromosome abnormalities, I am not aware of any agents known to induce nondisjunction in experimental animals, with the exception of ionizing irradiation. Radiomimetic chemicals would presumably, have the same effect in experimental animals.

ASSOCIATION OF CHROMOSOME DISORDERS WITH MORBIDITY AND MORTALITY

Embryonic and Fetal Deaths

The proportion of chromosome abnormalities associated with embryonic fetal deaths at various stages of gestation is given in Table 1-1. Although the presence of some of these abnormalities (e.g., XXY, XYY, and balanced translocations) is probably coincidentally associated with embryonic and fetal deaths, these groups represent considerably less than 5% of the total with cytogenetic abnormality. Distributions of abnormalities appear in Tables 1-3 and 1-4. Several factors of interest may be emphasized. The most prevalent single abnormality is 45,X, a genotype associated with Turner syndrome in those that survive to livebirth. Apparently about 99% of 45,X conceptuses alive at the fifth week do not survive gestation. Yet postnatal

Table 1-3. Percentage Distribution of Chromosome Abnormality in Six Cytogenetic Studies of Embryonic and Fetal Deaths up to Age 28 Weeks

	XO	Trisomy	Triploidy	Tetraploidy	*Gross structural abnormalities*	*Combination and mosaics*
Range in six studies	15.4–34.7	44.8–58.6	9.8–20.3	2.5–8.3	1.3–4.5	0.7–7.7
Mean in 1499 studied	22.9	52.5	14.6	4.3	3.6	4.0

Source: Calculated by Hook (1982) from data in Warburton (1980a).

14

Table 1-4. Distribution of Abnormalities in Livebirths[a]

Numerical		Structural	
47,+21	10	Interchange Down syndrome	0.5
47,+18	1	Interchange Patau syndrome	0.3
47,+13	1	Cri du chat, 5p-	0.2
47,XXY	5	46,X, iso X	0.2
47,XYY	5	Xq28 ("fragile")	5
47,XXX	5	All others including supernumerary	3
45,X	0.5		
46,XX/45,X	5[b]		
All others	0.2		
Total	32.7		9.2

[a] Estimated rates per 10,000.

[b] Not all clinically significant.

Source: Calculated from data in Hook and Hamerton (1977) and unpublished data.

mortality for 45,X individuals (Turner syndrome) is relatively normal. Perhaps those surviving to livebirth are cryptic 45,X/46,XX mosaics. The most frequent trisomy is 47,+16, but all those affected die during gestation. Trisomies for every chromosome except number one have been observed, but only trisomies X, 21, 18, 13, and the XXY and XYY conditions are viable. (Occasionally trisomies 8, 9, 11, 12, and 22 do survive to birth.) However, even trisomy 21 is associated with a fetal mortality of about 70%, and it is likely that embryonic mortality for trisomy 13 and 18 is even higher. (See Warburton et al., 1980a, for data on specific trisomies.) Triploidy is frequently associated with partial hydatidiform moles (Chapter 13).

Deaths in Infancy and Early Childhood

Although relatively few studies exist, it is of interest that the overall proportion of abnormalities in children dying in the first year of life is about 5–7%, the same as the observed rate in "stillbirths" (≥28 weeks). At least 95% of those infants with 47,+13 and 47,+18 genotypes expire in the first year of life, as do a significant proportion of those with Down syndrome. The mortality rate of Down syndrome infants depends on the vigor with which infections are treated and on the likelihood of these individuals receiving surgical correction of congenital heart defects, duodenal atresia, and other associated malformations. The mortality rate of Down syndrome children has decreased markedly since 1950, and it is difficult to establish any "stable" predictive life table for such individuals. A study of individuals in Massachusetts who were born between 1950 and 1967 with

Down syndrome estimated that survival to the age of ten was about 65% in this group (Fabia and Drolette, 1970). The survival rate was about 76% in those of both sexes without congenital heart defects, 45% in males with congenital heart defects, but only 32% in females with congenital heart defects. This reverses the usual male–female relationship in childhood mortality.

Congenital Defects

Most chromosome abnormalities are associated with a spectrum of congenital structural abnormalities that are often specific for the cytogenetic aberration. Some exceptions to this are balanced rearrangements, and the XYY and XXX genotypes. The specific patterns are noted in detail elsewhere (deGrouchy and Turleau, 1977). It has been estimated that about 4–8% of all children with a serious malformation have a chromosome abnormality (Hook, 1983a). This approach assumes that the phenotype of Down syndrome is itself a morphologic defect. If one includes only those who have some defined structural abnormality in addition (e.g., duodenal atresia), then the proportion is about 2.5–5%. It has also been estimated that 6–7.5% of all livebirths with a congenital heart defect present in infancy or diagnosed in childhood have Down syndrome. This proportion is 10% if those with all chromosome abnormalities are included (Hook, 1983a).

Mental Retardation

Among "severe" retardates—those with IQ under 50—about 20–30% have been found to have Down syndrome, and probably 1–2% have other chromosome abnormalities as well. Among those with moderate retardation (IQ 50–69), tentative indirect estimates suggest that 7–8% of females and perhaps a higher proportion (10–12%) of males have some chromosome abnormality. This includes, among other categories, 2–3% with Down syndrome, about 1% with sex chromosome abnormality, and an estimated 4% of females and possibly even higher proportion of males with the "fragile" X chromosome (a tendency to break at the Xq28 site). The greatest uncertainty is for the last estimate. (See references and discussion in Hook, 1983a.)

Studies in those with retardation and three independent malformations, but without a known syndrome, by the Wisconsin group found 11% (15 of 140) with cytogenetic abnormality compared to 0.7% (1 of 140) in a control group (Summitt, 1969; Doyle, 1976; Magnelli, 1976).

16

Infertility and Multiple Spontaneous Abortions

The proportion of all infertile men who have a chromosome abnormality is about 2–3%; about half of these have the 47,XXY genotype. In those with complete oligospermia, 15% have an abnormality, most (13%) with XXY genotype (Chandley et al., 1976).

In couples who experience multiple miscarriages, great variation has been reported in the literature, with rates of chromosome abnormalities, usually balanced translocations, varying from 15% to less than 1%. Almost certainly this variation is related to differences in the selective criteria of populations studied. (See references and discussion in Hook, 1983a.)

Abnormalities of Sexual Differentiation

The only survey of phenotypic females with pubertal anomalies of which I am aware noted about 23% of females with 45,X (or other genotypes producing Turner syndrome) and 5% with 45,X/46,XY mosaic pattern, often associated with mixed gonadal dysgenesis. If attention is limited to hypergonadotropic hypogonadism, the proportions are 53% and 12%, respectively (Reindollar et al., 1981).

In males there are no similar data to my knowledge, but the XXY genotype is responsible for a significant proportion of hypogonadism, perhaps as much as 10%.

Other Developmental Disabilities and Behavioral Abnormalities

The only extensive data on this subject pertain to antisocial behavior, defined operationally as presence in a security setting. Among psychologically disturbed or retarded male prisoners, 3% have a chromosome abnormality (about 2% XYY and 1% XXY). Among other male criminals about 0.4% have the XYY and 0.4% the XXY genotype. The comparable rate in newborn white males is about 0.1% for each genotype. In females in security settings, about 0.3% have the XXX genotype, compared to a newborn rate of 0.1%, but this difference is not statistically significant. There is also provocative evidence from recent studies of individuals identified and followed up from the newborn period that speech abnormalities are prominent in affected individuals (Ratcliffe et al., 1981). In addition, some workers have reported evidence for behavioral difficulties and temper tantrums early in childhood (Ratcliffe et al., 1981). There are also provocative data suggesting EEG abnormalities in XYYs as compared to controls. (For review and references see Hook, 1979.)

17

Malignancy

A detailed analysis of the association of *somatic* cytogenetic abnormalities with malignancy is beyond the scope of this chapter, but there are some data of interest on *germinal* cell abnormalities. Of the numerical chromosome abnormalities, Down syndrome has the most notable association with malignancy. There is about a 30-fold increased risk of a primitive stem cell leukemia. The 45,X/46,XY pattern associated with gonadal dysgenesis has a marked association with gonadoblastoma and dysgerminoma. It has been shown that several germinal structural chromosome abnormalities predispose to specific malignancies, for instance deletion of 11p to Wilms' tumor (in association with aniridia) and deletion of 13q to retinoblastoma. Association of structural and numerical somatic chromosome rearrangements with malignancy are discussed extensively elsewhere. (See for references and discussion German, 1974; Yunis, 1981.)

Autoimmunity

There are some provocative observations of the possible association of autoimmune with chromosome disorders. Women with thyroid autoantibodies, or at least thyroid disorders, appear to be at higher risk for having offspring with Turner syndrome and with Down syndrome. Moreover, individuals with Turner syndrome appear to be at higher risk to develop autoimmune thyroiditis. Whether autoimmunity is a factor that predisposes to nondisjunction or results from some other factor that is independently associated with chromosome abnormality is not yet known. (See discussion and references in Fialkow, 1969; Fialkow et al., 1971; McDonald, 1972.) Recently Mottironi et al. (1981) reported increased sharing of HLA-A and HLA-B antigens by parents of children with Down syndrome. This may reflect a relative protective effect of HLA-A and HLA-B maternal–fetal compatibility upon Down syndrome fetuses, but these observations are not yet confirmed.

REFERENCES

Alberman, E., Polani, P.E., Fraser Roberts, J.A., Spicer, C.C., Elliot, M., and Armstrong E. (1972). Parental exposure to X-irradiation and Down's syndrome. *Ann. Hum. Genet.* 36, 195–208.

Alfi, O.S., Chang, R., and Azen, S.P. (1980). Evidence for genetic control of non-disjunction in man. *Am. J. Hum. Genet.* 32, 477–483.

Awa, A. (1981). Personal communication.

Ayme, S. and Lippman-Hand, A. (1982). Maternal age effect in aneuploidy: Does altered embryonic selection play a role? *Am. J. Hum. Genet. 34*, 558–565.

Blumberg, B.S. (1978). Characteristics of the hepatitis B virus. In *Genetic epidemiology*, edited by N.E. Morton and C.S. Chung. New York: Academic Press, pp. 529–538.

Bracken, M.B. and Vita, K. (1983). Frequency of non-hormonal contraception around conception and association with congenital malformations in offspring. *Am. J. Epidemiol. 117*, 281–291.

Brewen, J.G., Preston, R.J., and Gergozian, N. (1975). Analysis of x-ray induced chromosomal translocations in human and marmoset spermatogonial cells. *Nature 253*, 468–470.

Carothers, A.D., Collyer, S., DeMey, R., and Frackiewicz, A. (1978). Parental age and birth order in the aetiology of some sex chromosome aneuploidies. *Ann. Hum. Genet. 41*, 277–287.

Chandley, A.C., Maclean, N., Edmond, P., Fletcher, J., and Watson, G.S. (1976). Cytogenetics and infertility in man II. *Ann. Hum. Genet. 39*, 231–252.

Cohen, B. H , Lilienfeld, A.M., Kramei, S., and Hyman, L.C. (1977). Parental factors in Down's syndrome: Results of the second Baltimore case-control study. In *Population cytogenetics: Studies in humans*, edited by E.B. Hook and I.H. Porter. New York: Academic Press, pp. 301–352.

deGrouchy, J. and Turleau, C. (1977). *Atlas of chromosome abnormalities*. New York: Wiley, p. 355.

Doyle, C.T. (1976). The cytogenetics of 90 patients with idiopathic mental retardation/malformation syndromes and of 90 normal subjects. *Hum. Genet. 33*, 131–146.

Fabia, J. and Drolette, M. (1970). Life tables up to age 10 for mongols with and without congenital heart defect. *J. Ment. Defic. Res. 14*, 235–242.

Fialkow, P.J. (1969). Genetic aspects of autoimmunity. *Prog. Med. Genet. 11*, 117–167.

———, Thulme, H.C., Hecht, F., and Bryant, J. (1971). Familial predisposition to thyroid disease in Down's syndrome: Controlled immunoclinical studies. *Am. J. Hum. Genet. 23*, 67–85.

German, J. (1974). *Chromosomes and cancer*. New York: Wiley, p. 737.

Hamerton, J.L. (1971). *Human cytogenetics*. Vol. 2, *Clinical cytogenetics*. New York: Academic Press.

Hara, S., Sherell, M.V., Davis, K.K., and Crump, E.P. (1976). Chromosome studies on 944 black newborn infants. *J. Natl. Med. Assoc. 68*, 14–15.

Harlap, S. (1973). Down's syndrome in West Jerusalem. *Am. J. Epidemiol. 97*, 225–232.

Hecht, F. (1977). The non-randomness of human chromosome abnormalities. In *Population cytogenetics: Studies in humans*, edited by E.B. Hook and I.H. Porter. New York: Academic Press, pp. 237–250.

Heston, L.L. (1977). Alzheimer's disease, trisomy 21, and myeloproliferative disorders: Associations suggesting a genetic diathesis. *Science 196*, 322–323.

Hook, E.B. (1974). Racial differentials in the prevalence rate of males with sex chromosome abnormalities (XXY, XYY) in security settings in the USA. *Am. J. Hum. Genet. 26,* 504–511.

—— (1979). Extra sex chromosomes and human behavior: The nature of the evidence regarding XYY, XXY, XXYY and XXX genotypes. In *Genetic aspects of sexual differentiation,* edited by H.L. Vallet and I.H. Porter. New York: Academic Press, pp. 437–463.

—— (1981). Down syndrome: Frequency in human populations and factors pertinent to variation in rates. In *Trisomy 21 (Down syndrome): Research perspectives,* edited by F. de la Cruz and P.S. Gerald. Baltimore, Md.: University Park Press, pp. 3–67.

—— (1981a). Prevalence rate of chromosome abnormalities during human gestation and implications for studies of environmental mutagens. *Lancet 2,* 169–172.

—— (1981b). Rates of chromosomal abnormalities at different maternal ages. *Obstet. Gynecol. 58,* 282–285.

—— (1983a). Contribution of chromosome abnormalities to human morbidity and mortality and some comments upon surveillance of chromosome mutation rates. *Mutation Research 114,* 393–423.

—— (1983b). Chromosome abnormalities and spontaneous fetal death following amniocentesis: Further data and associations with maternal age. *Am. J. Hum. Genet. 35,* 110–116.

—— (1983c). The epidemiology of Down's syndrome. In *Down syndrome: Advances in biomedicine and the behavioral sciences,* edited by S.M. Pueschel. New York: Garland—SPMM Press.

—— and Cross, P.K. (1982a). Interpretation of recent data pertinent to genetic counseling for Down syndrome: Maternal age-specific rates, temporal trends, adjustments for paternal age, recurrence risks, risks after other cytogenetic abnormalities, recurrence risk after remarriage. In *Clinical genetics: Problems in diagnosis and counseling,* edited by A.M. Willey, T.P. Carter, S.M. Kelly, and I.H. Porter. New York: Academic Press, pp. 119–145.

—— and ——. (1982b). Paternal age and Down's syndrome genotypes diagnosed prenatally: No association in New York State data. *Hum. Genet. 62,* 167–174.

——, ——, Lamson, S.H., Regal, R.R., Baird, P.A., and Uh, S.H. (1981). Paternal age and Down syndrome in British Columbia. *Am. J. Hum. Gen. 33,* 123–128.

—— and Harlap, S. (1979). Differences in maternal-age-specific rates of Down syndrome between Jews of European origin and North African or Asian origin. *Teratology 20,* 243–248.

—— and Porter, I.H. (1977). Human population cytogenetics: Comments on racial differences in frequency of chromosome abnormalities, putative clustering of Down's syndrome, and radiation studies. In *Population cytogenetics: Studies in humans,* edited by E.B. Hook and I.H. Porter. New York: Academic Press, pp. 353–365.

Huether, C.A. and Gummere, G.R. (1982). Influence of demographic factors on annual Down's syndrome births in Ohio 1970–1979 and the United States 1920–1979. *Am. J. Epidemiol. 115,* 846–860.

Huggins, G., Vessey, M., Flavel, R., Yeates, D., and McPherson, K. (1982). Vaginal spermicides and outcome of pregnancy. *Contraception* 25, 219–230.

Jacobs, P.A. (1974). Correlation between euploid structural chromosome rearrangements and mental subnormality in humans. *Nature 249*, 164–165.

———— (1979). Recurrence risks for chromosome abnormalities. *Birth Defects* 15(5C), 71–80.

Jick, H., Walker, A.M., Rothman, K.J., Hunter, J.R., Holmes, L.B., Watkins, R.N., D'Ewart, D.C., Danford, A., and Madsen, S. (1981). Vaginal spermicides and congenital disorders. *J.A.M.A.* 245, 1329–1332.

Lamson, S.H. and Hook, E.B. (1980). A simple function for maternal age-specific rates of Down's syndrome in the 20–49 age interval and its biological implications. *Am. J. Hum. Genet. 32*, 743–753.

———— and ———— (1981). Comparison of mathematical models for the maternal age dependence of Down's syndrome rates. *Hum. Genet. 59*, 232–234.

Lejeune, J., and Prieur, M. (1979). Contraceptifs orauz et trisomie 21. Etude retrospective de sept cent trois cas. *Ann. Genet. 22*, 61–66.

Lilienfeld, A. (1969). *Epidemiology of Down's syndrome.* Baltimore, Md.: Johns Hopkins University Press, p. 145.

Magnelli, N.C. (1976). Cytogenetics of 50 patients with mental retardation and multiple congenital malformations and 50 normal subjects. *Clin. Genet. 9*, 169–182.

Martin, R.H., Lin, C.C., Balkan, W., and Burns, K. (1982). Direct chromosomal analysis of human spermatozoa: Preliminary results from 18 normal men. *Am. J. Hum. Genet. 34*, 459–468.

Mavor, J.W. (1922). The production of non-disjunction by x-rays. *Science 55*, 295–297.

McDonald, A.D. (1972). Thyroid disease and maternal factors in mongolism. *Can. Med. Assoc. J. 106*, 1085–1089.

McKusick, V.A. (1978). *Mendelian inheritance in man.* Baltimore, Md.: Johns Hopkins University Press, p. 975.

Mottironi, V.D., Hook, E.B., Willey, A.M., Porter, I.H., Swift, R.V., and Hatcher, N.H. (1981). Restricted HLA heterogeneity in parents of Down syndrome children. *Am. J. Hum. Genet. 33*, 141A.

Penrose, L.S. and Smith, G.F. (1966). *Down's anomaly.* London: Churchill, p. 218.

Polednak, A.P., Janerich, D.T., and Glebatis, D.M. (1982). Birth weight and birth defects in relation to maternal spermicide use. *Teratology 26*, 27–38.

Ratcliffe, S.G., Tierney, I., Smith, L., and Callan, S. (1981). Psychological and educational progress in children with sex chromosome abnormalities in the Edinburgh longitudinal study. In *Human behavior and genetics,* edited by W. Schmid and J. Nielson. Amsterdam: Elsevier-North Holland, pp. 31–43.

Reindollar, R.G., Byrd, J.R., and McDonough, P.G. (1981). Delayed sexual development: A study of 252 patients. *Am. J. Obstet. Gynecol. 140*, 371–380.

Rothman, K.J. (1982). Spermicide use and Down's syndrome. *Am. J. Public Health 72*, 399–401.

Schreinemachers, D.M., Cross, P.K., and Hook, E.B. (1982). Rates of trisomies 21, 18, 13 and other chromosome abnormalities in about 20,000 prenatal studies compared with estimated rates in live births. *Hum. Genet. 61*, 318–324.

Schull, W.J. and Neel, J.V. (1962). Maternal radiation and mongolism. *Lancet 1*, 537–538.

Sever, J.L., Gilkeson, M.R., Chen, T.C., Ley, A.C., and Edmunds, D. (1970). Epidemiology of mongolism in the collaborative project. *Ann. N.Y. Acad. Sci. 171*, 328–340.

Stark, C.R. and White, N.B. (1977). Cluster analysis and racial differences in risk of Down's syndrome. In *Population cytogenetics: Studies in humans*, edited by E.B. Hook and I.H. Porter. New York: Academic Press, pp. 275–283.

Stein, Z., Kline, J., Susser, E., Shrout, P., Warburton, D., and Susser, M. (1980). Maternal age and spontaneous abortion. In *Human embryonic and fetal death*, edited by I.H. Porter and E.B. Hook. New York: Academic Press, pp. 107–127.

Stene, J., Stene, E., Stengel-Rutkowski, S., and Murken, J-D. (1981). Paternal age and Down's syndrome. Data from prenatal diagnoses (DFG). *Hum. Genet. 59*, 119–124.

Summitt, R.L. (1969). Cytogenetics in mentally defective children with anomalies: A controlled study. *J. Pediatr. 74*, 58–66.

———— (1981). Chromosome 21: Specific segments that cause the phenotype of Down syndrome. In *Trisomy 21 (Down syndrome): Research perspectives*, edited by F.F. de la Cruz and P.S. Gerald. Baltimore, Md.: University Park Press, pp. 225–235.

Uchida, I.A. (1977). Maternal radiation and trisomy 21. In *Population cytogenetics: Studies in humans*, edited by E.B. Hook and I.H. Porter. New York: Academic Press, pp. 285–289.

Warburton, D., Stein, Z., Kline, J., and Strobino, B. (1980a). Environmental influences on rates of chromosome anomalies in spontaneous abortions. *Am. J. Hum. Genet. 32*, 27.

————, Kline, J., Stein, Z., and Susser, M. (1980b). Monosomy X: A chromosomal anomaly associated with young maternal age (letter). *Lancet 1*, 167–169.

————, Stein, Z., Kline, J., and Susser, M. (1980c). Chromosome abnormalities in spontaneous abortion: Data from the New York City study. In *Human embryonic and fetal death*, edited by I.H. Porter and E.B. Hook. New York: Academic Press, pp. 261–287.

Yunis, J.J. (1981). Specific fine chromosomal defects in cancer: An overview. *Human Pathology 12*, 503–515.

2

Spontaneous Abortion (Miscarriage)

Jennie Kline and Zena Stein

We review here the epidemiology of spontaneous abortion, a common outcome of pregnancy. We begin with estimates of incidence, then consider the heterogeneity observed among spontaneous abortions, particularly with respect to the chromosomal characteristics of the aborted conceptus, and next discuss the processes that may underlie abortions of different types. Finally, we review studies that have related parental characteristics and exposures, whether to spontaneous abortion overall or to specific types of abortions in particular.

ESTIMATES OF INCIDENCE

Epidemiologic studies provide a range of estimates of the frequency of spontaneous abortion. Those studies concerned only with pregnancies surviving to at least four weeks from the last menstrual period have generally found that 10–20% end in miscarriage. By contrast, studies seeking to ascertain all pregnancy losses, including those occurring soon after conception, have showed higher frequencies, but these estimates must be regarded as far more tenuous, as they are based on studies of small and selected samples of women. Thus Hertig et al. (1959), in a unique study of 34 fertilized ova retrieved by hysterectomy, estimated that as many as 80% of fertilized ova might have morphologic characteristics that are incompatible with survival

This work was supported by grants from The National Institutes of Health (1 R01 HD 12207, 1 R01 DA 02090) and The Environmental Protection Agency (R 807355). Some of the material in this chapter is taken from: *Epidemiology in human reproduction*. Kline, J., Paneth, N., Stein, Z., and Susser, M. (forthcoming). New York: Oxford University Press.

to term. Miller et al. (1980) and Kline et al. (1981a) attempted to diagnose pregnancy around the time of the first missed menses, using sensitive assays for human chorionic gonadotropin (hCG); both series indicate that about 40% of pregnancies surviving to three weeks gestation (the time of implantation) may abort spontaneously.

Leaving aside for the moment these less traditional approaches, we have listed 15 studies in Table 2-1 that provide estimates of incidence. Even these estimates vary considerably. Some of the variation is undoubtedly a result of differences in the distribution of risk factors between study populations, and these will be explored in the next section. However, some of the variation results from methodologic factors, and we examine below the most important of these: the definition of spontaneous abortion, the method of ascertaining pregnancies, and the statistic used to measure the incidence of spontaneous abortion.

Definitions

The World Health Organization (WHO, 1970) defined spontaneous abortion as any nondeliberate interruption of an intrauterine pregnancy before the twenty-eighth week of gestation (since the last menstrual period) in which the fetus is dead when expelled. Epidemiologic studies of the frequency and determinants of spontaneous abortion have departed from this definition in a variety of ways, for example:

1. By including bleeding episodes where it is not possible to confirm pregnancy by pathologic examination of the aborted products of conception.
2. By excluding fetal deaths occurring after the eighteenth, twentieth, or twenty-fourth week of gestation
3. By including extrauterine pregnancies
4. By including terminations in which the fetus is alive on expulsion
5. By including terminations after 28 weeks (missed abortions)

Only the first two of these departures from the WHO definition are likely to produce substantial variations in estimates of the frequency of spontaneous abortion; the numbers of extrauterine pregnancies, livebirths before 28 weeks, and missed abortions are small relative to the number of spontaneous abortions that would be counted using the WHO definition.

Each of the studies listed in Table 2-1 has included, among spontaneous abortions, some episodes where it was not possible to confirm pregnancy by pathologic examination of the aborted conceptus. The proportion of abortions of this type will vary with the study design.

24

Table 2-1. Estimates of the Frequency (%) of Spontaneous Abortion[a]

Study	Design	Fetal death ratio[b]	Probability of fetal death[c]	Cutoff point in gestation (in weeks)
French and Bierman (1962)	Prospective	7.8	19.5 (22.7)[d]	28
Erhardt (1963)	Prospective	8.0	14.8	28
Pettersson (1968)	Prospective	9.7	13.3	28
Taylor (1969)	Prospective	3.6	11.8	28
Harlap et al. (1980a)	Prospective	4.8	9.5	28
Stevenson et al. (1959)	Cross-sectional	11.8		28
Shapiro et al. (1970)	Cross-sectional	14.3		28
Leridon (1976)	Cross-sectional	~11.5		Not given
Yerushalmy et al. (1956)	Retrospective	5.7		20
Stevenson et al. (1959)	Retrospective	16.8		28
Warburton and Fraser (1964)	Retrospective	14.7		26
Jain (1969)	Retrospective	7.5		Term
Naylor (1974)	Retrospective	12.6		20
Leridon (1976) (Creteil)	Retrospective	15.3		Not given
Leridon (1976) (Martinique)	Retrospective	12.1		Not given

[a] In order to improve the comparability of rates, we have recalculated incidence rates for spontaneous abortions up to 28 weeks gestation when data were provided in the published literature.

[b]

$$\text{Fetal death ratio} = \frac{\text{number of spontaneous abortions up to 28 weeks gestation}}{\text{number of spontaneous abortions, stillbirths, and livebirths}} \times 100$$

We have excluded induced abortions from the denominators of the fetal death ratios because not all studies presented data on the numbers of induced abortions. In populations where induced abortion is prevalent, the fetal death ratio, as defined above, overestimates the rate of spontaneous abortion. Susser and Kline (1982) provide a method of adjusting the fetal death ratio for the presence of induced abortions in the population.

[c] We have recalculated the probabilities of fetal death for the prospective studies in order to facilitate comparisons across studies. The probability of fetal death up to 28 weeks gestation was calculated using the method set out by French and Bierman (1962). These recalculated probabilities derive from monthly gestation-specific probabilities of fetal death, rather than from the daily or weekly gestation-specific probabilities that were used in several of the published studies (Pettersson, 1968; Taylor, 1969; Harlap et al., 1980a). Leridon (1977) provides a detailed discussion of the methods that have been used to analyze fetal life tables.

[d] The number in parentheses includes extrauterine pregnancies; the number outside of parentheses was estimated excluding extrauterine pregnancies.

Thus at one extreme, cross-sectional studies of pregnancies ascertained at termination in a medical facility will tend to include only a small proportion of episodes where pathologic confirmation was not available; in contrast, studies that rely on interview data regarding the outcome of previous pregnancies will include an unknown proportion of episodes where a delay in menses was interpreted, perhaps incorrectly, as a pregnancy. Even in cross-sectional studies, pathologic confirmation of spontaneous abortion will usually not be possible when the products of conception have been expelled before a woman seeks medical attention. In these cases, if pregnancy had been diagnosed earlier in gestation, by a positive pregnancy test or by clinical examination of the woman, it is reasonable to assume that a miscarriage did in fact occur.

It seems likely, then, that differences in diagnostic criteria among studies affect estimates of the frequency of spontaneous abortions, but it is not clear how much of the variation in estimates of incidence may be a result of such differences. Some sense of the extent of variation that might be produced by differences in the definition of pregnancy and of spontaneous abortion, is given by two recent studies (Miller et al., 1980; Kline et al., 1981a), both based on small volunteer samples. These studies attempted to diagnose pregnancy at the time of implantation. An assay of human chorionic gonadotropin (hCG) was done either before or shortly after the expected menses. In both of these studies, a low level of hCG might indicate that conception had occurred, because this hormone is specific to pregnancy and to a few rare neoplasms (Vaitukaitis, 1979). If episodes in which a low level of hCG that is followed by bleeding are considered pregnancies, the estimates of spontaneous abortion from these studies are 42.4% and 34.5%, respectively; if only confirmed episodes are counted as pregnancies, the estimates of spontaneous abortion are 13.9% and 18.2%, respectively. Confirmation of pregnancy requires identification of fetal or placental tissue at abortion, or an infant at later gestations.

Table 2-1 indicates the gestational end point that was used to define spontaneous abortion; for those studies that included terminations after 28 weeks of gestation, the rate of spontaneous abortion up to 28 weeks gestation has been recomputed. It is unclear from this table whether the variations between studies are attributable to differences in the gestational definition of spontaneous abortion. Furthermore, it is possible that the proportion of spontaneous abortions occurring at 20–28 weeks gestation may vary among populations. For example, in the two studies based on prepaid health plan facilities, the proportion of fetal deaths occurring at 20–28 weeks gestation was 6% (Shapiro et al., 1970) and 27% (Harlap et al., 1980a).

Ascertainment and Statistics

The incidence of spontaneous abortion can be estimated from three types of studies: prospective, cross-sectional, and retrospective. Each is represented in Table 2-1.

In prospective studies, women are identified prior to the termination of pregnancy and followed until delivery. The probability of spontaneous abortion is estimated from a life table analysis, which applies the gestation-specific rates of fetal death observed for all women identified prior to or during the gestation interval to a hypothetical cohort of pregnancies. The assumption underlying this calculation is that the characteristics of women identified early in pregnancy are similar to those of women identified at later stages in gestation. Although each of the five prospective studies summarized in Table 2-1 enrolled women beginning four weeks after the last menstrual period, the numbers of women enrolled at this early phase were small, and there is some evidence to suggest that the demographic and reproductive characteristics of women enrolling early in pregnancy differ from those of women enrolling later in pregnancy (French and Bierman, 1962; Taylor, 1964; Harlap et al., 1980a).

In cross-sectional studies, women are identified at the termination of pregnancy (spontaneous abortion, induced abortion, viable pregnancy), generally in a medical facility.

In retrospective studies, obstetric histories are obtained; the majority of such studies have collected histories from women ascertained in a medical facility at the time of a pregnancy. In both the latter types of studies, the measure of incidence is the *fetal death ratio*, which relates the number of spontaneous abortions to the total number of pregnancies identified.

For the five prospective studies summarized in Table 2-1, we have set out both the probabilities of fetal death, as calculated from a life table analysis, and the fetal death ratio. The fetal death ratios from these prospective studies tend to be lower than those obtained from cross-sectional and retrospective studies, because in prospective studies it is usual to exclude from the count of abortions those pregnancies that became known to the investigator at or around the time of termination.

The study carried out by French and Bierman (1962) on the island of Kauai probably provides the best single estimate of the probability of fetal death from 4 to 28 weeks of gestation. The estimate obtained from this study is higher than that obtained from the four other prospective studies. This disparity is largely explained by the unique method of ascertaining pregnancies on the island of Kauai: not only were pregnancies identified by the medical facilities, but in addition,

27

women with delayed menses were encouraged to notify the study team. Among the 273 pregnancies that ended in fetal death, 45% were identified by reports to the study team. In contrast, the four other prospective series (Erhardt, 1963; Pettersson, 1968; Taylor, 1969; Harlap et al., 1980a) relied solely on samples of women seeking care at medical facilities. It might be argued that a larger proportion of the spontaneous abortions identified by French and Bierman (1962), in contrast to those ascertained in the four other series, were actually episodes of amenorrhea unassociated with pregnancy. Although this possibility cannot be rigorously evaluated, the size of this inflation is unlikely to be substantial, because a delay in menses of more than three days appears rare among women who are not pregnant (Latz and Reiner, 1937). These and other methodologic issues producing variation in spontaneous abortion rates have been considered in detail elsewhere (Kline 1977; Leridon, 1977).

HETEROGENEITY AMONG SPONTANEOUS ABORTIONS

Spontaneous abortion is a heterogeneous outcome of pregnancy, comprising conceptions with chromosomal and morphologic anomalies, and conceptions that are apparently normal. Table 2-2 compares the frequencies of selected chromosomal anomalies among spontaneous abortions up to 28 weeks gestation (Warburton et al., 1982) and among livebirths (reviewed by Hook and Hamerton, 1977). Approximately 35% of spontaneous abortions up to 28 weeks gestation are chromosomally abnormal, the majority of these being anomalies that are incompatible with survival to term (Creasy et al., 1976; Warburton et al., 1980a). The frequency of chromosomal anomalies among abortions decreases with advancing gestational (Carr, 1967; Lauritsen, 1976; Hassold et al., 1980a) and developmental (Creasy et al., 1976; Takahara et al., 1977; Warburton et al., 1980a) age. For this reason, karyotyped series of spontaneous abortions where the cutoff for gestation is earlier than 28 weeks (Lauritsen, 1976; Hassold et al., 1980a), and series in which abortuses are selected for study on the basis of early developmental age (Boué and Boué, 1973a; Kajii et al., 1980), show higher rates of chromosomal anomalies than series that include all abortions up to 28 weeks gestation.

Assuming that about 15% of recognized pregnancies end in spontaneous abortion, we estimate that approximately 91% of all chromosomally abnormal conceptions are aborted spontaneously. For some anomalies like trisomy 16 and tetraploidy, the probability of abortion is 100%; for others, the probability is well over 98%; for trisomy 21 the probability is 70%, the remainder ending in stillbirth or livebirth, and

Table 2-2. Frequency (per 1000) of Chromosomal Anomalies Among Spontaneous Abortions and Livebirths

Type of anomaly	Spontaneous abortions[a]	Livebirths[b]
Autosomal trisomies		
13	12.98	.10
16	58.06	.00
18	7.51	.16
21	12.30	1.08
Other	88.11	.00
Mosaic	15.03	.00
Double	4.78	.00
Sex chromosomes		
45,XO	59.69	.06
47,XXX	.00	.48
47,XXY	3.42	.54
47,XYY	.00	.44
Mosaic	4.10	.38
Other	.00	.13
Triploids	58.74	.00
Tetraploids	18.44	.00
Rearrangements	13.66	2.51
Other	10.93	.16
Total abnormal	364.75	6.03
Number abnormal	534	190
Number karyotyped	1464	31,521

[a] Data derive from the New York City study of spontaneous abortions up to 28 weeks gestation (Warburton et al., personal communication, 1982).

[b] Data from four studies of consecutive livebirths identified in Aarhus County, Denmark; London, Ontario, Canada; Winnipeg, Manitoba, Canada; New Haven, Connecticut, United States. Summarized by Hook and Hamerton (1977).

for trisomies of some sex chromosomes, the probabilities may be as low as 20–40% (Stein et al., 1975).

For those chromosomal anomalies that are incompatible with survival to term, spontaneous abortions provide the only source in which a search for the causes of anomaly may be carried out. For the few anomalies that survive with measurable frequencies to term, spontaneous abortions provide a parsimonious source in terms of the number of pregnancies that need to be studied (Kline et al., 1977a). The ascertainment of chromosomal anomalies that are compatible with survival to term among abortions also affords an opportunity to distinguish those factors that influence the probability of anomaly from those that influence the probability of abortion (Fig. 2-1). Because infants with anomalies born at term have survived insults that increase the risk of fetal death, associations observed among births may result either from factors that influence intrauterine

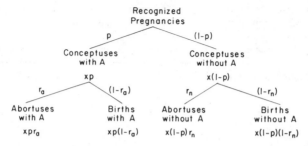

Fig. 2-1. Diagram showing relationships between incidence of anomalies, fetal loss, and birth defects among recognized pregnancies. p, the probability of anomaly A arising, could vary with gestational time; A, Anomaly or abnormality; r_a, probability of aborting an abnormal conceptus; r_n, probability of aborting a normal conceptus. For the purpose of this diagram, only one anomaly per conceptus is assumed; Anomaly A is assumed to arise at only one time in gestation.
Source: Stein et al. (1975).

survival or from factors that increase the probability of anomaly in the conceptus. These two different processes (p and r_a in Fig. 2-1) can be disentangled by comparing the epidemiology of anomalies identified among abortions with that of anomalies identified among births. For example, maternal age shows a similar association with trisomies identified among abortions and among births. It seems likely, then, that for the most part, the association of maternal age with trisomy reflects a change in the probability of a trisomic conception with maternal age.

Among spontaneous abortions up to 28 weeks gestation, about two-thirds are chromosomally normal. These conceptions vary, not only in the gestational age at which they are aborted, but also in morphologic characteristics. The aborted conceptus may consist of fragments, of an empty sac where an embryo is not retrieved, of a disorganized embryo, of an apparently normal embryo or fetus or of an embryo or fetus with focal malformations. Fantel et al. (1980) provide a review of the several large series in which the morphologic characteristics of aborted conceptions have been described. We conjecture that the processes leading to the abortion of conceptions that show an early cessation of development or focal malformation are different from those which occur where morphologic development appears normal. An example of the former situation, in which abnormal organogenesis apparently causes intrauterine death and hence abortion, is the abortion of chromosomally normal conceptions with neural tube defects. It appears that half of all recognized conceptions with this anomaly are aborted spontaneously (Creasy and Alberman, 1976). The latter situation supposes that abortion may result from a disturbance to the pregnancy without the induction of anomaly (Kline et al., 1980a), and certainly many aborted fetuses appear anatomically flawless. In practice, we can rarely distinguish between these two processes in any one particular case. We have estimated that approximately 10% of chromosomally normal conceptions are aborted spontaneously (Stein et al., 1980).

CAUSES AND RISKS

The preceding discussion points to the heterogeneity represented among spontaneous abortions; it is likely that the determinants of spontaneous abortion are equally heterogeneous. A first concern of the epidemiologist might be to refine the dependent variable, spontaneous abortion; unless this is done, it is likely that variations in the frequency of pregnancy loss will reflect only the variation of the largest component of spontaneous abortions, chromosomally normal abortions. However, refining the dependent variable can be a difficult and expensive undertaking. Categorizing by gestational age at abortion (e.g., less than 12 weeks, 13–16 weeks, and >17 weeks) may provide an indirect measure of the frequency of chromosomal anomaly, particularly for abortions of later gestation, which are unlikely to be abnormal. It will not, however, provide even an indirect measure of the frequency of specific chromosomal anomalies.

Table 2-3 lists the factors that have been considered as possible determinants or predictors of spontaneous abortion. For the great

Table 2-3. Possible Predictors of Spontaneous Abortion

1. Parental age
2. Previous spontaneous abortions and gravidity
3. Maternal smoking
4. Maternal alcohol drinking
5. Oral contraceptives, conception with intrauterine device in place, use of spermicidal agents
6. Induced abortion and/or dilatation and curettage
7. Parental occupational or environmental exposures
8. Irradiation
9. Maternal medication and drug use
10. Gynecologic conditions
11. Maternal illness (e.g., diabetes, infection)
12. Socioeconomic characteristics
13. Stress
14. Nutrition, including consumption of specific substances such as caffeine-containing foods and beverages, saccharin
15. Hormonal factors
16. Paternal and maternal histocompatibility

majority of these there is little firm evidence, if any. [See, for instance, reviews by Leridon (1977), Lauritsen (1977), Strobino et al. (1978).] Even so, the list of possible determinants remains too long to treat here in full. In this chapter, we focus primarily on those factors that have been examined not only in relation to the risk of spontaneous abortion, but also in relation to the chromosomal characteristics of the aborted conceptus. We will comment on some of the methodologic issues that have arisen in these studies of cause, and we will point up gaps in our understanding of underlying mechanisms.

Parental Age

An association of parental age with a particular type of spontaneous abortion might be related to factors intrinsic to the biology of aging, to cumulative exposure, to exposures that are specific to particular age groups, or to exposures that affect particular age groups. We first consider age of the mother and then, briefly, age of the father.

AGE OF MOTHER

There is little doubt that the risk of spontaneous abortion increases with maternal age and that this increase is most marked beginning at age 30–35 years (Stevenson et al., 1959; Warburton and Fraser, 1964; Pettersson, 1968; Taylor, 1969; Shapiro et al., 1970; Naylor, 1974; Leridon, 1976; Harlap et al., 1980a; Stein et al., 1980). We discuss here four possible components of this association: the risk of aborting a monosomy X conceptus, the risk of a trisomic conception, the risk of aborting a trisomic conception, and the risk of aborting a chromosomally normal conceptus.

Monosomy X. Monosomy X, a rare chromosomal anomaly in which only one sex chromosome is present, is considerably more frequent among abortions than among births (a condition known as Turner syndrome). In spite of the similar cytogenetic appearance, the two conditions (i.e., that at abortion and that at birth) may be quite dissimilar. Mothers of monosomy X births are on average about the same age as mothers of unaffected births, although one study, based on a pooled series, suggested an association with firstborn status, or with young mother, or with young father (Carothers, 1980). However, women experiencing monosomy X abortions have been shown in several populations to be younger than those having other kinds of abortions, or than those having births after 28 weeks gestation (Lauritsen, 1976; Creasy et al., 1976; Kajii and Ohama, 1979; Warburton et al., 1980b). Not all series of abortions show the association (Lazar et al.,

32

1973; Hassold et al., 1980a). In one series that did show the association, the investigators were able to rule out the possibility that paternal age or gravidity explained the association (Warburton et al., 1980b).

If a disparity between the findings in livebirths and abortion is sustained, two different explanations could be involved: (1) as suggested above, the determinants of monosomy X among abortions and among births could be different; or (2) the probability of aborting an affected conceptus could be greater among younger women (r_a in Fig. 2-1) than among older women. Although neither of these possibilities has yet been explored, there are grounds for the conclusion that the determinants of monosomy X at birth may be different from those in abortion, because monosomy X is more often seen in the mosaic form (monosomy/normal) among births than among abortions.

Trisomy at Conception. Unlike monosomy X, an association between advanced maternal age and trisomy has been observed among abortions and among livebirths. Until the development of techniques to karyotype the abortus, the epidemiology of human trisomy was based on studies of births. Three autosomal trisomies (13, 18, and 21) occur with measurable frequency among births, and each is associated with advanced maternal age (Hook and Fabia, 1978; Hook and Lindsjo, 1978). Studies of spontaneous abortions have made it clear that trisomy of virtually every chromosome occurs (excepting number one) and that the majority of these trisomies are associated with increased maternal age; there is some evidence to suggest that the maternal age effect is more marked for the shorter chromosomes and less marked for trisomy 16, the most common trisomy among abortions (Hassold et al., 1980b).

The Risk of Aborting a Trisomic Conceptus. The probability of abortion for an abnormal conceptus (r_a in Fig. 2-1) may vary not only with characteristics of the conceptus, but also with characteristics of the woman. It has been suggested that the association of maternal age with trisomy among births is at least in part a result of a failure among older women to abort affected conceptions. This suggestion might be tested by comparing the r_a values for trisomies that are sometimes compatible with birth among women of different ages. Unfortunately, there are still insufficient data available from abortions to test this hypothesis.

There is some evidence to suggest that maternal smoking affects the age-specific rate of trisomy among abortions, but not among births (Kline et al., 1981b, 1983). An excess of smokers was noted among young women delivering at 28 weeks or later compared to young women aborting trisomic conceptions; this effect was not present in women over 30 years of age. These data have been interpreted to suggest that among young women smoking may act either to prevent trisomic conception or to facilitate the early expulsion of such conceptions. Among births, smokers showed a slightly lower rate of trisomy at all ages than nonsmokers. These associations have not been searched for in other populations, and must await confirmation.

Probability of Abortion for Chromosomally Normal Conceptions. When it emerged that trisomy accounted for a significant proportion of abortions (about 15% of abortions up to 28 weeks; about 35% of abortions up to 14 weeks), it was suggested that trisomy accounted for the association of maternal age with spontaneous abortion (Leridon, 1973). It has now been shown, however, that older women are in double jeopardy; in addition to the increased risk for a trisomic conception, they are also more likely to abort a chromosomally normal conceptus (Hassold et al., 1980a; Stein et al., 1980). In this respect, humans are similar to rodents and other mammals observed in the laboratory, where a maternal "nesting" effect has been distinguished from an "egg" effect (Biggers, 1969; Maurer et al., 1971). The quality of both "nesting" and "egg" declines steeply with age.

AGE OF FATHER

The evidence regarding the possible relation of paternal age to spontaneous abortion is inconsistent. Warburton and Fraser (1964) report an effect of paternal age independent of maternal age; indeed their data suggest that paternal age may have a stronger association with abortion than maternal age. In contrast, no independent effect of paternal age was observed in a case-control study of spontaneous abortions (Kline, 1977).

Thus far, studies of karyotyped abortions have not provided a possible explanation for the positive association observed by Warburton and Fraser (1964). Some studies of trisomy 21 diagnosed at amniocentesis or at birth suggest that very advanced paternal age may increase the risk of trisomy, although the findings are by no means consistent (Stene et al., 1977, 1981; Erikson, 1978, 1979; Matsunaga et al., 1978; Hook et al., 1981). This association has not yet been evaluated with the same rigor for trisomic abortions, although two series report that the mean paternal age for trisomic abortions was not increased once maternal age was controlled (Lazar et al., 1973; Hassold et al., 1980a). Hassold et al. (1980a) report a decreased mean paternal age for triploid abortions, particularly those resulting from dispermy.

Previous Spontaneous Abortions and Gravidity

Spontaneous abortions, when compared with term births, are associated with a greater frequency of spontaneous abortion in previous pregnancies (Stevenson et al., 1959; Shapiro et al., 1970; Alberman et al., 1975; Kline et al., 1978a) and with a raised risk of abortion among subsequent pregnancies (Warburton and Fraser, 1964; Leridon, 1976; Harlap et al., 1980a). The risk of recurrence is about 1.6 times that of a first spontaneous abortion (about 24%), and some data suggest that the risk of recurrence increases with increasing number of spontaneous abortions (Warburton and Fraser, 1964; Leridon, 1976; Kline, 1977; Harlap et al., 1980a).

It has been conjectured that only a small proportion of women who experience a first spontaneous abortion are at high risk of aborting each of their pregnancies and that this subgroup contributes the majority of recurrences in the population of women experiencing a first spontaneous abortion (James, 1963; Warburton and Fraser, 1964; Leridon, 1976, 1977). In this subgroup, the increased risk of spontaneous abortion in each pregnancy might be due either to an increased probability of aborting chromosomally normal conceptions (r_n in Fig. 2-1) or to an increased probability of anomalous conceptions, which are in turn at high risk of fetal death. Follow-up studies of women identified at the time of a spontaneous abortion suggest that although both of these phenomena operate, the former accounts for nearly all of the observed increase in risk. The risk of spontaneous abortion following a spontaneous abortion of a chromosomally normal conceptus is almost double the risk following the abortion of a chromosomally abnormal conceptus (Boué et al., 1975; Lauritsen, 1976); comparisons of the rates of previous spontaneous abortions among women aborting chromosomally normal and abnormal conceptions are consistent with this observation (Alberman et al., 1975; Strobino et al., 1980a). If women experiencing at least three spontaneous abortions are compared to those having a first abortion, the former group has an excess of chromosomally normal abortions occurring late in gestation and an increased risk of premature deliveries among previous livebirths (Strobino et al., 1980a). These comparisons suggest that a mechanism relating to premature initiation of labor, possibly incompetent cervix, often underlies the spontaneous abortions of women who experience multiple spontaneous abortions.

Couples where one parent is a balanced translocation carrier are at increased risk for conceptions with unbalanced translocations. Because such conceptions would be at high risk of intrauterine death, it has been argued that recurrent spontaneous abortions might be due to inherited genetic defects. Overall, however, balanced translocations are rare (0.19% of newborns, from Hook and Hamerton, 1977) and inherited structural defects account for only a small proportion of recurrent abortions (reviewed by Carr, 1971; Strobino et al., 1980a).

It has been suggested that the variability in risk of spontaneous abortion among women can account for the observation, in many series (Stevenson et al., 1959; Warburton and Fraser, 1964; Shapiro et al., 1970; Naylor, 1974; Naylor and Warburton, 1979), that the risk of spontaneous abortion increases with gravidity (James, 1963; Leridon, 1976). James (1963) argued that pregnancy compensation (a tendency of couples experiencing spontaneous abortions to undertake additional pregnancies until they reached their desired family size) was needed to produce an artifactual association of both maternal age and gravidity with spontaneous abortion. However, both Leridon (1976, 1977) and Kline (1978) have demonstrated that pregnancy compensation need not be posited in order to produce a spurious association between gravidity and spontaneous abortion risk. Models based either on an assumption of heterogeneity of risk among women or simply on the observed population recurrence risk are sufficient to produce an association of gravidity with spontaneous abortion resembling that which has been reported in several settings. Data presented by Roman et al. (1978) could be interpreted to indicate that, at least in some populations, pregnancy compensation may also operate. In the two studies that attempted to assess the effect of gravidity, independently of the number of prior spontaneous abortions (Leridon, 1976; Kline et al., 1978a), there was no association between parity (gravidity minus abortions) and spontaneous abortion.

Maternal Cigarette Smoking

Maternal smoking during pregnancy (Kline et al., 1977b; Himmelberger et al., 1978; Harlap and Shiono, 1980; Knill-Jones et al., 1981), but not before pregnancy (Stein et al., 1981), has been associated with spontaneous abortion. This association appears to be independent of maternal age (Kline et al., 1977b; Himmelberger et al., 1978), alcohol drinking during pregnancy (Harlap and Shiono, 1980; Kline et al., 1980b), or a history of previous spontaneous abortion (Kline et al., 1977b). The increase in risk of abortion is probably concentrated among chromosomally normal conceptions (Lazar et al., 1973; Kline et al., 1980a). The data of Alberman et al. (1976) also showed an increased frequency of chromosomally normal abortions among smokers, but the excess was not statistically significant when maternal age, social class, and oral contraceptive use were controlled. In the New York City study (Kline et al., 1980a, 1982), the association of smoking with chromosomally normal abortion held when maternal age, alcohol drinking, and education were controlled; the effects of oral contraceptive use on this association have not yet been fully assessed (Stein and Susser, 1978), and it remains to be seen whether the London and New York series will appear more compatible when a combined analysis of the two series is carried out.

Maternal Alcohol Drinking

Two studies have examined the association of maternal alcohol drinking during pregnancy with spontaneous abortion, and in both an association that increased with increasing frequency of drinking was detected. Harlap and Shiono (1980) report a twofold increase in the risk of second-trimester spontaneous abortion among women who drank daily compared to women who never drank. Although these prospective data give no evidence of an association between drinking and first-trimester abortion, the investigators urge caution in interpreting this finding because women who registered early in gestation, prior to first-trimester loss, were not representative of all women ascertained prospectively (Harlap and Shiono, 1980; Harlap et al., 1980a). In contrast, in a case-control study of women using the public facilities of three New York City hospitals, drinking was associated with both first- and second-trimester spontaneous abortion; the odds of drinking twice a week or more among women experiencing spontaneous abortions were 2.6 times the odds among controls (Kline et al., 1980b). In both studies, the association was independent of maternal age and smoking. The data of Kline et al. (1980a) indicate that the association is primarily confined to the abortion of chromosomally normal conceptions, although these data also suggest a possible association of alcohol drinking before pregnancy and chromosomal anomalies other than trisomy. There is, in addition, some evidence from this same series that the association may vary with socioeconomic characteristics of the mother; alcohol drinking shows only a slight association with the abortion of chromosomally normal conceptions among women whose education continued beyond high school (Kline et al., 1981c).

The two series suggest that spontaneous abortion may follow from moderate alcohol consumption. This observation is in marked contrast to the association of fetal alcohol syndrome with heavy alcohol consumption. The possible effects of timing of drinking and of variations in the amount consumed (i.e., binge drinking) have not yet been examined in relation to abortion, nor is it clear whether drinking before pregnancy is a necessary antecedent for the effects of drinking during pregnancy.

37

Oral Contraceptives, Intrauterine Devices, and Spermicides

Oral contraceptive use has been examined in relation to both the frequency of spontaneous abortion and characteristics of the aborted conceptus. The rate of spontaneous abortion is not increased among women who used oral contraceptives prior to conception (Royal College of General Practitioners, 1976; Vessey et al., 1976, 1979; Harlap et al., 1980b); indeed the rate of spontaneous abortion may be slightly decreased among users of oral contraceptives (Royal College of General Practitioners, 1976; Harlap et al., 1980b). Similarly, and contrary to an early observation connecting oral contraceptive use to triploidy among abortions (Carr, 1970), the preponderance of evidence indicates that oral contraceptive use is not associated with an increased frequency of any type of chromosomal anomaly (Boué and Boué, 1973b; Lauritsen, 1975; Alberman et al., 1976). In the London series (Alberman et al., 1976) there was a small but statistically significant increase in the overall frequency of chromosomal anomaly among the abortuses of oral contraceptive users as compared to nonusers. This observation is compatible with the hypothesis that oral contraceptive use decreases the risk of abortion for chromosomally normal conceptions (Alberman et al., 1976; Stein and Susser, 1978). It is not clear whether oral contraceptive failures are associated with an increased risk of abortion; if such an effect is present, it is probably slight (Harlap et al., 1980b).

The use of an intrauterine device before conception, but not at the time of conception, has not been associated with spontaneous abortion (Vessey et al., 1979; Harlap et al., 1980b). Conception with an intrauterine device in place is associated with a two- to threefold increase in the risk of spontaneous abortion (Vessey et al., 1974, 1979; Harlap et al., 1980b), and this risk may persist even if the device is removed early in gestation (Harlap et al., 1980b).

The relation of the use of a spermicidal agent to spontaneous abortion has not been evaluated fully. Two prospective studies (Vessey et al., 1979; Harlap et al., 1980b) evaluated spermicide use both before and at the time of conception, and found no association with spontaneous abortion. The data regarding spermicide conceptions from a large case-control study of spontaneous abortions also show no association (Strobino et al., 1980b); the data relating to use before conception have not yet been reported for this series. Strobino et al. (1980b) note, however, an association between conception with a spermicide and two rare chromosomal anomalies among abortions (i.e., tetraploidy, hypertriploidy); this association would be unlikely to result in a detectable increase in the overall risk of abortion. Jick et al. (1981) have recently reported an association between spontaneous

38

abortion and presumed spermicide use, defined by the filling out of a prescription for a spermicidal agent within 20 months of termination of pregnancy. The time period before conception covered by these histories is longer for women experiencing abortions than for women experiencing term births. It is unclear whether or not the finding would hold if the time periods covered were equivalent.

Induced Abortion

We discuss below three issues of epidemiologic interest relating induced abortion to the epidemiology of spontaneous abortion. The first is the obvious substantive question: Is induced abortion a determinant of subsequent spontaneous abortion, and if so, under what conditions? The second question relates to a procedure that is frequently used not only for induced abortion, but at the time of spontaneous abortion: Is cervical curettage a determinant of subsequent spontaneous abortion? The third question is statistical: To what extent does the inclusion or exclusion of induced abortions in the fetal death ratio alter estimates of the incidence of spontaneous abortion?

INDUCED ABORTION AND SUBSEQUENT SPONTANEOUS ABORTION

Numerous studies have examined whether induced abortion increases the risk of subsequent spontaneous abortion. Differences in the interpretations of these studies depend less on the method of study (cohort or case-control) than on definitions of both the independent variable (number of induced abortions; procedure used) and the dependent variables (the gestational definition of spontaneous abortion; the numbers of first- and second-trimester abortions studied).

Three studies—a case-control study of spontaneous abortions (Kline et al., 1978b), a cross-sectional study of pregnancy outcomes among women with and without previous induced abortions (Madore et al., 1981), and a prospective study (Harlap et al., 1979)—provide a sufficient number of first-trimester spontaneous abortions to give confidence to the conclusion that a single induced abortion is unlikely to raise the risk of subsequent first-trimester spontaneous abortion. In all three studies the numbers of women with multiple induced abortions were too few to permit inferences regarding the effects of repeated induced abortions.

It has proved more difficult to evaluate whether induced abortion raises the risk of subsequent second-trimester spontaneous abortion. Kline et al. (1978b) did not detect an association, but the numbers of second-trimester spontaneous abortions were too few to rule out a modest association. Madore et al. (1981) defined spontaneous abortion as fetal death occurring before 20 weeks, thus excluding about half of all second-trimester spontaneous abortions. The association between induced abortion and second-trimester spontaneous abortion can be examined in the data provided by Harlap et al. (1979). These data suggest that the risk of second-trimester spontaneous abortion varies with parity and with method of induction. No association was detected in parous women, but among nulliparous women who had undergone induced abortion prior to 1973 the risk of second-trimester spontaneous abortion was three times that of nulliparous women who had not experienced an induced abortion. The risk of second-trimester spontaneous abortion among nulliparous women who had undergone induced abortion between 1973 and 1976 was similar to that in nulliparae who had not experienced induced abortion. Harlap et al. (1979) interpreted these data to suggest that instrumental methods of dilatation, common in their population prior to 1973, may increase the risk of second-trimester spontaneous abortion, but that gradual dilatation, such as that which occurs with laminaria tents, has practically eliminated this adverse effect. Using extreme estimates, they calculated that fewer than 4% of spontaneous abortions could reasonably be attributed to induced abortion.

Several investigators have noted that the demographic and reproductive characteristics of women having induced abortions differ from those who have not, and that failure to control for these potentially confounding factors may lead to spurious inferences. For example, smoking, alcohol drinking, and older maternal age are each associated with an increased risk of spontaneous abortion and may distinguish women who opt for induced abortion. Because induced abortion presumably indicates that the woman does not want to be pregnant, she may become either a diligent user of contraceptives in the years that follow or a repeated user of induced abortion. For those women who choose oral contraceptives, the risk of spontaneous abortion may be decreased slightly; for those who choose an intrauterine device and conceive in spite of its use, the risk of spontaneous abortion may be increased; for those who experience multiple induced abortions, it is unclear whether the risk of spontaneous abortion will be increased. In spite of these complexities in evaluating the effects of induced abortion, it appears unlikely that this procedure increases the risk of subsequent spontaneous abortion.

DILATATION AND CURETTAGE

Dilatation and curettage is used inconsistently, from hospital to hospital, for the treatment of women admitted for spontaneous abortion. It was suggested that this procedure might increase the risk of subsequent spontaneous abortion and thus explain at least a part of the increased risk of a second spontaneous abortion following a first (Alberman, 1973).

Studies of pregnancies subsequent to induced abortion bear on this hypothesis. Several studies suggest that dilatation and curettage, either for induced abortion (Kline et al., 1978b; Madore et al., 1981; Harlap et al., 1979) or for spontaneous abortion (Liu et al., 1972), does not increase the risk of subsequent first-trimester spontaneous abortion. As discussed above, the data of Harlap et al. (1979) raise the possibility that instrumental dilatation may increase the risk of second-trimester spontaneous abortion.

ESTIMATES OF THE INCIDENCE OF SPONTANEOUS ABORTION

Populations and subpopulations differ widely in the proportion of pregnancies terminated by induced abortion. In New York City, for instance, approximately equal numbers of pregnancies terminate in induced abortion as in livebirth, and the ratio of induced abortion to livebirth is greater at the extremes of the maternal ages than in the middle years (Pakter and Nelson, 1971). Comparisons of the fetal death ratios from two populations can be misleading if the numbers and patterns of induced abortion differ between the populations. For example, in a population where all induced abortions take place early in gestation, around the eighth to tenth week, a greater proportion of pregnancies destined to abort spontaneously will have ended in induced abortion than in a population where most induced abortions take place late in gestation, after the period of greatest risk for spontaneous abortion. In the first example, the conventional fetal death ratio (number of spontaneous abortions as related to number of spontaneous abortions, stillbirths, and livebirths) will underestimate the true rate of spontaneous abortions; in the second population, this ratio will overestimate the true rate of spontaneous abortions by having excluded induced abortions from the denominator.

Hemminki et al. (1980a,b) have attempted to deal with this issue by examining two ratios: the conventional fetal death ratio and a fetal death ratio that includes induced abortions in the denominator. A preferable approach, in populations where the majority of induced and spontaneous abortions occur over the same period of gestation, is to define the fetal death ratio as:

$$\frac{\text{number of spontaneous abortions}}{\text{number of (spontaneous abortions} + \text{stillbirths} + \text{livebirths} + \frac{1}{2} \text{ induced abortions)}}$$

41

In spite of the fact that this formula provides only an approximation to the true rate of spontaneous abortion (Susser and Kline, 1982; Susser 1983, it is likely to be adequate for making comparisons of spontaneous abortion rates across populations.

Occupational Exposures

Spontaneous abortion, for the reasons discussed earlier, would seem to provide one useful end point for monitoring the workplace for hazards to reproduction. Numerous epidemiologic studies have now been undertaken covering a range of occupational experiences, but often the results have been difficult to explain or confirm (Strobino et al., 1978; Report of Panel II, 1981). We consider here some of the work examining the effects of parental exposure to anesthetic gases, lead, vinyl chloride, and dibromochloropropane (DBCP).

The effects of parental exposure to anesthesia through work have now been examined in several countries, often on more than one occasion and by more than one group of investigators (Vaisman, 1967; Askrog and Harvald, 1970; Knill-Jones et al., 1972, 1975; Rosenberg and Kirves, 1973; American Society of Anesthesiologists, 1974; Pharoah et al., 1977; Cohen et al., 1971, 1975, 1980). Data on both work history and pregnancy outcomes were usually obtained by mailed questionnaire. Some of these studies have distinguished between maternal and paternal exposure; none of them have rigorously distinguished between maternal pre- and postconception exposures; few provide data on the type and dose of anesthetic, although exposures are variable. In some studies, the range of reproductive outcomes examined has been wide, with no attempt to adjust for multiple tests in assessing statistical significance. Low and/or different response rates between exposed and unexposed samples have also plagued many of the studies, making interpretation of the results difficult. For these reasons it is not possible to make a firm statement regarding any relationship between either maternal or paternal occupational exposure to anesthesia and spontaneous abortion. The majority of both positive and negative findings are open to question.

Maternal exposure to lead has been considered hazardous to reproduction for nearly a century (Oliver, 1914), and it was previously in use as an abortifacient (Hamilton and Hardy, 1949). It is not clear, however, whether the levels currently encountered in the workplace pose a hazard. In Sweden (Nordstrom et al., 1978), the rate of spontaneous abortion was increased among women exposed to lead either through work or through proximity to a smelter. A dose–response gradient was described: the rates of spontaneous abortion were lower in women who left the job and area than in those who remained, suggesting that at least part of the association is due to postconception exposure. Interestingly, the rates of spontaneous abortion were highest in those couples where both members were exposed in the workplace, raising the possibility of preconception effects on the sperm, egg, or both.

Isolated studies suggesting a possible relation of paternal exposure to vinyl chloride and DBCP to spontaneous abortion have been of considerable interest in light of the other effects of these agents. Infante et al. (1976a,b) reported an increased frequency of spontaneous abortion in the wives of vinyl chloride monomer workers. Although this report has been criticized on several grounds (Hatch et al., 1981), the suggested association is intriguing because it has also been suggested that vinyl chloride monomer acts as a clastogen (Ducatman et al., 1975; Funes-Cravioto et al., 1975; Purchase et al., 1975). If the findings for spontaneous abortion are replicated (Buffler, 1979), it could be hypothesized that the excess fetal deaths are attributable to chromosomal errors in the zygote that arose from breaks in the chromosomes of the male germ cells. An assumption, untested, that underlies this hypothesis is that an agent that induces chromosomal breaks in lymphocytes can also induce breaks in the germ cell.

Male exposure to DBCP, a well-demonstrated cause of infertility (Whorton et al., 1977, 1979), has been linked to spontaneous abortion in the wives of exposed workers (Kharrazi et al., 1980). The findings on spontaneous abortion derive from a different population than those for infertility. Nonetheless, these observations raise the possibility that the same mechanism may underlie the decrease in sperm count and conception of a zygote that is not viable.

Irradiation

Irradiation exposure has been examined in relation to the chromosomal characteristics of the aborted conceptus on two occasions, with inconsistent results. Alberman et al. (1972) estimated the average life-time ovarian dose of irradiation in women experiencing abortions and women experiencing births. Exposure to irradiation was associated with triploid abortion and possibly with trisomic abortions among women of advanced maternal age. Lazar et al. (1973) failed to detect an association between maternal irradiation exposure and either triploidy or trisomy. In this study, women were classified as irradiated or not irradiated; information on dose, frequency, and timing of exposure were not provided, and so it is unclear whether these findings are inconsistent with those of Alberman et al. (1972), where very detailed descriptions of irradiation exposure were needed to detect an effect.

Lazar et al. (1973) report an excess of chromosomally abnormal abortions where men were exposed through their occupation to irradiation. This association has not been evaluated in other settings.

CONCLUSION

The descriptive epidemiology of spontaneous abortion is still far from complete. The pathogenesis has only recently begun to be clarified, and few determinants are yet firmly established. Nevertheless, it remains a challenging field of study, offering the epidemiologist ample opportunity to add to knowledge of the processes involved in human reproduction, normal and abnormal.

REFERENCES

Alberman, E. (1973). The epidemiology of spontaneous abortions and their chromosome constitution. In *Les accidents chromosomiques de la reproduction*, edited by A. Boué and C. Thibault. Paris: Institut National de la Santé et de la Recherche Médicale, pp. 305–316.

———, Creasy, M., Elliott, M., and Spicer, C. (1976). Maternal factors associated with fetal chromosomal anomalies in spontaneous abortions. *Br. J. Obstet. Gynaecol. 83*, 621–627.

———, Elliott, M., Creasy, M., and Dhadial, R. (1975). Previous reproductive history in mothers presenting with spontaneous abortions. *Br. J. Obstet. Gynaecol. 82*, 366–373.

———, Polani, P.E., Fraser, J.A., Spicer, C., Elliott, M., Armstrong, E., and Dhadial, R.K. (1972). Parental x-irradiation and chromosome constitution in their spontaneously aborted foetuses. *Ann. Hum. Genet. 36*, 185–194.

American Society of Anesthesiologists (1974). Occupational disease among operating room personnel: A national study. *Anesthesiology 41*, 321–340.

Askrog, V. and Harvald, B. (1970). Teratogen effekt af inhalations anaesthaetika. *Nord. Med. 16*, 498–500.

Biggers, J.D. (1969). Problems concerning the uterine causes of embryonic death, with special reference to the effects of ageing in the uterus. *J. Reprod. Fertil. (Suppl.) 8*, 27–43.

Boué, A. and Boué, J. (1973b). Actions of steroid contraceptives on gametic material. *Geburtshilfe Frauenheilk. 33*, 77–85.

Boué, J. and Boué, A. (1973a). Anomalies chromosomiques dans les avortements spontanes. In *Les accidents chromosomiques de la reproduction*, edited by A. Boué, and C. Thibault. Paris: Institut National de la Santé et de la Recherche Médicale, pp. 29–55.

———, ———, and Lazar, P. (1975). Retrospective and prospective epidemiological studies of 1500 karyotyped spontaneous human abortions. *Teratology 12*, 11–26.

Buffler, P.A. (1979). Some problems in recognizing teratogens used in industry. *Contrib. Epidemiol. Biostatist. 1*, 118–137.

Carothers, A.D., Frackiewicz, A., Demey, R., Collyer, S., Ostovics, M., Horvath, K., Papp, Z., May, H.M., and Ferguson-Smith, M.A. (1980). A collaborative study of the aetiology of Turner's syndrome. *Ann. Hum. Genet. 43*, 355–368.

Carr, D.H. (1967). Chromosome anomalies as a cause of spontaneous abortion. *Am. J. Obstet. Gynecol. 97*, 283–293.

——— (1970). Chromosome studies in selected spontaneous abortions. I, Conception after oral contraceptives. *Can. Med. Assoc. J. 103*, 343–348.

——— (1971). Chromosomes and abortion. In *Advances in human genetics*, edited by H. Harris and L. Hirschhorn. New York: Plenum, pp. 201–257.

Cohen, E.N., Bellville, J.W., and Brown, Jr., B.W. (1971). Anesthesia, pregnancy, and miscarriage: A study of operating room nurses and anesthetics. *Anesthesiology 35*, 343–347.

———, Brown, B.W., Bruce, D.L., Cascorbi, H.F., Corbett, T.H., Jones, T.W., and Whitcher, C.E. (1975). A survey of anesthetic health hazards among dentists. *J. Am. Dent. Assoc. 90*, 1291–1296.

———, ———, Wu, M.L., Whitcher, C.E., Brodsky, J.B., Gift, H.C., Greenfield, W., Jones, T.W., and Driscoll, E.J. (1980). Occupational disease in dentistry and chronic exposure to trace anesthetic gases. *J. Am. Dent. Assoc. 101*, 21–31.

Creasy, M.R. and Alberman, E.D. (1976). Congenital malformations of the central nervous system in spontaneous abortions. *J. Med. Genet. 13*, 9–16.

———, Crolla, J.A., and Alberman, E.D. (1976). A cytogenetic study of human spontaneous abortions using banding techniques. *Hum. Genet. 31*, 177–196.

Ducatman, A., Hirschhorn, K., and Selikoff, I.J. (1975). Vinyl chloride exposure and human chromosome aberrations. *Mutat. Res. 31*, 163–168.

Erhardt, C.L. (1963). Pregnancy losses in New York City, 1960. *Am. J. Public Health 53*, 1337–1352.

Erickson, J.D. (1978). Down's syndrome, paternal age, maternal age and birth order. *Ann. Hum. Genet. 41*, 289–298.

——— (1979). Paternal age and Down's syndrome. *Am. J. Hum. Genet. 31*, 489–497.

Fantel, A.G., Shepard, T.H., Vadheim-Roth, C., Stephens, T.D., and Coleman, C. (1980). Embryonic and fetal phenotypes: Prevalence and other associated factors in a large study of spontaneous abortion. In *Human embryonic and fetal death*, edited by I.H. Porter and E.B. Hook. New York: Academic Press, pp. 71–87.

French, F.E. and Bierman, J.M. (1962). Probabilities of fetal mortality. *Public Health Rep. 77*, 835–847.

Funes-Cravioto, F., Lambert, B., Lindsten, J., Ehrenberg, L., Natarajan, A.T., and Osterman-Golkar, S. (1975). Chromosome aberrations in workers exposed to vinyl chloride (letter). *Lancet 1*, 459.

Hamilton, A. and Hardy, H.L. (1949). *Industrial Toxicology* (2nd Ed.). New York: Hoeber.

Harlap, S. and Shiono, P. (1980). Alcohol, smoking, and incidence of spontaneous abortions in the first and second trimester. *Lancet 2*, 173–176.

——, ——, and Ramcharan, S. (1980a). A life table of spontaneous abortions and the effects of age parity and other variables. In *Human embryonic and fetal death*, edited by I.H. Porter and E.B. Hook. New York: Academic Press, pp. 145–164.

——, ——, and —— (1980b). Spontaneous foetal losses in women using different contraceptives around the time of conception. *Int. J. Epidemiol.* 9, 49–56.

——, ——, ——, Berendes, H., and Pellegrin, F. (1979). A prospective study of spontaneous fetal losses after induced abortions. *N. Engl. J. Med. 301*, 677–681.

Hassold, T., Chen, N., Funkhouser, T., Joss, T., Manuel, B., Matsuura, J., Matsuyama, A., Wilson, C., Yamane, J.A., and Jacobs, P.A. (1980a). A cytogenetic study of 1000 spontaneous abortions. *Ann. Hum. Genet.* 44, 151–178.

——, Jacobs, P., Kline, J., Stein, Z., and Warburton, D. (1980b). Effect of maternal age on autosomal trisomies. *Ann. Hum. Genet.* 44, 29–36.

Hatch, M., Kline, J., and Stein, Z. (1981). Power considerations in studies of reproductive effects of vinyl chloride and some structural analogs. *Environ. Health Perspect.* 41, 195–201.

Hemminki, K., Franssila, E., and Vainio, H. (1980a). Spontaneous abortions among female chemical workers in Finland. *Int. Arch. Occup. Environ. Health 45*, 123–126.

——, Niemi, M.L., Koskinen K., and Vainio, H. (1980b). Spontaneous abortions among women employed in the metal industry in Finland. *Int. Arch. Occup. Environ. Health 47*, 53–60.

Hertig, A.T., Rock, J., Adams, E.C., and Menkin, M.C. (1959). Thirty-four fertilized human ova, good, bad, and indifferent, recovered from 210 women of known fertility. *Pediatrics 23*, 202–211.

Himmelberger, D.U., Brown, Jr., B.W., and Cohen, E.N. (1978). Cigarette smoking during pregnancy and the occurrence of spontaneous abortion and congenital abnormality. *Am. J. Epidemiol. 108*, 470–479.

Hook, E.B., Cross, P.K., Lamson, S.H., Regal, R.R., Baird, P.A., and Uh, S.H. (1981). Paternal age and Down syndrome in British Columbia. *Am. J. Hum. Genet. 33*, 123–128.

—— and Fabia, J.J. (1978). Frequency of Down syndrome by single-year maternal age interval: Results of a Massachusetts study. *Teratology 17*, 223–228.

—— and Hamerton, J.L. (1977). The frequency of chromosome abnormalities detected in consecutive newborn studies. Differences between studies: Results by sex and by severity of phenotypic involvement. In *Population cytogenetics: Studies in humans*, edited by I.H. Porter and E.B. Hook. New York: Academic Press, pp. 63–79.

———— and Lindsjo, A. (1978). Down's syndrome in livebirths by single year maternal age interval in a Swedish study: Comparison with results from a New York State study. *Am. J. Hum. Genet. 30*, 19–27.

Infante, P.F., Wagoner, J.K., McMichael, A.J., Waxweiler, R.J., and Falk, H. (1976a). Genetic risks of vinyl chloride. *Lancet 1*, 734–735.

————, ————, ————, ————, and ———— (1976b). Genetic risks of vinyl chloride (letter). *Lancet 1*, 1289–1290.

Jain, A.K. (1969). Fetal wastage in a sample of Taiwanese women. *Milbank Mem. Fund Q. 47*(3), 297–306.

James, W.H. (1963). Notes towards an epidemiology of spontaneous abortion. *Am. J. Hum. Genet. 15*, 223–240.

Jick, H., Walker, A.M., Rothman, K.J., Hunter, J.R., Holmes, L.B., Watkins, R.N., D'Ewart, D.C., Danford, A., and Madsen, S. (1981). Vaginal spermicides and congenital disorders. *J.A.M.A.. 245*, 1329–1332.

Kajii, T., Ferrier, A., Niikawa, N., Takahara, H., Ohama, K., and Avirachan, S. (1980). Anatomic and chromosomal anomalies in 639 spontaneous abortuses. *Hum. Genet. 55*, 87–98.

———— and Ohama, K. (1979). Inverse maternal age effect in monosomy X. *Hum. Genet. 51*, 147–151.

Kharrazi, M., Potashnik, G., and Goldsmith, J.R. (1980). Reproductive effects of dibromochloropropane. *Isr. J. Med. Sci. 16*, 403–406.

Kline, J. (1977). *The epidemiology of spontaneous abortion: An analysis of selected factors.* Doctoral dissertation, Graduate School of Arts and Sciences, Columbia University, New York.

———— (1978). I. An epidemiological review of the role of gravidity in spontaneous abortion. *Early Hum. Dev. 1*, 337–344.

————, Lansky-Kiely, M., Santana, S., Saxena, B., and Stein, Z. (1981a). *Estimates of very early fetal loss.* Abstracts of the Ninth Meeting of the International Epidemiological Association, Edinburgh, Scotland, August 1981.

————, Levin, B., Shrout, P., Stein, Z., Susser, M., and Warburton, D. (1983). Maternal smoking and trisomy among spontaneously aborted conceptions. *Am. J. Hum. Genet. 35*, 421–431.

————, ————, Stein, Z., Susser, M., and Warburton, D. (1981c). Epidemiological detection of low dose effects on the developing fetus. *Environmental Health Perspectives 42*, 119–126.

————, Shrout, P., Stein, Z., Susser, M., and Weiss, M. (1978a). II. An epidemiological study of the role of gravidity in spontaneous abortion. *Early Hum. Dev. 1*, 345–356.

————, ————, ————, ————, and Warburton, D. (1980b). Drinking during pregnancy and spontaneous abortion. *Lancet 2*, 178–180.

————, Stein, Z., Strobino, B., Susser, M., and Warburton, D. (1977a). Surveillance of spontaneous abortions: Power in environmental monitoring. *Am. J. Epidemiol. 106*, 345–350.

————, ————, Susser, M., and Warburton, D. (1977b). Smoking: A risk factor for spontaneous abortion. *N. Engl. J. Med. 297*, 793–796.

————, ————, ————, and ———— (1978b). Induced abortion and spontaneous abortion: No connection? *Am. J. Epidemiol. 107*, 290–298.

——, ——, ——, and —— (1980a). Environmental influences on early reproductive loss in a current New York City study. In *Human embryonic and fetal death*, edited by I.H. Porter and E.B. Hook. New York: Academic Press, pp. 225–240.

——, ——, ——, and —— (1981b). New insights into the epidemiology of chromosomal disorders: Their relevance to the prevention of Down's syndrome. In *Frontiers of knowledge in mental retardation*. Vol. 2, *Biomedical aspects*, edited by P. Mittler. Baltimore, Md.: University Park Press, pp. 131–141.

Knill-Jones, R.R., Newman, B.J., and Spence, A.A. (1975). Anaesthetic practice and pregnancy. *Lancet 2*, 807–809.

——, Rodrigues, L.V., Moir, D.D., and Spence, A.A. (1972). Anaesthetic practice and pregnancy: Controlled survey of women anaesthetists in the United Kingdom. *Lancet 1*, 1326–1328.

——, Spence, A.A., and Lawrie, C. (1981). *Occupation of female doctors and outcome of pregnancy*. Abstracts of the Ninth Meeting of the International Epidemiological Association, Edinburgh, Scotland, August 1981.

Latz, L.J. and Reiner, E. (1937). Failures in natural conception control and their causes. *Illinois Med. J. 71*, 210–215.

Lauritsen, J.G. (1975). The significance of oral contraceptives in causing chromosome anomalies in spontaneous abortions. *Acta Obstet. Gynecol. Scand. 54*, 261–264.

—— (1976). Aetiology of spontaneous abortion. A cytogenetic and epidemiological study of 288 abortuses and their parents. *Acta Obstet. Gynecol. Scand. (Suppl.) 52*, 1–29.

—— (1977). Genetic aspects of spontaneous abortion. *Dan. Med. Bull. 24*, 169–189.

Lazar, P., Guegen, S., Boué, J., and Boué, A. (1973). Epidemiologie des avortements spontanes precoces: Apropos de 1,469 avortements caryotypes. In *Les accidents chromosomiques de la reproduction*, edited by A. Boué, and C. Thibault. Paris: Institut National de la Santé et de la Recherche Médicale, pp. 317–331.

Leridon, H. (1973). Demographie des echecs de la reproduction. In *Les accidents chromosomiques de la reproduction*, edited by A. Boué and C. Thibault. Paris: Institut National de la Santé et de la Recherche Médicale, pp. 13–27.

—— (1976). Facts and artifacts in the study of intra-uterine mortality: A reconsideration from pregnancy histories. *Popul. Studies 30(2)*, 319–336.

—— (1977). *Human fertility*. Chicago: University of Chicago Press.

Liu, D.T.Y., Melville, H.A.H., and Martin, T. (1972). Subsequent gestational morbidity after various types of abortion (letter). *Lancet 2*, 431.

Madore, C., Hawes, W.E., Many, F., and Hexter, A.C. (1981). A study of the effects of induced abortion on subsequent pregnancy outcome. *Am. J. Obstet. Gynecol. 139*, 516–521.

Matsunaga, E., Tonomura, A., Hidetsune, O., and Yasumoto, K. (1978). Reexamination of paternal age effect in Down's syndrome. *Hum. Genet. 40*, 259–268.

Maurer, R.R. and Foote, R.H. (1971). Maternal ageing and embryonic mortality in the rabbit. I. Repeated superovulation, embryo culture, and transfer. *J. Reprod. Fertil. 25*, 329–341.

Miller, J.F., Williamson, E., Glue, J., Gordon, Y.B., Grudzinskas, J.G., and Sykes, A. (1980). Fetal loss after implantation. *Lancet 2*, 554–556.

Naylor, A.F. (1974). Sequential aspects of spontaneous abortion: Maternal age, parity, and pregnancy compensation artifact. *Soc. Biol. 21*, 195–204.

—— and Warburton, D. (1979). Sequential analysis of spontaneous abortion. II. Collaborative study data show that gravidity determines a very substantial rise in risk. *Fertil. Steril. 31*, 282–286.

Nordstrom, I., Beckman, L., and Nordenson, I. (1978). Occupational and environmental risks in and around a smelter in northern Sweden. III. Frequencies of spontaneous abortion. *Hereditas 88*, 51–54.

Oliver, T. (1914). *Lead poisoning from the industrial, medical, and social points of view, lectures delivered at the Royal Institute of Public Health by Sir Thomas Oliver.* New York: Hoeber, pp. 176–184.

Pakter, J. and Nelson, F. (1971). Abortion in New York City: The first nine months. *Fam. Planning Perspect. 3*(3), 5–12.

Pettersson, F. (1968). *Epidemiology of early pregnancy wastage: Biological and social correlates of abortion. An investigation based on materials collected within Uppsala County, Sweden.* Stockholm: Svenska Bokförlaget.

Pharoah, P.O.D., Alberman, E., Doyle, P., and Chamberlain, G. (1977). Outcome of pregnancy among women in anesthetic practice. *Lancet 1*, 34–36.

Purchase, I.F.H., Richardson, C.R., and Anderson, D. (1975). Chromosomal and dominant lethal effects of vinyl chloride. *Lancet 2*, 410–411.

Report of Panel II (1981). Guidelines for reproductive studies in exposed human populations. In *Guidelines for studies in human populations exposed to mutagenic and reproductive hazards*, edited by A.D. Bloom. New York: March of Dimes Birth Defects Foundation, pp. 37–110.

Roman, E., Doyle, P., Beral, V., Alberman, E., and Pharoah, P. (1978). Fetal loss, gravidity, and pregnancy order. *Early Hum. Dev. 2*, 131–138.

Rosenberg, P. and Kirves, A. (1973). Miscarriage among operating theatre staff. *Acta Anaesthesiol. Scand. (Suppl.) 53*, 37–42.

Royal College of General Practitioners (1976). Oral contraception study: The outcome of pregnancy in former oral contraceptive users. *Br. J. Obstet. Gynaecol. 83*, 608–616.

Shapiro, S., Levin, H.S., and Abramovicz, M. (1970). Factors associated with early and late fetal loss. In *Advances in planned parenthood*, Vol. 6. Amsterdam: Excerpta Medica, pp. 45–63.

Stein, Z., Kline, J., Levin, B., Susser, M., and Warburton, D. (1981). Epidemiologic studies of environmental exposure in human reproduction. In *Measurement of risks*, edited by G.C. Berg and H.D. Maillie. New York: Plenum, pp. 163–188.

——, ——, Susser, E., Shrout, P., Warburton, D., and Susser, M. (1980). Maternal age and spontaneous abortion. In *Human embryonic and fetal death*, edited by I.H. Porter and E.B. Hook. New York: Academic Press, pp. 107–127.

—— and Susser, M. (1978). Epidemiologic and genetic issues in mental retardation. In *Genetic epidemiology*, edited by N.E. Morton and C.S. Chung. New York: Academic Press, pp. 415–461.

——, ——, Warburton, D., Wittes, J., and Kline, J. (1975). Spontaneous abortion as a screening device. The effect of fetal survival on the incidence of birth defects. *Am. J. Epidemiol. 102*, 275–290.

Stene, J., Fischer, G., Stene, E., Mikkelsen, M., and Petersen, E. (1977). Paternal age effect in Down's syndrome. *Ann. Hum. Genet. 40*, 299–306.

——, Stene, E., Stengel-Rutkowski, S., and Murken, J.D. (1981). Paternal age and Down's syndrome: Data from prenatal diagnoses. *Hum. Genet. 59*, 119–124.

Stevenson, A.C., Dudgeon, M.Y., and McClure, H.I. (1959). Observations on the results of pregnancies in women resident in Belfast. *Ann. Hum. Genet. 23*, 395–411.

Strobino, B., Kline, J., Shrout, P., Stein, Z., Susser, M., and Warburton, D. (1980a). Recurrent spontaneous abortion: Definition of a syndrome. In *Human embryonic and fetal death*, edited by I.H. Porter and E.B. Hook. New York: Academic Press, pp. 315–330.

——, ——, and Stein, Z. (1978). Chemical and physical exposures of parents: Effects on reproduction and the offspring. *Early Hum. Dev. 1*, 371–399.

——, ——, ——, Susser, M., and Warburton, D. (1980b). Exposure to contraceptive creams, jellies and douches and their effect on the zygote. (Abstract) *Am. J. Epidemiol. 112*, 434.

Susser, E. (1983). Spontaneous abortion and induced abortion: An adjustment for the presence of induced abortion when estimating the rate of spontaneous abortion from cross-sectional studies. *Am. J. Epid. 117*, 305–308.

Susser, E. and Kline, J. (1982). Effects of induced abortion on spontaneous abortion rates. In *Occupational hazards and reproduction*, edited by K. Hemminki, M. Sorsa, and H. Vainio. Washington, D.C.: Hemisphere Publishing Corp. In press.

Takahara, H., Ohama, K., and Fujiwara, A. (1977). Cytogenetic study of early spontaneous abortion. *Hiroshima J. Med. Sci. 26*, 291–296.

Taylor, W.F. (1964). On the methodology of measuring the probability of fetal death in a prospective study. *Hum. Biol. 36*, 86–103.

—— (1969). The probability of fetal death. In *Congenital malformations*, edited by F. Clarke-Fraser and V.A. McKusick. New York: Excerpta Medica, pp. 307–320.

Vaisman, A.I. (1967). Working conditions in surgery and their effect on the health of anesthesiologists. *Eksp. Khir. Anesteziol. 3*, 44.

Vaitukaitis, J.L. (1979). Human chorionic gonadotropin: A hormone secreted for many reasons. *N. Engl. J. Med. 301*, 324–325.

Vessey, M.P., Doll, R., Johnson, B., and Peto, R. (1974). Outcome of pregnancy in women using an intrauterine device. *Lancet 1*, 495–498.

——, ——, ——, ——, and Wiggins, P. (1976). A long-term follow-up study of women using different methods of contraception—an interim report. *J. Bio. Soc. Sci. 8*, 373–427.

————, Meisler, L., Flavel, R., and Yeates, D. (1979). Outcome of pregnancy in women using different methods of contraception. *Br. J. Obstet. Gynaecol. 86*, 548–556.

Warburton, D. and Fraser, F.C. (1964). Spontaneous abortion risks in man: Data from reproductive histories collected in a medical genetics unit. *Am. J. Hum. Genet. 16*, 1–24.

————, Kline, J., Stein, Z., and Susser, M. (1980b). Monosomy X: A chromosomal anomaly associated with young maternal age. *Lancet 1*, 167–169.

————, Stein, Z., Kline, J., and Susser, M. (1980a). Chromosome abnormalities in spontaneous abortions: Data from the New York City study. In *Human embryonic and fetal death*, edited by I.H. Porter and E.B. Hook. New York: Academic Press, pp. 261–287.

————, Susser, M., Stein, Z., and Kline, J. (1982). Personal communication.

Whorton, D., Krauss, R.M., Marshall, S., and Milby, T. (1977). Infertility in male pesticide workers. *Lancet 2*, 1259–1261.

————, Milby, T., Krauss, R., and Stubbs, H. (1979). Testicular function in DBCP exposed pesticide workers. *J. Occup. Med. 21*, 161–166.

World Health Organization (1970). *Spontaneous and induced abortion*, Tech. Rep. Series No. 461. Geneva: World Health Organization.

Yerushalmy, J., Bierman, J.M., Kemp, D., Connor, A., and French, F. (1956). Longitudinal studies of pregnancy on the island of Kauai: Analysis of previous reproductive history. *Am. J. Obstet. Gynecol. 71*, 80–96.

3

Anencephalus, Hydrocephalus, and Spina Bifida

Milton Alter

CASE SERIES AND POPULATION STUDIES

A clinician's impression of a disease may differ considerably from an impression based on epidemiologic studies of a population. Clinicians often have the advantage of following afflicted individuals through the entire course of illness, from diagnosis until death. They may even have known patients (and their families) before disease develops. However, their view of the natural history of the disorder may be biased because they are rarely able to describe the population from which their patients are drawn. Clinicians do not know if their patients are typical (representative) of all patients with the particular disease. Epidemiologists, by contrast, take a *population* as their point of departure and relate observations about individual cases to the "universe" of patients in the population studied. Therefore, epidemiologists can be expected to estimate the frequency of a disease and judge how typical or unusual a given case is based on all patients in that population. They can compare disease among different populations and recognize peculiarities that would not be apparent to a clinician. Change in frequency of the disease over time (e.g., secular or seasonal trends) can often be estimated more precisely by epidemiologists than by clinicians.

Mathematical (biostatistical) analyses of observations about a disease are important to both epidemiologists and clinicians, but clinicians rarely formulate their observations mathematically. They are unlikely to think about diagnostic possibilities in terms of rates, ratios, probabilities, and confidence intervals. Clinicians may have some informal idea of what an "average" observation is like, but they do not calculate the average observation or its standard deviation in any precise way.

52

Having mentioned certain disadvantages of clinical impressions, it is important to stress that good clinical information about individual cases is no less important to the epidemiologist than to the clinician. Individual cases of a disease are the units that the epidemiologist must enumerate in forming ideas about the disease in the population. Unsound clinical work will render the "precision" of the epidemiologist misleading, if not meaningless. Therefore, both clinicians and epidemiologists must make sophisticated clinical judgments. In the case of an epidemiologist, the judgments take into account the population from which individual cases are drawn, whereas clinicians base their conclusions on a case series. If the difference between a case series and a population can be appreciated, the conceptual difference between the data base of the clinician and that of the epidemiologist can be bridged.

POPULATION STUDIES OF ANENCEPHALUS, HYDROCEPHALUS, AND SPINA BIFIDA

As a clinician who has studied neurologic diseases in populations, I have used many epidemiologic concepts. Several of the diseases I have studied occur in the perinatal period. In this chapter, my own studies of three severe congenital malformations of the nervous system will be described. These malformations are anencephalus, hydrocephalus, and spina bifida.

Considerations

Even though these disorders are relatively easy to diagnose clinically, there are problems of classification. Some of these problems are outlined in the following paragraphs.

Greater precision in diagnosis can perhaps be achieved with autopsy control of the clinical information, but an autopsy verification of the malformation has its shortcomings, because hydrocephalus and spina bifida are not necessarily lethal conditions. Also, tissue preservation postmortem may not always be optimal, and diagnosis may be compromised by postmortem artifacts. Not all fatal cases of these malformations go to autopsy. For these reasons autopsy control was not required in the studies described below, although postmortem data were used when available. Instead, the diagnoses of anencephalus, hydrocephalus, and spina bifida were based on clinical criteria.

Because of the relative rarity of the three malformations, prospective collection of data would have taken a long time and been costly.

Therefore, cases were accumulated retrospectively and I had to rely on case notes in clinical protocols. Personal verification of the diagnosis through actual examination of the patient was impossible. It must be appreciated that clinical protocols may vary greatly in quality, and that incomplete clinical notes introduce errors in case findings. Some cases that were inadequately documented had to be excluded.

Anencephalus posed the fewest diagnostic problems because the malformation is dramatic and is readily recognizable at birth. It consists of absence of the calvarium and cerebrum above the supraorbital ridges. Anencephalus should be distinguished from hydranencephalus. In anencephalus there are no cortex or meninges. The hydranencephalic infant, however, has a rim of cortex, and meningeal coverings should be detectable, at least histologically. Histologic analysis was not always performed and some patients listed as "anencephalic" may have actually been hydranencephalic infants.

In a retrospective study the epidemiologic investigator may be forced to accept the diagnosis of anencephalus made by the attending physician even if histologic confirmation was lacking. Such concessions to practicality introduce errors and weaken the conclusions that can be drawn from the population study. The perinatal epidemiologist must appreciate this weakness.

Hydrocephalus posed greater diagnostic problems than anencephalus. In a straightforward case of hydrocephalus, the head circumference at birth is greater than 2 standard deviations above the mean of 34 cm. However, racial differences might affect the mean value in that, for example, black infants are somewhat smaller than whites at birth. Correction for racial differences in head circumference was not used in my population study. Moreover, the head circumference was not always recorded in the clinical protocol when the diagnosis of hydrocephalus was made.

Even if the hydrocephalus is due to a prenatal condition, it may not always be apparent at birth; it may become obvious only in the later neonatal and perinatal period or even in adolescence (Davidson, 1980). If birth records alone were used to find cases, the number of hydrocephalic infants in the population would be underestimated. Additional sources of data that pertain at a time span beyond birth should be tapped, for example, pediatricians' records or records of an association for crippled children.

One should not include infants with enlarged heads due to an intracranial mass, intraspinal tumor (Oi and Raimondi, 1981), or central nervous system infection, because in such cases the hydrocephalus is not the primary condition. The entity of hydrolethalus has only recently been delineated as separate from hydrocephalus. Patients with hydrolethalus have polydactyly as well as heart, lung, occipital, and mandibular defects (Salonen et al., 1981). Because not all cases of "hydrocephalus" list the underlying cause or associated anomalies, the diagnosis listed by the attending physician would have to be accepted by the investigator in a retrospective study.

Spina bifida presented the most difficult problems in classification. The malformation may occur with no external sign of abnormality (spina bifida occulta). The latter was excluded in the population study because an occult spina bifida would be apparent only after a roentgenographic examination, which is not routinely done at birth. X-Ray exposure of a sample of otherwise healthy infants to reveal possible occult spina bifida would certainly not be justified in an epidemiologic study if the purpose were simply to establish a more accurate estimate of frequency. However, "routine" spinal X-ray examinations do reveal an appreciable number of cases of occult spina bifida. It is impossible to estimate the frequency of spina bifida occulta from "routine" spinal films, because the population sampled is unknown.

Combinations of anencephalus, hydrocephalus, and spina bifida can occur in individual patients. An infant with spina bifida, for example, could also have anencephalus. If this occurred, the patient was classified as "anencephalus." If a meningeal sac protruded through the spina bifida (meningocele) or if the meningeal sac contained spinal cord and nerve root elements (myelomeningocele), the patient was still classified as "spina bifida" in the study to be described. In a few cases the defect affected the brain cavity (encephalocele) instead of the spine, but for purposes of the population study, such defects in closure of the neural tube were all listed as "spina bifida." Rachischisis, which is a particularly severe form of nonclosure of the neural tube usually incompatible with life, was likewise listed as "spina bifida" in the population study. The classification described is modified slightly from the widely used conventions recommended by Record and McKeown (1949).

Choosing the Population

The study was conducted in Charleston, South Carolina. Several considerations entered into the choice of this population: size, dispersion, stability, and composition of the population as well as the availability of medical facilities.

POPULATION SIZE

In the case of a rare disease, the investigator has two options for ensuring that sufficient cases are available for analysis. Either a large population can be studied for a few years, or a smaller population can be studied over a longer period of time. Charleston County had about 200,000 inhabitants when the study was planned, and data were collected retrospectively for a ten-year period. Because the defects studied were usually present at birth or perinatally, the population at risk included individuals born during the study interval rather than the whole population. There were about 55,000 livebirths during the decade studied. Most investigators prefer to use *live* births as a standard reference population rather than *all* births.

POPULATION DISPERSION AND STABILITY

It is worth considering the dispersion of the population in the community. The population may be concentrated in one community or scattered in small towns and villages. In Charleston County, the city of Charleston is the major population center. However, an almost equal number of inhabitants live in rural enclaves and farms. Data collected in a population with a mixture of urban and rural inhabitants might be generalized more accurately than if the study were based solely on a rural or urban population. However, medical care in the outlying areas might be less accessible if not less adequate, and this factor might influence results. In comparing data from different populations, the dispersion of the population should be considered.

It is difficult to conduct an epidemiologic study if many new people are moving into the community, or emigration is appreciable. Charleston County had a stable population with low rates of immigration and emigration.

POPULATION COMPOSITION

A population is not a homogeneous entity but is composed of diverse elements. Analysis of data from the population must take this diversity into account. The age distribution, proportion of men and women, and racial and ethnic characteristics are some of the ways a population may be classified. The age distribution is clearly important if one is interested in perinatal problems, in that a disproportionate number of elderly people may mean fewer births. Racial factors are important primarily because of genetic and cultural differences among races that may influence the frequency of occurrence of various diseases. Dietary habits, for example, could alter the risk of congenital malformations of the nervous system. About half the population in Charleston County was black, there were approximately equal numbers of men and women, and the number of births for each racial group was nearly equal. The urban–rural residence ratio was about equal as already noted.

MEDICAL FACILITIES

Charleston is the site of the Medical University of South Carolina, so that patients with unusual or serious illnesses may be referred there for treatment. Malformations of the nervous system certainly fall into the category of serious illnesses, but some cases are so severe that death occurs before transfer can be made, or the infant is stillborn. Therefore, not all infants with malformations of the nervous system were referred to hospitals in Charleston County.

In a community served by a medical school, medical records would be expected to be superior to those in an ordinary community. Because anencephalus is obvious at birth, the number of cases recorded in birth records is likely to be relatively complete for the population. The disorder is sufficiently well recognized so that even stillborn infants and infants delivered before the mother can reach a medical facility are likely to be diagnosed and recorded. Obstetricians in Charleston County were complemented by trained midwives who helped with rural deliveries. These midwives were familiar with severe malformations, and it is unlikely that one as obvious as anencephalus or spina bifida would be missed. If a home delivery occurred and the mother was embarrassed or frightened by the malformation, a stillborn malformed infant could conceivably go unrecorded and therefore undetected in the population study. The amount of "loss" of such cases in a population study would, of course, be unknown.

Because anencephalic infants are stillborn or die early in the perinatal period, death certificates become an important source of data on this malformation. The death certificates for Charleston County were therefore searched for primary and secondary causes of death, and some cases of anencephalus were found to be recorded only on death certificates.

Patients with spina bifida tend to die of infection, and the latter may be recorded as the cause of death. In such instances, "spina bifida" might be listed only as a secondary or contributory cause of death. If the underlying defects were also not listed and the patients were not located independently through hospital or physician records, these cases would be lost, and the observed frequency of spina bifida would be an underestimation of the true frequency in the population.

Because death certificates alone could not be relied on to yield all cases of spina bifida or hydrocephalus, physicians' records were also reviewed. It is worth noting the number of physicians in the community in relation to the size of the population. Such an estimate is often expressed as a physician–population ratio and gives a rough index of the availability of medical care. In Charleston County, for example, the ratio was 1:810 (Alter, 1962).

57

It is often awkward and certainly time consuming to visit each physician in the community with a request to review records. Moreover, physicians are understandably reluctant to open their records to medical researchers—indeed, some are outright opposed. Considerations of confidentiality virtually preclude a direct search of physicians' records. Physicians rarely maintain a diagnostic index, so that a direct search would also be tedious and expensive. To avoid these problems, investigators usually resort to a questionnaire mailed to physicians with a request for cooperation in the study. Including a stamped, self-addressed return envelope would make it easier for physicians to cooperate in the study. Confidentiality must of course be assured in the explanatory letter that accompanies the questionnaire. A respected physician in the community rather than the investigator should ideally write the letter to the physicians. If this is not possible, however, and physician cooperation is not secured, it might be necessary to forego the data on malformations available in physicians' files. Although this might not pose a problem for identifying cases of anencephalus, it would possibly result in loss of the less severe cases of hydrocephalus and spina bifida.

RESULTS OF THE CHARLESTON STUDY

The population study in Charleston County was a retrospective study encompassing the decade 1946 through 1955 (Alter, 1962). A respected neurologist practicing in Charleston County headed the research team. Medical records of all hospitals, the Crippled Children's Program, death certificates, as well as records of the two neurosurgeons and the neurologist then serving the community were reviewed for cases involving anencephalus, spina bifida, and hydrocephalus.

Meningocele, meningomyelocele, encephalocele, and rachischises were recorded as "spina bifida." Infants with both spina bifida and hydrocephalus, a common combination, were recorded separately. Patients recorded as "hydrocephalic" whose head circumference was less than 2 standard deviations above the norm were not included. Patients with an underlying cause of hydrocephalus such as prior infection or tumor were excluded.

A total of 164 cases were identified with a diagnosis of anencephalus, hydrocephalus, or spina bifida between January 1, 1946 and December 31, 1955. Of these, 140 were residents of Charleston County. Livebirths in Charleston County during the study interval numbered 55,156 according to official publications of vital statistics for Charleston County.

Table 3-1. Anencephalus, Hydrocephalus, and Spina Bifida, Charleston County, S.C., 1946–1955

Source of cases	No. of cases	Percentage of total
Hospital records		
Inpatients	45	28
Autopsy	9	6
Mortality data		
Death certificates	24	15
Stillbirths	48	29
Clinic records	12	6
Physicians' records	6	4
Several sources combined	20	12
Total	164	100
No. who were residents of Charleston Co.	140	

The sources of the cases identified are shown in Table 3-1. Based on the 140 resident cases, the number of new cases (incidence) occurring per year for each 1000 livebirths is recorded in Table 3-2 by race and sex. Of the three malformations, hydrocephalus was the most common. The incidence of hydrocephalus was even higher if cases with hydrocephalus and spina bifida were added to those with hydrocephalus alone.

Hydrocephalus alone occurred more often in blacks than in whites and in males more often than females in both races. However, when hydrocephalus combined with spina bifida was considered, whites

Table 3-2. Average Annual Incidence by Race and Sex of Anencephalus, Hydrocephalus, and Spina Bifida, Charleston County, S.C., 1946–1955[a]

Race and sex	Total live births	Anencephalus		Hydrocephalus		Spina bifida		Spina bifida and hydrocephalus	
		N	I	N	I	N	I	N	I
White									
Male	15,262	8	0.52	15	0.98	14	0.92	8	0.52
Female	13,993	16	1.14	9	0.64	15	1.07	8	0.50
Black									
Male	13,244	2	0.15	16	1.21	5	0.38	2	0.16
Female	12,657	3	0.24	13	1.03	5	0.40	2	0.16
Total	55,156	29	0.53	53	0.96	39	0.71	19	0.34

[a] N, Number of cases; I, incidence per 1000 livebirths.

had a higher incidence and the sex difference disappeared. The relatively small number of cases with combined hydrocephalus and spina bifida warrants caution in accepting these observations. Unlike hydrocephalus alone, spina bifida was more common in whites than blacks, and there was virtually no difference in incidence for males and females.

Anencephalus afflicted 0.53 infants per 1000 livebirths in Charleston County, occurring about half as often as hydrocephalus alone. Comparing incidence by race and sex, anencephalus was more common in whites and in females. The incidence in females was twice as high as in males.

When all three of these severe malformations of the nervous system were combined, their average annual incidence was 2.5 per 1000 livebirths, or about 1 in 400 livebirths.

The incidence for each year of the study is shown in Table 3-3. Incidence varied in the narrow range of 1.8 to 3.5 per 1000 livebirths for all three malformations combined. Given the relatively small number of cases per year, the frequency of the malformations over the decade studied was remarkably constant. This suggests that whatever the environmental factors that influenced incidence may have been, they did not vary greatly over the time interval studied.

Seasonal incidence was examined only for anencephalus because month of birth was incomplete for hydrocephalic infants and those with spina bifida. The numbers of anencephalic births each month during the ten years of the study are shown in Table 3-4. The frequency varied from none to six cases per month. However, total livebirths also varied seasonally in Charleston County. The peaks in total livebirths matched the peaks in anencephalic births. Therefore, the conclusion should not be drawn from these data that seasonal fluctuations in anencephalic births are real or due to some environmental factors (e.g., ambient temperature) or to viral infections, which may vary seasonally.

The number of anencephalic births by age of mother in Charleston is shown in Table 3-5 for the 21 cases for which such information was available. Although most anencephalic births occurred among mothers who were 24 years of age and younger, it must be understood that the number of livebirths is greater in younger mothers. The cluster occurring in mothers 35 years of age and older is therefore noteworthy in that fewer older women give birth. It would be important to calculate age-specific incidence rates of anencephalus; however, the number of livebirths by age of mother was unavailable at the time of the study.

Anencephalus was noted in two black female twins, but it is uncertain whether they were monozygotic or dizygotic.

60

Table 3-3. Annual Incidence per 1000 Livebirths of Anencephalus, Hydrocephalus, and Spina Bifida, Charleston County, S.C., 1946–1955[a]

Year	Livebirths	Total N	Total I	Anencephalus N	Hydrocephalus N	Spina bifida N	Spina bifida and hydrocephalus N
1946	5249	11	2.1	2	5	3	1
1947	5429	14	2.5	—	8	5	1
1948	4833	14	2.9	1	7	4	2
1949	5015	14	2.8	4	3	4	3
1950	5143	16	3.1	4	4	8	—
1951	5492	10	1.8	—	3	3	4
1952	5585	14	2.5	4	7	1	2
1953	5845	12	2.0	3	5	2	2
1954	6283	13	2.1	4	2	5	2
1955	6282	22	3.5	7	9	4	2

[a] N, Number of cases; I, incidence per 1000 livebirths.

61

Table 3-4. Anencephalic Births per Month, Charleston County, S.C., 1946–1955[a]

Month	N	Month	N
January	6	July	2
February	2	August	2
March	2	September	6
April	—	October	4
May	1	November	1
June	—	December	2

[a] The month of birth is unknown in one case.

Table 3-5. Anencephalic Births by Age of Mother, Charleston County, S.C., 1946–1955

Maternal age (years)	N[a]
≤14	0
15–24	14
25–34	2
35–44	5
Total	21

[a] For eight infants, maternal age is unknown.

COMPARISON OF CHARLESTON COUNTY WITH OTHER COMMUNITIES

In order to compare the frequency of anencephalus, hydrocephalus, and spina bifida in Charleston County with the frequency in other communities, the method of case finding must be taken into account. The characteristics of the population are also important, as already discussed. Some studies use only mortality data, others rely on data collected from hospitals alone, and still others use a population survey technique in which several sources of information are reviewed—as was done in Charleston.

Mortality for anencephalus and spina bifida varied from about 0.5 to 2.5 patients per 1000 births, whereas hydrocephalus varied from 0.5 to 1.5 patients per 1000 births. Hospital surveys were the most common type of study, and these yielded incidence ratios that varied even more. Some investigators reported incidence ratios of over 5 per 1000 births for anencephalus, whereas ratios for hydrocephalus and spina bifida ranged from 0.3 and 0.2 to over 4 and 3 per 1000 births, respectively. Population studies in which several sources of data were used gave incidence ratios close to those in which only hospital data were used. Charleston County fell near the middle of the incidence range reported from various communities.

POSSIBLE RISK FACTORS FOR ANENCEPHALUS, HYDROCEPHALUS, AND SPINA BIFIDA

It was noted that many of the communities with a high incidence of these severe neurologic malformations included populations with large numbers of Irish and Scottish ethnic groups (Alter, 1962). However, the incidence of malformations of the nervous system in Britain (Editorial, 1980; Bound et al., 1981) and the northeastern United States (Stein et al., 1982) has been decreasing.

Among the ideas advanced to account for the decreasing incidence is introduction of effective birth control, which allowed increased intervals between pregnancies. The longer interpregnancy interval presumably enhanced the possibility that the uterus would recover from any adverse conditions leading to an increased risk of malformation. This hypothesis assumes that the intrauterine environment is an important risk factor. Clarke et al. (1975) showed that mothers of infants with a major malformation of the nervous system tended to have abnormal reproductive histories. For example, spontaneous abortion was twice as likely to precede birth of a neurologically malformed infant as it was to follow such a birth. They postulated that trophoblastic material from the abortion might induce the subsequent malformation. However, David et al. (1980) noted that half the women in their study who had aborted before giving birth to a child with anencephaly or spina bifida had had curettage of the uterus, which should have removed trophoblastic material. Therefore, David et al. (1980) considered unlikely the trophoblastic induction hypothesis as a cause of neurologic malformation in the subsequent pregnancy.

Occurrence of anencephalic fetuses in women with a copper-bearing intrauterine contraceptive device (Graham et al., 1980) raised the possibility that heavy metals were related to risk of malformation of the nervous system. Zinc levels were higher in the hair of newborn infants with spina bifida, and in their mothers, compared to control offspring and their mothers, according to Bergmann et al. (1980). They suggested abnormal zinc availability or impaired zinc metabolism as possible causes. Elwood and Coldman (1981), however, failed to find an association between risk of anencephalus and zinc or 13 other elements in the drinking water of the mother of an affected infant. Measurement of elements in drinking water is not as direct a method as analysis of the hair of affected individuals. Hard water has come under suspicion in the development of malformations (Bergmann et al., 1980; Elwood and Coldman, 1981).

According to Sever and Emanuel (1981), the mother's low socioeconomic status when she was growing up was thought to play a role in increasing risk of malformation of the nervous system in offspring. Baird (1980) and Nevin et al. (1981) also noted an association between lower social class and increased risk of anencephalus and spina bifida. Offspring of foreign workers in Vienna had a high occurrence of severe malformations (Spernol et al., 1981). These workers occupied the lower strata of the socioeconomic scale. However, Elwood and Coldman (1981) found no association between mean income of mothers with anencephalic offspring or with the proportion of women employed.

Gestational fever during the first trimester was significantly increased in mothers of offspring with neural tube defects (Layde et al., 1980) compared to mothers of Down syndrome and cleft palate offspring. Coffey and Jessop (1957) implicated influenza A as being teratogenic.

Although environmental factors are deemed important in determining a risk of central nervous system malformation, genetic factors are also suspected. In isolated families, clustering of anencephalus may be observed (Toriello et al., 1980), as it was in one black family in Charleston County. Farb et al. (1980) have recently reviewed the literature on anencephaly in twins. Hydrocephalus in some families appears to follow autosomal recessive or sex-linked inheritance (Mochizuki et al., 1981; Petrus et al., 1981). Various genetic syndromes with hydrocephalus as one feature are described with some frequency (Waaler and Aarskog, 1980). A single gene defect appeared to account for the four cases of anencephalus or spina bifida in one family (Toriello et al., 1980).

Even the decline of cases of severe congenital neurologic malformation in Britain and in areas of the United States such as Brooklyn, New York, and the Northeast in general might be reconciled with a genetic cause by assuming that the gene expression was environmentally influenced. Associations of HLA with anencephalus and spina bifida might have such significance in that the HLA complex is widely believed to influence immune responses, for example, the immune response to infection. Feingold et al. (1980) reported a positive association between HLA types A1 and B8, and spina bifida and anencephalus. However, B5 and Bw35 were negatively associated with these malformations. Experimentally, respiratory syncytial virus

(Lagac'e-Simard et al., 1982), mouse hepatitis virus (Hirano et al., 1980), and measles virus (Norrby et al., 1980) have all been implicated, especially in hydrocephalus.

Pietrzyk (1980), despite complex segregation analysis, was unable to discriminate clearly between a single-locus genetic model and multifactorial inheritance of neural tube defects. The possibility that the cases studied were due to a variety of causes would certainly make genetic analysis difficult. Phenocopies could easily confound the genetic studies.

James (1981) noted that concordance ratios of spina bifida and anencephalus in monozygotic twins increased on a continuum running from dichorionic to monochorionic–diamniotic to monochorionic–monoamniotic to conjoined pairs. This suggested to him that the timing of embryonic events rather than a specific gene action accounted for the concordance rates.

The preponderance of females among anencephalic infants has been widely noted. Ratios as high as three females to one male are sometimes seen. The malformation may be more lethal in males, who are aborted disproportionately early and "missed." Study of abortuses would be needed to confirm this, but the fetus is not always found in early abortions, or the tissue is usually badly macerated.

Among hydrocephalics there may be a slight male preponderance (Murphy, 1947; Record and McKeown, 1949; Alter, 1962). Risk of recurrence is of great concern to parents who have given birth to a malformed child. Empiric risk figures for the severe congenital malformations discussed in this chapter are not precisely known. Nevin and Johnston (1980) visited 226 sets of parents of 360 patients with anencephalus or spina bifida or both, born in Belfast, Northern Ireland. Among sibs of index cases with spina bifida, 10.4% had anencephalus or spina bifida. Among index cases with anencephalus, the proportion of sibs affected was 6.4%. For sibs born *after* the index patients, the proportions were 12.2% and 6.4%, respectively, whereas overall incidence of either malformation among sibs was 8.8%. With such high risks of recurrence, assay for alpha-fetoprotein level, which is correlated with presence of the malformation, should be advocated (U.K. collaborative study, 1982).

CONCLUSION

Epidemiologic approaches to the study of severe congenital malformations differ from clinical approaches in that the former involve well-defined populations whereas the latter rely on case series drawn from ill-defined sources. Both approaches require sophisticated clinical information. The malformations discussed in this chapter—anencephalus, hydrocephalus, and spina bifida—seem superficially easy to diagnose, but each entity presents complexities that confound analyses and cause the cases studied to be classified as a heterogeneous group rather than a single disorder.

The choice of a population suitable for study of the three malformations was described. Size, dispersion, composition, and stability of the population are important considerations, as are access to and quality of medical facilities.

An epidemiologic study of the incidence of anencephalus, hydrocephalus, and spina bifida in Charleston County, South Carolina is described. Race-specific incidence in whites and blacks, respectively, per 1000 livebirths was 1.2 and 0.2 for anencephalus, 1.4 and 1.7 for all hydrocephalics, and 1.5 and 0.6 for all individuals with spina bifida. These incidence rates were compared with results in other communities. The possible causes of the malformations were also discussed.

REFERENCES

Alter, M. (1962). Anencephalus, hydrocephalus and spina bifida: Epidemiology with special reference to a survey in Charleston, S.C. *Arch. Neurol.* 7, 411–422.

Baird, D. (1980). Environment and reproduction. *Br. J. Obstet. Gynaecol.* 87, 1057–1067.

Bergmann, K.E., Makosch, G., and Tews, K.H. (1980). Abnormalities of hair zinc concentration in mothers of newborn infants with spina bifida. *Am. J. Clin. Nutr.* 33, 2145–2150.

Bound, J.P., Harvey, P.W., Brookes, D.M., and Sayers, B.M. (1981). The incidence of anencephalus in the Fylde peninsula 1956–76 and changes in water hardness. *J. Epidemiol. Community Health* 35, 102–105.

Clarke, C.A., Hobson, D., McKendrick, O.M., Rogers, S.C., and Sheppard, P.M. (1975). Spina bifida and anencephaly: Miscarriage as a possible cause. *Br. Med. J.* 4, 743–746.

Coffey, V.P. and Jessop, W.J.E. (1957). A study of 137 cases of anencephalus. *Br. J. Prev. Soc. Med.* 11, 174–180.

David, T.J., Townley, P.A., and Goldstein, A.R. (1980). Prior abortions and neural tube defects. *Clin. Genet.* 18, 201–202.

Davidson, R.I. (1980). Primary hydrocephalus in adolescence. *Surg. Neurol.* 14, 137–140.

Editorial (1980). The uncertainty principal. *Lancet 2*, 784.

Elwood, J.M. and Coldman, A.J. (1981). Water composition in the etiology of anencephalus. *Am. J. Epidemiol.* 113, 681–690.

Farb, H.F., Thomason, J., Carandang, F.S., Sampson, M.B., and Spellacy, W.N. (1980). Anencephaly, twins and HLA-B27. *J. Reprod. Med.* 25, 166–170.

Feingold, J., Feingold, N., and Bois, E. (1980). Spina bifida and anencephaly: Geographic correlation with the HLA system. *Tissue Antigens 15*, 318–324.

Graham, D., Enkin, M., and deSa, D. (1980). Neural tube defects in association with copper intrauterine devices. *Int. J. Gynaecol. Obstet. 18*, 404–405.

Hirano, N., Goto, N., Ogawa, T., Ono, K., Murakami, T., and Fujiwara, K. (1980). Hydrocephalus in suckling rats infected intracerebrally with mouse hepatitis virus, MHV-A59. *Microbiol. Immunol. 24*, 825–834.

James, W.H. (1981). Differences between events preceding spina bifida and anencephaly. *J. Med. Genet. 18*, 17–21.

Lagac'e-Simard, J., Descoteaux, J.P., and Lussier, G. (1982). Experimental pneumovirus infections. 2. Hydrocephalus of hamsters and mice due to infection with human respiratory syncytial virus. *Am. J. Pathol. 107*, 36–40.

Layde, P.M., Edmonds, L.D., and Erickson, J.D. (1980). Maternal fever and neural tube defects. *Teratology 21*, 105–108.

Mochizuki, Y., Suyehiro, Y., Ihara, Y., Tomimoto, K., Saito, A., and Ito, T. (1981). Congenital hydrocephalus and clasped thumbs: Two cases of brothers in a family. *Brain Dev. 3*, 407–409.

Murphy, D.P. (1947). *Congenital malformations: A study of parental characteristics with special reference to the reproductive process.* Philadelphia: Lippincott.

Nevin, N.C. and Johnston, W.B. (1980). A family study of spina bifida and anencephalus in Belfast, Northern Ireland (1964 to 1968). *J. Med. Genet. 17*, 203–211.

Nevin, N.C., Johnston, W.P., and Merrett, J.D. (1981). Influence of social class on the risk of recurrence of anencephalus and spina bifida. *Dev. Med. Child. Neurol. 23*, 155–163.

Norrby, E., Swoveland, P., Kristensson, K., and Johnson, K.P. (1980). Further studies on subacute encephalitis and hydrocephalus in hamsters caused by measles virus from persistently infected cell cultures. *J. Med. Virol. 5*, 109–116.

Oi, S. and Raimondi, A.J. (1981). Hydrocephalus associated with intraspinal neoplasms in childhood. *Am. J. Dis. Child. 135*, 1122–1124.

Petrus, M., Dutau, G., and Rochiccioli, P. (1981). Autosomal recessive inheritance of hydrocephalus with stenosis of the duct of Sylvius. *J. Genet. Hum. 29*, 155–160.

Pietrzyk, J.J. (1980). Neural tube malformations: Complex segregation analysis and recurrence risk. *Am. J. Med. Genet. 7*, 293–300.

Record, R.G., and McKeown, T. (1949). Congenital malformations of the central nervous system: I. A survey of 930 cases. *Br. J. Prev. Soc. Med. 3*, 183–219.

Salonen, R., Herua, R., and Norio, R. (1981). The hydrolethalus syndrome: delineation of a "new" lethal malformation syndrome based on 28 patients. *Clin. Genet. 19*, 321–330.

Sever, L.E. and Emanuel, I. (1981). Intergenerational factors in the etiology of anencephalus and spina bifida. *Dev. Med. Child. Neurol. 23*, 151–154.

Spernol, R., Endler, M., and Schaller, A. (1981). Incidence of congenital malformations among births of foreign workers. *Wien. Med. Wochenschr.* *131*, 319–324.

Stein, S.C., Feldman, J.G., Friedlander, M., and Klein, R.J. (1982). Is myelomeningocele a disappearing disease? *Pediatrics 69*, 511–514.

Toriello, H.V., Warren, S.T., and Lindstrom, J.A. (1980). Brief communication: Possible X-linked anencephaly and spina bifida—report of a kindred. *Am. J. Med. Genet. 6*, 119–121.

U.K. Collaborative Study (1982). Third report on alpha-fetoprotein in relation to neural-tube defects. Survival of infants with open spina bifida in relation to maternal serum alpha-fetoprotein level. *Br. J. Obstet. Gynaecol. 89*, 3–7.

Waaler, P.E., and Aarskog, D. (1980). Syndrome of hydrocephalus, costo-vertebral dysplasia and Sprengel anomaly with autosomal dominant inheritance. *Neuropaediatrie 11*, 291–297.

4

Prematurity

Bea J. van den Berg and Frank W. Oechsli

Premature or preterm birth is the most important single cause of perinatal death and neonatal morbidity. An international comparison shows that differences in the incidence of premature birth, in large part, explain differences in the national rates of neonatal and late fetal mortality. The incidence of preterm birth in the United States is relatively high, and the reduction in the neonatal death rate of the last decade has been achieved without reducing the incidence of premature birth. To attain a minimum rate of perinatal mortality requires a reduction in the incidence of premature birth. Preventive measures at a local level and specialized obstetric management indicate that a reduction is feasible. It is therefore important to investigate factors bearing on preterm delivery as a basis for further improving obstetric practice and for planning public health programs to reduce preterm birth and, indirectly, perinatal death and neonatal morbidity.

DEFINITION

Preterm birth as defined by the World Health Organization (WHO, 1975) is a birth that occurs at a gestational age of less than 37 completed weeks (<259 days). The duration of gestation is measured from the first day of the last normal menstrual period and expressed in completed days or completed weeks. It is further recommended in the same WHO source that national perinatal statistics should include all delivered fetuses and infants weighing at least 500 g, or having a

From the Child Health and Development Studies, School of Public Health, University of California, Berkeley. Supported by grants HD07256 and HD15622 from the National Institutes of Health.

gestational age of 22 weeks, or having a body length of 25 cm crown–heel, whether alive or dead. For international comparisons, standard perinatal statistics should be restricted to fetuses and infants weighing 1000 g or more, or having a gestational age of 28 weeks, or having a body length of 35 cm crown–heel.

UNITED STATES CRITERIA

In most states, the minimum period of gestation for which fetal death registration is required is 20 completed weeks or more, calculated from the date of the last menstrual period; a few states require registration of all periods of gestation, however (National Center for Health Statistics, 1981). A distribution by length of gestation from 20 weeks onward is presented in Table 4-1. It shows that 63% of the dead fetuses had a gestational age of less than 37 completed weeks. The table also shows that the number of registered fetal deaths with unknown duration of gestation amounts to 18% of the number with known duration of gestation.

Livebirths must be registered in the United States irrespective of gestational age (National Center for Health Statistics, 1981a). A distribution by period of gestation is provided in Table 4-2. The proportion of preterm livebirths (<37 weeks' gestation) is shown to be 8.9% of all livebirths. Here the number with unknown gestation amounts to 24% of the total with known length of gestation.

Table 4-1. Fetal Deaths by Period of Gestation, United States, 1977[a,b]

Period of gestation (weeks)	No. of deaths	Percentage distribution	Cumulative percentage
20–23	4,128	14.8	14.8
24–27	3,830	13.7	28.5
28–31	3,566	12.7	41.2
32–35	4,476	16.0	57.2
36	1,589	5.7	62.9
37–39	4,628	16.5	79.4
40	2,476	8.8	88.2
⩾41	3,292	11.8	100.0
Total known	27,985	100.0	
Not stated	5,068	18.1	

[a] Fetal deaths include only those with stated or presumed period of gestation of 20 weeks or more.
[b] Excluded are Arkansas, Maine, and New York City.
Source: National Center for Health Statistics (1981).

Table 4-2. Livebirths by Period of Gestation,
United States, 1979[a]

Period of gestation (weeks)	No. of livebirths	Percentage distribution	Cumulative percentage
<28	15,872	.61	.61
28–31	25,673	1.00	1.61
32–35	110,065	4.30	5.91
36	76,098	2.97	8.88
37–39	923,383	36.07	44.95
40	572,388	22.36	67.31
41	410,834	16.05	83.36
≥42	426,094	16.64	100.00
Total known	2,560,407	100.00	
Not stated	615,201	24.03	

[a] Excludes data for Connecticut, New Mexico, and Texas, which did not require reporting of first day of last menstrual period.

Source: National Center for Health Statistics (1981a).

Because ascertaining the length of gestation depends on the mother's recall of the date of her last menstrual period, vital statistics reports list it as unknown more often than they do birthweight (e.g., 2 per 1000 of the livebirths in 1979 had unknown birthweight). Therefore, epidemiologic studies sometimes utilize incidence rates of low birthweight (<2500 g) as indicators of preterm birth. There is only partial overlapping of these two measures, however: approximately half of low-birthweight infants have gestations of less than 37 weeks, and about 40–50% of preterm infants weigh less than 2500 g at birth (Yerushalmy et al., 1965; Hemminki and Starfield, 1978).

INTERNATIONAL COMPARISONS

An international comparison of length of gestation of fetal deaths and livebirths is fraught with difficulties. Even when these statistics are collected, the completeness of the registration is difficult to assess. Furthermore, the difficulties are most often the result of differences in d finitions of livebirth and fetal death, in the definition of gestational a e, in the minimum length of gestation required for registration, in the level of compliance with the stated requirements, and in the processing and presentation of the data. Nevertheless, undertaking international comparative studies could be a significant contribution, because such studies may stimulate improvements in the collection and publication of standard perinatal statistics and promote the use of these statistics for social and medical intervention programs.

Under the auspices of the World Health Organization, eight countries participated in an international collaborative study of social and biologic effects on perinatal mortality. The extensive findings have been reported in two volumes (WHO, 1978), and a third volume is in preparation. The procedures for collecting and processing the vital statistics in these countries are not exactly the same, but efforts have been made to make the data comparable.

Five of the participating countries provided information on length of gestation of fetal deaths and of livebirths calculated from the date of the last menstrual period and expressed in completed weeks. These countries were Cuba, Hungary, New Zealand, Sweden, and the United States. For the United States the data relate to the births in 1973 in six states with linked birth and neonatal death records. These are Hawaii, Rhode Island, Utah, Vermont, Oklahoma and Washington. For other countries all births in each country during 1973 are included.

The data in Tables 4-3 to 4-6 are calculated from the raw data provided in Vol. 2 of the WHO report. Table 4-3 shows the distribution of late fetal deaths (≥28 weeks of gestation) and of livebirths (all gestational ages) by period of gestation. First, it is important to

Table 4-3.   Percentage Distributions of Late Fetal Deaths and Livebirths by Period of Gestation in Selected Countries, 1973

Country	Period of gestation (weeks)				Total known		Not stated (% of known)
	<28	28–36	37–41	≥42	Number	%	
1. Fetal deaths: ≥28 weeks' gestation (%)							
Cuba		49.0	41.5	9.5	2,620	100.0	10.9
Hungary		58.0	40.0	2.0	1,291	100.0	0.2
New Zealand							
(1972 + 1973)		47.6	43.2	9.2	1,124	100.0	1.3
Sweden		45.5	46.3	8.2	706	100.0	3.0
United States							
(five states)[a]		44.7	41.4	13.9	432	100.0	38.9
2. Live births: all gestations							
Cuba	0.5	10.1	80.3	9.1	156,102	100.0	43.1
Hungary	0.8	18.7	77.0	3.5	152,983	100.0	0.0
New Zealand	0.1	3.9	83.8	12.2	59,425	100.0	0.2
Sweden	0.1	4.6	79.6	15.7	105,703	100.0	1.8
United States							
(five states)[a]	0.4	6.7	74.8	18.1	82,961	100.0	18.1

[a] Includes Hawaii, Rhode Island, Utah, Vermont, and Washington. Weeks of gestation not available on Oklahoma data.

Source: World Health Organization (1978), Vol. 2.

note that the proportion of fetal deaths and of livebirths with un-known gestational age expressed in the table as percentage of the total with known gestation is rather large in some countries. These figures are low for Hungary, New Zealand, and Sweden—at most, 3% for fetal deaths and 2% for livebirths. Cuba and the United States have considerably higher percentages with unknown gestational length. These quantities warn against a detailed international com-parison. Table 4-4 summarizes the data of Table 4-3 by providing the proportion of preterm births (<37 weeks' gestation) among late fetal deaths and livebirths, and the proportion of preterm births among the first-week neonatal deaths. Except for the somewhat higher per-centages for Hungary, the percentages for the other countries are not far apart. The percentages for late fetal deaths range between 45 and 49, and for livebirths between 4 and 10. For early neonatal deaths, the percentage of preterm births is quite high, ranging between 61 and 69 in four of the five countries; for Hungary the proportion is indicated as 81%.

Table 4-5 provides the incidence rates for late fetal deaths per 1000 births, first-week neonatal death rates per 1000 livebirths, and peri-natal death rates per 1000 births. The rates for Sweden are the lowest in all three categories; Cuba has the highest rate for fetal death and Hungary for neonatal death. A comparison of Tables 4-4 and 4-5 indicates that countries with a high proportion of preterm livebirths (Table 4-4) also have a high early neonatal mortality rate (Table 4-5). This is to be expected because the proportion of preterm infants among neonatal deaths is high, more than 60% in all countries.

The neonatal mortality rate reflects the distribution of births by length of gestation and also the gestation-specific death rates. The

Table 4-4. Percentage of Late Fetal Deaths, Livebirths, and Early Neonatal Deaths with Length of Gestation Less Than 37 Weeks in Selected Countries, 1973[a]

Country	Percentage with length of gestation <37 weeks		
	Late fetal deaths	*Livebirths*	*Early neonatal deaths*
Cuba	49.1	10.5	60.7
Hungary	58.0	19.4	81.2
New Zealand			
(1972–1973)	47.6	3.8	66.2
Sweden	45.5	4.7	61.3
United States (part)	44.7	7.2	69.0

[a] Late fetal deaths of ≥28 weeks of gestation, livebirths of any gestational length, early neonatal deaths of any gestational length where death occurred in the first week of life.

Source: World Health Organization (1978), Vol. 2.

Table 4-5. Rates of Late Fetal Deaths, Early Neonatal Deaths, and Perinatal Deaths in Selected Countries, 1973[a]

Country	Late fetal deaths per 1000 births	Early neonatal deaths per 1000 livebirths	Perinatal deaths per 1000 births
Cuba	12.8	14.2	26.9
Hungary	8.4	20.8	29.0
New Zealand (1972–1973)	9.4	8.0	17.3
Sweden	6.6	6.1	12.6
United States (part)	6.7	8.3	14.9

[a] Late fetal deaths of ≥28 weeks of gestation, early neonatal deaths of any gestational length where death occurred in the first week of life.

Source: World Health Organization (1978), Vol. 2.

relative importance of the gestational age distribution may be demonstrated by direct standardization, a method by which the gestational age-specific death rates of each country are applied to a standard distribution of gestational ages of livebirth, and the resulting standardized neonatal death rates are compared with the original crude neonatal death rate. Table 4-6 shows the crude early neonatal mortality rates and the standardized rates, utilizing as standard the gestational age distribution of Sweden. To avoid the very small and inconsistent values of the very immature births, Table 4-6 is limited to births of ≥22 weeks of gestation. The differences between countries are much reduced after standardization, indicating that most of the differences among crude rates are due to differences in the proportion of preterm births.

A similar comparison for Sweden and the State of Massachusetts of the crude neonatal mortality with standardized neonatal mortality

Table 4-6. Crude and Standardized Early Neonatal Mortality Rates for Five Countries, 1973[a]

Country	Early neonatal mortality rates per 1000 livebirths[b]	
	Crude	Standardized
Cuba	18.2	12.7
Hungary	20.4	8.2
New Zealand (1972–1973)	7.7	8.5
Sweden	5.9	—
United States (part)	7.6	5.4

[a] Standard is the Swedish distribution of livebirths by gestational age of ≥22 weeks.
[b] Neonatal mortality rates in first week of life.

Source: World Health Organization (1978), Vol. 2.

was recently published by Guyer et al. (1982). The standard was the *birthweight* distribution of Swedish livebirths. The birthweight-specific neonatal death rates of Massachusetts were applied to this standard. The excess in the crude neonatal mortality of the United States disappeared after standardization. These two sets of comparisons indicate that the relative frequency of preterm deliveries and the closely related relative frequency of low birthweight are key issues in the level of neonatal mortality.

Assuming that the data of the states involved in these two studies approximately represent the United States, it can be concluded that the difference between the relatively high neonatal mortality rate in the United States and the favorable rates in countries such as Sweden could be leveled by a reduction in the incidence of preterm birth and low birthweight.

We standardized to show what hypothetically would happen if the gestational age distributions were shifted to the Swedish pattern, assuming that the gestation-specific mortality rates would not change. This assumption is not entirely realistic. Some of the "hard core" high-risk infants would not benefit from a slightly longer gestation and hence the improvements in neonatal mortality suggested by standardization are slightly exaggerated.

HISTORIC TRENDS IN THE UNITED STATES

In the United States the early neonatal death rate decreased during the last decade, but the proportion of preterm liveborn neonates changed very little. The neonatal death rate decreased from 13.6% in 1970 to 8.4% in 1977 (National Center for Health Statistics 1981), an average yearly reduction of 0.7%. The proportion of preterm births among livebirths was 9.3% in 1970 (National Center for Health Statistics, 1974) and 8.8% in 1977 (National Center for Health Statistics, 1981b), an average yearly reduction of 0.07%. It seems unlikely that the decrease in preterm births contributed much to the decrease in the early neonatal mortality, but from this comparison we cannot conclude whether the neonatal mortality has decreased among both the preterm infants and the term infants, or among only one of these groups. This cannot be studied because gestation-specific neonatal death rates (and birthweight-specific neonatal death rates) are generally not available.

Birthweight-specific death rates were assembled, in 1950 and 1960, from a national U.S. sample of vital statistics (National Center for Health Statistics, 1972, 1972a). These data have been used to evaluate the effect of birthweight distribution of livebirths on the recent decrease in neonatal mortality. Lee et al. (1980) utilized the

75

birthweight-specific neonatal mortality rates of the 1950 national sample and applied these rates to the birthweight distribution in each of the years 1951–1975. By this indirect standardization method, Lee and co-workers came to the conclusion that the decrease in the neonatal death rate from 20.0 per 1000 livebirths in 1950 to 11.6 per 1000 livebirths in 1975 (deaths within 28 days) was due to a decline in birthweight-specific neonatal mortality and very little, or not at all, to changes in the birthweight distribution. There was no evidence that a shift in gestational age within the same birthweight categories had occurred to contribute to the decline in the neonatal death rate.

Kleinman et al. (1978) directly compared the birthweight-specific early neonatal mortality rates of five states (Oklahoma, Rhode Island, Utah, Vermont, and Washington) of the United States, all participants in the WHO Collaborative Study mentioned earlier (1978), with the last national study of linked birth and death records of 1960. The early (first week) neonatal death rate in the five states declined from 15.5 per 1000 livebirths in 1960 to 9.8 per 1000 livebirths in 1973, a reduction of 37%. The authors showed that the reduction ratio was equal for all birthweight groups from 1000 to 4500 g. The decline in mortality among low-birthweight infants (<2500 g) accounted for more than half of the overall decline in early neonatal mortality. The proportion of infants with low birthweight among all liveborn infants changed only minimally, from 6.7% to 6.2%, and this change made only a small contribution to the overall decline in first-week neonatal mortality. This study also indicated that the gestational age of low-birthweight infants did not vary. It is therefore reasonable to conclude that gestation-specific neonatal mortality rates have declined fairly equally among the preterm infants and the term infants, and that a change in the percentage of preterm births did not materially contribute to the decline in early neonatal mortality.

FACTORS ASSOCIATED WITH PRETERM BIRTH

The recent downward trend in neonatal mortality does not preclude further reductions in the neonatal mortality of preterm infants. On the contrary, differences between states and between ethnic groups indicate that much improvement is possible. However, a decline in the incidence of preterm delivery would make a major contribution. Several variables have been identified that are associated with preterm delivery, some of which are accessible for prevention.

We utilized the data of the Child Health and Development Studies (CHDS, designed and initiated by J. Yerushalmy) to examine a variety of variables in relation to the rate of preterm births. The

CHDS program is a prospective, longitudinal study of pregnancy and of the subsequent development of the offspring. The study population consists of women who resided in the San Francisco East Bay area of California and who were members of the Kaiser Foundation Health Plan. This prepaid medical insurance plan provides comprehensive medical care to the family in any of the Kaiser Foundation clinics. Subscribers to the health plan constitute a predominantly employed, urban population representing a wide variety of economic and social characteristics deficient only in extremes. The mothers enrolled in CHDS early in their pregnancies and delivered at Kaiser Hospital during the years 1959–1967. They were interviewed extensively early in pregnancy, and the complete medical records relating to pregnancy, labor, and delivery are abstracted in detail. The data for Table 4-7 are derived from information obtained during the pregnancy interviews and from the abstracted medical records pertaining to 10,947 white pregnant women whose single pregnancies progressed beyond 22 weeks after their last menstrual period.

Table 4-7 presents the characteristics that were found to be statistically significantly related to premature delivery and shows the percentage of premature deliveries for subgroups of each characteristic. With maternal age the relationship is U-shaped, with the highest percentage of premature deliveries among the two extreme age groups. Inverse relationships between the proportion of premature deliveries and the duration of education of both mother and father are evident. The percentage of short-gestation births is lower where the father has a professional or managerial occupation.

Women who smoked cigarettes during pregnancy had a higher risk of premature delivery than women who never smoked or who stopped smoking either before or in the beginning of pregnancy. The percentage of preterm births was lower when the parents had planned the pregnancy in advance and when they had used contraceptives prior to conception.

The number of previous pregnancies was not related to preterm delivery; however, those multigravidas with one or more prior fetal deaths experienced an increased risk to deliver prematurely. Significantly more infants were born prematurely when the immediately preceding pregnancy ended in a fetal death and/or had less than 37 weeks' gestation, when the interpregnancy interval was less than four months, or when a preceding liveborn infant weighed 2500 g or less.

First-trimester bleeding and low weight gain (less than half a pound per week after 20 weeks' gestation) increased the risk of premature delivery. Male infants were more often born at gestational ages of less than 37 weeks than were female infants.

Table 4-7. Percentage of Pregnancies Terminating Before 37 Completed Weeks of Gestation by Selected Characteristics

Factor	Level	No. of pregnancies	Percentage terminating ≤37 weeks	Probability of significant difference[a]
Demographic				
Maternal age (years)				.0000
	<20	567	11.46	
	20–24	3202	6.28	
	25–34	4860	5.21	
	≥35	1329	8.95	
Mother's education				.0000
	Less than high school	1426	9.26	
	High school	3858	6.87	
	Some college	2360	5.51	
	College graduate	2300	4.78	
Father's education				.0002
	Less than high school	1337	8.45	
	High school	2806	6.81	
	Some college	2195	6.56	
	College graduate	3501	5.14	
Father's occupation				.0019
	Professional, managerial	4393	5.44	
	Office, sales	1269	7.09	
	Crafts, operator	2794	6.69	
	Blue collar	1224	8.17	
Maternal habits				
Cigarette smoking				.0012
	Never	4306	5.43	
	Stopped before pregnancy	1069	5.89	
	Stopped beginning of pregnancy	767	6.78	
	Smoker	3780	7.57	
Use of contraception				.0000
	No	2522	8.60	
	Yes, but stopped before LMP	3434	5.04	
	Continued	3108	5.79	

[a] Probability of significant difference tested with F-ratio of analysis of variance. No statistically significant association was found between premature birth and mother's height, weight, profession, alcohol consumption, attitude toward pregnancy, or father's cigarette smoking habits. Also, no significant association was found with infections of the genitourinary tract before or after 22 weeks' gestation, or with third-trimester elevated blood pressure.

[b] Premarital conception.

Source: Child Health and Development Studies.

Factor	Level	No. of pregnancies	Percentage terminating ≤37 weeks	Probability of significant difference[a]
Pregnancy was planned in advance				.0009
	No	4817	6.71	
	Yes	3222	5.02	
	Not asked[b]	1072	7.74	
Previous pregnancies				.4506
Number	0	2961	6.45	
	1–2	4495	5.74	
	≥3	1132	6.01	
Previous fetal deaths				.0001
	0	4817	5.61	
	≥1	2180	8.12	
Immediately preceding pregnancy				
Outcome				.0001
	Liveborn	5871	5.86	
	Fetal death	1067	9.00	
Length of pregnancy (weeks)				.0000
	<37	1342	11.40	
	≥37	5557	5.18	
Birthweight of liveborn (grams)				.0000
	≤2500	311	11.90	
	>2500	5563	5.55	
Interval between preceding and current pregnancy (months)				.0007
	>4	638	9.25	
	4–7	1064	6.77	
	≥8	5213	5.85	
Current pregnancy				
First-trimester bleeding				.0002
	No	9117	6.13	
	Yes	841	9.39	
Weight gain (pounds) per week, from 20 weeks to termination				.0000
	$<\frac{1}{2}$	1020	7.94	
	$\frac{1}{2}$ to <1	4076	4.59	
	≥1	1535	4.56	
Sex of infant				.0321
	Male	5059	6.46	
	Female	4850	5.44	

Table 4-7 analyzes relationships of single variables to premature delivery; however, because some of these variables are interrelated, a multivariate regression analysis was used to calculate whether the association between premature birth and single variables remains statistically significant after controlling for other variables. The variables were recoded to obtain dichotomies for comparing the categories in each variable with the strongest association of preterm birth with all others. The exception was maternal age, where the group under 20 years old and that over 34 years old were each compared with all other ages. The dichotomized variables entered in the analysis were mother's education, father's occupation, mother's smoking, length of gestation of preceding pregnancy, interval between preceding and current pregnancy, weight gain, first-trimester bleeding, and sex of infant. Controlling for all other variables, only father's occupation and sex of infant failed to maintain a statistically significant relationship with premature birth.

Several of these variables have also been found to be associated with preterm birth by other investigators, for example, maternal age and social class (Fedrick and Anderson, 1976; Berkowitz, 1981); maternal cigarette smoking (Meyer, 1977; van den Berg, 1977); previous history of perinatal loss, of low birthweight, and short gestation (Yerushalmy, 1967; Hemminki and Starfield, 1978; Bakketeig and Hoffman, 1981).

The characteristics of pregnant women that have been shown to be significantly associated with preterm birth have been used to identify women at high risk of premature delivery. If high-risk pregnancies could be identified early in pregnancy, the nature and intensity of prenatal care might be adjusted to maximize the possibility of preventing preterm delivery (or other unfavorable pregnancy outcomes). The concept of identifying high-risk pregnancies is an important issue in obstetrics and in public health, and many attempts have been made to develop a scoring system for categorizing pregnant women according to their predicted risk of an unfavorable pregnancy outcome. However, disappointment with the clinical usefulness of the developed risk-screening tests has also been expressed (Lesinski, 1975; Ledger, 1980).

The effectiveness of a screening test depends for the most part on two measures: the *sensitivity* or the probability of a correct diagnosis of positive cases, and the *specificity* or the probability of a correct diagnosis of negative cases (Yerushalmy, 1947). Several workers have examined the effectiveness of several published scoring systems that identify high-risk pregnancies (Newcombe and Chalmers, 1981; Fortney and Whitehorne, 1982). Fortney and Whitehorne (1982) copied or calculated the sensitivity, specificity, and other measures of effectiveness of several systems and concluded that no index is completely satisfactory; the sensitivity and the specificity are too small. It is not possible to minimize the proportion of infants classified as being at high risk and at the same time to predict a large percentage of jeopardized infants.

The method shown by Fortney and Whitehorne to predict preterm birth best was that used by Creasy et al. (1980), a modification of the method developed by Papiernik-Berkhauer (1969). By this method factors associated with premature delivery are grouped in four categories, three of which relate to information obtainable early in pregnancy during the initial interview (socioeconomic status, past fertility history, daily habits). The fourth category relates to data obtained from the examination later in the pregnancy. Each factor received a rather arbitrary score, ranging from 1 to 10.

Utilizing the CHDS data, we developed two scoring systems, keeping data separate for multigravidas and primigravidas. The first scoring method relates to all the variables of Table 4-7. One point was assigned to each mother if she was represented in the category having the strongest association with preterm birth. The total score for each woman was obtained by simple addition of the scores. The results were similar to the results of most of the more complicated systems reviewed by Fortney and Whitehorne.

The second scoring method duplicated the scoring of socioeconomic status variables, past history, and daily habits utilized by Creasy et al. (1980). The most important findings of both methods are provided in Table 4-8. Both methods yielded very similar results. With about a quarter of the pregnancies assessed as being "at risk," the sensitivity was about .40 and the specificity about .75. These results are, obtained solely from the sociomedical history, however, and may improve if information obtained from examinations at later stages of gestation is included in the score as shown by Creasy et al. (1980).

PREVENTION

In most scoring systems, women of unfavorable socioeconomic status are overrepresented in the high-risk groups. It is unclear through what mechanism socioeconomic variables are causally related to premature delivery. Working on the assumption that deficiencies in the quality of nutrition are of major importance, programs have often been instituted to supplement the nutrition of low-income pregnant women in order to promote both the health of the mother and a favorable outcome of pregnancy. One such program, administered with careful medical evaluation, is the Special Supplemental Food

Table 4-8. Results of Two Risk-Screening Methods[a,b]

| | Method I | | | | | | Method II | | | | | |
| | *Multigravidas* | | | *Primigravidas* | | | *Multigravidas* | | | *Primigravidas* | | |
A	B	C	A	B	C	A	B	C	A	B	C
0	1.8	2.4	0	3.2	4.2	0–3	7.5	3.3	0–3	11.5	4.1
1	8.8	3.4	1	13.9	5.3	4	18.7	3.9	4	40.9	5.8
2	18.5	3.8	2	26.1	4.7	5	15.6	4.1	5	7.1	7.1
3	24.3	5.3	3	27.4	6.4	6–7	22.6	5.8	6	26.7	7.0
4	19.9	7.1	4	17.2	8.5	8–9	7.6	7.4	7–8	8.8	12.1
5	13.9	7.8	5	8.9	6.4	10–14	7.2	8.5	9–10	3.1	13.3
6	7.8	10.0	6+	3.3	17.3	15–16	7.3	9.1	11+	1.9	11.5
7	3.2	11.8				17–19	7.8	8.5			
8+	1.8	20.0				20+	5.7	16.1			
	100.0	6.4		100.0	6.5		100.0	6.4		100.0	6.5
	6944	441		2961	191		6944	441		2961	191

	Score	Percentage assessed at risk	Sensitivity	Specificity	Percentage of preterm birth
Method I					
Multigravidas	5+	26.8	.41	.74	9.78
Primigravidas	4+	29.4	.40	.71	8.84
Method II					
Multigravidas	10+	28.0	.45	.73	10.2
Primigravidas	6+	39.9	.51	.61	8.78

[a] Method I is based on all variables in Table 4-7, dichotomized. Method II duplicates method described by Creasy et al. (1980). Separate results are given for multigravidas and primigravidas.
[b] A, Score; B, percentage distribution of pregnancies; C, percentage of preterm births.
Source: Child Health and Development Studies.

Program for Women, Infants, and Children (WIC). Nineteen projects in 14 U.S. states participated in this program, reaching about 700,000 people. One of the conclusions was that the program was associated with an increase in the mean birthweight. This was ascribed partly to an average of five days' increase in gestational duration; a smaller proportion appeared to be due to an increase in fetal growth (Select Committee on Nutrition and Human Needs, 1976).

A randomized controlled study of prenatal nutritional supplementation in New York City by Rush et al. (1980) yielded ambiguous results. The participants in this study were about 800 low-income women with unfavorable fertility histories. It was concluded that balanced protein–calorie supplements did increase the length of gestation (with borderline significance). With high-protein supplementation, however, the results were negative and suggested an increase in very early preterm births. The publication of this study increased interest in and intensified discussions about the nutrient needs of pregnant women (Barness, 1980; Hegsted, 1980; Jacobson, 1980). Thus it is clear that much still has to be learned about the nutritional requirements of pregnancy.

Besides these general efforts to prevent preterm birth by trying to improve women's health and nutritional status, more specific approaches have aimed at delaying the delivery of women for whom such a delay was obstetrically desirable. Pharmacologic agents play an increasing role among the obstetric measures used to inhibit preterm labor. The recently introduced beta sympathomimetics are not without their problems, but they do seem especially promising (Fuchs, 1980). However, these drugs may only be effective if preterm labor is recognized at an early enough stage to allow intervention.

The preliminary report of an extensive study on the prevention of premature birth by Herron et al. (1982) indicates that it is possible to recognize the early stages of preterm labor and to postpone delivery until the chances of the fetus have improved. Their preliminary program included a risk scoring of some 900 patients, education of the women who were at medium or high risk with regard to the early signs and symptoms of beginning labor, and intensive specialized care of patients who presented themselves in the early stages of labor. The report indicated a considerable reduction in preterm births since the implementation of the program.

A reduction in the incidence of preterm births may be achieved if public health programs are implemented to improve the health and nutritional status of those pregnant women who are at increased risk of preterm delivery, and if intensified prenatal care, including patient education, is achieved. Such intervention efforts should, however, be accompanied by intensive medical monitoring and statistical analysis of the data.

REFERENCES

Barness, L.A. (1980). Moderation, the noblest gift of heaven. *Pediatrics 65*, 834.
Bakketeig, L.S. and Hoffman, H.J. (1981). Epidemiology of preterm birth: Results from a longitudinal study of births in Norway. In *Preterm labor. Obstetrics and Gynecology 1*, edited by M.G. Elder and C.H. Hendricks. Woburn, Mass.: Butterworth.

Berkowitz, G.S. (1981). An epidemiologic study of preterm delivery. *Am. J. Epidemiol. 113*, 81–92.

Creasy, R.K., Gummer, B.A., and Liggins, G.C. (1980). System for predicting spontaneous preterm birth. *Obstet. Gynecol. 55*, 692–695.

Fedrick, J. and Anderson, A.B.M. (1976). Factors associated with spontaneous preterm birth. *Br. J. Obstet. Gynaecol. 83*, 342–350.

Fortney, J.A. and Whitehorne, E.W. (1982). The development of an index of high-risk pregnancy. *Am. J. Obstet. Gynecol. 143*, 501–508.

Fuchs, F. (1980). Prevention of premature birth. In *Symposium on neonatal intensive care*, edited by P.A.M. Auld. *Clin. Perinatol. 7*, 3–15.

Guyer, B., Wallach, L.A., and Rosen, S.L. (1982). Birth-weight-standardized neonatal mortality rates and the prevention of low birth weight: How does Massachusetts compare with Sweden? *N. Engl. J. Med. 306*, 1230–1233.

Hegsted, D.M. (1980). Prenatal nutritional supplementation. *Pediatrics 65*, 842–843.

Hemminki, E. and Starfield, B. (1978). Prevention of low birth weight and pre-term birth: Literature review and suggestions for research policy. *Milbank Mem. Fund Q. 56*, 339–361.

Herron, M.A., Katz, M., and Creasy, R.K. (1982). Evaluation of a preterm birth prevention program: Preliminary report. *Obstet. Gynecol. 59*, 452–456.

Jacobson, H.N. (1980). A randomized controlled trial of prenatal nutritional supplementation. *Pediatrics 65*, 835–836.

Kleinman, J.C., Kovar, M.G., Feldman, J.J., and Young, C.A. (1978). A comparison of 1960 and 1973–1974 early neonatal mortality in selected states. *Am. J. Epidemiol. 108*, 454–469.

Ledger, W.J. (1980). Identification of the high risk mother and fetus—does it work? *Clin. Perinatol. 7*, 125–134.

Lee, K.S., Paneth, N., Gartner, L.M., Pearlman, M.A., and Gruss, L. (1980). Neonatal mortality: An analysis of the recent improvement in the United States. *Am. J. Public Health 70*, 15–21.

Lesinski, J. (1975). High-risk pregnancy, unresolved problems of screening, management and prognosis. *Obstet. Gynecol. 46*, 599–603.

Meyer, M.B. (1977). Effects of maternal smoking and altitude on birth weight and gestation. In *The epidemiology of prematurity*, edited by D.M. Reed and F.J. Stanley. Baltimore, Md.: Urban and Schwarzenberg, pp. 81–101.

National Center for Health Statistics (1972). A study of infant mortality from linked records: Comparison of neonatal mortality from two cohort studies—United States. *Vital Health Stat.* (20), No. 13, DHEW Publication No. HSM 72-1056.

National Center for Health Statistics (1972a). A study of infant mortality from linked records: By birth weight, period of gestation, and other variables—United States. *Vital Health Stat.* (20) No. 12, DHEW Publication No. HSM 72-1055.

National Center for Health Statistics (1974). Final natality statistics, 1970. *Monthly Vital Statistics Report 22*, 12 (Suppl.).

National Center for Health Statistics (1981). *Vital statistics of the United States, 1977.* Vol. 2, *Mortality, Part A.* Washington, D.C.: U.S. Department of Health and Human Services, Public Health Service.

National Center for Health Statistics (1981a). Advance report of final natality statistics, 1979. *Monthly Vital Statistics Report 30*(6), (Suppl. 2), DHHS Publication No. (PHS) 81-1120.

National Center for Health Statistics (1981b). *Vital statistics of the United States, 1977.* Vol. 1, *Natality.* Washington, D.C.: U.S. Department of Health and Human Services, Public Health Service.

Newcombe, R.G. and Chalmers, I. (1981). Assessing the risk of preterm labour. In *Preterm labor. Obstetrics and Gynecology 1,* edited by M.G. Elder and C.H. Hendricks. Woburn, Mass.: Butterworth.

Papiernik-Berkhauer, E. (1969). Coefficient de risque d'accouchement prématuré (C.R.A.P.). *La Presse Médicale 77,* 793–794.

Rush, D., Stein, Z., and Susser, M. (1980). A randomized controlled trial of prenatal nutritional supplementation in New York City. *Pediatrics 65,* 683–697.

Select Committee on Nutrition and Human Needs (1976). *United States Senate: Medical evaluation of the special supplemental food program for women, infants and children.* Washington, D.C.: U.S. Government Printing Office.

van den Berg, B.J. (1977). Epidemiologic observations of prematurity: Effects of tobacco, coffee and alcohol. In *The epidemiology of prematurity,* edited by D.M. Reed and F.J. Stanley. Baltimore, Md.: Urban and Schwarzenberg, pp. 157–176.

World Health Organization (1975). *Manual of the international statistical classification of diseases, injuries, and causes of death.* Vol. 1 (9th rev.), Geneva: World Health Organization.

—— (1978). *Social and biological effects on perinatal mortality: Report on an international comparative study,* Vols. 1, 2. Geneva: World Health Organization.

Yerushalmy, J. (1947). Statistical problems in assessing methods of medical diagnosis with special reference to X-ray techniques. *Public Health Rep.* 62, 1432–1449.

—— (1967). Biostatistical methods in investigations of child health. *Am. J. Dis. Child. 114,* 470–476.

——, van den Berg, B.J., Erhardt, C.L., and Jacobziner, H. (1965). Birth weight and gestation as indices of "immaturity." *Am. J. Dis. Child. 109,* 43–57.

5

Low Birthweight

Eva Alberman

The weight of a fetus at any stage in pregnancy reflects an exceedingly complex interaction between time elapsing since fertilization, timing and site of implantation, and rate of fetal cell multiplication. The latter is itself influenced by characteristics inherent in the fetus and the mother—some genetically, some hormonally, and some environmentally determined—and by the availability to the fetus of nutrient agents. Fetal infection or the fetal exposure to a toxin or teratogen will generally slow down fetal growth, although the risk of retardation will depend on the agent and on the stage fetal development has reached. It follows that the epidemiology of "low" birthweight, however defined, must be complex, and despite a vast literature on the subject much of it is still not fully understood.

COMMONLY USED DEFINITIONS BASED ON BIRTHWEIGHT ONLY

A time-honored definition of low birthweight has been *2500 g (or 5.5 pounds) and below,* although the ninth revision of the *International Classification of Diseases* of the World Health Organization (1978) has changed this to *less than 2500 g.* In the recent literature concerned with the survival of low-birthweight infants, further subdivisions of low birthweight have been commonly used, though not always consistently. "Very low birthweight" has been the term used for infants weighing 2000 g or less, and also for those weighing 1500 g or less. "Extremely low birthweight" has been applied to infants weighing 1000 g or less. There is as yet no universally agreed on nomenclature for these groups.

86

PROBLEMS OF MEASURING BIRTHWEIGHT

The measurement of birthweight is probably the most universally reliable indicator of fetal maturity available. Even so it must be recognized that there are numerous problems inherent in its measurement and definition.

First, there is the question of "subject variation." The birthweight of an infant can vary with the amount of placental blood infused, and this will vary with local policy on the time the cord is clamped. The birthweight will also vary considerably with the time the infant is weighed, whether immediately after birth or a day or so later, for there can be substantial weight losses in the first days of life. The rate of these weight losses varies with the maturity and nutritional status of the fetus, as well as with feeding policies. The World Health Organization recommends that birthweight be considered the first weight recorded, preferably within the first hours of life.

"Observer variation" can also be a problem. This includes the errors introduced by the use of inaccurate scales, by inaccurate reading of the scales, and by the rounding up or down of the reading. On a worldwide basis it is extremely rare for weighing, if carried out at all, to be performed using scales that are accurate to the nearest gram. Even in the developed countries, only a minority of maternity units are likely to have such scales available and to have them regularly calibrated. Where scales of this level of accuracy are not available, or staff training is poor, the tendency is to round readings up or down to the nearest 5 or 10g, or larger round number, but this is often not done at random. All studies of birthweight distribution reveal a tendency to digit preference, and this affects the change from a definition of 2500 g or less to one of less than 2500 g, and all the other groupings chosen. A recent analysis of data from England and Wales showed that a change in classification from 2500 g or less to one of less than 2500 g decreased the percentage of low birthweight in 1978 from 7.09 to 6.74 (Office of Population Censuses and Surveys, 1981). Such changes become increasingly important at the lower end of the birthweight range, particularly at the 1000- or 500-g cutoff points, which many countries use as the lower level of legal viability and registerability. Errors introduced by rounding up or down become even larger when birthweight is expressed in pounds and ounces.

The other problem that can cause serious difficulties in comparability is absence of a lower limit of birthweight. It is left to the individual attendant at the birth to decide whether a neonate shows any signs of life, but at the low end of the birthweight range it can be difficult to decide whether a neonate showing such signs that subsequently dies should be counted as a livebirth or as an abortion.

VALIDITY OF LOW-BIRTHWEIGHT CUTOFF POINTS

In spite of these problems of definition, measurement, and recording, even these crude subdivisions have been shown to have considerable validity in terms of predicting survival and, it will be shown later, handicapping disorders. In England and Wales 68.5% of perinatal deaths in 1979 were attributable to the 6.9% of total births weighing less than 2500 g; 39.0% of perinatal deaths were attributable to the 0.97% of total births weighing less than 1500 g. With accelerating social and medical progress and the subsequent reduction in the more easily preventable deaths of infants of normal birthweight, the contribution of low birthweight to perinatal mortality is increasing in importance.

COMMONLY USED DEFINITIONS OF LOW BIRTHWEIGHT ALLOWING FOR GESTATIONAL AGE

Definitions that do not allow for gestational age as well as birthweight render it impossible to make the important distinction between low birthweight resulting from retarded fetal growth, and low birthweight due only to preterm labor (see Chapter 4).

There have been several attempts to agree on definitions for infants who are small for dates (SFD), or low birthweight but appropriate for dates (AFD). The problem is to find a consistent cutoff point at the lower end of the distribution of birthweight for given gestational ages. Cutoff points that have been commonly used are 1 or 2 standard deviations below the mean birthweight for that gestational age, or percentiles: the 3rd, 5th, or 10th percentiles of birthweight have all been used for this purpose.

PROBLEMS OF USING DEFINITIONS BASED ON BIRTHWEIGHT FOR GESTATIONAL AGE

Figure 5-1 (derived from Hoffman et al., 1974) shows that even at 40 weeks of gestation for a very large sample of 95,806 births, the distribution of birthweight is somewhat skewed. This tends to be even more marked at lower gestational ages, and for this reason it is probably better to use a percentile cutoff point rather than the multiple of a standard deviation.

The use of gestational age in these definitions brings with it the further difficulties of defining and assessing gestational age that have

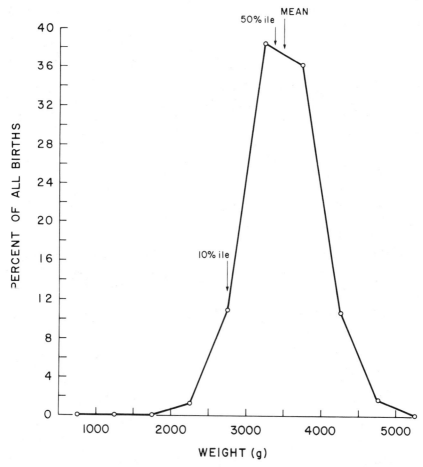

Fig. 5-1. Percentage distribution by birthweight group, 1968: U.S. white males of 40 weeks gestational age (95,806 births).

been considered in Chapter 4. It also raises the question of the validity of using as a standard, birthweight distributions derived from preterm births. Preterm births, virtually by definition, are abnormal in some way. Unfortunately we have no way of accurately measuring the weight of all fetuses still in utero during the early weeks of the third trimester and thus obtaining longitudinal rather than cross-sectional distribution of birthweight for gestation. However, recent developments in ultrasound techniques suggest that it may soon become possible to obtain good estimates for longitudinal growth (Shepard et al., 1982).

VALIDITY OF CUTOFF POINTS OF BIRTHWEIGHT FOR GESTATIONAL AGE

Reference to mortality rates confirms that even within gestational age bands, low birthweight—however defined—entails an increased risk of stillbirth and neonatal mortality. This is rather more difficult to demonstrate than for the crude low-birthweight cutoff points, but it has been illustrated diagrammatically by the use of contour charts and statistically by the use of multiple variance analyses. Figure 5-2 (Goldstein and Peckham, 1976) is derived from the 1958 British Perinatal Mortality Study and shows clearly how, at all gestational ages, infants with a weight below the 6th percentile run more than an average risk. Outside the range 38–42 weeks this risk is always more

Fig. 5-2. Late fetal neonatal mortality rates by birthweight and gestation (1958 Perinatal Mortality Survey). Continuous lines, contours of constant mortality rate with mean rate of 100; broken lines, percentiles of birthweight for gestational age.
Source: Goldstein and Peckham (1976).

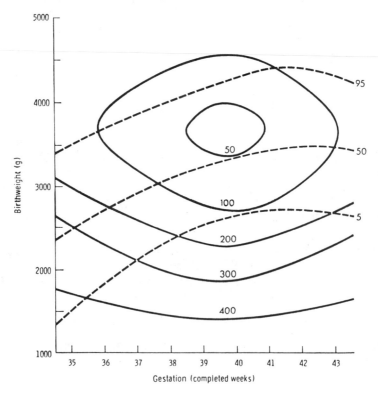

Table 5-1. Observed Percentages in Need for Special Schooling in the British National Child Development Study by Gestational Age and Birthweight

	35	36	37	38	39	40	41	42	≥43	Total
					Length of gestation (weeks)					
Percentage needing special schooling	8.1	9.0	6.0	4.2	4.0	4.4	3.5	4.9	5.8	4.5

	≤1999	2000 –2499	2500 –2999	3000 –3499	3500 –3999	≥4000	Total
				Birthweight (grams)			
Percentage needing special schooling	20.0	9.5	5.3	4.0	3.7	4.0	4.5

Source: Goldstein and Peckham (1976).

than twice, and up to four times, the average for the whole sample.

In contrast to gestational immaturity, retarded fetal growth is more marked for its association with morbidity than mortality. The association with morbidity depends on the cause for the retardation, which either may have inflicted or may be associated with irreversible damage to the fetus before delivery. Preterm births with a weight appropriate for dates are more likely to be potentially normal and, if they survive, to be intact, than term births of low weight who have often been damaged in utero.

Thus the British National Child Development Study revealed a weak association between gestational age at delivery and 11-year-old mental and physical status but a stronger association for birthweight even after allowance was made for associated social and biologic factors (Goldstein and Peckham, 1976). Table 5-1 shows only the more extreme outcome of children reported to be in need of special (remedial) education by birthweight and gestational age separately, and demonstrates the greater importance of birthweight than gestational age in this respect.

THE VARIABILITY OF FETAL GROWTH RATE WITH SOCIAL AND BIOLOGIC FACTORS

The introduction to this chapter stated that many factors—some inherent in the fetus and mother, some stemming from the external

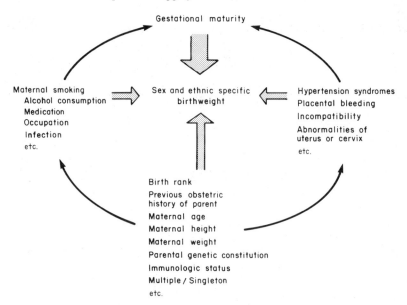

Fig. 5-3. Interrelationship of factors affecting length of gestation and fetal growth.

environment—influenced rate of fetal growth. Some of the ways these factors can affect fetal growth and length of gestation are illustrated diagrammatically in Fig. 5-3.

There are many bodies of data now available that illustrate the associations of sociobiologic factors with low birthweight. Data in Table 5-2 taken from the 1958 British Perinatal Mortality Survey (Butler and Alberman, 1969) show how the proportions of infants weighing 2500 g or less at birth vary with maternal parity, social class, height, smoking habit, and the presence or absence of preeclamptic toxemia. Similar findings could be produced from many different countries and at other times. Table 5-2 also shows the association of these factors with gestational age. Wherever an association is seen with low birthweight, an increase in preterm labor is also seen, but to a considerably reduced extent, and for each of these associations a relationship with birthweight can be demonstrated even after allowing for the reduction in gestational age. The associations do not always take a simple form. Thus low birthweight is more common in first and in third and later births, than in second births, at least in cross-sectional studies (Butler and Alberman, 1969). The relationship between gravidity and birthweight becomes more complex still and is discussed below.

Low Birthweight

Table 5-2. Percentage Low-Birthweight and Preterm Deliveries by Parity, Social Class, Maternal Height, Preeclampsia, and Smoking

Characteristic and level	Birthweight ≤2500 g (%)	Gestation <37 weeks (%)
Parity		
0	7.6	4.7
1	5.4	3.9
2,3	6.8	5.2
4	7.4	5.5
Social class (father)		
Professional, managerial, and supervisory	4.9	3.9
Skilled worker	6.6	4.6
Semiskilled worker	7.2	4.8
Unskilled	8.2	5.3
No husband	10.8	5.9
Maternal height (inches)		
≥65	4.7	3.9
62–64	6.1	4.4
<62	9.3	5.3
Preeclampsia		
None or mild	5.4	5.1
Moderate	5.8	3.5
Severe	18.0	8.5
Smoking		
Nonsmoker	5.4	4.1
Smoker	9.3	5.9

Source: Butler and Alberman (1969).

There are close interrelationships among many of these factors. For example, reduced maternal height, high parity, and social disadvantage may be related, as may preeclampsia and primiparity. In order to study their joint and independent effects, and their relationship with gestational age, multivariate analyses are necessary. The results of such an analysis of the 1958 British Perinatal Mortality Survey (Butler and Alberman, 1969) data showed that the relationship of birthweight with social disadvantage was largely explained by the excess of short mothers in the disadvantaged social classes. Low maternal height remained significantly associated with low birthweight even after allowing for gestational age, however. Similarly, severe preeclampsia and maternal smoking were shown to have independent and highly significant associations with low birthweight (Butler and Alberman, 1969).

93

FUNDAMENTAL CAUSES OF FETAL GROWTH RETARDATION

Despite the considerable knowledge we now have on the relationship of sociobiologic variables with low birthweight, the more fundamental nature of the causes of fetal growth retardation remain poorly understood. In order to study them further it is necessary to distinguish between genetic, physiologic, and environmental effects on birthweight, and this can be a very difficult exercise.

Genetic Effects

These can take several forms. The Y chromosome, for example, has the effect of increasing the rate of fetal growth. An abnormal chromosomal constitution is known to affect fetal growth; fetuses affected by Down syndrome, for example, are usually growth retarded. Similarly, reduced birthweight has been reported in infants with certain autosomal recessive conditions such as cystic fibrosis and phenylketonuria. It has been demonstrated with twin and family studies that there are other genetic effects on fetal growth related to both the fetal and the maternal genotypes, although these seem to be relatively unimportant compared with environmental effects. Almost certainly there are genetically determined differences that account for some of the observed ethnic variations in fetal growth rate, although these are currently largely accounted for by the nutritional and socioeconomic differences existing among ethnic groups. All these considerations have been discussed by Robson (1978). Multiple births are also associated with a reduced fetal growth rate, although there are many different causes for this (Falkner, 1978).

Nutritional Effects

Certainly the nutritional status of the fetus, its oxygenation, and probably the combination of these have important effects on fetal growth rate. Nourishment of the fetus depends on placental function and must also depend to some extent on maternal nutritional status. It is probable that the association of hypertensive disease of pregnancy with fetal growth retardation is caused, at least in part, by placental insufficiency secondary to this condition. The best epidemiologic evidence for the association of maternal nutrition in pregnancy with fetal growth comes from situations where the maternal diet is at or near starvation levels. Stein and colleagues have shown how birthweight was reduced in mothers in the third trimester of pregnancy during the Dutch famine in 1945 (Stein et al., 1975), and others have

94

maintained that dietary supplementation in pregnancy to malnourished mothers will lead to an increase in birthweight, although
this has not been demonstrated in the developed countries. However,
there is a well-established positive relationship between maternal
weight gain within and between pregnancies and birthweight. This
complex subject has been reviewed elsewhere (Metcoff, 1978; Dobbing, 1981).

Hypoxia

The relationship between fetal hypoxia and low birthweight has
also been investigated. Meyer (1977) has shown how in two situations where the supply of oxygen is decreased—high altitudes and
maternal smoking—the whole birthweight distribution is shifted
downward. In the case of smoking the weight reduction is directly
proportional to the number of cigarettes smoked by the mother
during pregnancy, and in the case of altitude it appears that mean
birthweight is also inversely proportional to elevation. In both cases
adaptation of the placenta has been demonstrated, with a high
placental–infant weight ratio and a greater area of attachment. The
increased risk of antepartum bleeding in mothers who smoke may be
related to these changes.

Infection

Fetal infections such as rubella and cytomegalovirus have also been
shown to be associated with increases in low birthweight, mostly
because of fetal growth retardation (Alberman and Peckham, 1977).
The effect on birthweight of maternal infections, such as urinary tract
infection, is probably more closely related to a curtailment of length of
gestation, possibly sometimes due to an amnionitis or chorionitis
(Naeye et al., 1971).

LONGITUDINAL STUDIES

Thus far only measures of low birthweight in cross sectional studies
of births in a given population have been described, that is, in births
occurring to different women within a limited time period usually less
than a year. This method points up differences in births between
different women who have been exposed to a variety of circumstances. Interest has been increasing in the study of birth events
studied longitudinally within women. Such studies have shown that
low birthweight, preterm delivery, and retarded fetal growth rate

tend to be repeated in successive pregnancies in the same women. These repetitions are only partly accounted for by a tendency to repeat pathologic events such as placenta praevia or preeclamptic toxemia, and much of the repetitive nature of low-birthweight births remains unexplained (Bakketeig et al., 1979).

Also intriguing is the finding that low birthweight is associated with early fetal loss to the same parents, livebirths occurring both before and after an early fetal loss having a lower than average birthweight (Alberman et al., 1980). All these findings point to an inherent heterogeneity among women in so far as their risk of reproductive disadvantage is concerned.

The relationship of previous induced abortion to birthweight in subsequent deliveries is very complex and depends on many factors including methods used and the gestational age at abortion. This problem has been recently reviewed by Bracken (1978) and Grimes and Cates (1979).

TRENDS OVER TIME IN BIRTHWEIGHT

In general, birthweight data from many different countries testify to the remarkable stability of birthweight distributions over time, a stability that is surprising in view of short-term demographic changes in births and behavior such as smoking (Alberman, 1977). This stability is almost certainly related to the tendency for mothers to repeat in successive pregnancies birthweight and gestational maturity patterns at birth, probably because of the persisting influence of factors such as maternal stature and socioeconomic status. Japan is one exception to this generalization, for there was a fundamental change over a short time in standard of living, and the most rapid rise ever documented in mean adult height in the decade after the 1939–1945 war. In that country it appears that the birthweight distribution also shifted to the right, with a rise in mean birthweight for gestational age in males and females at all birthweights (Gruenwald et al., 1967). The changes in standard of living were also accompanied by a massive program of legal abortion, which may also have affected this change, by altering the age, parity, and social class distribution of livebirths in a favorable direction. Certainly the change in birthweight distribution was accompanied by an extraordinarily rapid fall in perinatal mortality.

With the exception of Japan, the stability of the birthweight distribution and the strong correlation between low birthweight and mortality have tended to maintain over time the relative positions of different countries and of different regions within countries, if they

are ranked by level of perinatal mortality. The changes that have
occurred in Japan are an example of the extent of social change that is
necessary to bring about a substantial reduction in low-birthweight
proportions over a short period of time.

AREAS FOR FURTHER RESEARCH

Perhaps one of the most important areas for future action is in the
further refinement of the definitions of low birthweight. It would be a
great advance if an infant were to be thus classified only after
allowing for its gestational age, sex, birth rank, and maternal stature.
At least two nomograms (Tanner and Thomson, 1970; Brenner et al.,
1976) have been published to help classify birthweight after allowing
for such factors, and it is to be hoped that these will come into
common use. Descriptions of such high quality will enable us to
identify more precisely specific environmental or even genetic causes
of fetal growth retardation.

An area sorely in need of further research is the identification of
the exact pathways—biochemical, physical, or metabolic—through
which environmental factors act on fetal growth. Interventional
studies, such as nutritional programs before and during pregnancy,
may become helpful methods of pursuing such research, but can
carry their own hazards and need to be conducted with great caution.
Controlled trials attempting to reduce obvious risks such as maternal
exposure to smoking, alcohol, or occupational hazards probably
entail no hazards, however, and are likely to be beneficial.

Another area that may merit further research is the role of maternal
and fetal infection. Indications are that this may be an even more
important field of investigation than was previously thought.

REFERENCES

Alberman, E.D. (1977). Sociobiologic factors and birthweight in Great Britain.
In *The epidemiology of prematurity*, edited by D.M. Reed and F.J.
Stanley. Baltimore, Md.: Urban and Schwarzenberg, pp. 145–156.
—— and Peckham, C. (1977). Long term effects following infections in
pregnancy. In *Infections and pregnancy*, edited by C. Coid. New York:
Academic Press, p. 37.
——, Roman, E., Pharoah, P.O.D., and Chamberlain, G. (1980). Birth-
weight before and after a spontaneous abortion. *Br. J. Obstet. Gynaecol.*
87, 275–280.
Bakketeig, L.S., Hoffman, H.J., and Harley, E.E. (1979). The tendency to
repeat gestational age and birthweight in successive births. *Am. J.
Obstet. Gynecol.* 135, 1086–1103.

Bracken, M.B. (1978). Induced abortion as a risk factor for perinatal complications: A review. *Yale J. Biol. Med. 51,* 539–548.

Brenner, W.E., Edelman, D.A., and Hendricks, C.H. (1976). A standard of fetal growth for the USA. *Am. J. Obstet. Gynecol. 126,* 555–564.

Butler, N.R. and Alberman, E.D. (1969). *Perinatal problems. The second report of the British perinatal mortality survey.* Edinburgh and London: E & S Livingstone Ltd.

Dobbing, J. (1981). *Maternal nutrition in pregnancy—eating for two?* London: Academic Press.

Falkner, F. (1978). Implications for growth in human twins. In *Human growth,* Vol. 1, *Principles and prenatal growth,* edited by F. Falkner and J.M. Tanner. London: Bailliere Tindall, pp. 397–413.

Goldstein, H. and Peckham, C. (1976). Birthweight, gestation, neonatal mortality and child development. In *The biology of human fetal growth,* edited by D.F. Roberts and A.M. Thomson. London: Taylor and Francis, pp. 81–103.

Grimes, D.A. and Cates, Jr., W. (1979). Complications from legally-induced abortion: A review. *Obstet. Gynecol. Surv. 34,* 177–191.

Gruenwald, P., Funakawa, H., Mitaui, S., Nishimura, T., and Takenchi, S. (1967). Influence of environmental factors on foetal growth in man. *Lancet 1,* 1026–1028.

Hoffman, H.J., Stark, C.R., Lundin, F.E., Jr., and Ashbrook, J.D. (1974). Analysis of birthweight, gestational age, and fetal viability US births 1968. *Obstet. Gynecol. Surv. 29,* 651–681.

Metcoff, J. (1978). Association of fetal growth with maternal nutrition. In *Human growth.* Vol. 1, *Principles and prenatal growth,* edited by F. Falkner, and J.M. Tanner. London: Bailliere Tindall, pp. 415–460.

Meyer, M.B. (1977). Effects of maternal smoking and altitude on birthweight and gestation. In *The epidemiology of prematurity,* edited by D.M. Reed and F.J. Stanley. Baltimore, Md.: Urban and Schwarzenberg, pp. 81–104.

Naeye, R.L., Dellinger, W.S., and Blane, W.A. (1971). Fetal and maternal features of antenatal bacterial infections. *Pediatrics 48,* 733–739.

Office of Population Censuses and Surveys (1981). Birthweight statistics 1980. *Monitor* DH3 *81*(4).

Robson, E.B. (1978). The genetics of birthweight. In *Human growth.* Vol. 1, *Principles and prenatal growth,* edited by F. Falkner and J.M. Tanner. London: Bailliere Tindall, pp. 285–297.

Shepard, M.J., Richards, V.A., Berkowitz, R.L., Warsof, S.L., and Hobbins, J.C. (1982). An evaluation of two equations for predicting fetal weight by ultrasound. *Am. J. Obstet. Gynecol. 142,* 47–54.

Stein, Z., Susser, M., Saenger, G., and Marolla, F. (1975). *Famine and human development: The Dutch hunger winter of 1944–5.* New York: Oxford University Press.

Tanner, J.M. and Thomson, A.M. (1970). Standards for birthweight at gestation periods from 32 to 42 weeks allowing for maternal height and weight. *Arch. Dis. Child. 45,* 566.

World Health Organization (1978). *International classification of diseases 1975* (9th rev.). Geneva: World Health Organization.

6

PERINATAL MORTALITY

Leiv S. Bakketeig, Howard J. Hoffman,
Ann R. Titmuss Oakley

The term "perinatal period" was introduced in 1936 by the German pediatrician Pfaundler. He defined this period as the time interval just prior to, during, and after birth, arguing that the period was characterized by a peak in the mortality of the fetus and newborn infant. Earlier an Austrian pediatrician named Peller (1923, 1965) had suggested that stillbirths and deaths during the first week of life should be treated as one statistical entity in the analysis of causes of death, reasoning that these deaths have in common a complex of causes that differ from the pattern in older infants.

The term "perinatal mortality" was increasingly used in the 1940s and 1950s (Wallgren, 1942; Baird et al., 1953, 1954; WHO, 1957). By the end of the 1960s, a number of comprehensive studies of perinatal mortality had been carried out (Kaern, 1960; Erhardt, et al., 1964; Hammoud, 1965; Butler and Alberman, 1969; Rantakallio, 1969). The impetus for the increasing attention being paid to perinatal mortality was the observation that the fall in infant mortality derived mainly from the reduction in deaths for infants surviving beyond the first few days of life (Taylor, 1954). It appeared that the progress being made was almost entirely a result of the success in combating those causes

The authors wish to thank Professor Tor Bjerkedal and his staff at the Medical Birth Registry of Norway for having made available for analysis many of the data presented here. Also, we want to thank Director Anders Ericson of the Swedish Medical Birth Registry, National Board of Health and Welfare of Sweden, for providing data for use in this chapter.

Dr. Heinz Berendes, Dr. Iain Chalmers, Dr. Olav Meirik, and Dr. Karl-Erik Larssen have given valuable comments on the several drafts of the chapter, and Dr. Larssen has also provided considerable assistance in searching the literature.

Mrs. Brit Fladvad and Miss Dorothy Day have provided outstanding secretarial assistance during the preparation of the chapter.

of death that were linked to infectious diseases in early infancy. Mortality among infants shortly after birth, as well as fetal mortality, had decreased far less markedly and more slowly by comparison (WHO, 1957; Chase, 1967).

The "perinatal" mortality rate supplemented the traditional mortality measures already in use such as the "stillbirth," "neonatal," and "infant" mortality rates, and proved to be increasingly more valuable as a measure for comparisons between populations on a national and international scale. Perinatal deaths had been defined as the number of stillbirths (fetal deaths of 28 weeks or more of gestation) and the number of deaths within the first week of life per 1000 births (livebirths plus stillbirths). In 1977, the World Health Organization (WHO) recommended a broadening of the term to include all fetuses and infants who are delivered weighing at least 500 g. If birthweight is unavailable, then the WHO report recommends including births at or above the corresponding gestational age (22 weeks) or crown–heel length (25 cm). This broader definition was suggested for use in compiling national perinatal mortality statistics. For international comparisons, the WHO report recommends the use of "standard perinatal statistics" in which both the numerator and denominator of the rate are restricted to fetuses and infants weighing 1000 g or more (or the corresponding gestational age of 28 weeks, or crown–heel length of 35 cm).

The epidemiology of perinatal death involves the associations with such general factors as time and space, the behavioral and social milieu surrounding mothers and their pregnancies, as well as the biologic factors and the medical conditions that affect the health of mothers and the outcomes of their births. Advances in medical treatments and the improved delivery of medical care also have an impact on the epidemiology of perinatal mortality.

DATA SOURCES

Ten years of Norwegian births (1967–1976) comprise a major part of the results presented in this chapter. Selected figures are presented for the longer period 1967–1979. This information was collected through the Medical Registration of Births, a notification system in operation in Norway since 1967 that covers all livebirths and fetal deaths with gestational age of 16 weeks or more (Bjerkedal and Bakketeig, 1975; Bakketeig et al., 1979). The information on births was linked to information on infant deaths that was provided by the Norwegian Central Bureau of Statistics. A unique identification number is assigned to each individual shortly after birth, facilitating

100

the linkage between births and deaths. This number also allows for linkage between a mother and all of her births since 1967 (Bakketeig et al., 1979; Lunde et al., 1980).

Other results presented in this chapter are based on births in Sweden, 1977–1978 (Official Statistics of Sweden, 1981). In addition, perinatal mortality data are given for England and Wales, including information on behavorial, social, and environmental factors. Data from the United States were provided by the National Center for Health Statistics.

Perinatal mortality is defined throughout this chapter as the number of stillbirths (fetal deaths of 28 weeks or more of gestation) plus first-week deaths per 1000 births. However, in some of the analyses based on Norwegian data, perinatal death is defined as the number of fetal deaths of 16 weeks or more of gestation and neonatal deaths within the first week of life (less than seven days) per 1000 births. The reason for this variation is that medical birth registration in Norway covers fetal deaths from 16 weeks of gestation. In the United States, the outcomes of pregnancy are usually registered beginning with 20 weeks of gestation, but for purposes of this presentation, U.S. perinatal mortality rates are presented in accordance with the conventional WHO definition.

OCCURRENCE IN TIME AND PLACE

The decreases in perinatal mortality rates in recent decades, the differences in the declining rates between selected developed nations, and the fluctuations that occur on a seasonal, weekly, or daily time scale are examined in the following sections.

Time Trends

Perinatal mortality has been markedly reduced since 1950. In Fig. 6-1 the time trends in perinatal mortality rates are shown for each consecutive five-year period from 1950 through 1980 for a number of developed countries. The most striking feature of this figure is the relative fall in the perinatal mortality rate for Japan, which parallels similar strides in the post-World War II growth of the Japanese economy. Japan is now among the top five countries having the lowest perinatal mortality rates (United Nations, 1981). More modest relative gains have been accomplished by Denmark, Finland, Sweden, and, most recently, Scotland during this 30-year time span. Perhaps the most impressive finding for the countries shown in this figure is the steady and continuing decline in perinatal mortality rates, especially since 1960 (Weatherall, 1975).

101

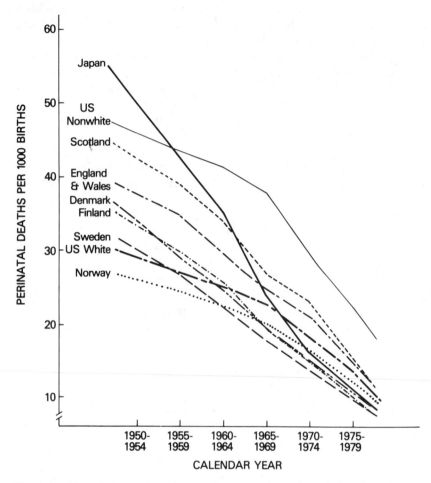

Fig. 6-1. Trends in perinatal mortality rates for selected developed countries covering the most recent 30-year time span. These rates were computed as averages for each consecutive five-year period. (Data were abstracted from the United Nations Demographic Yearbooks, the Nordic Statistical Yearbooks, or from national sources directly.)

Interpretations of these reported statistics should not be carried too far without considering much additional information on the differences in definitions and reporting routines that may have existed in the various countries and over time. Even though this important documentation may be lacking or difficult to ascertain, there is often an opportunity for fruitful investigations into the causes of a slower decline in one country or state, compared to neighboring countries or states. For example, recent studies by Larssen et al. (1981, 1982) have

102

been carried out in Norway to identify the numbers of potentially preventable perinatal deaths in selected areas of the country. This research may help to elucidate the reasons Norway no longer has the lowest perinatal mortality rate in the world as was the case in 1950–1959, and instead is currently ranked sixth among developed nations. The trend for the United States is very similar to that of Norway. The United States has been displaced from a position among the best three countries in the decade of the 1950s to a relative ranking of only thirteenth among developed nations.

Seasonality

Perinatal mortality has been shown to vary by calender month of birth. In a Norwegian study (Bjerkedal and Bakketeig, 1972), the mortality was shown to be lower in late spring and early fall, and higher during late fall and winter months, the range being from 17.0 per 1000 in September to 23.2 per 1000 in January. The seasonal variation in perinatal mortality was shown in this study to be weakly associated with a corresponding variation in preterm birth and the frequency of low birthweight. Similar seasonal patterns in perinatal mortality have been shown by other authors (Hewitt, 1962; Backer and Aagenes, 1966; Janerich and Garfinkel, 1970; Erhardt et al., 1971).

In the United States there is a seasonal pattern in the monthly birth rate that is the inverse of the pattern found in northern Europe (Rosenberg, 1966; Parkes, 1976). The peak number of U.S. births occur between July and October, whereas in Europe it is more common for the peak number of births to occur from February through May. Secondary, or minor, peaks in the occurrences of births also occur about six months out of phase both in northern Europe and in the United States. In a detailed study of New York City births and linked perinatal deaths from 1960 to 1967 (Erhardt et al., 1971), it was shown that the highest perinatal mortality rates were associated with conceptions occurring during the spring. As with the Norwegian data, births occurring in the late fall or winter months carried the highest risk of perinatal death. The study by Erhardt and colleagues showed that the rate of low-weight and preterm births was also somewhat seasonal (higher mean birthweight in spring deliveries, and lower for both summer and winter), but it was not sufficient to account for much of the variation in perinatal mortality rates by month of birth. These authors did suggest, based on their data, that if conception occurs when the risks of the common viral and bacterial infections are least, then fetal growth and development may be more nearly optimal. Other researchers have concluded to the contrary, that the seasonal

103

interaction with infection is more directly linked to the third trimester of pregnancy (Keller and Nugent, 1982).

No firm conclusions can be drawn as to the mechanisms by which the seasonal pattern in perinatal mortality is generated. Pure climactic factors are not likely to account for any major part of the variation (Hare et al., 1981). However, behavioral and social variables with regularly occurring changes over the year may partially explain the patterns (Parkes, 1976).

Variations by Day of the Week

Variations in the frequency of birth and associated perinatal mortality by day of the week are shown in Table 6-1. The data in this table are based on births in Norway (Bjerkedal and Bakketeig, 1972) and in England and Wales (MacFarlane, 1978). The total number of births is higher in the middle of the week and lower on weekends, especially Sundays. Data from the United States (1979 births) show a pattern similar to the Norwegian data, with a relative rate of only .87 for Sunday births (Heuser, 1982).

As shown in Table 6-1, perinatal mortality rates in England and Wales have an inverse relationship to day of the week: lower during the week and higher on weekends. Hendry (1981) also confirmed this finding in Scotland and further analyzed his data by cause of death, maternal complications, and obstetric emergencies. The Norwegian study by Bjerkedal and Bakketeig (1972) showed a less marked variation over the week: Perinatal mortality was not particularly

Table 6-1. Relative Number of Births and Perinatal Mortality by Day of Week

Day of week	Norway, 1967–68[a]		England and Wales, 1978[b]	
	Relative number of births	Perinatal mortality	Relative number of births	Perinatal mortality
Monday	1.02	20.9	0.97	15.9
Tuesday	1.06	18.8	1.07	17.5
Wednesday	1.03	20.7	1.08	17.1
Thursday	1.03	19.4	1.09	17.4
Friday	1.02	20.9	1.08	17.2
Saturday	0.96	20.4	0.93	19.2
Sunday	0.89	18.5	0.77	20.0

[a] Data from Bjerkedal and Bakketeig (1972).

[b] Data from MacFarlane (1978).

higher on weekends compared to the rest of the week. When spontaneous births were examined separately, the variation by day of the week was practically nonexistent. The one exception was a slight increase on Mondays. Other authors have noted variations in the perinatal mortality rate over the week, especially for induced births, and have associated the increased rate with staffing problems and the dictates of medical convenience (Stanley and Alberman, 1978; Rindfuss et al., 1979).

Variations by Hour of Day

A number of studies have shown trends in different countries toward a consistent relationship between the hour of birth and perinatal mortality (Malek, 1952; Charles, 1953; Kaiser and Halberg, 1962). Yerushalmy (1938) compared several data sets from New York State and England and concluded that the highest rate of perinatal mortality occurred for infants born between noon and midnight. Yerushalmy noted that this time period also coincided with the highest rate of induced births. He also reiterated DePorte's observation (1932) that births do not occur uniformly throughout the day but instead are more likely to occur between midnight and noon than between noon and midnight.

In Fig. 6-2 perinatal mortality rates are shown by hour of birth for 1967–1968 Norwegian births (Bjerkedal and Bakketeig, 1972) and 1978 Swedish births (Ericson, 1981). For example, the Swedish data show that the perinatal mortality rate is lower from midnight to noon and that the rate increases during the day and evening until it reaches a peak between 6:00 PM and midnight (the variation ranges from a low of 6.4 per 1000 births between 3:00 and 5:00 AM to a high of 12.3 per 1000 births between 9:00 PM and midnight). Although the general level or baseline of perinatal mortality is considerably lower in the Swedish data as compared to the Norwegian data, the same pattern of variation across the day is found for both data sets. Patterns similar to these were reported nearly 50 years earlier (DePorte, 1932; Hill, 1937; Yerushalmy, 1938), despite the fact that the baseline perinatal mortality rate then was almost sixfold higher than the current rates.

The Norwegian data set also permits a distinction to be made between births with spontaneous and induced mode of onset. Figure 6-3 and Table 6-2 display these mortality rates by mode of onset and hour of day. The mortality by hour of day for births with spontaneous onset is similar to that of the general mortality rates shown in Fig. 6-2, although the total variation is somewhat less. Together these two figures illustrate that births occurring between 3:00 AM and 6:00 AM have the best outcome in terms of perinatal

105

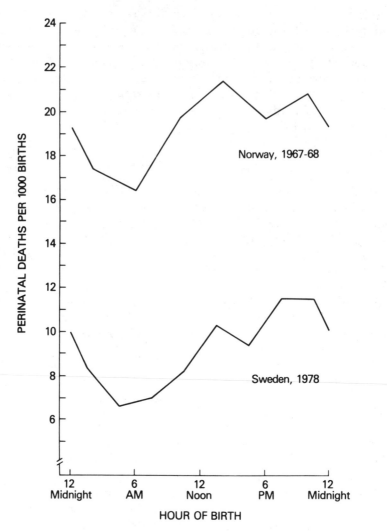

Fig. 6-2. Perinatal mortality rates by hour of birth. These rates were derived from two separate national medical birth registries using all 135,731 births in Norway, 1967–68, and all 93,156 births in Sweden, 1978.

mortality, a result that does not seem to have been widely appreciated. However, Kaiser and Halberg (1962) have attempted to focus attention on the association with underlying biologic rhythms, which must somehow be responsible for this mortality pattern. Glattre and Bjerkedal (1982) have also demonstrated that the minimum perinatal mortality is achieved with births occurring in the early morning hours. It is possible to argue from an evolutionary biologic point of view that this is in fact the finding that should be expected. The chances of survival for the newborn during the first critical 12 hours after birth should be maximized if maternal care can be provided during a period of daylight and increased individual alertness.

Fig. 6-3. Perinatal mortality rates by hour of birth and by mode of labor onset, induced or spontaneous. The data were derived from the Medical Birth Registry of Norway, 1968, and are based on 7320 induced and 61,087 spontaneous births (see Table 6-2 for numerical data).

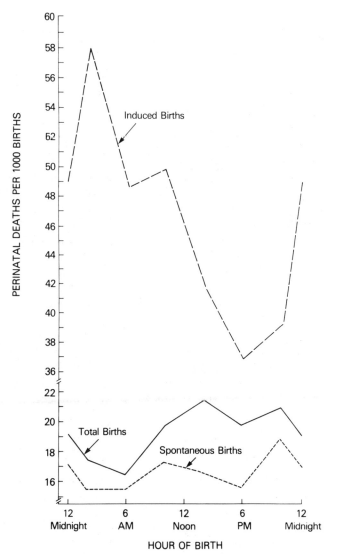

107

Table 6-2. Number of Births and Perinatal Mortality for Induced and Spontaneous Onset of Birth by Hour of the Day Born, Norway, 1968[a]

Hour of day born	Induced		Spontaneous	
	Number of births	*Perinatal mortality*	*Number of births*	*Perinatal mortality*
Midnight–4 AM	504	58.1	10,810	15.5
4 AM–8 AM	292	48.6	10,798	15.5
8 AM–noon	910	49.9	11,020	17.2
Noon–4 PM	2382	41.8	10,104	16.6
4 PM–8 PM	2200	37.0	9,150	15.5
8 PM–midnight	1027	39.2	9,005	18.9
Unknown	5	–	200	45.9
Total	7320	42.2	61,087	16.6

[a] Data from Bjerkedal and Bakketeig (1972).

Reports have more commonly focused on the issue of quality of care in relation to hour of birth (Tyson et al., 1979). In the results based on the Norwegian data, the mortality for induced births is approximately 2.5 times higher than that for spontaneous-onset births. Also, the mortality pattern by hour of day for induced births is reversed, with the lowest perinatal mortality rates occurring in the afternoon. In fact, the majority of induced births are terminated in the time period from noon to 6:00 PM (Table 6-2), which does contribute to the generally higher perinatal mortality rate from noon to midnight shown in Fig. 6-2. In Fig. 6-3, the better outcome of the induced births terminated in the afternoon can be attributed to the fact that these high-risk pregnancies were elected for induction at the most appropriate time. The induced births at other hours of the day, that have higher mortality rates, are more likely either to be emergency inductions or those elected inductions that do not respond as appropriately to the induction process. Stanley and Alberman (1978) have also suggested that low hospital staffing during early morning hours may partially account for the higher mortality of induced births at this time.

Birthweight-specific Comparisons

Perinatal mortality has since the 1950s been used increasingly as a basis for international comparisons (WHO, 1957). Infant mortality has also been widely used for comparison purposes. Difficulties with standardized definitions of what constitutes a livebirth or a fetal death have made international comparisons of infant mortality rates conceptually difficult. For example, Hoffman et al. (1978) have used twin births in Minnesota and Norway to show that the criteria used for labeling a birth as a livebirth can vary, with considerable consequences for the infant mortality rate but not for the perinatal mortality rate. The lower limit of gestational age used in defining the stillbirths to be included among perinatal deaths can also create problems of comparability. Many birth notification systems now include fetal deaths with gestations less than 28 weeks, so that the underreporting of stillbirths (28 weeks or more of gestation) has become less problematic.

The overall perinatal mortality rate has been criticized because no allowance is made for the varying incidence of low-weight births among populations. The need for the analysis of more refined mortality measures, especially birthweight-specific perinatal mortality rates, has been stressed by Chalmers (1979) and Macfarlane (1981). Figure 6-4 compares birthweight-specific perinatal mortality rates of Norway and Sweden for 1979 births. In these two countries, the birthweight distributions are nearly identical, yet Norway has a higher birthweight-specific perinatal mortality rate than does Sweden, particularly for average-sized infants weighing between 2500 and 4000 g. These mortality differences most likely reflect real differences in the chances of survival, because the birthweight distributions are comparable. There is a tendency for more very-low-birthweight deliveries to be registered in Norway, which surely reflects the fact that in Norway all deliveries are reported for gestational ages reaching 16 weeks or more.

The comparison of birthweight-specific perinatal mortality rates among populations can be very misleading, however, if proper allowance has not been made for differing birthweight distributions. As a rule, in a population where low birthweight is common, the perinatal mortality rate among low-weight births will tend to be lower than for a population where low birthweight is less common. For example, a simple comparison of birthweight-specific perinatal mortality rates between U.S. whites and blacks would suggest that low-weight black newborns fare much better than low-weight white newborns. However, the overall perinatal mortality rate for blacks is 75% higher than that for whites. The problem is that, relatively speaking, there are many more low-weight black births than low-weight white births. Several methods have been suggested that can adjust for the differences in birthweight distributions (Mallett and Knox, 1979; Rooth, 1980). These further adjustments of birthweight-specific perinatal mortality rates are necessary whenever the underlying birthweight distributions of the two or more populations being compared are different.

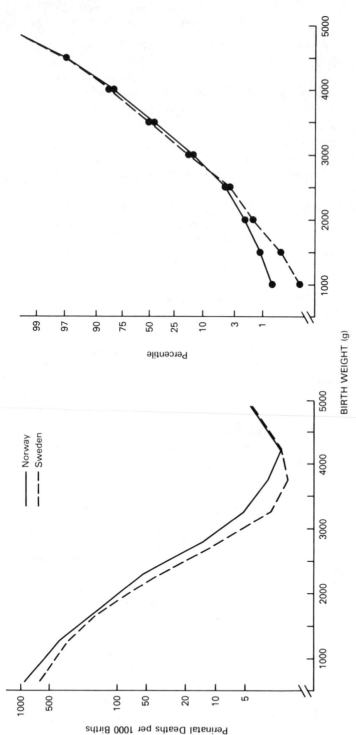

Fig. 6-4. Birthweight-specific perinatal mortality rates for Norway and Sweden in 1979 (*left*), and the cumulative birthweight distributions for these two countries in 1979 (*right*). The disparity below 2500 g may be ascribed in part to the differing birth registration rules: the Norwegian registry includes all births of gestational ages of 16 weeks or more, while the Swedish registry includes only births of 28 weeks or more. The differences in birthweight-specific perinatal mortality rates above 2500 g appear to be real, especially in view of the similarity in the cumulative birthweight distributions above 2500 g.

BEHAVIORAL, SOCIAL, AND ENVIRONMENTAL FACTORS

"There is no clear distinction between social and biological factors" (WHO, 1978). This statement applies to health and illness generally, but it is especially relevant in the perinatal field, where social differences between groups of mothers and infants have been noted for many years in many countries to be associated with varying risks of mortality and morbidity. Socioeconomic status and perinatal mortality showed such an association in all countries covered by the *WHO Report on Social and Biological Effects on Perinatal Mortality* (1978). For example, gradients were shown in the perinatal mortality rates by father's occupation, more or less continuously from the professional, technical, and administrative groups to the agricultural, production, and service groups.

Social Class

In Fig. 6-5, perinatal mortality rates from congenital malformations and other causes are shown by social class strata for England and Wales in 1977. Table 6-3 provides the distribution of births by birthweight in each of the social class strata in England and Wales in 1980. Together these data indicate that the risks of perinatal death and low birthweight increase from social classes I and II through to social class V. Similar findings have been noted in the United States by MacMahon et al. (1972) and Paneth et al. (1982), although "social class" was determined by a combination of factors in these studies. Dowding (1981) has recently demonstrated similar associations with birthweight and social class strata in Ireland.

Interpreting these associations is a controversial problem, in that researchers have a tendency to reify social class into a simple explanatory, if not causal, phenomenon. An association between social class (however defined) and perinatal or infant mortality does not constitute an explanation. Rather, as Illsley (1980) has stated, the social class effects suggest the existence of socioeconomic influences whose origins, nature, and mode of transmission need to be separated out and identified.

Because social class differences in perinatal mortality are consistently found in different countries, and in the same country over a period of many years, the differences noted may, to some extent, represent an artifact of measurement. The social class differences tend to persist throughout periods when there have been substantial changes in the definition and status of occupations and in the distribution of the employed population among the different occupations. Because of changing fertility patterns, the proportion of total

111

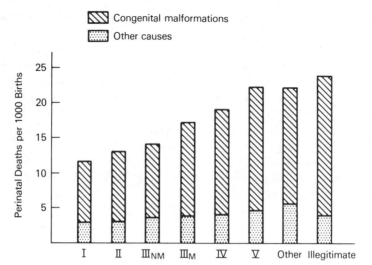

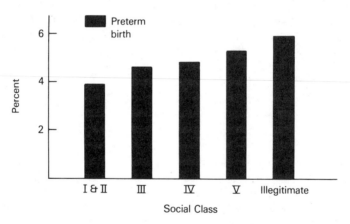

Fig. 6-5. Perinatal mortality rates in association with congenital malforma-tions and all other causes are shown by social class for England and Wales in 1977 at the top (MacFarlane and Chalmers, 1981). (Bottom) The incidence of preterm birth, 28–36 weeks of gestation, is shown by social class for Great Britain. From Butler and Alberman, 1969.

births contributed by different social classes has also been altered (Fig. 6-6). In addition, movement between classes is highly selective. Illsley (1980) has shown that women brought up in social classes I and II who marry into social classes IV and V are shorter, have poorer physiques, have dietary intakes lower in protein, calcium, and vita-mins A, B, and C, leave school earlier, achieve lower scores on IQ

Table 6-3. Percentage[a] Distributions of Births (Live and Still) by Birthweight in Each Social Class, England and Wales, 1980[b]

Birthweight, g	Social class of father							
	I Profess-ional	II Intermed-iate	III Skilled	IV Partly skilled	V Unskilled	Other legitimate	Illegi-timate	Total
<1500	0.9	0.7	0.9	1.0	1.0	0.9	1.4	1.0
1500–1999	0.9	1.2	1.2	1.5	1.4	1.0	1.9	1.3
2000–2499	3.8	3.7	4.6	5.3	6.3	4.6	6.7	4.8
2500–2999	15.8	15.7	18.6	20.8	23.1	18.7	23.2	19.0
3000–3499	39.8	39.2	39.0	39.8	39.8	40.0	39.4	39.3
3500–3999	30.3	29.9	27.1	24.7	22.6	26.9	22.0	26.7
4000+	8.5	9.6	8.4	7.0	5.8	7.9	5.5	7.9
Total %	100.0	100.0	100.0	100.0	100.0	100.0	100.0	100.0
No. stated	35,643	108,478	236,118	75,565	28,454	16,860	72,041	573,159
% not stated	13.1	12.8	14.5	14.5	13.7	16.0	7.7	13.3
Total	41,007	124,331	276,144	88,407	32,982	20,068	78,068	661,007

[a] Percentage of total where birthweight was stated.
[b] Data from Office of Population Censuses and Surveys (1981) and reproduced with permission of the Controller of Her Majesty's Stationery Office.

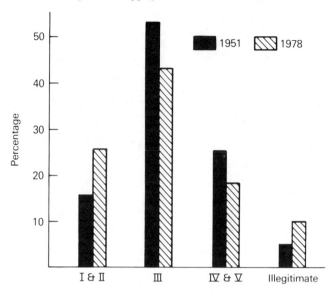

SOCIAL CLASS

Fig. 6-6. Proportions of total births contributed by different social classes in England and Wales in 1951 and 1978. Department of Health and Social Security, HMSO, 1980.

tests, enter less prestigious occupations, and run a higher risk of perinatal loss than those who marry within their social class group. The overall contribution of this "biologic drift" must be to maintain the social class gradient, yet this factor probably does not provide the whole explanation. There is considerable evidence linking patterns of perinatal mortality with socioeconomic indices both contemporaneously and intergenerationally (Sjolin, 1975; Alberman, 1977, 1978; Baird, 1980; Knox et al., 1980).

In addition, there is a considerable body of evidence linking particularly social and behavioral factors with perinatal mortality. The following paragraphs review each of these factors separately.

Occupation

Although categorizations of social class based on male occupation are associated with different risks of perinatal mortality, as yet very little information is available about the mechanisms underlying this association. It is known that some types of occupations can exert a direct effect on a person's chances of health or illness. Also, there are some data linking certain illness conditions in women (e.g., cervical cancer) with their husbands' occupations (Robinson, 1982). Thus it is possible that the occupation in which a fetus's father is employed could have a direct, adverse effect on perinatal survival. However, it seems more probable that the effect is indirect, that is, mediated by the different socioeconomic conditions of the different occupational groups.

Maternal employment has been a favored issue in research on the epidemiology of poor perinatal outcome. Many studies have indicated an apparent association between the two (Douglas, 1950; Stewart, 1955; McDowall et al., 1982). Attention to the methodology of these studies suggests that this is normally an association accounted for by the disadvantaged social circumstances of the women who must continue to be employed throughout pregnancy.

Some recent research in France (I.N.S.E.R.M., 1980) has identified certain features of employment that appear to be associated with poor perinatal outcome. These features include a long working week, standing during work, having few work breaks, having a lengthy and difficult journey to and from work, and performing especially tiring work. Overall, however, this research suggested a generally more favorable outcome (specifically a lower rate of preterm delivery) for economically active women. This does not mean that maternal employment necessarily has a directly positive effect (although it does raise family income and expose women to public discussion of health care issues); rather, it indicates the relevance of the entire work and family situation of pregnant women.

One striking aspect of perinatal researchers' interest in maternal employment is their failure to take into account the unpaid work that women perform at home. Studies of housework show that unemployed women put in at least the equivalent of a 40-hour working week on housework. For employed women, housework counts as a second job. The possible effect of the physical activity of housework on fetal health has scarcely been examined. For example, only one of the epidemiologic surveys of perinatal mortality in Britain (Joint Committee, 1948) considered the mother's domestic work. Analyzing the data collected in this survey, Douglas (1950) found an apparent beneficial effect on birthweight of having household help during the last trimester of pregnancy for two groups of women: primiparas and multiparas giving birth after an interval following the last birth of two years or less.

Education

In so far as membership of different social class groups is predictive of different rates of educational experience, one would expect an association between parental education and perinatal mortality.

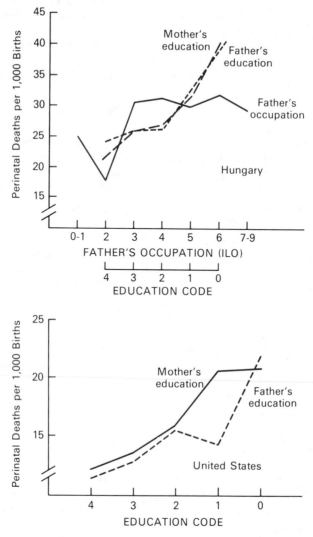

Fig. 6-7. Perinatal mortality rates by parental occupational and educational levels in Hungary in 1973, top, and by parental educational levels for six selected states from the United States in 1973, the bottom (World Health Organization, 1978).

There is evidence from some countries that such an association exists. For example, the *WHO Report on Social and Biological Effects on Perinatal Mortality* (1978) described a consistent inverse relationship between educational level and perinatal mortality for Hungary and the United States (Fig. 6-7). Maternal education produced a slightly

Table 6-4. Perinatal Mortality*a* in the Total Series by Mother's School Attendance*b*

Schooling	Number of perinatal deaths	All cases	Rate per 1000
1. University level	9	468	19.2
2. Secondary school	29	1,325	21.9
3. At least 6 months vocational school	48	2,160	22.2
4. 5–8 years	186	6,958	26.7
5. Less than 5 years	34	1,104	30.8
6. Not known	12	216	55.6
Total	318	12,231	26.0

a All births with minimum birth weight of 600 g, stillbirths, and deaths up to age of 28 days.
b Data from Rantakallio (1979).

steeper gradient in Hungary, and paternal education in the United States. Table 6-4 gives perinatal mortality by mother's school attendance for a sample of Finnish mothers in 1966; the figures show a pronounced gradient in perinatal mortality with decreasing levels of school attendance.

The degree of differentiation between the educational backgrounds of parents in different social classes (and thus the extent to which education is linked with perinatal mortality) clearly depends on the structure of, and access to, the educational system in any society. In a society where length of education does not vary to any great extent among different groups of mothers, as is the case in Britain, there will not be the same marked association with perinatal mortality as exists for social class. It is interesting to note that none of the three national perinatal mortality surveys (Joint Committee, 1948; Butler and Alberman, 1969; Chamberlain et al., 1978) analyzed perinatal mortality in relation to parental education. In the United States and in Scandinavia, parental education is a much more useful variable for explaining differences in outcome (Rantakallio, 1969; Kessner et al., 1973).

Education of a more specific kind—that is, educational classes for childbirth and motherhood during the antenatal period—does not appear to be of itself associated with improved perinatal mortality (Enkin, 1982). So far, only one of the very considerable number of studies carried out on the possible effect (beneficial or hazardous) of antenatal education on perinatal outcome has met the requirement of random assignment of subjects to experimental and control groups (Chalmers and Enkin, 1982).

117

Housing

Membership of different social classes is associated with different types of housing tenure, conditions, and amenities. Figure 6-8 shows shared or no inside toilet as an indicator of housing quality by social class for Great Britain in 1971, 1976, and 1980. In 1980, 5% of all households lacked this facility, but the proportion varied from 1% of those homes owned with a mortgage or loan, to 54% of those rented and privately furnished (Office of Population Censuses and Surveys, 1981). Data that would help to establish whether or not there is a relationship between housing (tenure, density, etc.) and perinatal mortality are not available. However, it is worth noting that over-crowding has been implicated as a factor in poor pregnancy outcome in many animal studies (Christian and Davis, 1964; Fryer et al., 1979). Myers (1979) has suggested that overcrowding may be the key factor underlying the class difference in a whole range of pregnancy outcomes. Analysis of the 1946 national survey of British maternities demonstrated an increase in stillbirth and neonatal death rates in

Fig. 6-8. Trends in the proportion of homes lacking certain amenities by social class of the head of the household for 1971, 1976, and 1980 (Office of Population Censuses and Surveys, 1982).

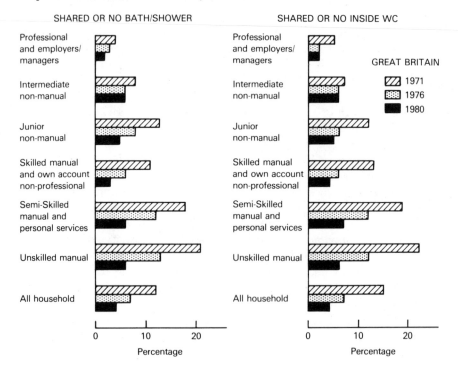

118

both home and hospital confinements as housing density increased, a fact suggesting, as the Joint Committee phrased it (1948), "that increasing povery is the causative factor."

Income

The variable of income is also linked with social class, and, as in the case of housing, adequate data have not been assembled for testing the hypothesis of a direct relationship with perinatal mortality. Occupationally defined social class is not an especially good index of real disposable income (Illsley, 1956). It is a particularly poor guide to the actual division of income within the family, that is, to the amount of money available to pregnant women themselves (Young, 1975). Several British studies have highlighted the fact that income is not shared equally between many couples, and the wife/mother's share does not necessarily rise with inflation and wage/salary increases obtained by the husband/father (Young and Syson, 1974; Land, 1977). It is possible that women and children can live in poverty while their men do not, a fact that points to an important distinction between two types of inequality characterizing modern industrialized societies. On the one hand there are inequalities associated with what might be termed "economic class", on the other, there are those associated with what could be called "gender class." The latter type of inequality that exists between men and women should be addressed in future research in the perinatal field.

Ethnicity

Several studies have shown that ethnicity is associated with variation in rates of low birthweight and perinatal mortality (Shapiro et al., 1968; Weatherall, 1975; Davies, 1980). An exception is a recent study of immigrants in Sweden that does not confirm the usual pattern (Smedby and Ericson, 1979). Table 6-5 shows perinatal mortality in 1977 by birthplace of the mother for England and Wales. Birthplace is only a crude indicator of ethnic group, a notoriously difficult topic on which to obtain reliable information. Different communities exhibit different birthweight distributions so that the association between low birthweight and perinatal mortality may be mediated by the biologic differences among women. Some communities may be responsible for a higher rate of small babies.

Marital Status

Tables 6-3 and 6-5 also show a poorer perinatal outcome for the "illegitimate" category of births, which supports an association that has been known for some time, and that apparently holds for many countries (WHO, 1978). The birthweight distribution of the illegitimate

Table 6-5. Perinatal Mortality in England and Wales, 1977, by Birthplace of Mother[a]

Place of birth of mother	*All legitimate* Number of perinatal deaths	Rate per 1000	*Illegitimate* Number of perinatal deaths	Rate per 1000
All	8411	16.2	1306	23.3
United Kingdom	7076	15.7	1160	23.7
Irish Republic	143	15.7	30	21.6
Australia, Canada, New Zealand	26	13.1	7	35.5
New Commonwealth				
Bangladesh, India	305	21.8	5	34.0
Africa	177	24.3	4	11.1
West Indies	87	25.2	66	18.7
Malta, Gibraltar				
Cyprus	29	11.5	3	19.0
Remainder	67	18.3	3	15.3
Pakistan	242	25.2	1	16.7
Remainder of Europe	113	13.8	12	18.4
Not stated or at sea	35	60.6	12	250.0
Other	111	13.6	3	6.9

[a] Data from Adelstein et al., (1980).

group is shifted toward the lower end of the range, and the incidence of preterm birth is also increased (Bakketeig and Hoffman, 1981, 1983).

Because it is unlikely that the legal status of the mother could have a direct impact on her fetus's growth and thereby affect the chances of survival, there must be mediating factors having to do with social and economic support. In many developed countries there are now probably two distinct groups within the "illegitimate" category: mothers who are living in a stable union with the father of their child and who choose not to be married, and those who are living on their own or in otherwise generally nonsupportive circumstances. Pettersson (1968) has discussed this issue in terms of a "marriage late in pregnancy" bias using Swedish data in the 1960s.

Sexual Activity

All forms of sexual activity decline progressively throughout pregnancy (Morris, 1975; Lumley, 1978; Grudzinskas et al., 1979). It has been suggested that continuation of sexual activity in late pregnancy is a factor predisposing toward poor perinatal outcome, especially preterm delivery and amnionitis (Naeye and Ross, 1982), and fetal distress in labor (Grudzinskas et al., 1979). Still other studies do not find this type of association (Pugh and Fernandez, 1953; Solberg et al., 1973; Perkins, 1979; Rayburn and Wilson, 1980; Mills et al., 1981). As Lumley and Asbury (1982) observe in their discussion of this literature, the methodology of these studies so far has not been adequate to the task of disentangling the following crucial questions: Are different rates of sexual activity per se associated with different perinatal outcomes? What kind of sexual activity is implicated?

Interpregnancy Interval

Many authors have suggested that short and long intervals between pregnancies are associated with an increased risk of perinatal death and other adverse outcomes of pregnancy (Yerushalmy, 1945; Bishop, 1964; Day, 1967). It has been suggested that an optimal interval exists that will minimize the risk of adverse perinatal outcomes (Day, 1967; Spiers and Wang, 1976). Fedrick and Adelstein (1973), using the British Perinatal Mortality Survey of 1958 to examine these relationships, found that the most important factors influencing pregnancy spacing were outcomes of the preceding pregnancy, social class, and maternal age. When these variables were taken into account they found that the length of interpregnancy interval was not associated with the stillbirth rate. However, they were able to show that very short interpregnancy intervals (less than six months) were associated with higher neonatal mortality. Long intervals were not shown to be associated with higher mortality rates.

Erickson and Bjerkedal (1978) examined pairs of Norwegian births to determine the association between interpregnancy interval and perinatal mortality rates. They found that the association between interpregnancy interval and low birthweight was the same for births that precede the interval as for births that follow an interval. Even though the authors were able to demonstrate some association between long intervals and the risk of stillbirth, and between short intervals and increased neonatal mortality, they concluded that manipulation of the interval between pregnancies is unlikely to have any marked beneficial or detrimental effect on outcomes of pregnancy. Alberman et al. (1980) and Roman and Alberman (1980) have also examined the relationships between pregnancy spacing and outcome for women of varying gravidity. They found that long intervals were more likely to precede miscarriages, but the effect was not large and could be due in part to the fact that the women were older.

Diet

The importance of nutrition to successful pregnancy outcome relates not only to pregnancy itself but to prepregnancy nutritional status, including that in the mother's own childhood (Baird, 1977b); an indicator of the latter effect is the significance of both height and prepregnancy weight as a predictor of pregnancy outcome. The investigation of nutrition during pregnancy and its relationship with outcome is not a new theme in perinatal research (see Burke et al., 1943; Thomson, 1958, 1959). It is apparent that dietary restriction can cause a marked decrease in mean birthweight. During famine conditions, such as those that existed during the siege of Leningrad in 1941–1943, during the 1944–1945 winter in Holland, and during the period of severe food shortages in the German city of Wuppertal in 1945–1946, mean birthweight may be depressed by more than 550 g (Antonov, 1947; Dean, 1951; Stein et al., 1975); and perinatal survival may be correspondingly jeopardized.

Little is known about which dietary elements are important in guaranteeing fetal health and survival. Practically the only available evidence comes from intervention studies designed to change dietary habits during pregnancy. These have not always had the predicted effect. For example, in the study by Rush et al. (1974), 1000 women at high risk of low birthweight were randomly assigned to three groups: (1) high-protein supplement, (2) balanced protein and calorie supplement, and (3) normal clinic care (routine supplements of vitamin and mineral tablets). There was no significant variation in birthweight among the three groups, but the group receiving the high-protein supplement appeared to do worse than the others in terms of curtailed gestation and fetal growth retardation. The exception to this was that among women with low prepregnancy weight who smoked, the high-protein supplement provided a significant birthweight increment at term. There is some evidence that the weight of male fetuses is more responsive to dietary supplementation than is that of female fetuses (Mora et al., 1981).

However, it is not clear whether birthweight increments achieved via programs of nutritional supplementation are associated with decreased perinatal mortality and morbidity or, indeed, with improved long-term child development. There is also the methodologic problem of determining whether it is dietary advice or dietary supplementation or the generally supportive effect of inclusion in such a research program that accounts for improved outcome, where such improvement is found. The conclusion reached by Susser and Stein in their discussion of "Prenatal Nutrition and Subsequent Development" (1977) would seem appropriate: "We can be sure," they say, "that prenatal nutrition affects fetal growth viability and vitality, but only under certain conditions. We need to know more about these conditions and the specifics of the nutrients involved."

Smoking and Alcohol

The relationship between smoking during pregnancy and reduced birthweight has been shown clearly and consistently in a large number of studies. The mean shift downward is in the region of 150–250 g and is not due to a mean shift in gestational age. The weight reduction is proportional to the number of cigarettes smoked and is independent of many other factors (Meyer, 1977).

The question as to the relationship between maternal smoking and perinatal mortality is more difficult to answer. Some studies (Butler and Alberman, 1969; Bailey, 1970; Meyer and Tonascia, 1971; Meyer et al., 1974; Rush and Kass, 1972) find increased mortality, whereas others (O'Lane, 1963; Rantakallio, 1969; Yerushalmy, 1974) do not. The debate hinges on whether the apparent differences in mortality are due to the act of smoking or to characteristics of those who smoke. However, it does seem that, if the relationship between smoking and perinatal mortality is indeed causal, the effect is smallest when the mother is relatively young, of low parity, and of high social class (Butler and Alberman, 1969; Goldstein, 1977; Rantakallio, 1979).

Much less is known about the effect of maternal alcohol consumption than about smoking on the fetus, because it is only recently that epidemiologists and others have begun to consider the possibly deleterious effects of alcohol on perinatal survival. Chronically alcoholic women may give birth to offspring with a specific set of anomalies, known as the fetal alcohol syndrome (Streissguth, 1978; Kaminski et al., 1976; Olegaard et al. 1979; Newman and Correy, 1980). It has been estimated that the level of alcohol consumption needed to produce these developmental abnormalies is approximately 30 ml of alcohol per day. Relatively low levels of consumption may cause spontaneous abortion (Kline et al., 1980). The association with increased mortality has been demonstrated only for animal populations (Streissguth, 1978).

Stress

The idea that socially generated stress affects reproduction receives support from many fields, including experimental work on animals and humans. Developments in biochemical measurements of "stress hormones" have made it possible to show a direct biologic effect of social and biologic stressors. Low birthweight, preterm labor, the need for obstetric intervention in delivery, and disturbed early mother–child relationships are among those pregnancy outcomes in which stress has been implicated (Shaw et al., 1970; Cohler et al., 1975; Erickson, 1976; Yang et al., 1976; Lederman et al., 1978; Newton et al., 1979; Wolkind, 1981).

One approach to documenting the importance of stress is the intervention study, of which several have been done. Sosa et al. (1980) provided a supportive companion for the mother during childbirth and found a reduced incidence of adverse outcomes as compared with a control group. Sokol et al. (1980) evaluated the effects of inclusion in a maternity and infant care project in which underprivileged pregnant women received a "package" consisting of health education, nutritional counseling, parenting guidance, and home visits. When compared with a similar group not included in the project, they were found to experience 60% less perinatal mortality.

The processes whereby support and information may reduce stress and lower perinatal mortality are not clear. Childbearing is a social and psychologic exercise as much as a biologic and medical one. Although it seems obvious that a mother's mental and emotional state is not unrelated to the condition of her fetus, very few studies have addressed this question with an adequate research design. Most studies are descriptive, anecdotal, retrospective, and uncontrolled. For the most part, childbearing studies do not examine the outcome of perinatal survival.

With regard to the relationship between stress and social class, it would seem important to bear in mind the fact that the class structure impinges on the distribution of life stresses in two ways: (1) The incidence of potentially negative life events is greater with descending social class; but (2) resources and skills relevant to coping with such stress are also unevenly distributed, with lower class individuals possessing fewer of these resources and skills than those in positions higher up the social scale (Brown and Harris, 1978; Oakley et al., 1982). It is unlikely that any given psychosocial process or stressor is etiologically specific for any particular reproductive difficulty. Rather it would seem that the effect of "stress" is to alter the endocrine balance of the body, thereby making a range of pathologies more likely to occur. Stress may also be associated with more directly noxious effects if, for example, it depresses nutrition, causes insomnia, or raises smoking and alcohol consumption. There is some evidence that both maternal smoking and maternal alcohol consumption are responses to, or attempts to cope with, stress (Graham, 1977; Farrant, 1980).

124

MATERNAL BIOLOGIC FACTORS

This section discusses the relation of perinatal mortality to factors that can to a great extent be considered biologic ones. However, such associations are not fully understood and might operate partially through behavioral pathways. This is one of the reasons researchers find it so difficult to distinguish between biologic, and behavioral and social, factors in perinatal mortality.

Parity

The association generally accepted in perinatal epidemiology between parity and perinatal mortality is based on the analysis of data from cross-sectional studies. In such studies the mortality rates are derived after combining all first births in the data set, all second births, all third births, and so forth. The association that emerges using this approach is a U-shaped one, as shown in Fig. 6-9a, the mortality being higher for first births, lower for second births, and then increasing for third and fourth births (dotted-lined curve in the figure).

If, however, the relationship between parity and perinatal death is examined within groups of women based on their attained size of sibship, a very different pattern emerges, as also shown in Fig. 6-9a. The solid lines in the figure are based on 137,919 mothers who delivered either their first two births, first three births, or first four births in Norway within the ten-year study period. Within each sibship group the perinatal mortality decreases by increasing parity. Also, the mortality is generally higher among births of mothers with larger sibships.

The U-shaped cross-sectionally derived relationships and the longitudinally derived relationships between parity and perinatal death shown in Fig. 6-9a are based on exactly the same data set. In the cross-sectional analysis the perinatal mortality is lower for second births compared with higher order births, largely because the dominant contribution to second births comes from women having only two births, who have lower overall perinatal mortality rates. Because the mortality of third and fourth births necessarily must be based on women with larger sibships, who have generally higher perinatal mortality rates, a selection phenomenon occurs that accounts for the discrepancy between the cross-sectional and longitudinal results.

Although the longitudinal analysis discloses artifacts of cross-sectional studies, there are also methodologic issues associated with the longitudinal results. It is well known that mothers with perinatal deaths tend to have larger sibships by replacement of their adverse

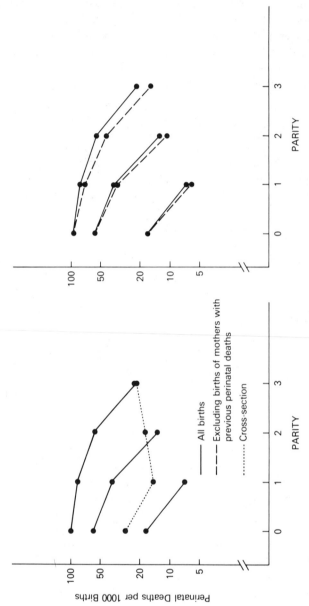

Fig. 6–9. Perinatal mortality rates by parity and size of sibship based on all 137,919 births to mothers having two, three, or four singleton deliveries in Norway during the ten-year study period, 1967–76. (Left) Longitudinal and cross-sectional analyses of the data. (Right) Total longitudinal analysis compared to the longitudinal analysis after sibships containing previous perinatal deaths were excluded.

126

outcomes (Billewicz, 1973; Record and Armstrong, 1975; Ressequie, 1976; Bakketeig and Hoffman, 1979). Also, there is a tendency for mothers to stop their childbearing after a success. These "self-selections for pregnancy" may have some confounding influences on the results obtained through longitudinal analyses (Bakketeig and Hoffman, 1979, 1980). In Fig. 6-9b, there are three stippled curves showing the associations between parity and perinatal death that exist after mothers with previous perinatal deaths have been removed from the analysis. Exclusion of mothers who have had previous perinatal deaths lowers the overall mortality, but the decline in mortality by increasing parity is not much changed. This provides support for the "biologic" as opposed to the "behavioral" interpretation of the longitudinal analysis results.

If the observational interval for a longitudinal study is too short, then the results based on attained sibship size may not reflect the results based on completed sibship size. This possible confounding factor has been examined in a study of preterm birth based on the longitudinal analysis method (Bakketeig and Hoffman, 1981). In this study, the relative truncation of the time period to seven years was shown not to have changed the basic association with parity when compared to a ten-year time span. A longitudinal study covering a much longer span of time is more likely to be affected by secular trends in the perinatal mortality rates. The point to be stressed, then, is that some of the possible biases cannot be fully eliminated or controlled for in any longitudinal analysis. The same biases also are operating when a cross-sectional analysis is used. The difference is that it is far less obvious that such biases exist in cross-sectional studies. In particular, the bias introduced by pooling across sibship groups is completely missed by the cross-sectional approach.

To conclude, births within larger sibships have a higher overall perinatal mortality rate, and within each sibship group, the perinatal mortality rate decreases with increasing parity. There is no evidence that the perinatal mortality rate increases with increasing parity for moderate-sized sibships (less than five siblings).

Maternal Age

Because parity and maternal age are closely interrelated, the association between these two variables in combination and perinatal mortality is examined in Table 6-6 and Fig. 6-10. The U-shaped association between maternal age and perinatal mortality that was found in the cross-sectional analysis is not present here. For first births there is a steady increase in perinatal mortality from maternal age of under 20 years to age 35 years or over, the mortality being nearly three times

Table 6-6. Number of Births and Rates of Perinatal Death per 1000 Births by Maternal Age and Parity. Based on 26,923 Mothers with Their First Three Singleton Births, Norway, 1967–76

Parity	Total number of births	Maternal age (years)				
		<20	20–24	25–29	30–34	35+
0	26,923	4875	15,624	5410	854	160
	(59.5%)	(53.3%)	(55.7%)	(67.3%)	(86.7%)	(143.8%)
1	26,923	1011	13,460	10,006	2078	368
	(36.6)	(45.5)	(30.5)	(41.0)	(47.6)	(57.1)
2	26,923	47	5575	13,928	6231	1142
	(12.6)	(42.6)	(12.0)	(12.2)	(13.8)	(12.3)
Total	80,769	5933	34,659	29,344	9163	1670
	(36.2%)	(51.9%)	(38.9%)	(32.2%)	(28.3%)	(34.7%)

Fig. 6-10. Perinatal mortality rates by parity and maternal age groups based on all 26,923 mothers with their first three singleton births in Norway during the ten-year study period, 1967–76.

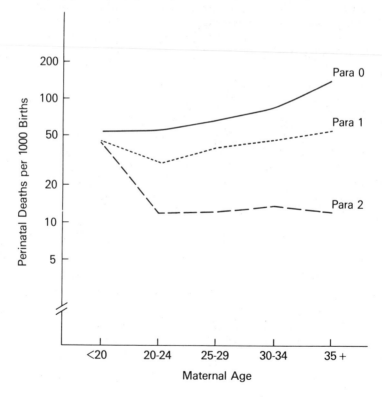

128

higher in the older as compared to the younger age group. For second births, the mortality is lowest for mothers aged 20–24 years. Above that age the mortality increases only moderately. For third births there is virtually no change in mortality with increasing age.

Meirik et al. (1979) have analyzed what proportion of the decline in perinatal mortality rates from the mid-1950s through the mid-1970s occurring in Sweden could be attributed to the changing maternal age and parity distributions. They concluded that only 9% of the decline was attributable to a shift toward a more favorable age and parity composition of the mothers. Results from Scotland (Billewicz, 1973) and the United States (Morris et al., 1975) have suggested a much higher proportion of the decline could be attributed to shifting age and parity distributions, from 50 to 27%, respectively.

The discrepancy may exist because these demographic factors have contributed comparatively much less to the decline in perinatal mortality in Sweden since the 1950s. Scotland and the United States may have lagged behind Sweden in the demographic transition toward more favorable age and parity distributions (Meirik et al., 1979). However, this situation may have changed in the past decade. A recent study by Forbes et al. (1982) found that only 7% of the decline in perinatal mortality in the 1970s in Scotland could be attributed to a more favorable age, parity, and social class composition of the obstetric population. Given the continuing reduction in the perinatal mortality rate in Scotland, it is clear that many other factors are now contributing to this improvement.

The Tendency to Repeat Perinatal Death

The risk of perinatal death by perinatal survival of previous birth or births is shown in Table 6-7. The results are based on 107,495 mothers

Table 6-7. The Risk of Perinatal Death (PND) in Subsequent Births by Perinatal Survival of Previous Birth(s). Based on 134,418 Mothers with Their First Two or Three Singleton Births, Norway 1967–76

			Subsequent perinatal death		
First birth	Second birth	Number of mothers	Numbers	Per 1000	Relative risk
Not PND		131,004	1543	11.8	1.0
PND		3,414	180	52.7	4.5
Not PND	Not PND	24,438	259	10.6	0.9
PND	Not PND	1,499	34	22.7	1.9
Not PND	PND	893	38	42.6	3.6
PND	PND	93	8	86.0	7.3

with their first two singleton births and 26,923 mothers with their first three singleton births only. From the table, we note that if the first birth survived the perinatal period, then only 11.8 per 1000 second births died perinatally. If, however, the first birth died, then 52.7 per 1000 second births were perinatal deaths. Comparing the latter rate with the previous one, mothers with a perinatal death at first birth have a relative risk for a subsequent perinatal death of 4.5. From this table it also appears that the risk of a subsequent perinatal death was further increased if the mother had had two previous perinatal deaths. Thus the relative risk for these mothers increased to 7.3 (86.0 per 1000). However, for each birth that survived the perinatal period, the risk of a subsequent perinatal death decreased. Among mothers with one previous perinatal death and one infant who survived, the risk of a perinatal death among their third births was higher if the previous death was the adjacent birth.

Maternal Diseases During Pregnancy

Table 6-8 shows the perinatal mortality rates for the offspring of mothers suffering from some major diseases during pregnancy. The data presented in the table are based on births in Sweden, 1977–1978. Whereas the overall perinatal mortality rate during this two-year period was 9.6 per 1000, births of diabetic mothers had a perinatal mortality rate of 41.3 per 1000. Preeclampsia was associated with a less dramatically increased perinatal mortality risk, namely 14.1 per 1000. A common complication during pregnancy such as urinary tract infection does not seem to be associated with any increased mortality risk. These observations are generally in agreement with those made in other studies (Chamberlain et al., 1975). It should be noted,

Table 6-8. Perinatal Mortality by Maternal Diseases During Pregnancy. Based on 189,228 Births in Sweden, 1977–78

Maternal diseases during pregnancy	Number of births	Perinatal deaths	
		Number	*Per 1000*
Diabetes	727	30	41.3
Blood incompatibility	857	19	22.2
Urinary infections	1,969	20	10.2
Renal disease	263	10	38.0
Pre-eclampsia and eclampsia	15,099	213	14.1
All births	189,228	1,822	9.6

however, that these data need to be interpreted cautiously because the quality of reporting information to the Swedish Medical Birth Registry ultimately depends on hospital-based records. Such information varies from hospital to hospital in such areas as the propensity to note various diagnoses and the use of varying criteria for classifying underlying conditions.

Complications During Delivery

Similar data are shown for complications during delivery in Table 6-9. Where there was no complication, the perinatal mortality was 6.0 per 1000. The mortality risk was dramatically increased if there were placental complications like placenta praevia or abruptio placentae, but also where there were reported complications of the umbilical cord. Uterine rupture was associated with the highest perinatal mortality risk, but this complication is fortunately very rare. Prolonged labor was not associated with any markedly increased mortality risk. Similar findings also have been reported by other authors (Chamberlain et al., 1978). Reservations about accepting the actual incidence rates in the table should be borne in mind for the same reasons as mentioned in the previous paragraph. These data will vary somewhat, depending on the quality of the systems for maintaining medical records in different hospitals.

Table 6-9. Perinatal Mortality by Some Obstetric Diagnoses (Complications During Delivery). Based on 189,228 Births in Sweden, 1977–78

Complications during delivery	Number of births	Perinatal deaths	
		Number	Per 1000
Placenta praevia/abruptio placentae	2,061	203	98.5
Pelvis anomalies and discrepancy between pelvis and fetus	7,335	53	7.2
Malpresentation of the fetus	2,969	53	17.9
Prolonged duration of labor	14,276	112	7.8
Uterine rupture	51	11	215.7
Complications of the umbilical cord	391	38	97.2
Fetal complications	11,703	327	27.9
No complications	125,440	757	6.0

131

FETAL AND INFANT FACTORS

Fetal Age and Birthweight

Perinatal mortality is most closely related to fetal age and weight. Table 6-10, which is based on all births in Sweden in 1978, shows that perinatal mortality was the lowest if the birth was delivered at term (40–41 weeks) and weighed between 4000 and 4500 g, namely 1.2 per 1000 births. If the baby weighed less than 1500 g, perinatal mortality was 400 times higher.

Examination of the totals in the table reveals that although the perinatal mortality varies from 309.1 at 28–29 weeks of gestation to 2.7 per 1000 at term (114:1), the mortality by birthweight varies from 461.1 to 1.7 per 1000 (271:1). This affirms the conclusion of several studies that the association of perinatal mortality with birthweight is stronger than that with fetal age (Susser et al., 1972; Hoffman et al., 1974, 1977; Lee et al., 1980; Bakketeig and Hoffman, 1983).

Crown–Heel Length

Table 6-11 relates perinatal mortality to fetal crown–heel length. This has been done for selected birthweight groups in order to simplify the presentation of the data. Within each weight group, crown–heel length

Table 6-10. Perinatal Mortality by Gestational Age and Birthweight. Based on 93,156 Births in Sweden, 1978

Gestational age (weeks)	Birthweight								
	<1500	1500–1999	2000–2499	2500–2999	3000–3499	3500–3999	4000–4499	4500+	Total
28–29	376.8	375.0	428.6	250.0	–	58.8	–	–	309.1
30–31	447.2	195.9	206.9	–	–	–	–	–	248.7
32–33	458.8	99.5	61.5	30.8	23.3	28.6	–	–	116.7
34–35	333.3	141.5	47.8	18.8	3.7	–	–	–	56.4
36–37	451.6	136.1	57.5	16.2	7.4	4.6	–	29.4	21.4
38–39	444.4	131.6	22.9	8.6	3.0	1.4	2.5	2.9	4.4
40–41	500.0	125.0	58.6	7.7	2.5	1.5	1.2	1.9	2.7
42–43	–	125.0	52.6	13.1	5.1	2.0	1.7	1.6	3.8
44–45	–	500.0	83.3	28.0	6.8	3.5	14.2	–	9.3
>45	–	–	285.7	30.8	–	–	–	–	5.7
Unknown[a]	250.0	333.3	125.0	33.3	27.8	29.4	–	–	45.5
Total	461.1	146.2	50.3	11.3	3.6	1.7	1.7	2.3	9.1

[a] Only 0.1% of all births.

Table 6-11. Perinatal Mortality by Birthweight and Crown–Heel Length. Based on 138,192 Second Births to Mothers with Their First and Second Singleton Births, Norway, 1967–76

Births weight groups	Total number of births	By crown–heel length[a]							
		Short		Medium		Long		Unknown	
		No. of births	Perinatal deaths per 1000	No. of births	Perinatal deaths per 1000	No. of births	Perinatal deaths per 1000	No. of births	Perinatal deaths per 1000
2501–3000	14,001	1451	22.7	10,496	8.3	1994	38.1	60	50.0
3001–3500	44,699	5376	5.0	35,009	2.7	4126	15.5	188	26.6
3501–4000	50,160	2763	5.4	38,372	1.4	8818	4.4	207	0

[a] 2501–3000: short:<47 cm long:>49 cm
3001–3500: ” :<49 ” ” :>51 ”
3501–4000: ” :<50 ” ” :>52 ” .

133

has been characterized as short, medium, and long according to the actual distribution of lengths within that weight group of second births. For these weight groups, "short" corresponds approximately to the lower decile and "long" to the upper decile of the crown–heel length distributions. The pattern turns out to be similar within each of these weight groups: Crown–heel length is closely related to perinatal mortality. The short and long babies had quite dramatically higher perinatal mortality. In particular, the "long and skinny" births had markedly reduced chances of survival. This observation underlines the importance of paying attention to birth length—as well as birthweight—of the fetus and the infant as a predictor of perinatal health. Further information on this topic is available from the literature (Gruenwald, 1969; Miller and Hassanein, 1971; Fryer et al., 1977; Bakketeig and Hoffman, 1983).

Cause-specific Perinatal Mortality

Table 6-12, based on Norwegian births between 1967 and 1976, shows perinatal mortality by primary cause of death for three weight groups. For the lowest weight group (1500 g or lower), the two predominant

Table 6–12. Perinatal Mortality Rate by Birthweight and Primary Cause of Death. Based on 138,182 second births to Mothers with Their First and Second Single Births, Norway, 1967–76

Primary cause of death	Birthweight (grams)		
	≤1500 (n = 1251)	1501–2500 (n = 3688)	>2500 (n = 133,253)
Maternal complications during pregnancy	63.9	13.8	0.3
Placenta previa, abruptio placenta, complications of umbilical cord	243.0	40.4	1.5
Other complications of delivery including birth injury	252.6	26.8	0.7
Congenital malformations	48.0	23.0	1.0
Asphyxia (unspecified)	54.4	13.8	0.1
"Premature" birth (unspecified)	80.7	3.3	—
Other causes	35.2	13.8	0.5
Total perinatal mortality rate	777.8	134.8	4.1

causes of perinatal death are placental complications and other complications during delivery, including birth injury. These two causes, together with congenital malformations, are also the predominant causes for the births weighing between 1500 and 2500 g. Congenital malformations and placental complications are the main causes of deaths within the highest weight group. Of all perinatal deaths resulting from congenital malformations, nearly half of them weighed more than 2500 g.

Causes of perinatal death reported in the literature vary according to whether the diagnoses are based on death certificates or clinical diagnoses with or without autopsy findings reported in hospital records, or alternatively, whether the study is based on autopsy findings with or without adequate consideration of clinical information (Nakamura et al., 1981). However, most studies show that for all births taken together, the most common cause of stillbirth is anoxia/asphyxia with or without known association with maternal complications such as placental conditions. The principal causes of neonatal death are hyaline membrane disease (or respiratory distress syndrome) and congenital malformations (Nakamura et al., 1981).

MEDICAL CARE

It is hard to establish to what extent the recent decline in perinatal mortality in developed countries has been influenced by improvements in antenatal, intrapartum, and neonatal care, and to what extent it may be due to other factors, such as improvements in the health of the population or changes in the structure of the childbearing population itself.

Since the late 1960s there have been tremendous changes in perinatal practice and service provision; in particular, new technology has to an increasing extent been introduced in obstetrics and neonatology. Obstetric practice has become more active with a steady increase in the use of induction of labor and interventions during delivery. For example, in Norway the use of induction of labor increased by 70% from the late 1960s through the end of the 1970s (Bjerkedal, 1982). Perinatal mortality among induced births did not, however, decrease more rapidly than mortality among births spontaneously delivered, as shown in Fig. 6-11. This might be taken to indicate that the increased use of induction has not contributed much to the overall decline in perinatal mortality.

Operative deliveries have also become more and more common since 1970. For example, the use of cesarean section in Norway

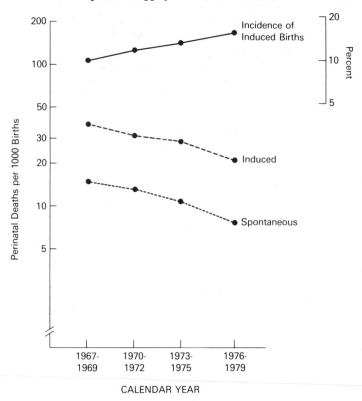

Fig. 6-11. Frequency of the induction of labor and the associated perinatal mortality rates among induced or spontaneous onset births by calendar year in Norway, 1967–79. Newborns weighing less than 1000 g have been excluded.

increased from 1.8% in 1967 to 8.0% in 1979. In the United States, cesarean deliveries increased from 4.5% in 1965 to 16.5% in 1980. Considerable regional variations also exist in the United States: In 1980, the Northeast region had a cesarean section rate of 19.2%, whereas the North Central region had a rate of only 14.9%.

The decline in perinatal mortality among births delivered by cesarean section compared with births delivered by other interventions and those delivered without the use of any interventions is shown in Fig. 6-12 based on Norwegian data. The decline in perinatal mortality among cesarean section births is apparently steeper than among any of the other categories. Similar observations have been documented by other authors. For example, Williams and Chen (1982) have shown that the perinatal mortality rate among cesarean section

136

births in California in the late 1970s was equal to that of vaginally delivered births. The cesarean section rate in California, as is true for the United States generally, was twice that in Norway.

Several authors have focused on the recent decline in perinatal mortality rates after a period of relative stability in the 1950s and early 1960s (Kleinman et al., 1978; MacFarlane, 1979; Lee et al., 1980; Williams and Chen, 1982). In their study from California, Williams and Chen (1982) demonstrated that neonatal mortality from 1960 to 1977 had decreased twice as rapidly as fetal mortality. They concluded that more than 80% of the decline in perinatal mortality was due to reduced birthweight-specific perinatal mortality rates. In part because of such results, it has been suggested that birthweight-specific perinatal mortality rates are a sensitive measure of the potential

Fig. 6-12. Perinatal mortality rates for different types of obstetrical intervention at delivery by calendar year in Norway, 1967–79. Newborns weighing less than 1000 g have been excluded.

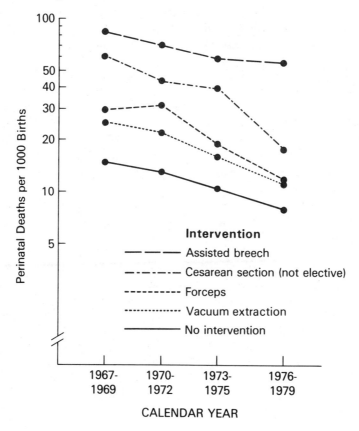

influences of perinatal care on pregnancy outcome (Chalmers et al., 1978; MacFarlane, 1981; Dowding, 1982). It is worth noting, however, that the recent improvements in perinatal mortality rates have not only occurred in low-weight groups, but are even more marked for average-weight births (Bakketeig et al., 1978; Roberton, 1979; Chalmers, 1979). These authors also have suggested that the mortality among average-weight births may often be a better indicator of the quality of perinatal care than the mortality among low-weight births.

In spite of the results cited above, the focus in this field has been mainly on low-weight births, especially the very-low-weight infants (less than 1500 g at birth). Most authors claim that a considerable proportion of the decline in the perinatal mortality rates among low-weight births is likely to be due to improved perinatal care, particularly to the increased provision and use of neonatal intensive care units (Stewart and Reynolds, 1974; Berger et al., 1976; Lee et al., 1976; Usher, 1977; Brown and Taeusch, 1978; Stanley and Alberman, 1978; Gamsu et al., 1979; Nelson et al., 1979; Reynolds and Stewart, 1979; Roberton, 1979; Sinclair et al., 1981). However, others are more skeptical about the beneficial effects of perinatal care on survival (Davis, 1976, 1980; Jones et al., 1979).

Most of the studies on these issues are based on hospital data. Few of the studies have been truly population based. In Sweden, Falk and Wranne (1973) showed that perinatal mortality was lower for offspring of mothers living within the vicinity of a highly specialized central county hospital in comparison to mothers living within the vicinity of less specialized hospitals in the same county. Ritter et al. (1977) investigated the disparity in infant mortality between urban and rural areas, and postulated that the lower mortality rates for urban areas were at least partly attributable to the greater accessibility of perinatal care facilities.

Bakketeig et al. (1978) used a scoring system based on the available equipment and staffing of each maternity institution in Norway. Each county was assigned an average score weighted by the number of births in each institution. The counties were then divided into three groups: a high-score, median-score, and low-score county group. A strong association was demonstrated between the quality of care (as reflected in the staffing and equipment score) and perinatal mortality within each birthweight class. The relative difference in mortality was greater for average- and high-weight births compared to low-weight births. Thus two-thirds of the additional perinatal deaths in the "low-score" county group weighed 3000 g or more.

Nearly all studies of the associations between perinatal care and outcome are observational ones, and very few controlled trials have been conducted to assess the impact of medical care on perinatal mortality. Electronic fetal monitoring, however, has been studied using randomized controlled trials (Renou et al., 1976; Havercamp et al., 1976; Kelso et al., 1978). These studies were unable to show differences in the outcome for the groups being monitored versus the controls, illustrating well the dilemma faced in attempting to examine outcomes such as perinatal death. In order to demonstrate any substantial effects (i.e., reduction in mortality), an unmanageable number of randomized patients are often required. For this reason, randomized controlled trials in perinatal medicine must often rely on measures of outcome other than perinatal death. It is fair to conclude that many processes and treatments applied within antenatal, intra-partum, and neonatal care have not been carefully evaluated in terms of actual benefits and potential hazards. Unfortunately, it is often considered unethical to do a randomized controlled trial in order to evaluate the effects of a procedure. Still, whenever this is not the case, and particularly before new procedures and treatments become widely accepted, researchers should be encouraged to evaluate the possible benefits and hazards through randomized controlled trials so that this field of medicine can advance on a rational and scientific basis. Several authors have recently discussed the historical development of controlled clinical trials and their proper use and importance for the scientific evaluation of new medical therapies (Mosteller et al., 1980; Chalmers, 1981; McKinley, 1981; and Chapter 17).

Finally, it should not be forgotten that much more information can still be gleaned from observational studies, particularly as more complete population-based data sets become available for analysis. This, in combination with new indices for the quality of care (Dennis and Chalmers, 1982), should prove to be valuable tools in analyzing the effects of changes in the provision of perinatal care.

CONCLUSION

Perinatal and infant mortality rates are indicators of the general health of a population. Perinatal mortality is presumably also a good indicator of the medical care offered to pregnant women, their deliveries, and their newborns. For these purposes, the overall perinatal mortality rate is a fairly crude measure and needs to be supplemented by birthweight-specific comparisons. In this respect, differences in the birthweight distributions of the populations being compared also need to be examined in any detailed epidemiologic study.

It should be evident from the material presented in this chapter that even though much is known about the associations between perinatal survival and biologic, social, and environmental factors, many more questions remain to be answered and therefore much more epidemiologic work is waiting to be done. As to the impact of social factors on perinatal mortality, it is far easier to list what is *not* known than to be decisive about what is known. To illustrate this point, the term "social class" has been too often employed as a critical kind of explanatory variable. It is preferable to have available some knowledge of the relative contributions of a number of individual factors that collectively define the different social classes and their individual influences on perinatal survival.

New methods of analysis that have exploited more comprehensive data sets have demonstrated that even well-established relationships are open to question, as for example, the association described in this chapter between perinatal mortality and parity as a function of different sibship sizes. The problems shown to exist through the conflicting results found by using the longitudinal rather than the cross-sectional method of analysis may indeed serve to stimulate much additional research in related areas of perinatal epidemiology. This projected research activity should flourish as new and larger data sets become available with the potential for undertaking longitudinal analyses on the obstetric careers of individual women.

In regard to what effects medical care or interventions have on perinatal mortality, a great deal more epidemiologic study remains to be done. Too few controlled intervention studies have been conducted as new technology and methodology have been introduced into the practice of perinatal medicine at an accelerating pace. In many instances, it has long since become impossible to conduct randomized trials. Many new methods that were introduced in the past 20 years have become so quickly established that they are now an integral and unquestioned part of accepted medical practice.

Still, whenever possible, epidemiologists and other scientists should encourage the use of controlled intervention studies before new methods become widely accepted as necessary parts of established medical care practices. Where such trials are impossible to conduct, it will be necessary to fall back on observational studies. Fortunately, much more knowledge can be gained from these studies than has been the case so far, particularly as more extensive and improved data sets become available for use within the field of perinatal epidemiology. As a specific example of an improvement of the observational study, the retrospective "perinatal audit" (Larssen et al., 1982) technique can be developed into a powerful tool for disentangling the effects of many different procedures on perinatal survival.

REFERENCES

Adelstein, A.M., McDonald, I.M., and Weatherall, J.A.C. (1980). *Perinatal and infant mortality, social and biological factors, 1975–1977*. London: Her Majesty's Stationery Office.

Alberman, E. (1977). Facts and figures. In *Benefits and hazards of the new obstetrics*, edited by T. Chard and M. Richards. *Clin. Dev. Med.*, No. 64. London: Heinemann.

—— (1978). Perinatal mortality rates. *Br. J. Hosp. Med. 20*, 439–443.

——, Roman, E., Pharoah, P.O.D., and Chamberlain, G. (1980). Birth weight before and after a spontaneous abortion. *Br. J. Obstet. Gynaecol. 87*, 275–280.

Antonov, A. (1947). Children born during the siege of Leningrad in 1942. *J. Pediatr. 30*, 250–259.

Backer, J. and Aagenes, Ø. (1966). *Infant mortality in Norway 1901–1963*. Oslo: Central Bureau of Statistics of Norway.

Bailey, R.R. (1970). The effect of maternal smoking on the infant birth weight. *N.Z. Med. J. 71*, 293–294.

Baird, D., Thomson, A.M., and Duncan, E.H.L. (1953). The causes and prevention of stillbirths and first week deaths. *J. Obstet. Gynaecol. Br. Emp. 60*, 17–30.

——, Walker, J., and Thomson, A.M. (1954). The causes and prevention of stillbirths and first week deaths, Part III. *J. Obstet. Gynaecol. Br. Emp. 61*, 433–448.

—— (1977a). Epidemiologic patterns over time. In *The epidemiology of prematurity*, edited by D.M. Reed and F.J. Stanley. Baltimore, Md.: Urban and Schwarzenberg, pp. 5–15.

—— (1977b). The perinatal mortality rate as a measure of the efficiency of the maternity services. *Health Bull. (Edinb.) 35*, 234–242.

—— (1980). Environment and reproduction. *Br. J. Obstet. Gynaecol. 87*, 1057–1067.

Bakketeig, L.S. and Hoffman, H.J. (1979). Perinatal mortality by birth order within cohorts based on sibship size. *Br. Med. J. 2*, 693–696.

—— and —— (1980). Pregnancy order and reproductive loss. *Br. Med. J. 1*, 716.

——, ——, and Sternthal, P.M. (1978). Obstetric service and perinatal mortality in Norway. *Acta Obstet. Gynecol. Scand. 58*, 129–134.

——, ——, and Harley, E.E. (1979). The tendency to repeat gestational age and birth weight in successive births. *Am. J. Obstet. Gynecol. 135*, 1086–1103.

—— and —— (1981). The epidemiology of preterm birth. In *Preterm labor*, edited by M.G. Elder and C.H. Hendricks. London: Butterworths, pp. 17–46.

—— and —— (1983). The tendency to repeat gestational age and birth weight in successive births related to perinatal survival. *Acta Obstet. Gynecol. Scand.* In press.

Berger, G.S., Gillings, D.B., and Siegel, E. (1976). The evaluation of regionalized perinatal care programs. *Am. J. Obstet. Gynecol. 125*, 924–932.

Billewicz, W.Z. (1973). Some implications of self-selection for pregnancy. *Br. J. Prev. Soc. Med. 27*, 49–52.

Bishop, E.H. (1964). Prematurity, etiology and management. *Postgrad. Med. 35*, 185–188.

Bjerkedal, T. (1982). Personal communication. Medical Birth Registry of Norway, Oslo.

—— and Bakketeig, L.S. (1972). *Medical registration of births in Norway, 1967–1968. Some descriptive and analytical aspects.* Institute of Hygiene and Social Medicine, University of Bergen, Bergen, Norway.

—— and —— (1975). *Medical registration of births in Norway during the 5-year period 1967–1971.* Institute of Hygiene and Social Medicine, University of Bergen, Bergen, Norway.

Brown, E.R. and Taeusch, H.W. (1978). Intensive care and the very low birth weight infant. *Lancet 2*, 362–363.

Brown, G.W. and Harris, T. (1978). *Social origins of depression.* London: Tavistock.

Burke, B.S., Beal, V.A., Kirkwood, S.B., and Stuart, H.C. (1943). Nutritional studies during pregnancy. *Am. J. Obstet. Gynecol. 46*, 38–52.

Burnham, D. (1982). Personal communication.

Butler, N.R. and Alberman, E.D. (1969). *Perinatal problems 1st report—2nd report.* Edinburgh: Churchill Livingstone.

Central Statistical Office (1982). *Social trends 12.* London: Her Majesty's Stationery Office.

Chalmers, I., Newcombe, R., West, R., Campbell, H., Weatherall, J., Lambert, P., and Adelstein, A. (1978). Adjusted perinatal mortality rates in administrative areas of England and Wales. *Health Trends 10*, 24–29.

—— (1979). The search for indices. *Lancet 2*, 1063–1065.

—— and Enkin, M. (1982). Miscellaneous interventions in pregnancy: Rhesus immunization, breast care, external cephalic version. In *Effectiveness and satisfaction in antenatal care,* edited by I. Chalmers and M. Enkin. London: Heinemann, Spastics International Medical Publications.

Chalmers, T.C. (1981). The clinical trial. *Milbank Mem. Fund Q. 59*, 324–339.

Chamberlain, G., Philip, E., Howlett, B., and Masters, K. (1978). *British births 1970.* Vol. 2, *Obstetric care.* London: Heinemann.

Chamberlain, R., Chamberlain, G., Howlett, B., and Claireaux, A. (1975). British births 1970. Vol. 1, *The first week of life.* London: Heinemann.

Charles, E. (1953). The hour of birth, a study of the distribution of times of onset of labour and of delivery throughout the 24-hour period. *Br. J. Prev. Soc. Med. 7*, 43.

Chase, H.C. (1967). Perinatal and infant mortality in the United States and six West European countries. *Am. J. Public Health 57*, 1735–1748.

Christian, J.J. and Davis, D.E. (1964). Endocrines, behaviour and population. *Science 146*, 1550–1560.

Cohler, B.J., Gallant, D.H., Grunebaum, H.U., Weiss, J.L., and Gamer, E. (1975). Pregnancy and birth complications among mentally ill and well mothers and their children. *Soc. Biol. 22*, 269–278.

Davies, I.M. (1980). Perinatal and infant deaths: Social and biological factors. *Popul. Trends 19*, 19–21.

Davis, P.A. (1976). Outlook for the low birth weight baby—then and now. *Arch. Dis. Child. 51*, 817–819.

——— (1980). Perinatal mortality. *Arch. Dis. Child. 55*, 833–837.

Day, R.L. (1967). Factors influencing offspring. Number of children, interval between pregnancies, and age of parents. *Am. J. Dis. Child. 113*, 179–185.

Dean, R.F.A. (1951). The size of the baby at birth and the yield of breastmilk. In *Studies of under-nutrition, Wuppertal 1956–1959*. Medical Research Council No. 275, pp. 346–378.

Dennis, J. and Chalmers, I. (1982). Very early neonatal seizure rate: A possible epidemiological indicator of the quality of perinatal care. *Br. J. Obstet. Gynaecol. 82*, 418–426.

Department of Health and Social Security (1980). *Enquiries in health.* London: Her Majesty's Stationery Office.

Deporte, J.V. (1932). The prevalent hour of stillbirth. *Am. J. Obstet. Gynecol. 23*, 31–37.

Douglas, J.W.B. (1950). Some factors associated with prematurity. *J. Obstet. Gynaecol. Br. Emp. 57*, 143–170.

Dowding, V. (1981). New assessment of the effects of birth order and socioeconomic status on birth weight. *Br. Med. J. 1*, 683–686.

——— (1982). Distributions of birth weight in seven Dublin maternity units. *Br. Med. J. 1*, 1901–1904.

Enkin, M. (1982). The effects of antenatal classes. In *Effectiveness and satisfaction in antenatal care*, edited by I. Chalmers and M. Enkin. London: Heinemann.

Erhardt, C.L., Joshi, G.B., Nelson, F.G., Kroll, B.H., and Weiner, L. (1964). Influence of weight and gestation on perinatal and neonatal mortality by ethnic group. *Am. J. Public Health 54*, 1841–1855.

———, Pakter, J., Nelson, F.G., Bigus, E.A., Laredo, C.D., and Jennings, E.P. (1971). *The influence of season of conception on obstetric problems and casualties*. New York: Health Services Administration, Department of Health, and Medical and Health Research Association.

Erickson, J.D. and Bjerkedal, T. (1978). Interpregnancy interval. Association with birth weight, stillbirth, and neonatal death. *J. Epidemiol. Community Health 32*, 124–130.

Erickson, M.T. (1976). The influence of health factors on psychological variables predicting complications of pregnancy, labour and delivery. *J. Psychosom. Res. 20*, 21–24.

Ericson, A. (1981). Personal communication. Medical Birth Registry of Sweden, Stockholm.

Falk, G. and Wranne, L. (1973). Perinatal mortality in Orebro county. *Läkartidningen 70*, 2539–2541.

Farrant, W. (1980). Stress after amniocentesis for high serum alpha-feto-protein concentrations. *Br. Med. J. 1*, 452.

Fedrick, J. and Adelstein, P. (1973). Influence of pregnancy spacing on outcome of pregnancy. *Br. Med. J. 2*, 753–776.

Forbes, J.F., Boddy, F.A., Pickering, R., and Wyllie, M.M. (1982). Perinatal mortality in Scotland: 1970–1979. *J. Epidemiol. Community Health 36*, 282–288.

Fryer, J.G., Harding, R.A., Ashford, J.R., and Karlberg, P. (1977). Some indicators of maturity. In *Fundamentals of mortality risks during the perinatal period and infancy*, edited by F. Falkner. Basel: Karger.

——, ——, MacDonald, M.D., Read, K.L.Q., Crocker, G.R., and Abernethy, J. (1979). Comparing the early mortality rates of local authorities in England and Wales. *J. R. Stat. Soc. (A) 142*, 181–198.

Gamsu, H.R., Light, F., Potter, A., and Price, I.F. (1979). Intensive care and the very-low-birthweight infant. *Lancet 2*, 736.

Glattre, E. and Bjerkedal, T. (1983). The 24 hour rhythmicity of birth. A population study, *Acta Obstet. Gynecol. Scand. 62*, 31–36.

Goldstein, H. (1977). Smoking in pregnancy: Some notes on the statistical controversy. *Br. J. Prev. Soc. Med. 31*, 13–17.

Graham, H. (1977). Smoking in pregnancy: The attitudes of expectant mothers. *Soc. Sci. Med. 10*, 399–405.

Gruenwald, P. (1969). Growth and maturation of the fetus and its relationship to perinatal mortality. In *Perinatal problems—the second report of the 1958 British Perinatal Mortality Survey*, edited by N.R. Butler and E.D. Alberman. Edinburgh: E. and S. Livingstone.

Grudzinskas, J.G., Watson, C., and Chard, T. (1979). Does sexual intercourse cause fetal distress? *Lancet 2*, 692–693.

Hammoud, E.I. (1965). Studies in fetal and infant mortality. A methodological approach to the definition of perinatal mortality. *Am. J. Public Health 55*, 1012–1023.

Hare, E.H., Moran, P.A.P., and MacFarlane, A. (1981). The changing seasonality of infant deaths in England and Wales 1912–1978 and its relation to seasonal temperature. *J. Epidemiol. Community Health 35*, 77–82.

Havercamp, A.D., Thomson, H.E., McFee, J.G., and Cetrulo C. (1976). The evaluation of continuous fetal heart rate monitoring in high risk pregnancy. *Am. J. Obstet. Gynecol. 125*, 310–317.

Hendry, R.A. (1981). The weekend—a dangerous time to be born? *Br. J. Obstet. Gynaecol. 88*, 1200–1203.

Heuser, R. (1982). Personal communication. Natality Statistics Branch, NCHS.

Hewitt, D. (1962). A study of temporal variations in the risk of fetal malformation and death. *Am. J. Public Health 52*, 1676–1688.

Hill, A.B. (1937). *Principles of medical statistics*. London: The Lancet, Ltd.

Hoffman, H.J. and Bakketeig, L.S. (1983). Fetal and perinatal mortality comparisons between the United States and Norway. *Int. J. Gynaecol. Obstet.* In press.

——, ——, and Stark, C.R. (1978). Twins and perinatal mortality: A comparison between single and twin births in Minnesota and in Norway, 1967–1973. In *Twin research.* (Part B), *Biology and epidemiology*, edited by N.E. Nance, G. Allen, and P. Parisi. New York: Alan R. Liss, pp. 133–142.

————, Lundin, F.E., Jr., Bakketeig, L.S., and Harley, E.E. (1977). Classification of births by weight and gestational age for future studies of prematurity. In *The epidemiology of prematurity*, edited by D.M. Reed and F.J. Stanley, Baltimore, Md.: Urban and Schwarzenberg, pp. 297–333.

————, Meirik, O., and Bakketeig, L.S. (1984). Methodological consideration in the analysis of perinatal mortality rates. In *Perinatal epidemiology*, edited by M.B. Bracken. Oxford: Oxford University Press.

————, Stark, C.R., Lundin, F.E., Jr., and Ashbrook, J.D. (1974). Analysis of birth weight, gestational age, and fetal viability, U.S.—births, 1968. *Obstet. Gynecol. Surv. 29*, 651–681.

Illsley, R. (1956). The social context of childbirth. I. *Nurs. Mirror*, Sept. 14, pp. 1709–1710.

———— (1980). *Professional or public health?* London: Nuffield Provincial Hospitals Trust.

Institut National de la Santé et de La Recherche Médicale (1980). Service de presse information. Grossesse et environment. *Medicin et Hygiene 38*, 2409–2426.

Janerich, D.T. and Garfinkel, J. (1970). Season of birth and birth order in relation to prenatal pathology. *Am. J. Epidemiol. 92*, 351–356.

Joint Committee of the Royal College of Obstetricians and the Population Investigation Committee (1948). *Maternity in Great Britain*. Oxford: Oxford University Press.

Jones, R.A.K., Cummins, M., and Davies P.A. (1979). Infants of very low birth weight: A 15 year analysis. *Lancet 1*, 1332–1335.

Kaern, T. (1960). Perinatal mortality. *Acta Obstet. Gynecol. Scand. 39*, 392–437.

Kaiser, I.H. and Halberg, F. (1962). Circadian periodic aspects of birth. *Ann. N.Y. Acad. Sci. 98*, 1056–1068.

Kaminski, M., Rumeau-Rouquette, C., and Schwartz, D. (1976). Alcohol consumption among pregnant women and outcome of pregnancy. *Rev. Epidemiol. Med. Soc. Sante Publique 24*, 27–40.

Keller, C. and Nugent, R. (1983). Seasonal patterns in perinatal mortality and premature delivery. *Am. J. Epidemiol.* In press.

Kelso, I.M., Parsons, R.G., Lawrence, G.F., Arora, S.S., Edmonds, D.K., and Cooke, I.D. (1978). An assessment of continuous fetal heart rate monitoring in labour. A randomized trial. *Am. J. Obstet. Gynecol. 131*, 526–532.

Kessner, D.M., Singer, J., Kalk, C.E., and Schlesinger, E.R. (1973). *Infant death: an analysis by maternal risk and health care*. Washington, D.C.: Institute of Medicine, National Academy of Sciences.

Kleinman, J.C., Kovar, M.G., Feldman, J.J., and Young, C.A. (1978). A comparison of 1960 and 1973–1974 early neonatal mortality in selected states. *Am. J. Epidemiol. 108*, 454–469.

Kline, J., Shrout, P., Stein, Z., Susser, M., and Warburton, D. (1980). Drinking during pregnancy and spontaneous abortion. *Lancet 2*, 176–180.

Knox, E.G., Marshall, T., Kane, S., Green, A., and Mallett, R. (1980). Social and health care determinants of area variations in perinatal mortality. *Community Med.* 2, 282–290.

Land, H. (1977). Inequalities in large families: More of the same or different? In *Equalities and inequalities in family life,* edited by R. Chester and J. Peel. London: Academic Press.

Larssen, K.E., Bakketeig, L.S., Bersjó, P., and Finne, P.H. (1981). *Perinatal service in Norway during the 1970's.* Trondheim, Norway: The Norwegian Institute for Hospital Research.

——, ——, ——, ——, Laurini, R., Knoff, H., Holt, J., Vogt, H., and Hafnes, C. (1982). *Perinatal audit in Norway, 1980.* Trondheim, Norway: The Norwegian Institute for Hospital Research.

Lederman, R.P., Lederman, E., Work, B.A., and McCann, D.S. (1978). The relationship of maternal anxiety, plasma catecholamines, and plasma cortisol to progress in labour. *Am. J. Obstet. Gynecol. 132,* 495–500.

Lee, K., Eidelman, A.I., Kandall, S.R., and Gartner, L.M. (1976). Quality of care vs neonatal mortality rate. *J. Pediatr. 89,* 161–162.

——, Paneth, N., Gartner, L.M., Pearlman, M.A., and Grus, L. (1980). Neonatal mortality: An analysis of the recent improvement in the United States. *Am. J. Public Health 70,* 15–21.

Lumley, J. (1978). Sexual feelings in pregnancy and after childbirth. *Aust. N.Z. J. Obstet. Gynaecol. 18,* 114–117.

—— and Asbury, J. (1982). Perfect remedies, imperfect science: Advice in pregnancy. In *Effectiveness and satisfaction in antenatal care,* edited by I. Chalmers, and M. Enkin. London: Heinemann.

Lunde, A.S., Lundeborg, S., Lettenstróm, G.S., Thygesen, L., and Huebner, J. (1980). The person-number systems of Sweden, Norway, Denmark, and Israel. *Vital Health Stat. (2),* No. 84, DHHS Publication No. (PHS) 80–1358. Hyattsville, Md.: National Center for Health Statistics.

Macfarlane, A. (1978). Variations in number of births and perinatal mortality by day of the week in England and Wales. *Br. Med. J. 2,* 1670–1673.

—— (1979). Perinatal mortality. *Lancet 2,* 255–256.

—— (1981). The derivation and uses of perinatal and neonatal mortality rates. *J. Pediatr. 98,* 61–62.

—— and Chalmers, I. (1981). Some problems in the interpretation of perinatal mortality statistics. In *Recent advances in paediatrics,* edited by D. Hull. Edinburgh: Churchill Livingstone.

MacMahon, B., Kovar, M.G., and Feldman, J.J. (1972). Infant mortality rates: Socioeconomic factors. *Vital Health Stat. (22),* No. 14, DHEW Publication No. (HSM) 72-1045. Washington, D.C.: U.S. Government Printing Office.

Malek, J. (1952). The manifestation of biological rhythms in delivery. *Gynaecologia 133,* 365–372.

Mallett, R. and Knox, E.G. (1979). Standardized perinatal mortality rates: Technique, utility and interpretation. *Community Med. 1,* 6–13.

McDowall, M., Goldblatt, P., and Fox, J. (1982). Employment during pregnancy and infant mortality. *Popul. Trends 26,* 12–15.

McKinley, S.M. (1981). Experimentation in human populations. *Milbank Mem. Fund Q. 59,* 308–323.

Meirik, O., Smedby, B., and Ericson, A. (1979). Impact of changing age and parity distributions of mothers on perinatal mortality in Sweden, 1953–1975. *Int. J. Epidemiol. 8,* 361–364.

Meyer, M.B. (1977). Effects of maternal smoking and attitude on birth weight and gestation. In *The epidemiology of prematurity,* edited by D.M. Reed and F.J. Stanley. Baltimore, Md.: Urban and Schwarzenberg, pp. 81–104.

――― and Tonascia, J.A. (1971). Maternal smoking pregnancy complications, and perinatal mortality. *Am. J. Obstet. Gynecol. 128,* 494–502.

―――, ―――, and Buck, C. (1974). The interrelationship of maternal smoking and increased perinatal mortality with other risk factors: Further analysis of the Ontario Perinatal Mortality Study 1960–1961. *Am. J. Epidemiol. 100,* 443–452.

Miller, H.C. and Hassanein, K. (1971). Diagnosis of impaired fetal growth in newborn infants. *Pediatrics 48,* 511–522.

Mills, J., Harlap, S., and Harley, E. (1981). Should coitus late in pregnancy be discouraged? *Lancet 2,* 136–138.

Mora, J.O., Sanchez, R., Deparedes, B., and Herrara, M.G. (1981). Sex related effects of nutritional supplementation during pregnancy on fetal growth. *Early Hum. Devel. 5,* 243–251.

Morris, N.M. (1975). The frequency of sexual intercourse during pregnancy. *Arch. Sex. Behav. 4,* 501–507.

―――, Udry, J.R., and Chase, C.L. (1975). Shifting age-parity distribution of births and the decrease in infant mortality. *Am. J. Public Health 65,* 359–362.

Mosteller, F., Gilbert, J.P., and McPeek, B. (1980). Reporting standards and research strategies for controlled trials: Agenda for the editor. *Controlled Clinical Trials 1,* 37–58.

Myers, R.E. (1979). Maternal anxiety and fetal death. In *Psychoneuroendocrinology in reproduction,* edited by L. Zichella and P. Pancheri. Amsterdam: Elsevier-North Holland.

Naeye, R.L. and Ross, S. (1982). Coitus and chorioamnionitis—a prospective study. *Early Hum. Devel. 6,* 91–97.

Nakamura, Y., Yano, H., Nakashima, T., Nakashima, H., Knyama, M., Nagasue, N., and Kabashima, S. (1981). Primary causes of perinatal death. An autopsy study of 1000 cases in Japanese infants. *Hum. Pathol. 13,* 54–61.

Nelson, R.M., Resnick, M.B., and Eitzman, D.V. (1979). Intensive care and the very-low-birth weight infant. *Lancet 2,* 737.

Newman, N.M. and Correy, J.F. (1980). Effects of alcohol in pregnancy. Clinical review. *Med. J. Aust. 2,* 5–10.

Newton, R.W., Webster, P.A.C., Binu, P.S., Maskrey, N., and Phillips, A.B. (1979). Psychosocial stress in pregnancy and its relation to the onset of premature labour. *Br. Med. J. 2,* 411–415.

Oakley, A., MacFarlane, A., and Chalmers, I. (1982). Social class, stress and reproduction. In *Disease and environment,* edited by A.R. Rees and H. Purcell. New York: Wiley.

Office of Population Censuses and Surveys (1981). *Mortality statistics: Childhood and maternity* London: Her Majesty's Stationery Office.

Official Statistics of Sweden (1981). *Medical birth registration in 1977–1978. Statistics of the National Board of Health and Welfare.* Central Bureau of Statistics, Statistical Reports, HS 1981: 2, Stockholm.

O'Lane, J.M. (1963). Some fetal effects of maternal cigarette smoking. *Obstet. Gynecol.* 22, 181–184.

Olegaard, R., Sabel, K-G., Aronsson, M., Sandin, B., Johansen, P.R., Carlson, C., Kyllerman, M., Iversen, K., and Horbek, A. (1979). Effects on the child of alcohol abuse during pregnancy. *Acta Paediatr. Scand. (Suppl.)* 275, 112–121.

Paneth, W., Wallenstein, S., Keily, J.L., and Susser, M. (1982). Social class indicators and mortality in low birth weight infants. *Am. J. Epidemiol.* 116, 364–375.

Parkes, A.S. (1976). *Patterns of sexuality and reproduction.* London: Oxford University Press.

Peller, S. (1923). Die Saenglingsterblichkeit nach dem Kriege. *Wein. Klin. Wochenschr.* 36, 799–801.

——— (1965). Proper delineation of the neonatal period in perinatal mortality. *Am. J. Public Health* 55, 1005–1011.

Perkins, R.P. (1979). Sexual behavior and response in relation to complications of pregnancy. *Am. J. Obstet. Gynecol.* 134, 498–505.

Pettersson, F. (1968). *Epidemiology of early pregnancy wastage.* Stockholm: Scandinavian University Books, Nordstedts.

Pfaundler, M. (1936). Studien über Frühtod, Geschlechtsverhältnis und Selection. In *Zur intrauterinen Absterbeordnung*, edited by M. Heilung. *Z. Kinderheilk.* 57, 185–227.

Pugh, W.E. and Fernandez, F.L. (1953). Coitus in late pregnancy. *Obstet. Gynecol.* 2, 636–642.

Rantakallio, P. (1969). *Groups at risk in low birth weight infants and perinatal mortality.* Acta Paediatr. Scand. (Suppl.) 193 (entire issue).

——— (1979). Social background of mothers who smoke during pregnancy and influence of these factors on the offspring. *Soc. Sci. Med.* 13A, 423–429.

Rayburn, W.F. and Wilson, E.A. (1980). Coital activity and premature delivery. *Am. J. Obstet. Gynecol.* 137, 972–974.

Record, R.G. and Armstrong, E. (1975). The influence of the birth of a malformed child on the mother's further reproduction. *Br. J. Prev. Soc. Med.* 29, 267–273.

Renou, P., Chang, A., Anderson, I., and Wood, C. (1976). Controlled trial of fetal intensive care. *Am. J. Obstet. Gynecol.* 126, 470–475.

Ressequie, L.J. (1976). Comparison of longitudinal and cross-sectional analysis: Maternal age and stillbirth ratios. *Am. J. Epidemiol.* 103, 551–559.

Reynolds, E.O.R. and Stewart, A.L. (1979). Intensive care and the very-low-birth weight infant. *Lancet 2,* 254.

Rindfuss, R.R., Ladinsky, J.L., Coppock, E., Marshall, V.W., and MacPherson, A.S. (1979). Convenience and the occurrence of births: Induction of labour in the United States and Canada. *Int. J. Health Serv.* 9, 439–460.

Ritter, H., Byrne, P.A., Domke, H.R., and Stockbauer, J.W. (1977). *Disparity in infant mortality between nonmetropolitan and metropolitan Missouri.* Jefferson City: Missouri State Health Department.

Roberton, N.R.C. (1979). Intensive care and the very-low-birth weight infant. *Lancet 2*, 362.

Robinson, J. (1982). *Cancer of the cervix: Occupational risks of husbands and wives and possible preventive strategies.* Proceedings of the Ninth Study Group, Royal College of Obstetricians and Gynaecologists, London.

Roman, E. and Alberman, E. (1980). Spontaneous abortion gravidity, pregnancy order, age, and pregnancy interval. In *Human embryonic and fetal death,* edited by E.B. Hook and I.H. Porter. New York: Academic Press.

Rooth, G. (1980). Low birth weight revised. *Lancet 1*, 639–641.

Rosenberg, H.G. (1966). Seasonal variation of births, United States, 1933–63. *Vital Health Stat. (21)*, No. 9. Washington, D.C.: U.S. Government Printing Office.

Rush, D. and Kass, E.H. (1972). Maternal smoking: A reassessment of the association with perinatal mortality. *Am. J. Epidemiol. 96*, 183–196.

————, Stein, Z., Christakis, G., and Susser, M. (1974). The prenatal project: The first 20 months of operation. In *Malnutrition and human development,* edited by M. Winick. New York: Wiley.

Shapiro, S., Schlesinger, E.R., and Nesbitt, R.E.L., Jr. (1968). *Infant, perinatal, maternal, and childhood mortality in the United States.* Cambridge, Mass.: Harvard University Press.

Shaw, J.A., Wheller, P., and Morgan, D.W. (1970). Mother-infant relationship and weight gain in the first month of life. *J. Am. Acad. Child Psychiatry 9*, 428–444.

Silverman, W.A. (1980). *Retrolental fibroplasia: A modern parable.* New York: Grune and Stratton.

Sinclair, J.C., Torrance, G.W., Boyle, M.H., Horwood, S.P., Saigal, S., and Sackett, D.L. (1981). Evaluations of neonatal-intensive care programs. *N. Engl. J. Med. 305*, 489–494.

Sjolin, S. (1975). Infant mortality in Sweden. In *Health care of mothers and children in National Health Services,* edited by H. Wallace. Cambridge, Mass.: Ballinger.

Slatis, H.M., and Decloux, R.J. (1967). Seasonal variance in stillbirth frequencies. *Hum. Biol. 39*, 284–294.

Smedby, B. and Ericson, A. (1979). Perinatal mortality among children of immigrant mothers in Sweden. *Acta Paediatr. Scand. (Suppl.) 275*, 41–46.

Social Services Committee (1980). *Perinatal and neonatal mortality. Second Report from the Social Services Committee 1979–80.* London: Her Majesty's Stationery Office.

Sokol, R.J., Woolf, R.B., Rosen, M.G., and Weingarden, K. (1980). Risk, antepartum care, and outcome: Impact of a maternity and infant care project. *Obstet. Gynaecol. 56*, 150–156.

Solberg, D.A., Butler, J., and Wagner, N.N. (1973). Sexual behavior in pregnancy. *N. Engl. J. Med. 288*, 1098–1103.

Sosa, R., Kennell, J., Klaus, M., Robertson, S., and Urruha, J. (1980). The effect of a supportive companion on perinatal problems, length of labour and mother-infant interaction. *N. Engl. J. Med. 303*, 597–600.

Spiers, P.S. and Wang, L. (1976). Short pregnancy interval, low birth-weight, and the sudden infant death syndrome. *Am. J. Epidemiol. 104*, 15–21.

Stanley, F.J. and Alberman, E. (1978). Infants of very low birth weight. I. Perinatal factors affecting survival. *Dev. Med. Child Neurol. 20*, 300–312.

Stein, Z., Susser, M., Saeneger, G., and Marolla, F. (1975). *Famine and human development: The Dutch hunger winter of 1944–45.* New York: Oxford University Press.

Stewart, A.L. and Reynolds, E.O.R. (1974). Improved prognosis of infants of very low birth weight. *Pediatrics 54*, 724–735.

Stewart, A.M. (1955). A note on the obstetric effects of work during pregnancy. *Br. J. Prev. Soc. Med. 9*, 159–161.

Streissguth, A.P. (1978). Fetal alcohol syndrome: An epidemiologic perspective. *Am. J. Epidemiol. 107*, 467–478.

Susser, M., Marolla, F.A., and Fleiss, J. (1972). Birth weight, fetal age and perinatal mortality. *Am. J. Epidemiol. 96*, 197–204.

—— and Stein, Z. (1977). Prenatal nutrition and subsequent development. In *The epidemiology of prematurity*, edited by D.M. Reed and F.J. Stanley. Baltimore, Md.: Urban and Schwarzenberg, pp. 177–192.

Taylor, W. (1954). The changing pattern of mortality in England and Wales. I. Infant mortality. *Br. J. Prev. Soc. Med. 8*, 1–9.

Thomson, A.M. (1958). Diet in pregnancy. *Br. J. Nutr. 12*, 446–461.

—— (1959). Diet in pregnancy. *Br. J. Nutr. 13*, 190–204.

Tyson, J., Schultz, J.C., and Gill, G. (1979). Diurnal variation in the quality and outcome of newborn intensive care. *J. Paediatr. 95*, 277–280.

United Nations (1981). *Demographic yearbook 1980.* New York: Department of Economic and Social Affairs, Statistical Office.

Usher, R. (1977). Changing mortality rates with perinatal intensive care and regionalization. *Semin. Perinatol. 1*, 309–319.

Wallgren, A. (1942). The neonatal mortality in Sweden, from a pediatric point of view. *Acta Paediatr. Scand. 29*, 372–386.

Weatherall, J.A.C. (1975). Infant mortality: International differences. *Popul. Trends 1*, 9–12.

Williams, R.L. and Chen, P.M. (1982). Identifying the sources of the recent decline in perinatal mortality in California. *N. Engl. J. Med. 306*, 207–214.

Wolkind, S. (1981). Prenatal emotional stress—effects on the fetus. In *Pregnancy—a psychological and social study*, edited by S. Wolkind and E. Zajicek. London: Academic Press.

World Health Organization (1957). *Epidemiological and vital statistics. Report* 57, pp 506–511.

—— (1977). *Manual of the international statistical classification of diseases, injuries and causes of death.* Geneva: World Health Organization.

—— (1978). *A WHO report on social and biological effects on perinatal mortality*, Vol, 1, p. 177. Budapest, Hungary: World Health Organization.

Yang, R., Zweig, A.R., Ponthitt, T.C., and Federmann, E.J. (1976). Successive relationships between maternal attitudes during pregnancy, analgesic medication during labour and delivery and newborn behaviour. *Dev. Psychobiol. 12*, 6–14.

Yerushalmy, J. (1938). Hour of birth and stillbirth and neonatal mortality rates. *Child Dev. 9*, 373–378.

—— (1945). On the interval between successive births and its effect on survival of infant. I. An indirect method of study. *Hum. Biol. 17*, 65–106.

—— (1974). The relationship of parents' cigarette smoking to outcome of pregnancy implications as to the problem of inferring causation from observed associations. *Am. J. Epidemiol. 93*, 443–445.

Young, M. (1975). *The poverty report.* London: Temple Smith.

—— and Syson, L. (1974). Women: The new poor. *Observer*, January 20.

7

Multiple Births

Gordon Allen

Twinning deserves consideration by epidemiologists not as pathology but as a rare event that is associated with increased obstetric hazards. Single births are the rule in all higher primates, including Old World monkeys and anthropoid apes. Multiple births in humans therefore represent the failure of established regulatory mechanisms. Multiple births also interest epidemiologists because they afford insights into fetal and child development and sometimes permit differentiation between environmental and constitutional factors in disease.

The phenomenon of twinning comprises two quite different processes that must generally be considered independently: monozygotic (MZ) twinning, in which two or more embryos develop from a single zygote, and dizygotic (DZ) twinning, in which two ova are fertilized by two sperms. The difference is fundamental for the embryologist and the epidemiologist, but it also has obstetric implications: The genetic identity of MZ infants, their lower birthweight, and in most cases their common circulation through the placenta.

Monozygotic twinning is almost constant in frequency and offers few promising clues to its biologic basis. In contrast, the frequency of DZ twinning varies significantly in relation to demographic variables, and study of these effects helps to define and elucidate the central phenomenon. Multiple ovulation can now be induced; its elective prevention is not imminent but may reasonably be anticipated. Monozygotic twinning appears to be subject to no natural or artificial controls.

STATISTICAL METHODS

Collection of Twin Statistics

Accurate birth statistics can be generated only in a developed country, and twin births are especially difficult to count completely and in a standard manner. To illustrate, twins attract special cultural interest in Italy, so that twin birth statistics have been collected there at least since 1868. Around 1930 the Italian twinning rate suddenly and implausibly increased by 10%. The change was not noticed immediately but has now been traced (Parisi and Caperna, 1983) to the initiation of the linking of twins on the original birth reports.

In the United States multiple births have been a standard reporting item on birth certificates since 1900, but the two reports of a twin pair are not internally linked. Extracting information about sex concordance or about livebirth status of the partner necessitates finding the matching certificates. This has not been done on a routine basis since 1958, but complete and valuable twin statistics were assembled for the year 1964 (Heuser, 1967).

Hospital records provide the best available twin statistics in less developed countries and the only data anywhere on placental relationship. Hospital series lack a geographic population base and may be suspect because difficult pregnancies and difficult deliveries tend to occur in hospitals where research is conducted (Nylander, 1971). This bias may increase the apparent twinning rate in less developed countries and distort the relative frequencies of the different types of multiple births and of complicated deliveries.

Large twin registries, so useful in epidemiologic studies of twin children and adults, are assembled retrospectively from birth certificates of specified years and areas. They provide little systematic information about perinatal phenomena.

Standardization of Twinning Rates

The frequency of twin births is usually expressed as the number of twin maternities per 1000 maternities. The time-honored rate in Caucasians of 1 twin gestation per 86 confinements (Strandskov, 1945) becomes 11.2 per 1000, but the rate has declined and there is so much variation even within one country that 10 per 1000 or 1% is a more useful reference figure. Of the 10 per 1000, about 4 are MZ twins and 6, DZ twins. The frequency of DZ twinning varies by a factor of about four between 18-year-old and 38-year-old mothers. This expresses the effect of parity as well as of age.

Table 7-1. Estimated Relative Effects of Maternal Age and Parity on the DZ Twinning Rate, all births, United States, 1941–1948

Year	Mean maternal age	DZ Twinning rate at mean age	Mean parity	DZ Twinning rate at mean parity
1941	29.18	6.94	2.63	5.75
1942	29.08	6.90	2.51	5.57
1943	29.31	7.00	2.59	5.69
1944	29.62	7.13	2.69	5.84
1945	29.94	7.27	2.71	5.87
1946	29.58	7.12	2.51	5.57
1947	29.19	6.94	2.39	5.39
1948	29.10	6.90	2.47	5.51

Sources: U.S. Bureau of the Census (1946); National Office of Vital Statistics (1950). Rates based on those given by Heuser (1967), by interpolation.

The effect of maternal age on twinning is often considered more important than that of parity, but in the United States the effects seem to be nearly equal (Yerushalmy and Sheerar, 1940; Stocks, 1953; Heuser, 1967). This is illustrated in its relevance to standardization in Table 7-1, which gives a sample of the annual variation imparted to the DZ twinning rate by maternal age and parity, respectively. By mean maternal age, the standard deviation of expected annual twinning rates is .134; by mean parity, it is .167. Corresponding standard deviations based on medians are .147 and .161.

Not only may the effect of parity sometimes be the larger of the two; the effects may also be opposite and offsetting. In Table 7-2, four of

Table 7-2. Some Regional and Temporal Differences in the Total Twinning Rate and the Effects of Standardizing by Maternal Age and Birth Order[a]

Geographic division	Central year	Crude rate	Adjusted for maternal age	Adjusted for maternal age and birth order
Middle Atlantic	1937	10.0	—	—
New England	1937	10.3	10.1	10.0
East South Central	1937	12.3	13.0	11.9
West South Central	1937	13.0	13.9	13.1
East South Central	1954	9.9	10.6	9.9
West South Central	1954	9.8	10.5	9.8

[a] Regional rates calculated from three-year blocks of data and adjusted to the age and/or parity composition of the Middle Atlantic states in 1937.

Source: Reproduced by permission from Allen and Schachter (1970). Original source: *Vital Statistics of the United States.*

the five rates fully adjusted to standard were better approximated by the crude rates than by those adjusted for maternal age alone. Thus adjusting for age alone can be misleading. Although parity and maternal age are correlated within a population, this is not necessarily true between populations.

Adjustment for maternal age and parity usually confirms differences observed in the crude rates, but differences by specific maternal age and parity are much more informative than the crude difference. Ideally, therefore, any comparison of twinning rates should consider rates that are specific for both maternal age and parity. Lilienfeld and Pasamanick (1955) illustrate a method attributed to Cochrane (1954) for pooling the specific comparisons over all ages and parities when a test of significance is needed.

When age-specific and parity-specific twinning rates are available and a single summarizing rate is desired, age and parity effects can be largely eliminated either by regression methods (Mosteller et al., 1981) or more precisely by direct standardization (Fleiss, 1973). When age-specific or parity-specific rates are unknown for one or both populations, but total births can be classified by either variable, indirect standardization is useful (Fleiss, 1973). If one population is known, its rates are applied to the general birth distribution of the other. If specific rates are not available for either population, those of a third population are applied to both birth distributions. The predicted rates are then compared with the crude rates to assess the effects of difference in age and parity, or they are used to adjust the crude rates. The third population should be similar in racial and cultural characteristics to the populations being compared, but reliability of the rates is also important. Heuser's data (1967) are currently the best for the United States.

Zygosity Classification

Blood types and other genetic traits are preferable for diagnosing zygosity in any twin study, but short-cut methods of diagnosing or simply counting the zygosity types are available and often adequate for epidemiologic analyses. For example, classification by sex concordance and, if possible, by chorion type, can be valuable: Opposite-sex pairs are all DZ, and monochorionic pairs, all MZ.

Chorion type is available only from hospital series, but sex concordance is sometimes given even in nationwide twin birth statistics. From the frequency of sex concordance one can estimate frequencies of the zygosity types by the difference method of Weinberg (1901). The relative frequencies provide a valuable index even in the absence of a population denominator. When one is not studying

155

the frequencies per se, they may still be useful in detecting biased ascertainment of twins or of same-sex twins when the estimated MZ rate is much above 4 per 1000.

In Weinberg's method, the number of MZ pairs is estimated very simply by subtracting the number of opposite-sex pairs from the number of same-sex pairs. This assumes, accurately enough for sex ratios in the usual range, that DZ twins are equally divided among same-sex and opposite-sex pairs. Although the method is sometimes evidently in error (Nylander and Corney, 1969; James, 1979), this may reflect sampling or bias rather than failure of the above assumption (Bulmer, 1976; Allen, 1981a). Weinberg's method is the basis on which norms have been established, so it should not be rejected without decisive evidence.

The method can be extended to estimating type frequencies in triplets (Allen, 1960) and quadruplets (Bulmer, 1970) among sufficiently large numbers of births.

When sex concordance is given, Weinberg's method permits the analysis of frequency phenomena such as mortality in terms of the zygosity classes. Even means or variances of metric traits can be estimated for the two zygosity types on the assumption that same-sex and opposite-sex DZ pairs have the same values. The mean and variance for opposite-sex pairs is taken as that of all DZ twins. For MZ twins the mean and variance are obtained by subtracting the sum, and sum of squares, respectively, of all opposite-sex pairs from the sum and sum of squares of all same-sex pairs, and dividing by the estimated number of MZ twins. In the case of weight, as will be illustrated in the discussion of birthweight, if SS refers to same-sex and OS to opposite-sex pairs,

$$\frac{\text{mean weight of}}{\text{MZ individuals}} = \frac{\text{sum of SS weights} - \text{sum of OS weights}}{2(\text{SS pairs} - \text{OS pairs})}$$

Conclusions based on Weinberg's method, other than population rates, should be conservative. The estimated frequencies within a sample of twins, as opposed to frequencies in the whole population, appear to be subject to a large standard error that has not yet been exactly formulated (Allen, 1981a). Significance tests concerning Weinberg difference estimates should, in any event, be based on numbers of same-sex and opposite-sex pairs, not on the estimated zygosity proportions.

In the absence of zygosity diagnosis, other traits besides sex may be useful for genetic analysis (Selvin, 1970; Gedda et al., 1979). As a last resort in the study of twinning rates per se, one may have to assume that the MZ rate is constant and attribute all variation to the DZ rate.

Analysis of Clustering

The clustering in space or time of twin births (or of conjoined twins, triplets, etc.) is often reported in the press, and can usually be dismissed as anecdotal. An illustration would be an excess of twinning that is statistically significant only when one combines MZ and DZ pairs without regard to their independent origins. A recent report from Brno, Czechoslovakia (Zahálková, 1979) of spatial clustering employed a faulty statistical analysis that is influenced by concentration of population in towns and cities.

Nevertheless, clustering of twins on a larger scale is sometimes significant, and such observations provide the basis for much of this chapter.

Measures of Heritability

The most rigorous epidemiologic use of twins is to exclude a purely genetic cause when one or more MZ twin pairs are found to be discordant for the disease in question (Cederlof et al., 1971). Quantitative epidemiologic evidence can also be extracted from large series of twins, however, (Cederlof et al., 1971; White, 1981). Qualitative observations on twin pairs are usually analyzed within a conventional model of concordance (Smith, 1974; Allen and Hrubec, 1979), but other methods have been explored (Selvin, 1970; Vollmer, 1972) and logit analysis appears to be appropriate but untried.

Measures of exposure or morbidity are often quantitative and therefore not expressible in terms of concordance. Applications of analysis of variance to epidemiologic twin data of this kind are well developed (Christian et al., 1974; Havlik et al., 1979; Rose et al., 1980).

The objective of most quantitative methods of twin data analysis is to assess the relative roles of inheritance and environment measurable as heritability or, more accurately, as degree of genetic determination. It must be recognized that these terms are applicable only on the assumption that the environments experienced by members of a DZ pair are as similar as those experienced by members of an MZ pair. The most obvious violation of this assumption in perinatal epidemiology is the fact that most MZ pairs and no DZ pairs share a common placenta and chorion. Origin of MZ twins from a single egg cell is also of major developmental importance.

RARER TYPES OF MULTIPLE BIRTHS

Although ordinary MZ and DZ twins probably account for 98% of all multiple gestations reaching term, the remainder may be more important in some respects. About 1% of multiple births in the United States are triplets or quadruplets (Strandskov, 1945; Heuser, 1967). Another small proportion of gestations, not yet even estimated, are known to originate in other ways related to twinning and to end in an abnormal single birth.

Higher Order Multiple Births

In most large collections of birth statistics, the frequency of triplets is close to the squared frequency of twins, and quadruplets come close to the cube of the same frequency (Hellin, 1895). Among 10,389,800 white U.S. maternities in the years 1952–1954 there were about 105,000 sets of twins (the counting of stillbirths introduces some ambiguity), a rate of .0101. There were 970 sets of triplets, a rate of 0.000093. In the eight-year period from 1947 to 1954 the frequency of quadruplets was about 1.02 per million maternities, or 0.00000102 (Allen, 1960).

This nearly perfect geometric relation among the frequencies is known as Hellin's law. Its accuracy and the proportions of sex types among triplets and quadruplets support the simple principle of random combination and repetition of the two twinning mechanisms (Bulmer, 1970). For example, by random combination, the frequencies of triplets arising from one, two, or three zygotes, respectively, should be represented by $2m^2$, $2md$, and d^2, where m and d are the frequencies of MZ and DZ twinning. This exceeds Hellin's prediction, $(m + d)^2 = m^2 + 2md + d^2$, by the small value m^2, approximately 10% of the triplet rate. The logical explanation for the coefficient 2 in the first two terms is that the presence of two embryos doubles the chance that an embryo will divide (Allen and Firschein, 1957).

Small discrepancies indicate, however, that even this formulation is too simple. The most serious complication is probably uncounted prenatal loss. Another is the change in twinning frequency with maternal age, emphasized in this connection by Jenkins (1929) and Jenkins and Gwin (1940). The most twin-prone, older women, contribute a minority of births, which would raise the frequency of triplets and quadruplets above the value calculated from twins. Still another inaccuracy is the improbable assumption that second or third divisions of embryo are as probable as primary division. However, if the conditional probabilities of division and ovulation decrease in the higher ranks, this may offset the age effect.

The use of fertility drugs would multiply the higher order births more than twins even if Hellin's law applied nicely to gestations resulting from fertility drugs. If 1 in 200 maternities resulted from use of ovulation inducers (a rate of .005) and 10% of those were twins, then by Hellin's law the frequency of higher multiple births among those maternities would be 1% triplets and 0.1% quadruplets. The last figure would amount to $0.001 \times 0.005 = 0.000005$, five times the natural frequency of quadruplets, whereas the twinning rate would be incremented by only 5%. Actually, among these pregnancies quadruplets and quintuplets greatly exceed the geometric proportions (Gemzell et al., 1975). It is therefore unlikely that future birth statistics will follow Hellin's law.

Variants of DZ Twinning

If double ovulation ordinarily occurs within a span of minutes, one would expect both ova to be fertilized by a single insemination or by spermatozoa from different inseminations both preceding ovulation. The latter circumstance would constitute superfecundation, fertilization by spermatozoa from each of two inseminations in one cycle, and could be detected if the inseminations were by two men of different blood types or skin color. The babies would share the uterus and be born together like twins, but would be related as half-sibs. Such an event has been documented (Andreassi, 1947).

A more extraordinary phenomenon, superfetation, is apparently also possible and does not require different fathers to be detected. Many women report spotting in the first month of pregnancy, and this suggests the possibility of ovulation at that time. If a second ovum were released and fertilized, two sibs conceived a month apart would occupy the uterus together. There would be a large disparity in their birthweights or, in the rare case of twins in a bicornuate uterus, a long interval between the two births (Bhagwat, 1953).

Apparent superfetation indicated by a wide difference in stage of development of the fetuses has been reported at least twice (Scrimgeour and Baker, 1974; Rhine and Nance, 1976). Rhine and Nance described pedigrees of familial twinning in which there was a consistently large weight difference and in which the twinning tendency often appeared to be transmitted through the twins' father. The authors suggest that these families may have a genetic endocrine defect in the placenta that permits continued cycling of the maternal pituitary. However, this trait is too rare to account for many twin pairs with large weight differences. In a systematic study, Nance et al. (1978b) did not find an association between large birthweight difference in twins and familial twinning.

Another set of anomalies results when circulatory anastomosis occurs between the placentas of DZ twins. Such anastomosis is usual in monochorionic MZ twins, but quite exceptional for dichorionic twins, whether MZ or DZ (Benirschke and Driscoll, 1967; Cameron,

1968; Benirschke and Kim, 1973). The connecting vessels are generally too small to be identified, but they permit stem blood cells to establish mixed populations in both fetuses. Race and Sanger (1975—see their addenda) have collected reports of 21 blood group chimeras, but their failure to find cases by systematic search of a large series of blood donors sets a low upper limit on its frequency.

Variants of MZ Twinning

The placental membranes do not provide a ready diagnosis of zygosity as was once believed. Not only may dichorionic pairs be either MZ or DZ, but when the placentas of dichorionic pairs are fused, the septum between the sacs may be so thin that only careful dissection can differentiate it from a purely amniotic septum (Corney, 1975). The twin placenta is nevertheless of considerable interest (Benirschke and Driscoll, 1967), and its relation to twin characteristics is still under investigation (Corey et al., 1979; Feinleib et al., 1981).

Over two-thirds of MZ twins share one chorion. Of these, about 1 in 20, or 3.4% of all MZ twins, also share a single amnion (Bulmer, 1970; Myrianthopoulos, 1970). All conjoined twins must belong to this relatively rare type, of which they may constitute as many as a fourth (Boklage, 1981). From the relative frequencies of monochorionic, monoamnionic, and conjoined twins, Boklage (1981) estimated the average time of determination of MZ twinning at just under five days after fertilization. Very few MZ twin pairs, if any, are formed at the two-cell stage.

The implications of a shared chorion, circulation, or amnion may not be so far-reaching as suggested in 1950 by Price (Melnick and Myrianthopoulos, 1979), but some effects, for example the immunologic consequences, are not yet completely known. Even fused versus separate placentas may affect DZ twin development (Corey et al., 1979).

A Third Type of Twinning

The frequency of twin pairs that appear intermediate between MZ and DZ twins in degree of similarity keeps alive speculation that a third mechanisms of twinning may exist. However, Bulmer (1970) analyzed blood group data from several series of nonidentical twins and ruled out any important fraction of genetically intermediate types.

Large polar bodies have sometimes been observed in other species (Austin, 1961), suggesting that they might be fertilized and give rise to a second zygote. If the two zygotes formed a single cell mass, the result would be a "whole-body chimera," and the existence of such chimeras is well established (Gartler et al., 1962; Race and Sanger, 1975). Whether the second zygote ever separates from the first and gives rise to twins is not known, and the differentiation of one such pair from ordinary DZ twins by study of genetic markers would be difficult (Nance, 1981).

VARIABLES AFFECTING TWINNING RATES

The MZ Twinning Rate

The only variable shown unquestionably to influence the MZ twinning rate is maternal age. When MZ twinning is estimated within maternal age groups by Weinberg's difference method, the rate in the United States ranges from about 3 pairs per 1000 maternities under age 20 to around 4.5 over age 40 (Heuser, 1967). Most studies have shown no effect of race (Morton et al., 1967) or parity (Heuser, 1967), and temporal trends are not discernible (Jeanneret and MacMahon, 1962). Inouye and Imaizumi (1981) reported a negative relation between MZ twinning and the square of parity in Japan, and a greater seasonal variation in MZ than in DZ twin births. These isolated findings require confirmation.

The remainder of this section will deal only with variation in the DZ twinning rate, or will assume that variation in the total twinning rate is due to the DZ component.

Maternal Age and Parity

The separate effects of maternal age and birth order are shown in Fig. 7-1 for 1964 births in the United States. The lowest DZ rate, in first births to young women, is considerably lower than that for MZ twinning in the same age group (1.9 vs 3.2). At parity six in mothers between 35 and 39, the DZ rate is three times the MZ rate at that age. The upward trend with parity appears to continue linearly at least to birth order 14 (Mosteller et al., 1981).

Race and Heredity

The DZ twinning rate is much lower in Mongoloid peoples than in Europeans. Data for Japan place the DZ rate lower than the MZ rate at every parity and maternal age represented by more than 100 twin deliveries (Inouye and Imaizumi, 1981). American Indians have a twinning rate intermediate between Japanese and Caucasians.

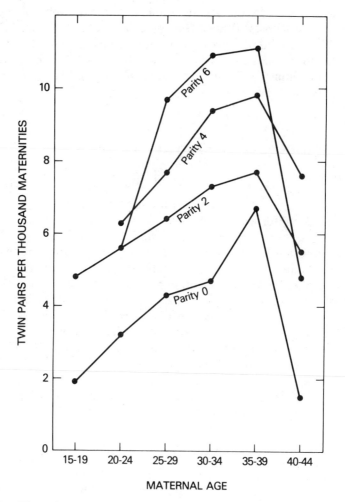

Fig. 7-1. The relations of the dizygotic twinning rate to maternal age and parity (birth order). United States white births, 1964.
Source: Heuser (1967).

In American blacks the DZ twinning rate is about half again as great as in American whites over all maternal ages and parities (Strandskov, 1945; Heuser, 1967). In African blacks the rate is higher still (Jeffreys, 1953; Nylander, 1971), even when some allowance is made for biased ascertainment (Nylander and Corney, 1969).

The racial differences in twinning suggest a genetic factor, which also finds support in the reproductive histories of mothers of twins. Women with opposite-sex twins are more likely to have twins in a subsequent pregnancy than mothers of singletons (Bulmer, 1970).

However, this elevated "repeat frequency" of twinning might be explained by social or physical factors in the woman's history, or by sexual behavior patterns.

Stronger evidence for genetic transmission comes from family data. The twinning rate is significantly increased among female relatives of women who have borne DZ twins (Weinberg, 1909). It is commonly assumed that any genetic factor for DZ twinning must act only on the female reproductive system, although Greulich (1934) reported increased twinning in relatives of fathers of twins.

Wyshak and White (1965) concluded from family data that inheritance was recessive. Morton et al. (1967) found that twinning was inherited recessively in marriages between Caucasians and Mongoloids and between Caucasians and Negroes. Nylander (1978) found no increased twinning tendency in Nigerian mothers who were themselves members of opposite-sex twin pairs. This is not necessarily incompatible with recessive inheritance in Caucasians or in Negro–Caucasian crosses, because nearly all Nigerians might have the genes for twin-proneness.

The hypothesis that nearly all Nigerian women are twin prone would require one or at most two major gene loci, certainly if the trait is recessive. Twin proneness must, however, be measured quantitatively, probably as the frequency of double ovulation, and this suggests a continuous distribution of twin proneness and dependence on multiple genes. Evidence for a single locus and two distinct ovulation patterns among women would be the finding that a single DZ twin birth to a woman indicates as much twin-proneness for that woman as two DZ twin births. One attempt, on rather small numbers, to measure the double-repeat frequency of twinning found no greater twinning rate after two than after one twin delivery (Allen, 1978).

Regardless of the number of genes involved, family data like those of Wyshak and White (1965) ought to be reanalyzed by threshold methods (Falconer, 1965; Reich et al., 1972), as appropriate for a quantitative trait that is detected by a qualitative phenomenon.

Geographic Variation

In addition to racial variation in twinning, there is geographic variation that may represent environmental effects, an explanation that is supported by temporal variations.

Twinning rates in the U.S. white population averaged over the five years 1933–1937 ranged from <10.2 per 1000 maternities in the New England and Middle Atlantic states to 13.1 in the West South Central states (Jeanneret and MacMahon, 1962). Table 7-2, covering nearly the same years, shows that adjustment for maternal age and parity would probably increase the spread. The most obvious environmental correlate of this distribution is urban–rural differentiation. Racial and ethnic factors are ruled out by the uniformity of the regional rates in 1954 (Table 7-2).

Regional differences in other countries are susceptible to genetic as well as environmental explanations. In Japan between 1955 and 1959, Kamimura (1976) found twinning rates significantly higher in the Northeast than in the Southwest; this does not correspond to urban–rural differences. Correlation of DZ twinning with air temperatures was highly significant and negative, whereas a negative correlation with recorded annual hours of sunshine was insignificant. Annual hours of sunshine have little relation to seasonal changes in length of day, so the latter factor remains unstudied in Japan.

In Nigeria all black populations have very high twinning rates, but a rate of 58 per 1000 maternities in the western region contrasts with 36 in the midwestern region after standardization for age and parity (Nylander, 1978). These rates are based on hospital births, but if elevation of the MZ rate is a measure of hospital bias toward twin deliveries, that bias is small and nearly equal in the two regions (4.4 and 4.6 per 1000, respectively).

Differences in twinning rates among the countries of Europe (Bulmer, 1960) also may be genetic as well as environmental. A positive association of twinning with frequency of blood group B in France by provinces was attributed by Bulmer to genetic differences between ethnic groups. However, Lazar et al. (1981) found the association to be negative within a French sample.

Short-term Temporal Variation

Temporal variation in twinning rates is one of the most provocative observations in twin biology, because it cannot be explained in genetic terms and seems to offer strong clues to reproductive physiology. Because the twinning rate is measured as a proportion of all births, it adjusts for variables like family planning unless they particularly affect twinning. Such particular effects offer clues to reproductive physiology that are complementary to and perhaps better than the complexities of total natality. Two known effects can be adjusted statistically: exaggerated perinatal mortality in twins and prematurity that offsets births relative to conceptions by three weeks.

A good illustration is seasonal variation, which is known for total births and conceptions to vary in a complex way and by country (Bailar and Gurian, 1967; Cohen and Bracken, 1977). Similar bimodal curves for twin births were reported from Liverpool, England (Edwards, 1938) and from Niigata City, Japan (Kamimura, 1976). The proportion of twin births was high in May, June, November, and December. A unimodal curve was reported from Finland (Timonen and Carpen, 1968), where the high spring birthrate of singletons is even higher for twins. The Finnish authors suggested that seasonality of both types of birth might reflect an influence of length of day on pituitary gonadotropin levels. One Finnish province is the most northern population for which twin birth statistics are available, and might show a length-of-day effect better than other countries. As in Japan, the highest annual twinning rates occur in the North, so that long summer days would appear to outweigh short winter days. However, the high proportion of ovulatory cycles in adult women (Vollman, 1977) may exclude ovulation as a physiologic common denominator in seasonality of twins and singletons.

Another example of short-term temporal variation is a decrease in twinning associated with wartime famine from 1941 to 1945 in France, Holland, and Norway (Bulmer, 1959a). Famine was not so severe in Sweden, where a wartime decrease occurred but persisted, or in Denmark, which showed only a postwar decrease. The temporary decreases appear to reflect malnutrition, whereas the permanent decreases were apparently part of a long-term trend.

The most dramatic short-term changes in twinning rates occurred immediately after World War I in Italy (Parisi and Caperna, 1981) and after both world wars in the United States. This phenomenon was first detected by Jeanneret and MacMahon (1962) in the U.S. twin birth statistics of the 1940s, but Fig. 7-2 also shows a peak in 1919. In two of these instances (apparently not in the United States after World War I) the peak in twinning rates occurred while total births were rising from a wartime low. In all three instances large numbers of men had been released from military service within a period of a few months (Allen and Schachter, 1970). Absence of a twinning peak in Italy at the end of World War II could be related to the fact that Italian demobilization was drawn out over a number of years (Parisi and Caperna, 1982). The observed peaks have been interpreted in two quite different ways, discussed in the section on causes.

Long-term Temporal Trends

A decline in twin births relative to single births has been observed in nearly all developed countries (James, 1972). Guttmacher (1953) noted a decline in U.S. twinning that he attributed to changes of mean maternal age and parity. Bulmer (1959a) observed a decline in northern Europe even after standardization for maternal age. The worldwide extent of the phenomenon was apparently first grasped by Jeanneret and MacMahon (1962). Some authors report a decline

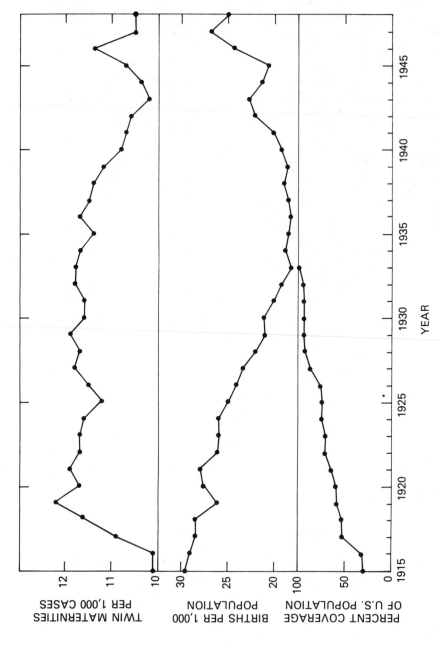

Fig. 7-2. Twinning rate and birthrate for all U.S. births reported from the registration area, 1915–1948, and additions to the registration area. Additions may have affected changes in the twinning rate from 1915 to 1917. Note relation of twinning peak in 1946 to birthrate peak in 1947.

Sources: U.S. Bureau of the Census (1946); National Office of Vital Statistics (1950).

mainly or wholly at older maternal ages (Jeanneret and MacMahon, 1962; Hémon et al., 1981; Inouye and Imaizumi, 1981), but they did not adjust fully for parity distributions within maternal age groups.

The period of decline varies from one country to another. In Sweden a decline was recorded between 1790 and 1850, and again, more marked, since 1930 (Eriksson et al., 1976). During the latter decline in Sweden twinning increased in Finland (Eriksson and Fellman, 1973). In Italy the decline started in the 1940s and accelerated in the late 1950s, presenting a nearly constant trend from >12 per 1000 in 1957 to <9 per 1000 in 1979 (Parisi and Caperna, 1982). In the United States (Fig. 7-2) the greatest decline, between 1936 and 1943 (Jeanneret and MacMahon, 1962), was followed by postwar stabilization or, in the black population, gradual increase until 1958. Data of 1964 showed some further decline in both white and black populations (Heuser, 1967). The crude twinning rate for 1977–1979, based on livebirths in twin deliveries, shows no further decline (National Center for Health Statistics, 1980, 1981, and unpublished), but adjustment for age and parity might alter this conclusion.

The reduction in twinning rates is seen by some writers (Lazar, 1976; James, 1978) as a sign of general decline in reproductive capacities. It can also be interpreted as a self-limiting type of phenomenon with few reproductive implications beyond twinning (Allen, 1981b).

Body Build, Social Class, and Nutrition

Despite some strong indications that these three variables affect twinning rates, the findings are inconsistent and the overall picture is confused.

The temporary drop in twinning in wartime Europe is probably a direct consequence of malnutrition (Bulmer, 1959a). An alternate explanation may be the psychosocial factors to be discussed below. Lilienfeld and Pasamanick (1955) found elevated twinning rates in Baltimore in the highest economic stratum among whites, but not among blacks, between 1941 and 1948. They attributed this finding tentatively to higher fetal losses in lower socioeconomic groups. Myrianthopoulos (1970) analyzed twin birth data in the Collaborative Perinatal Project that studied over 54,000 births between 1959 and 1966. He too found an excess of twins in the uppermost socioeconomic classes, both white and black, MZ and DZ. Morton et al. (1967) confirmed the positive association of DZ twinning with social class from Hawaiian data.

Studies in Aberdeen, Scotland found DZ twinning to be associated both with maternal stature and with maternal weight for height, but not with social class (MacGillivray and Campbell, 1978). Age and parity were not controlled. Nylander (1978) confirmed an effect of maternal stature in Nigerian blacks but found higher twinning in the lower social classes. He postulated that the native diet eaten by the lower classes might contain a natural substance that imitates or induces gonadotropins. Nylander measured serum gonadotropin (follicle-stimulating hormone, FSH) levels in mothers of twins and in mothers of singletons in Aberdeen and Ibadan. Levels of FSH were strongly related to twinning only in the Ibadan population, but were also elevated in the Ibadan mothers of singletons.

The high rate of twinning in American blacks would imply a still higher rate in native Africans, so a dietary explanation of the high Nigerian twinning rate is not needed except possibly to explain the class difference in twinning rate in Nigeria. Relevant to this hypothesis, but not directly supporting it, is the fact that yams contain steroid precursors of estrogens (Hardman, 1969; Nylander, 1978).

Pharmacologic Agents

Any hormonal or pharmacologic agent capable of restoring fertility in nonovulating women is likely to induce multiple ovulation (Gemzell et al., 1975). The frequency varies in different series, but is usually under 10% when clomiphene is used or between 10 and 40% when gonadotropins are used (Wyshak, 1978). These rates are so much higher than the normal rate that the use of the agents in as few as 1 of every 200 pregnancies could effect a detectable 5% increase in the twinning rate, or conceal a 5% decline. The actual extent of use of fertility drugs is undocumented.

Oral contraceptives also appear to be related to twinning, possibly in three ways. The best documented effect is an increase of twinning by a factor close to two in conceptions occurring within two or three months after termination of certain contraceptive regimens (Rothman, 1977; Bracken, 1979; Métneki and Czeizel, 1980). This is thought to result from a rebound in gonadotropin levels, thus resembling the effect of gonadotropin administration.

A second relation of oral contraceptives to twinning is opposite to the first. Some preparations or regimens would not be likely to induce a rebound of gonadotropins (Benirschke, 1974; Métneki and Czeizel, 1980), and in at least two studies oral contraceptives were negatively associated with later twinning (Vessey et al., 1976; Hémon et al., 1979). Hémon et al. (1979) found that the proportion of previous users of oral contraceptives was 52% among 622 mothers of singletons, 48% among 423 mothers of same-sex twins, and 38% among 199 mothers of opposite-sex twins. The probability of this was less than .01 and remained significant when age was controlled.

Finally, oral contraceptives, like any contraception, might influence the rate of twinning in a population by a differential effect on twin-prone women if they are more fertile than other women (Allen and Schachter, 1970).

PROPOSED CAUSES OF VARIATION IN THE TWINNING RATE

The causes of variation in twinning fit logically into two types. One type promotes double ovulation or division of the zygote or early embryo. The other acts negatively to prevent two ova or two products of one ovum from both developing into viable fetuses.

An agent or influence that by its nature eliminates both products in a twin pregnancy and terminates the pregnancy would generally be expected similarly to terminate singleton gestations, thus not affecting the twinning rate. In contrast, an agent that can eliminate one of two ova or embryos thereby reduces a potential twin gestation to a singleton gestation. Such incomplete action probably would not terminate all singleton gestations similarly exposed, so it would reduce the relative frequency of twins. Because MZ twins begin life as a single egg and embryo, and they share the same genes, they are more likely to be eliminated together than separately. Thus the negative factors in twinning would be expected to affect mainly the DZ twinning rate.

Positive factors proposed as causes of MZ twinning have included oxygen deprivation (Stockard, 1921) and overripeness of the egg (Schinzel et al., 1979). These ideas are derived from laboratory experiments in other species and are not easily reconciled with the diversity of stages at which MZ twins are known to originate or with the usual absence of other abnormalities.

Control Points in the Genesis of DZ Twins

The frequency of double ovulation is a primary limiting factor in DZ twinning if it varies significantly, but such variation is not easily established. Growth of primordial follicles is initiated continually even before puberty. During the reproductive years many primordial follicles are converted to Graafian follicles in each menstrual cycle. Block (1952) counted a minimum of 21 and a maximum of 136 Graafian follicles in women between 18 and 38 years old. Ordinarily, in the late follicular phase of the menstrual cycle, a single "dominant follicle" emerges that secretes 17α-hydroxyprogesterone (Goodman et al.,

1977) before releasing its ovum. Thus in human and other monotocous species the endocrine mechanisms are fine-tuned to eliminate many follicles in each cycle and permit only one to rupture. Dizygotic twinning is a measure of the imperfection of that fine-tuning. Deviations might originate in the pituitary gland, in the ovaries, in the hormones, or in the follicles as end organs.

Double ovulation is certainly more frequent than DZ twinning, so the negative factors play an important secondary role. Losses may include incompetence of ovulated ova, nonfertilization and non-implantation, early and late abortion. Such losses will affect the twinning rate, however, only if they can eliminate one ovum or embryo and allow the other to survive. This condition is satisfied by random elimination of embryos, as in genetic mutation, or by any physiologic mechanism that tends to regulate litter size after ovulation.

Another more subtle control of twinning might act at the population level and is possible only if some women are more twin-prone than others. Thus racial and geographic differences in twinning may depend in part on the frequency of twin-prone women in each population. Even temporal changes could be explained in these terms if the representation of twin-prone women is not constant in the maternities of all seasons or years.

Gonadotropin Levels

The best documented cause of natural variation in DZ twinning is of the positive type: the progressive elevation of gonadotropin levels as women age (Albert et al., 1956). Congruence of this measurement with the direction of principal age change in twinning and the demonstrated relation of gonadotropins to multiple ovulation (Gemzell et al., 1975) leave little room to question this explanation of the increase in twinning up to the late 30s of maternal age.

The steep decline in twinning after age 37 or 38, while gonadotropins continue to rise, might be explained by the decreasing number of Graafian follicles at these ages (Block, 1952), resulting in diminished response to gonadotropins or diminished probability of two follicles reaching ripeness just at the same time. Lazar (1976), however, attributes the decrease after age 37 to lethal mutations that usually cause early abortion of one rather than both of DZ embryos. Many chromosomal aberrations found in early abortions involve an extra chromosome (also see Chapter 2), and this type of anomaly, illustrated in Down syndrome, is age dependent.

The increase of twinning with parity is probably to be explained on the same endocrine basis as the age effect. The anterior pituitary enlarges with age and, more dramatically, with each pregnancy by cell multiplication (Russell, 1966), producing a 'ratchet" effect. Direct evidence of increasing secretory activity is lacking, however.

If the frequency of multiple ovulation varies widely, then the pituitary gland may be the mediating variable for some of the other proposed influences (Milham, 1964), including genetic variation and psychoendocrine effects. It remains possible, however, that these other influences could act as negative agents in postovulatory stages.

Failure of Implantation

Women of reproductive age are believed to ovulate in nearly every menstrual cycle (Vollman, 1977). The average delay of several months to conception in cohabiting couples (Westoff et al., 1961; Jain, 1969) may therefore represent, in large part, failures of implantation or very early abortions. The same phenomena would probably pose greater obstacles for DZ twin conceptions.

In 1941 Brewer and Jones reported that about 10% (5 in 40 cases) of ovulatory cycles produced two or more ova, but they relied on a count of corpora lutea. At the same time it was discovered by Corner (1940) that some follicles give rise to corpora lutea without having released an ovum. It is therefore likely that Brewer and Jones included some of these accessory corpora lutea, although no subsequent study has clearly refuted their finding. Kratochwil et al. (1979), in a series of unspecified size, observed no instances of two ripe Graafian follicles in natural menstrual cycles, but several instances in women treated with ovulation inducers. Edwards et al. (1972) observed an *average* of five or six follicles secreting steroids in treated women. Even in these cases, however, a majority of resulting pregnancies are single.

Current immunologic investigations in sheep (e.g., Scaramuzzi et al., 1981) are pointing to a microenvironment of each follicle that may doom an ovum, even if it is ovulated, not to implant or not to be fertilizable. This seems to be particularly frequent when more than one ovum is released, and it may therefore be viewed as a post-ovulatory control of litter size initiated before ovulation. However, because implantation depends on the endometrium and the post-ovulatory endocrine environment, other physiologic controls may be initiated at that stage.

Failure of Fertilization and Coital Frequency

Fertilization is a prerequisite of implantation, and some early losses of ova despite timely coitus may represent failure of fertilization. James (1981) points out that the elevation of twinning rates in early post-marital conceptions and upon return of soldiers and sailors from war

171

would coincide with times of high coital frequency. He postulates that if double ovulation consists of two events separated by an interval sometimes as great as the fertile period, frequent coitus would often be a requirement for fertilization of both ova. Further, if ova are released simultaneously but each fertilization has a low probability, frequent coitus would increase that probability. The increase would be squared for two ova, increasing the relative frequency of DZ twins.

If fertilization is an efficient process, two ova released simultaneously should be fertilized together or not at all. That the ova are released nearly simultaneously appears to be a safe assumption. The efficiency of fertilization is more problematic. In humans, insemination timing is not physiologically controlled but depends on repeated inseminations in each cycle. When coitus is widely spaced and timing poor, there will be few or no viable spermatozoa in the female tract at the time of ovulation. This would reduce the likelihood of all conceptions but would reduce the proportion of twins among such conceptions only during the interval when there was a small residual population of sperms, so that the square of the probability of one ovum being fertilized was much less than unity. The length of this interval—that is, the variance in longevity of spermatozoa, or even the mean—is undocumented, but if the standard deviation is not greater than half the mean longevity, infrequent coitus would not significantly reduce the frequency of DZ twinning (Allen, 1982).

Spontaneous Abortion

Other evidence for a rate of double ovulation much greater than the twinning rate derives from cytogenetic studies in early abortions. Many of these embryos have severe chromosome anomalies (Hassold et al., 1980). If anomalies similar to those observed in several small chromosomes occur in the other chromosomes and cause earlier terminations, as many as half of all conceptions are subject to early lethal genetic defects (Boué et al., 1975). Such lethals would eliminate half of all MZ pairs (both members), but from the binomial formula they would eliminate three-fourths of DZ gestations either completely or by converting them to singletons.

The early diagnosis of twin pregnancy by ultrasound indicates that about half of such pregnancies end in singleton births (Robinson and Caines, 1977; Schneider et al., 1979). These losses would overlap only partly with the early losses as estimated by Boué and co-workers. Moreover, it is not clear whether the later losses are shared by singleton fetuses or are in some way peculiar to multiple pregnancy. Like the "doomed" accessory ova of sheep, these resorptions might be one of the mechanisms that regulate litter size. There is certainly

172

individual variation in tendency to abort (Hassold et al., 1980), and losses occurring after diagnosis of twin pregnancy may be subject to physiologic control. In the series of Schneider et al. (1979), "early ovular resorption" occurred in 34 of 54 spontaneous twin pregnancies and in 7 of 11 clomiphene-induced twin pregnancies, but in none of 12 induced by a combination of gonadotropins (HMG and HCG).

Population Structure: Inbreeding

It was stated earlier that twin-proneness seems to be inherited as a recessive trait (Wyshak and White, 1965). Rare recessive traits are expressed particularly in the progeny of cousin marriages, and such marriages are promoted in isolated or subdivided populations (Cavalli-Sforza and Bodmer, 1971). However, the gene or genes for twinning are far from rare, and Morton and Schull (1953) found no effect of inbreeding on twinning in Japan. Regional isolates could, nevertheless, present a pattern of heterogeneity in the twinning rate, because they promote genetic drift and consequent variation in trait frequency.

Both population heterogeneity and inbreeding would be diminished or erased with the advent of modern transportation and the breakup of isolates (Sutter and Tabah, 1954). Whether this effect would be strong enough to explain much of the secular decline in twinning is problematic. Eriksson (1962) has made a strong case for this explanation of twinning decline in the Åland Islands in the Baltic Sea (see also Eriksson et al., 1973). In France, however, geographic distribution of the decline in twinning is not correlated with variables thought to measure isolate breakup (Hémon et al., 1981).

Demographic Selection

If twin-prone women differ in reproductive patterns from other women, their relative contribution to total births may vary over time, and this would be reflected in annual or seasonal twinning rates. Mothers of twins have been reported to have shorter average menstrual cycles and an earlier menarche (Wyshak, 1981). If they are also more fecund (i.e., become pregnant more promptly when exposed to conception), this would explain several observations: the elevated twinning rate seen in some series of illegitimate pregnancies (Eriksson and Fellman, 1967), in the earliest conceptions after marriage (Bulmer, 1959b), and the peaks of twinning among postwar births in Italy and the United States.

Higher fecundity in twin-prone women might also explain some long-term changes in twinning rates. Twinning rates would rise with

173

increasing use of inefficient contraception, and fall with introduction of highly efficient methods like the pill or the IUD (Allen, 1978). The negative effect of contraception has been proposed as a likely explanation of the midcentury decline in twinning rates (Allen and Schachter, 1970; Elwood, 1973; Parisi and Caperna, 1981). The greater decline reported for older maternal age groups in some countries strengthens the hypothesis, because older mothers are more likely to limit their childbearing.

The main evidence for high fertility in mothers of DZ twins is the association of twinning with larger families and with higher birth orders (Weinberg, 1901; Renkonnen, 1966). Weinberg recognized that this association might be due to other factors, either the biased selection of large families whenever a particular type of birth is sought (see also Record et al., 1978) or a direct effect of parity on the tendency to bear twins. The parity effect has recently been detected independently of family size (though short of statistical significance; Allen, 1978), weakening the evidence for high fertility.

The main evidence against the theory that twin-prone women are unusually fecund is that such women do not conceive more promptly than women without twins as measured by the interval between births (Weinberg, 1901; Record et al., 1978). Another difficulty is that the large fertility difference needed to explain the recent decline in twinning (James, 1975) would affect all birth ranks for mother's age in families containing twins. Twins have a high birth rank relative to their sibs (Allen, 1978), and the birth order effect observed in twinning can hardly accommodate an additional large increment from fertility (Allen, 1981b).

Psychoendocrine Effects

A more direct explanation of high twinning rates immediately after marriage and after sudden demobilization would be a neural influence on gonadotropin levels (Allen, 1981b). The stimulus might be frequent coitus or simply the emotional state of sexual arousal. The latter would be more likely than frequent coitus in illegitimate conceptions, found in some series to carry a high risk of twinning (Eriksson and Fellman, 1967; James, 1981). The high frequency of twinning among early conceptions after marriage is apparently just that, and not a consequence of generally prompt conception by twin-prone women. Comparing twin-prone women whose twins occurred at different birth orders, Allen (1981b) found an adjusted mean interval of 76 days to conception for 273 mothers of DZ twins whose first child was a singleton, and 30 days for 89 such women who bore twins in their first confinement. If twin-prone women happen to conceive very soon after marriage, the probability of twins is enhanced.

There is published evidence that sexual arousal (i.e., anticipation of intercourse) raises gonadotropin levels in men (Anonymous, 1970; LaFerla et al., 1978), and evidence presented at a meeting for the same phenomenon in women (LaFerla et al., 1980).

The possibility of psychologic induction of double ovulation has far-reaching implications for the epidemiology of multiple births. For example, changes in women's social status, either in their roles as wives or in their relations with men, might account for the secular decline in twinning.

Noxious Environmental Effects

The long-term decline in twinning is likely to find its explanation in some aspects of modern living. In Italian data, a negative regional correlation has been demonstrated between twinning and industrial development (Parisi and Caperna, 1982). The early twinning data for the United States show lower twin frequencies in the industrial northeastern states than elsewhere (U.S. Bureau of the Census, 1925). Jeanneret and MacMahon (1962) found this to be true as late as 1937 (also see Table 7-2), and the decline between 1937 and 1950 that they reported occurred mainly in the central and southern parts of the country, perhaps because of accelerated urbanization associated with World War II.

Contraception and changing sex roles, mentioned above as possible causes of the twinning decline, do not seem to impair voluntary childbearing. Of greater concern is the possibility that toxic substances in air, water, or food are responsible for the decline and are really impairing human reproduction.

One hypothesis (James, 1978) takes note of reported decreases in average human sperm counts (Nelson and Bunge, 1974; Rehan et al., 1975) and infers a diminished probability of both ova being fertilized after double ovulation. Lower sperm counts could be attributed to dietary stilbestrol in beef and poultry, or to pesticide residues. Decreased spermatogenesis might also be a psychoendocrine effect.

James cites good evidence for declining sperm counts, from a mean around 100 million per milliliter a generation ago to less than half that now. As measured by a history of fatherhood, however, male function is unimpaired at sperm counts as low as 20 million, and counts below 10 million are compatible with fertility (Smith and Steinberger, 1977). The lower sperm counts might, nevertheless, influence the twinning rate. An appreciably lowered probability of fertilizing any given ovum might not be detected in a couple already controlling their fertility, and this lowered probability would be squared for fertilization of two ova in the same cycle.

Another hypothesis to account for the decline in the twinning rate is an increased frequency of early lethal mutations (Lazar, 1976). These would reduce the frequency of DZ twins relative to singletons and MZ twins. One large group of these anomalies, with an extra chromosome, increases notably with maternal age (Hassold et al., 1980), and some studies of the secular decline in twinning find it most marked in older age groups. However, an environmentally caused increment might be unrelated to age. In fact, the incidence of abortions due to chromosomal lethals seems to be increasing in younger mothers (Uchida, 1979). Environmental explanations are not needed to account for the baseline chromosomal anomalies, but the secular decline in twinning may indicate an environmental increment.

SOME USES OF TWINS IN PERINATAL EPIDEMIOLOGY

In addition to the light that multiple births can shed on reproduction and development, they provide a set of natural experiments for studying heredity and environment. However, the special circumstances of twin development make it hazardous to generalize from twin data to singletons, particularly as regards perinatal phenomena (Benirschke and Kim, 1973). For example, the majority of MZ twin pairs, unlike DZ pairs, share a single placenta and circulation, creating some of the problems that have appropriately been characterized as "primary biases" (Price, 1950).

Congenital Anomalies

Because twins constitute only 2% of all Caucasian births, and MZ twins less than half that, it is difficult to assemble a series of twins that are thoroughly examined at birth and numerous enough to provide useful statistics even on relatively commonplace anomalies. Many pairs, and especially those in which one is stillborn or dies neonatally, cannot be classified as to zygosity, necessitating analysis in terms of sex concordance. In a small series sex concordance tells only a little about MZ–DZ differences. Nevertheless, many studies of congenital anomalies in twins have been attempted (MacGillivray, 1975).

ILLUSTRATIVE STUDIES

Twin studies of congenital anomalies have employed a spectrum of sources and methods. The National Cleft Lip and Palate Intelligence

Service collected birth certificate reports of malformations in the United States for the years 1962–1965 (Hay and Wehrung, 1970). This series includes about 2000 individual twins with malformations. Birth certificates do not provide complete ascertainment, but major malformations are not likely to be missed, and the denominator population of singletons is clearly specified and perhaps equally well ascertained.

A more recent report covers 4490 individual twins found to have malformations in any examination during the first year. All births were studied in metropolitan Atlanta, Georgia, from 1969 to 1976 (Layde et al., 1980). In this series ascertainment should be virtually complete, and the denominator population is probably representative. However, conclusions must, as in the first study, be based on sex concordance and the Weinberg difference method.

Two large studies have been conducted by collaborating hospitals (Stevenson et al., 1966; Myrianthopoulos, 1975), so that diagnosis of zygosity was possible for most pairs. The source population and the twins may not be wholly representative, but comparisons within each sample are likely to yield useful relative frequencies.

FINDINGS

These studies all arrive at similar principal conclusions, some of which are summarized in the last two lines of Table 7-3 from Myrianthopoulos (1975). Among some 54,000 deliveries, malformations were found in 219 twin individuals, 181 of whom belonged to pairs of known zygosity. The outstanding findings concern incidence. Malformations are no more frequent in DZ twins than in singletons, but in MZ twins there is an excess of more than 50%.

Concordance rates were significantly higher in MZ pairs for both major and minor malformations, and only a little of this difference was due to the higher frequency in MZ twins. The musculoskeletal system, with the most numerous malformations, also had the highest concordance rate of all anatomic systems and was the only one in which the MZ–DZ difference in concordance was significant. The concordance rate was .59 in MZ pairs and .09 in DZ pairs.

Significant differences in concordance did not occur for any one defect; only for three forms of clubfoot taken together: 6 concordant among 8 MZ pairs and 2 concordant among 12 DZ pairs. Even metatarsus adductus, the single defect for which the largest number of pairs were concordant, occurred discordantly in two MZ pairs, showing that genetic factors are not decisive in its genesis. However, quantitative inferences about heritability are precluded by the difference between MZ and DZ twins in incidence of the defects.

177

Table 7-3. Distribution of Malformations in Twins by Zygosity, and in Singletons

	Twins				Singletons
	Monozygotic	Dizygotic	Zygosity undetermined	Total	
Total number of malformations	119 (44)[a]	112 (36)	63 (35)	294 (115)	10,480 (3,574)
Total number of malformed cases	90 (15)	91 (15)	38 (10)	219 (40)	8,288 (1,382)
Total number of individuals	373	617	205	1,195	53,257
Frequency (mean number) of malformations	0.319	0.181	0.307	0.246	0.197
Frequency of malformed cases (%)	24.13 (4.02)	14.75 (2.43)	18.54 (4.88)	18.33 (3.35)	15.56 (2.59)

[a] Numbers in parentheses are multiple malformations, included in the accompanying numbers.

Source: Myrianthopoulos (1975), in part.

SIGNIFICANCE

The MZ–DZ difference in incidence may be more informative than the difference in concordance rates. Schinzel et al. (1979) inferred that MZ twinning is an indicator of a general tendency toward malformation. This hypothesis requires an association, within individuals if not within families, among all the malformations that are so greatly increased in MZ twins, and the authors do not cite evidence for this.

A more plausible and perhaps very important suggestion is made by Melnick and Myrianthopoulos (1979). They observe that division of the early embryo temporarily halves the number of cells in each individual, presumably setting back development. Such a setback may affect the developmental time of some processes more than of others. Thus disturbed, the embryo is less able to maintain developmental homeostasis in the presence of other disturbing factors, genetic or environmental, and is therefore more subject to most malformations than are singletons or DZ twins. The higher concordance rate of MZ pairs would be due to genetically similar vulnerabilities, not to the twinning process.

Birthweight

A DELIBERATELY SIMPLIFIED ANALYSIS

In contrast to the rarity of congenital anomalies, birthweight is available on every infant, and relatively small series of twins can yield crude statistics. Such data illustrate both the method and the pitfalls of applying Weinberg's difference method to quantitative data. The essential datum needed, but often not obtained, is sex concordance of each pair associated with other information to be analyzed.

Table 7-4 is based on the Weinberg difference method and the formula given in the Statistical Methods section. The resulting estimated individual weight of MZ twins is about 80 g less than that of DZ twins. This value is just a little less than the difference of approximately 100 g given or implied in two studies where zygosity was individually diagnosed (Corney et al., 1972; Corey et al., 1979; see also Wilson, 1979, and Asaka et al., 1980). The estimated weight difference within MZ pairs is also close to the only observed value found in the literature, 278 g (Corey et al., 1979).

Agreement between estimates obtained by Weinberg's difference method and results of studying true zygosity classes appears, in this instance, to be fortuitous. Weinberg's method assumes that opposite-sex and same-sex DZ twins have the same average value of any trait that is being studied. An earlier report by Karn (1952) suggested that males were heavier in opposite-sex pairs than in same-sex DZ pairs.

179

Table 7-4. Birthweight of Twins and Estimates of Numbers of MZ Twins, Their Mean Weight, and Their Mean Intrapair Weight Difference by Weinberg's Difference Method (in Grams)

	Total	Opposite-sex pairs	Same-sex pairs	Estimated MZ pairs
Number	574	178	396	218
Summed weight	2,739,450	860,407	1,879,043	1,018,636
Mean weight (individuals)	2,386	2,417	2,373	2,336
Summed absolute differences	174,168	60,369	113,799	53,430
Mean intrapair weight difference	303	339	287	245

Source: Keith et al. (1980) and Keith (unpublished data). Sex concordance information had been collected but not originally used. Dr. Keith and Mark Binstock assisted with the reanalysis.

The data of Corey et al. are consistent with this finding, but those of Corney et al. (1972) are not. The approximation also escapes another hazard. Because male babies weigh more than female babies, it might be anticipated that opposite-sex twins would have a larger weight difference than same-sex DZ twins. Actually the study of Corey and co-workers belies this expectation.

MEANING OF THESE DATA FOR PERINATAL EPIDEMIOLOGY

These findings emphasize the fact that mean birthweights are rather uninformative. Birthweight in twins varies not only with zygosity, but perhaps also with maternal age, weight, and stature (Karn, 1952; Anderson, 1956; Hémon et al., 1981), and also as in singletons with sex of the infant, birth order, and, of course, length of gestation (Selvin and Janerich, 1971). A thorough study of birthweight in twins must include these variables, and thus requires a sample size almost as great as does the study of malformations. Even the best studies to date appear to be flawed by uncontrolled variation, so that the figures given in Table 7-4 provide, fortuitously, about as good a brief summary of the statistics as any available.

In the case of birthweight, as with malformations, twin data are likely to mislead if used to estimate heritability. In a more complicated study design, however, the *progeny* of MZ twins are more informative. Babies born to MZ twin sisters are found to be more alike in birthweight than the babies of MZ twin brothers. Nance et al. (1978a) infer that about 40% of the variance in birthweight, after adjustment for sex and gestational age, may be attributable to maternal effects.

The most general insight to be gained from the study of twin birthweights per se may emerge from investigation of the two most surprising findings: the greater weight of infants in opposite-sex compared to DZ same-sex pairs if confirmed in other studies, and the greater weight of DZ pairs compared to MZ pairs. The latter fact, although not matched in studies in mice (Corney et al., 1972), tends to support the hypothesis of Melnick and Myrianthopoulos (1979) that division of the early embryo significantly sets back the developmental clock or otherwise impedes development.

REFERENCES

Albert, A., Randall, R.V., Smith, R.A., and Johnson, C.E. (1956). The urinary excretion of gonadotrophin as a function of age. In *Hormones and the aging process*, edited by E.T. Engle and G. Pincus. New York: Academic Press, pp. 49–62.

Allen, G. (1960). A differential method for estimation of type frequencies in triplets and quadruplets. *Am. J. Hum. Genet. 12*, 210–224.

—————— (1978). The parity effect and fertility in mothers of twins. In *Twin research: Biology and epidemiology*, edited by W.E. Nance. New York: Alan R. Liss, pp. 89–97.

—————— (1981a). Errors of Weinberg's difference method. In *Twin research 3: Twin biology and multiple pregnancy*, edited by L. Gedda, P. Parisi and W.E. Nance. New York: Alan R. Liss, pp. 71–74.

—————— (1981b). The twinning and fertility paradox. In *Twin research 3: Twin biology and multiple pregnancy*, edited by L. Gedda, P. Parisi and W.E. Nance. New York: Alan R. Liss, pp. 1–13.

—————— (1982). Reply to W.H. James. *Acta Genet. Med. Gemellol. (Rome) 31*, 121–126.

—————— and Firschein, I.L. (1957). The mathematical relations among plural births. *Am. J. Hum. Genet. 9*, 181–190.

—————— and Hrubec, Z. (1979). Twin concordance: A more general model. *Acta Genet. Med. Gemellol. (Rome) 28*, 3–13.

—————— and Schachter, J. (1970). Do conception delays explain some changes in twinning rates? *Acta Genet. Med. Gemellol. (Rome) 19*, 30–34.

Anderson, W.J.R. (1956). Stillbirth and neonatal mortality in twin pregnancy. *J. Obstet. Gynaecol. Br. Emp. 63*, 205–215.

Andreassi, G. (1947). Problemi e considerazioni sulla gravidanza multipla. *Medicus, Vatican City 3*(2), 41. Cited by Bulmer (1970).

Anonymous (1970). Effects of sexual activity on beard growth in man. *Nature 226*, 869–870.

Asaka, A., Imaizumi, Y., and Inouye, E. (1980). Analysis of multiple births in Japan. I. Weight at birth among 12,392 pairs of twins. *Jpn. J. Hum. Genet. 25*, 65–71.

Austin, C.R. (1961). *The mammalian egg*. Oxford: Blackwell.

Bailar, J.C. and Gurian, J. (1967). The medical significance of date of birth. *Eugen. Q. 14*, 89–102.

Benirschke, K. (1974). Twinning and oral contraceptives. *N. Engl. J. Med. 290*, 346.

—— and Driscoll, S.G. (1967). The pathology of the human placenta. In *Handbuch der speziellen pathologischen Anatomie und Histologie*, Vol. 7, Part 5, edited by O. Lubarsch and F. Henke. Berlin: Springer-Verlag, pp. 97–571.

—— and Kim, C.K. (1973). Multiple pregnancy. *N. Engl. J. Med. 288*, 1276–1284 and 1329–1336.

Bhagwat, S.A. (1953). Twin pregnancy in bicornuate uterus. *J. Indian Med. Assoc. 22*, 330–331.

Block, E. (1952). Quantitative morphological investigations of the follicular system in women. *Acta Anat. (Basel) 14*, 108–123.

Boklage, C.E. (1981). On the timing of monozygotic twinning events. In *Twin research 3: Twin biology and multiple pregnancy*, edited by L. Gedda, P. Parisi and W.E. Nance. New York: Alan R. Liss, pp. 155–156.

Boué, J., Boué, A., and Lazar, P. (1975). Retrospective and prospective epidemiological studies of 1500 karyotyped spontaneous human abortions. *Teratology 12*, 11–26.

Bracken, M.B. (1979). Oral contraception and twinning: An epidemiologic study. *Am. J. Obstet. Gynecol. 133*, 432–434.

Brewer, J.J. and Jones, H.O. (1941). A study of the corpora lutea and the endometrium in patients with uterine fibroids. *Am. J. Obstet. Gynecol. 41*, 733–751.

Bulmer, M.G. (1959a). Twinning rate in Europe during the war. *Br. Med. J. 1*, 29–30.

—— (1959b). The effect of parental age, parity and duration of marriage on the twinning rate. *Ann. Hum. Genet. 23*, 454–458.

—— (1960). The twinning rate in Europe and Africa. *Ann. Hum. Genet. 24*, 121–125.

—— (1970). *The biology of twinning in man*. Oxford: Clarendon Press.

—— (1976). Is Weinberg's method valid? *Acta Genet. Med. Gemellol. (Rome) 25*, 25–28.

Cameron, A.H. (1968). The Birmingham twin survey. *Proc. R. Soc. Med. 61*, 229–234.

Cavalli-Sforza, L.L. and Bodmer, W.F. (1971). *Genetics of human populations*. San Francisco: W.H. Freeman.

Cederlof, R., Epstein, F.H., Friberg, L.T., Hrubec, Z., and Radford, E.P., Editors (1971). Twin registries in the study of chronic disease. *Acta Med. Scand. (Suppl. 523)* (entire issue).

Christian, J.C., Kang, K.W., and Norton, J.A. (1974). Choice of an estimate of genetic variance from twin data. *Am. J. Hum. Genet. 26*, 154–161.

Cochrane, W.G. (1954). Some methods for strengthening the common chi-square tests. *Biometrics 10*, 417–451.

Cohen, I.C. and Bracken, M.B. (1977). Monthly variation in conceptions leading to induced abortion. *Soc. Biol. 24*, 245–250.

Corey, L.A., Nance, W.E., Kang, K.W., and Christian, J.C. (1979). Effects of type of placentation on birthweight and its variability in monozygotic and dizygotic twins. *Acta Genet. Med. Gemellol. (Rome) 28*; 41–50.

Corner, G.W. (1940). Accessory corpora lutea in the ovary of the monkey Macaca rhesus. *Ann. Fac. Med. Montevideo 25*, 553–560.

Corney, G. (1975). Placentation. In *Human multiple reproduction*, edited by I. MacGillivray, P.P.S. Nylander, and G. Corney. London: W.B. Saunders, pp. 40–76.

——, Robson, E.B., and Strong, S.J. (1972). The effect of zygosity on the birth weight of twins. *Ann. Hum. Genet. 36*, 45–59.

Edwards, J. (1938). Season and rate of conception. *Nature 142*, 357.

Edwards, R.G., Steptoe, P.C., Abraham, G.E., Waltus, E., Purdy, J.M., and Fotherby, K. (1972). Steroid assays and preovulatory follicular development in human ovaries primed with gonadotrophins. *Lancet 2*, 611–615.

Elwood, J.M. (1973). Changes in the twinning rate in Canada 1926–1970. *Br. J. Prev. Soc. Med. 27*, 236–241.

Eriksson, A.W. (1962). Variations in the human twinning rate. *Acta Genet. (Basel) 12*, 242–250.

——, Eskola, M.R., and Fellman, J.O. (1976). Retrospective studies on the twinning rate in Scandinavia. *Acta Genet. Med. Gemellol. (Rome) 25*, 29–35.

—— and Fellman, J.O. (1967). Twinning and legitimacy. *Hereditas 57*, 395–402.

—— and —— (1973). Differences in the twinning trends between Finns and Swedes. *Am. J. Hum. Genet. 25*, 141–151.

——, ——, Workman, P.L., and Lalouel, J.M. (1973). Population studies in the Åland Islands. I. Prediction of kinship from migration and isolation by distance. *Hum. Hered. 23*, 422–433.

Falconer, D.S. (1965). The inheritance of liability to certain diseases estimated from the incidence among relatives. *Ann. Hum. Genet. 29*, 51–76.

Feinleib, M., Christian, J.C., Ingster-Moore, L., Garrison, R.J., Breckenridge, W.C., and Uchida, I. (1981). The Hamilton twin study: Comparison of serum lipid levels in monozygotic and dizygotic twins by chorion type. In *Twin research 3: Epidemiological and clinical studies*, edited by L. Gedda, P. Parisi and W.E. Nance. New York: Alan R. Liss, pp. 149–161.

Fleiss, J.L. (1973). *Statistical methods for rates and proportions*. New York: Wiley.

Gartler, S.M., Waxman, S.H., and Giblett, E.R. (1962). An XX/XY human hermaphrodite resulting from double fertilization relevant to irregular twin types. *Proc. Natl. Acad. Sci. U.S.A. 48*, 332–335.

Gedda, L., Rossi, C., and Brenci, G. (1979). Twin azygotic test for the study of hereditary qualitative traits in twin populations. *Acta Genet. Med. Gemellol. (Rome) 28*, 15–19.

Gemzell, C., Roos, P., and Loeffler, F.E. (1975). Follicle-stimulating hormone extracted from human pituitary. In *Progress in infertility* (2nd ed.), edited by S.J. Behrman and R.W. Kistner. Boston: Little, Brown and Co., pp. 479–493.

183

Goodman, A.I.., Nixon, W.E., Johnson, D.K., and Hodgen, G.D. (1977). Regulation of folliculogenesis in the cycling rhesus monkey: Selection of the dominant follicle. *Endocrinology 100*, 155–161.

Greulich, W.W. (1934). Heredity in human twinning. *Am. J. Phys. Anthropol. 19*, 391–431.

Guttmacher, A.F. (1953). The incidence of multiple births in man and some other unipara. *Obstet. Gynecol. 2*, 22–35.

Hardman, R. (1969). Pharmaceutical products from plant steroids. *Trop. Sci. 11*, 196–228.

Hassold, T., Chen, N., Funkhouser, J., Jooss, T., Manuel, B., Matsuura, J., Matsuyama, A., Wilson, C., Yamane, J.A., and Jacobs, P.A. (1980). A cytogenetic study of 1000 spontaneous abortions. *Ann. Hum. Genet. 44*, 151–163.

Havlik, R.J., Garrison, R.J., Katz, S.H., Ellison, R.C., Feinleib, M., and Myrianthopoulos, N.C. (1979). Detection of genetic variance in blood pressure of seven-year-old twins. *Am. J. Epidemiol. 109*, 512–516.

Hay, S. and Wehrung, D.A. (1970). Congenital malformations in twins. *Am. J. Hum. Genet. 22*, 662–678.

Hellin, D. (1895). *Die Ursache der Multiparität der uniparen Tiere überhaupt und der Zwillingsschwangerschaft beim Menschen insbesondere*. Munich. Cited by Bulmer, M.G. (1970).

Hémon, D., Berger, C., and Lazar, P. (1979). The etiology of human dizygotic twinning with special reference to spontaneous abortions. *Acta Genet. Med. Gemellol. (Rome) 28*, 253–258.

——, ——, and —— (1981). Some observations concerning the decline of dizygotic twinning rate in France between 1901 and 1968. In *Twin research 3: Twin biology and multiple pregnancy*, edited by L. Gedda, P. Parisi and W.E. Nance. New York: Alan R. Liss, pp. 49–56.

Heuser, R.L. (1967). *Multiple births: United States 1964*. National Center for Health Statistics, Series 21, No. 14. Washington, D.C.: U.S. Department of Health, Education and Welfare.

Inouye, E. and Imaizumi, Y. (1981). Analysis of twinning rates in Japan. In *Twin research 3: Twin biology and multiple pregnancy*, edited by L. Gedda, P. Parisi and W.E. Nance. New York: Alan R. Liss, pp. 21–33.

Jain, A.K. (1969). Fecundability and its relation to age in a sample of Taiwanese women. *Popul. Studies 23*, 69–85.

James, W.H. (1972). Secular changes in dizygotic twinning rates. *J. Biosoc. Sci. 4*, 427–434.

—— (1975). The secular decline in dizygotic twinning rates in Italy. *Acta Genet. Med. Gemellol. (Rome) 24*, 9–14.

—— (1978). A hypothesis on the declining dizygotic twinning rates in developed countries. In *Twin research: Biology and epidemiology*, edited by W.E. Nance. New York: Alan R. Liss, pp. 81–88.

—— (1979). Is Weinberg's differential rule valid? *Acta Genet. Med. Gemellol. 28*, 69–71.

—— (1981). Dizygotic twinning, marital stage and status and coital rates. *Ann. Hum. Biol. 8*, 371–378.

Jeanneret, O and MacMahon, B. (1962). Secular changes in rates of multiple births in the United States. *Am. J. Hum. Genet. 14*, 410–425.

Jeffreys, M.D.W. (1953). Twin births among Africans. *S. Afr. J. Sci. 50*, 89–93.

Jenkins, R.L. (1929). Twin and triplet birth ratios. A further study of the interrelations of the frequencies of plural births. *J. Hered. 20*, 485–494.

—— and Gwin, J. (1940). Twin and triplet birth ratios. Rigorous analysis of the interrelations of the frequencies of plural births. *J. Hered. 31*, 243–248.

Kamimura, K. (1976). Epidemiology of twin births from a climatic point of view. *Br. J. Prev. Soc. Med. 30*, 175–179.

Karn, M.N. (1952). Birth weight and length of gestation of twins, together with maternal age, parity and survival rate. *Ann. Eugen. 16*, 365–377.

Keith, L., Ellis, R., Berger, G.S., and Depp, R. (1980). The Northwestern University multihospital twin study. I. A description of 588 twin pregnancies and associated pregnancy loss, 1971–1975. *Am. J. Obstet. Gynecol. 138*, 781–789.

Kratochwil, A., Kemeter, P., and Friedrich, F. (1979). Ultrasonics of Graafian follicles. In *Human ovulation*, edited by E.S.E. Hafez. Amsterdam: North-Holland Publishing, pp. 339–350.

LaFerla, J.J., Anderson, D.L., and Schalch, D.S. (1978). Psychoendocrine response to sexual arousal in human males. *Psychoso. Med. 40*, 166–172.

——, Labrum, A.H., and Tang, K. (1980). *Psychoendocrine response to sexual arousal in human females*, Presented at the Sixth International Congress of Psychosomatic Obstetrics and Gynecology, West Berlin, Sept. 2–6.

Layde, P.M., Erickson, J.D., Falek, A., and McCarthy, B.J. (1980). Congenital malformations in twins. *Am. J. Hum. Genet. 32*, 69–78.

Lazar, P. (1976). Effet des avortements spontanés sur la fréquence des naissances gémellaires. *C. R. Acad. Sci. (D) Paris 282*, 243–246.

——, Berger, C., and Hémon, D. (1981). Preconceptional prediction of twin pregnancies. In *Twin research 3: Twin biology and multiple pregnancy*, edited by L. Gedda, P. Parisi and W.E. Nance. New York: Alan R. Liss, pp. 175–181.

Lilienfeld, A.M. and Pasamanick, B. (1955). A study of variations in the frequency of twin births by race and socio-economic status. *Am. J. Hum. Genet. 7*, 204–217.

MacGillivray, I. (1975). Malformations and other abnormalities in twins. In *Human multiple reproduction*, edited by I. MacGillivray, P.P.S. Nylander and G. Corney. London: W.B. Saunders, pp. 165–175.

—— and Campbell, D.M. (1978). The physical characteristics and adaptations of women with twin pregnancies. In *Twin research: Clinical studies*, edited by W.E. Nance. New York: Alan R. Liss, pp. 81–86.

Melnick, M. and Myrianthopoulos, N.C. (1979). The effects of chorion type on normal and abnormal developmental variation in monozygous twins. *Am. J. Med. Genet. 4*, 147–156.

Métneki, J. and Czeizel, A. (1980). Contraceptive pills and twins. *Acta Genet. Med. Gemellol. (Rome) 29*, 233–236.

Milham, Jr., S. (1964). Pituitary gonadotrophin and dizygotic twinning. *Lancet 2*, 566.

Morgan, K. (in preparation). Population biology of twinning.

Morton, N.E., Chung, C.S., and Mi, M.P. (1967). *Genetics of interracial crosses in Hawaii. Monographs in human genetics*, 3. Basel: Karger.

———— and Schull, W.J. (1953). *Studies on consanguinity and heritability*. Atomic Bomb Casualty Commission, Hiroshima. Cited by Morton et al. (1967).

Mosteller, M., Townsend, J.I., Corey, L.A., and Nance, W.E. (1981). Twinning rates in Virginia: Secular trends and the effects of maternal age and parity. In *Twin research 3: Twin biology and multiple pregnancy*, edited by L. Gedda, P. Parisi and W.E. Nance. New York: Alan R. Liss, pp. 57–69.

Myrianthopoulos, N.C. (1970). An epidemiologic survey of twins in a large, prospectively studied population. *Am. J. Hum. Genet. 22*, 611–629.

———— (1975). Congenital malformations in twins: Epidemiologic survey. *Birth Defects 11*(8), 1–39.

Nance, W.E. (1981). Malformations unique to the twinning process. In *Twin research 3: Twin biology and multiple pregnancy*, edited by L. Gedda, P. Parisi and W.E. Nance. New York: Alan R. Liss, pp. 123–133.

————, Corey, L.A., and Boughman, J.A. (1978a). Monozygotic twin kinships: A new design for genetic and epidemiologic research. In *Genetic epidemiology*, edited by N.E. Morton and C.S. Chung. New York: Academic Press, pp. 87–132.

————, Winter, P.M., Segreti, W.O., Corey, L.A., Parisi-Prinzi, G., and Parisi, P. (1978b). A search for evidence of hereditary superfetation in man. In *Twin research: Biology and epidemiology*, edited by W.E. Nance. New York: Alan R. Liss, pp. 65–70.

National Center for Health Statistics (1980). Final natality statistics, 1978. *Monthly Vital Statistics Report 29*(1), (Suppl.), DHHS Publication No. (PHS) 80-1120.

———— (1981). Advance report of final natality statistics, 1979. *Monthly Vital Statistics Report 30*(6), (Suppl. 2), DHHS Publication No. (PHS) 81-1120.

National Office of Vital Statistics (1945–1958). *Vital statistics of the United States*. Washington, D.C.: U.S. Government Printing Office.

Nelson, C.M.K. and Bunge, R.G. (1974). Semen analysis: Evidence for changing parameters of male fertility potential. *Fertil. Steril. 25*, 503–507.

Nylander, P.P.S. (1971). Ethnic differences in twinning rates in Nigeria. *J. Biosoc. Sci. 3*, 151–157.

———— (1978). Causes of high twinning frequencies in Nigeria. In *Twin research: Biology and Epidemiology*, edited by W.E. Nance. New York: Alan R. Liss, pp. 35–43.

———— and Corney, G. (1969). Placentation and zygosity of twins in Ibadan, Nigeria. *Ann. Hum. Genet. 33*, 31–40.

Parisi, P. and Caperna, G. (1981). The changing incidence of twinning: One century of Italian statistics. In *Twin research 3: Twin biology and multiple pregnancy*, edited by L. Gedda, P. Parisi and W.E. Nance. New York: Alan R. Liss, pp. 35–48.

────── and ────── (1982). Twinning rates, fertility, and industrialization: A secular study. In *Proceedings of the Sixth International Congress of Human genetics part A*, edited by B. Bonne-Tamir. New York: Alan R. Liss, pp. 375–394.

Price, B. (1950). Primary biases in twin studies. A review of prenatal and natal difference-producing factors in monozygotic pairs. *Am. J. Hum. Genet.* 2, 293–352.

Race, R.R. and Sanger, R. (1975). *Blood groups in man* (6th ed.). Oxford: Blackwell.

Record, R.G., Armstrong, E., and Lancashire, R.J. (1978). A study of the fertility of mothers of twins. *J. Epidemiol. Community Health* 32, 183–189.

Rehan, N.E., Sobrero, A.G., and Fertig, J.W. (1975). The semen of fertile men. Statistical analysis of 1300 men. *Fertil. Steril.* 26, 492–502.

Reich, T., James, J.W., and Morris, C.A. (1972). The use of multiple thresholds in determining the mode of transmission of semi-continuous traits. *Ann. Hum. Genet.* 36, 163–184.

Renkonnen, K.O. (1966). The mothers of twins and their fertility. *Ann. Med. Exp. Fenn.* 44, 322–325.

Rhine, S.A. and Nance, W.E. (1976). Familial twinning: A case for superfetation in man. *Acta Genet. Med. Gemellol. (Rome)* 25, 66–69.

Robinson, H.P. and Caines, J.S. (1977). Sonar evidence of early pregnancy failure in patients with twin conceptions. *Br. J. Obstet. Gynaecol.* 84, 22–25.

Rose, R.J., Fulker, D.W., Miller, J.Z., Grim, C.E., and Christian, J.C. (1980). Heritability of systolic blood pressure. Analysis of variance in MZ twin parents and their children. *Acta Genet. Med. Gemellol. (Rome)* 29, 143–149.

Rothman, K.J. (1977). Fetal loss, twinning and birth weight after oral-contraceptive use. *N. Engl. J. Med.* 297, 468–471.

Russell, D.S. (1966). Pituitary gland (hypophysis). In *Pathology*, Vol. 2 (5th ed.), edited by W.A.D. Anderson. St. Louis: C.V. Mosby, pp. 1052–1073.

Scaramuzzi, R.J., Baird, D.T., Martinez, N.D., Turnbull, K.E., and Van Look, P.F.A. (1981). Ovarian function in the ewe after active immunization against testosterone. *J. Reprod. Fertil.* 61, 1–9.

Schinzel, A.A.G.L., Smith, D.W., and Miller, J.R. (1979). Monozygotic twinning and structural defects. *J. Pediatr.* 95, 921–930.

Schneider, L., Bessis, R., and Simonnet, T. (1979). The frequency of ovular resorption during the first trimester of twin pregnancy. *Acta Genet. Med. Gemellol. (Rome)* 28, 271–272.

Scrimgeour, J.B. and Baker, T.G. (1974). A possible case of superfetation in man. *J. Reprod. Fertil.* 36, 69–73.

Selvin, S. (1970). Concordance in a twin population model. *Acta Genet. Med. Gemellol. (Rome)* 19, 584–590.

────── and Janerich, D.T. (1971). Four factors influencing birth weight. *Br. J. Prev. Soc. Med.* 25, 12–16.

Smith, C. (1974). Concordance in twins: Methods and interpretation. *Am. J. Hum. Genet.* 26, 454–466.

Smith, K.D. and Steinberger, E. (1977). What is oligospermia? In *The testis in normal and infertile men*, edited by P. Troen and H.R. Nankin. New York: Raven Press, pp. 489–503.

Stevenson, A.C., Johnston, H.A., Stewart, M.I.P., and Goldring, D.R. (1966). Congenital malformations. A report of a study of series of consecutive births in 24 centres. *Bull. WHO 34* (Suppl.).

Stockard, C.R. (1921). Developmental rate and structural expression: An experimental study of twins, "double monsters" and single deformities, and the interaction among embryonic organs during their origin and development. *Am. J. Anat. 28,* 115–277.

Stocks, P. (1953). Multiple birth frequency according to parity and maternal age. *Acta Genet. Med. Gemellol. (Rome) 2,* 113–117.

Strandskov, H.H. (1945). Plural birth frequencies in the total, the "white" and the "colored" U.S. populations. *Am. J. Phys. Anthropol. 3,* 49–55.

Sutter, J. and Tabah, L. (1954). The break-up of isolates. Its genetic consequences in two French *départements. Eugen. Q. 1,* 148–154.

Timonen, S. and Carpen, E. (1968). Multiple pregnancies and photo-periodicity. *Ann. Chir. Gynaecol. Fenn. 57,* 135–138.

Uchida, I.A. (1979). Radiation-induced nondisjunction. *Environ. Health Perspect. 31,* 13–17.

U.S. Bureau of the Census (1925). *Birth, stillbirth and infant mortality statistics for the birth registration area of the United States 1923,* Ninth annual report. Washington, D.C.: U.S. Government Printing Office.

———— (1946). *Vital statistics of the United States 1944.* Washington, D.C.: U.S. Government Printing Office.

Vessey, M., Doll, R., Peto, R., Johnson, B., and Wigging, P. (1976). A long-term follow up study of women using different methods of contraception. An interim report. *J. Biosoc. Sci. 8,* 373–427.

Vollman, R.F. (1977). The menstrual cycle. In *Major problems in obstetrics and gynecology,* 7. Philadelphia: W.B. Saunders.

Vollmer, R.T. (1972). Twin concordance: A set theoretic and probability approach. *J. Theor. Biol. 36,* 367–378.

Weinberg, W. (1901). Beitrage zur Physiologie und Pathologie der Mehrlings-geburten beim Menschen. *Pfluegers Arch. ges. Physiol. 88,* 346–430.

———— (1909). Die Anlage zur Mehrlingsgeburt beim Menschen und ihre Vererbung. *Arch. Rass.-u. ges. Biol. 6,* 322–339, 470–482, and 609–630.

Westoff, C.F., Potter, Jr., R.G., Sagi, P.C., and Mishler, E.G. (1961). Fecundity. In *Family growth in metropolitan America.* Princeton, N.J.: Princeton University Press, pp. 45–69.

White, C. (1981). Matching in epidemiology as a paradigm for twin research on the etiology of disease. *Acta Genet. Med. Gemellol. (Rome) 30,* 77–86.

Wilson, R.S. (1979). Twin growth: Initial deficit, recovery, and trends in concordance from birth to nine years. *Ann. Hum. Biol. 6,* 205–220.

Wyshak. G. (1978). Statistical findings on the effects of fertility drugs on plural births. In *Twin research: Biology and epidemiology,* edited by W.E. Nance. New York: Alan R. Liss, pp. 17–33.

———— (1981). Reproductive and menstrual characteristics of mothers of multiple births and mothers of singletons only: A discriminant analysis.

In *Twin research 3: Twin biology and multiple pregnancy*, edited by L. Gedda, P. Parisi and W.E. Nance. New York: Alan R. Liss, pp. 95–105.

——— and White, C. (1965). Genealogical study of human twinning. *Am. J. Public Health* 55, 1586–1593.

Yerushalmy, J. and Sheerar, S.E. (1940). Studies on twins. I. The relation of order of birth and age of parents to the frequency of like-sexed and unlike-sexed twin deliveries. *Hum. Biol.* 12, 95–113.

Zahálková, M. (1979). Clustering of twin births in space and time. *Acta Genet. Med. Gemellol. (Rome)* 28, 259–260.

8

Congenital and Perinatal Viral Infections

Warren A. Andiman and Dorothy M. Horstmann

It has been estimated that maternal bacterial, protozoan, and viral infections affect about 2–8% of all livebirths in the United States. These infections are cumulatively responsible for a considerable amount of morbidity and mortality in infancy and childhood; they also may result in resorption of the embryo, abortion, stillbirth, intrauterine growth retardation, or persistent pre- and postnatal infection.

The outcome in a particular infant is the result of a complex interplay of epidemiologic factors, biologic attributes of the agent in question, and the immunologic status of the host. In this chapter some general epidemiologic and biologic principles as they apply to intrauterine and perinatal infections will be outlined, and certain viral infections that represent important clinical and public health problems will be discussed in more detail.

ASPECTS OF PATHOGENESIS

Primary and Recurrent Infection

Most viral infections during pregnancy are mild and limited to the upper respiratory or gastrointestinal tract; they pose no risk to the unborn child. However, in the course of *primary* infection with some agents, bloodstream invasion occurs. Virus particles, either free or associated with white blood cells, may infect the placenta, the fetus, or both. The fetus may be affected as a result of sequential replication of virus in all the layers of the placenta, or by spread of virus-infected maternal leukocytes into the fetal circulation (Driscoll, 1969; Plotkin, 1975). Also, infected chorionic cells may break off and act as emboli, carrying virus to various fetal tissues (Tondüry and Smith, 1966). In addition to viruses, *Treponema pallidum*, the etiologic agent of syphilis, and the protozoan parasite *Toxoplasma gondii* are other organisms that generally fit this pathogenetic model of potential fetal damage.

Recurrent infection occurs when host defenses are altered or when immunity—humoral, cell-mediated, or both—has declined. The result may be exogenous reinfection with the same agent, or reactivation of virus that has remained latent in an incomplete state in host cells. In both cases the second infection is apt to be a modified one, influenced by some residual immunity. For example, viremia may be prevented or greatly limited by circulating humoral antibodies. Reactivation of some viruses may nevertheless result in infection of the fetus even when the mother's primary infection occurred at some time in the past. This is especially true of the herpesviruses, a group of agents that includes herpes simplex (HSV), varicella-zoster (VZV), and the cytomegaloviruses (CMV). The herpes group of agents all share the biologic property of latency. Following primary infection, they persist in incomplete form in various host tissues, probably for life, even in the presence of high levels of circulating antibody. Reactivation may be induced by a number of factors, particularly immunosuppression. Recurrent virus shedding is from characteristic anatomic sites: HSV type 1 from the oropharynx and type 2 from the genital tract, CMV in the urine and from the uterine cervix, and VZV from the skin in the course of zoster. A mother experiencing recurrent infection of the genital tract is most apt to transmit the agent to her offspring at the time of birth, when the infant is exposed to virus-laden secretions during passage through the birth canal.

Local infection of the genital tract, whether primary or due to reactivation, may also involve the fetus by the ascending route. This is most likely to occur during prolonged rupture of the membranes and has been demonstrated most convincingly for HSV. There is little evidence that HSV or CMV can produce fetal infection by the ascending route through intact fetal membranes, although this is at least theoretically possible.

During primary maternal infection with agents such as CMV or rubella, the fetus is affected by direct invasion and continuous replication of the agent, even though the mother may not be very ill. In other instances, such as in the course of maternal influenza or measles, abortion may occur as a result of profound toxemia, fever, and metabolic disturbances associated with the disease (Hardy et al., 1961; Jespersen et al., 1977). Premature birth has been associated with maternal measles (Siegel and Fuerst, 1966).

191

Stage of Pregnancy When Maternal Infection Occurs

For each agent, the time during gestation when the infection occurs is critical with regard to outcome in the fetus. For rubella this is the first trimester, with the greatest risk of fetal malformations associated with maternal infection in the first eight weeks of pregnancy (Horstmann, et al., 1965; Peckham, 1972). Although not as clearly established as for rubella, there is some evidence that the most serious fetal CMV infections occur when the mother experiences primary infection in the first half of pregnancy. Late gestational infections with this agent apparently result in milder or completely silent infections.

In contrast to rubella, CMV, and toxoplasmosis, infections with herpes simplex, varicella-zoster, hepatitis B, and the enteroviruses pose risks to the fetus when infection is present in the mother at the end of the third trimester, in the days immediately preceding labor, or during parturition. Primary or recurrent infections with these agents jeopardize the infant in one of two ways: either by transplacental spread of infection in the days just prior to birth and before the modifying effects of maternal antibody can be transferred, or by heavy contamination of the infant with genital secretions or stool during birth.

Incidence of Congenital Infection: Influence of Geography, Socioeconomic Status, Age, and Sexual Behavior

There is great variation in the rate of maternal and fetal infection with individual agents. The frequency of infection with the more common viruses acquired in utero or around the time of birth is listed in Table 8-1. Cytomegalovirus infection is the most common congenital viral infection of humans; recurrent excretion in the maternal genital or urinary tract occurs in 2–10% of pregnant women, depending on the population examined (Hildebrandt et al., 1967; Feldman, 1969; Knox et al., 1979). Most transmission occurs peripartum. Although recurrent excretion of HSV is far less frequent, it appears to be increasing. Gestational rubella was also relatively common during the last great epidemic in 1964, but since the introduction of live attenuated rubella vaccines in 1969, the incidence of maternal infection and the congenital syndrome have declined.

The occurrence of some infections varies considerably depending on the population studied; genetic and environmental factors may play significant roles in some of these instances. For example, the rate of hepatitis B surface antigen (HBs Ag) carriage is at least 50 times more common in parts of the Far East than in the United States (Punyagupta et al., 1973; Anderson et al., 1975; Okada et al., 1975, 1976). In this instance, vertical transmission of surface antigen from

192

Table 8-1. Frequency of Maternal, Fetal, and Neonatal Viral Infections

Agent	Mother (per 1000 pregnancies)	Fetus[a] (per 1000 livebirths)	Neonates[a] (per 1000 livebirths)
Cytomegalovirus			
During pregnancy	10–130	6–34	—
At delivery	30–280	—	20–100
Herpes simplex	1–10	Rare	<0.1–0.5
Varicella-zoster	0.5–0.7	Very rare	Very rare
Rubella			
Endemic	0.1–1.0	0.2–0.5	None
Epidemic	20–40	4–30	None
Hepatitis B			
Acute infection[b]	Same as in general population	—	50–100% (United States)[c]
Antigen carrier state	1–3 (United States)	—	5–8% (United States)[c]
	50–200 (Far East)	—	40–73% (Far East)[c]
	~6 (Paris)	—	67% (Paris)[c]

[a] Number of infections acquired by the *fetus* in utero, or by the *neonate* at birth or in the early postpartum period.

[b] Acute hepatitis during third trimester or within two months postpartum.

[c] *Percentage* of exposed infants who become carriers of HBs Ag during the first six months of life.

Sources: Adapted from Klein et al. (1976); and Glasgow and Overall (1977).

large numbers of infected mothers to their offspring allows hepatitis B to persist in the Taiwanese through many generations. In addition, for reasons that are not clear, excretion of CMV occurs at least two to three times more frequently in Japan than in the United States.

Socioeconomic status also influences infection patterns with certain agents. Seroepidemiologic studies have shown that infection with HSV type 2 does not occur until puberty; thereafter, the incidence rises more rapidly in lower than in upper socioeconomic groups. On average, 50% of women of childbearing age from middle and upper income groups and 80–90% of those from lower income groups have antibodies to HSV type 2 (Nahmias, 1970; Nahmias et al., 1970a). Infection with CMV is acquired rapidly during childhood in populations living in developing countries, 80–100% being antibody-positive by 15 years of age (Li and Hanshaw, 1967; Krech et al., 1971). In contrast, in economically advanced countries, the comparable figure is 20–40%. Because both HSV type 2 and CMV infections are transmitted venereally, sexual promiscuity and early sexual activity influence the frequency of fetal and neonatal infection.

Many of the incidence figures shown in Table 8-1 are undoubtedly underestimates. There are several reasons for this. First, many congenitally infected infants are born with signs of disease that are so mild or nonspecific that congenital infection is not suspected and diagnostic tests are not performed. In addition, the majority of maternal viral infections are asymptomatic. In such instances, the physician may falsely assume that congenital infection is unlikely in the absence of a maternal history of illness during pregnancy. Also, diagnosis of congenital infection often requires a comprehensive set of virologic and serologic tests, many of which are unavailable except in large medical centers. Finally, signs of congenital infection such as nerve deafness and learning disability are often not recognized until the child is three or four years old. Although the pediatrician may consider these as possible sequelae of intrauterine or intrapartum infection, it is virtually impossible, in retrospect, to identify the responsible etiologic agent by using the available diagnostic tests.

Seasonal Influences

Some infections are endemic and occur with regularity throughout the year; others are seasonal, causing sharp outbreaks yearly or less often. As noted earlier, each agent generally causes damage at a more or less specific time during pregnancy. Therefore, the outcome of infection in each mother–infant pair depends to a large extent on the coincidence of the stage of gestation when the mother is most vulnerable and the season when particular agents predominate. For example, rubella is most prevalent in late winter and early spring. All seronegative women are at equal risk for rubella infection, but those who are in the first trimester of pregnancy during the spring are far more likely, if infected, to present a risk to their fetuses. In contrast, enterovirus circulation predominates in summer and early autumn. Because infections caused by these agents pose the greatest threat to the neonate when transmission occurs around the time of birth, mothers who deliver in the warm months are more apt to jeopardize their babies by exposure to Coxsackie and ECHO viruses. Herpes simplex, cytomegalovirus, and hepatitis B circulate year-round; there is therefore no seasonal influence on the outcome of pregnancies in mothers who have acquired these infections.

CYTOMEGALOVIRUS INFECTIONS

The cytomegaloviruses of humans belong to the herpesvirus group of agents and share with other members of this group the biologic property of latency. Following primary infection, the virus remains latent in several sites and is recurrently excreted at various times throughout life. The fetus is at risk for intrauterine infection when the mother experiences either primary or recurrent infection during pregnancy. Far more frequently, infection occurs during passage through the birth canal, or postpartum by exposure to contaminated breast milk or other maternal secretions.

The cytomegaloviruses occur in multiple antigenic types, and it is now clear that infection with one strain does not necessarily afford protection against another (Embil et al., 1970; Stagno et al., 1977b; Huang et al., 1980). Therefore, a pregnant woman who has been infected in the past is subject both to recurrent infection with her own endogenous strain, and to exogenous reinfection with other strains.

Rates of Infection in Women and Neonates

The cytomegaloviruses are ubiquitous in nature. Based on current knowledge, they are probably responsible for a greater number of congenital infections than any other microorganism. Studies of antibody prevalence indicate that there are two age ranges when acquisition of infection is most likely to occur: in the infant and toddler, and in the sexually active young adult. Because of this bimodal distribution, seroconversion rates vary widely in different populations. Between 65 and 90% of individuals living in Japan and in regions of East Africa are antibody-positive by early adolescence (Numazaki et al., 1970; Krech et al., 1971; Lang, 1975). In certain parts of the United States, Canada, and western Europe, the rates are not as high, but there appears to be a profound effect of socioeconomic status on the acquisition of CMV infection. Thus by age 21 about 60% of middle to high income groups in the United States are antibody-positive; this is approximately one-third lower than the rate in individuals of low income (Wentwerth and Alexander, 1971). Factors that may play a role in the different rates of seroconversion include poor sanitation, crowding, sexual promiscuity, breast-feeding, and the prevalence of certain early childrearing practices, such as extensive use of day-care facilities.

As noted above, socioeconomic status influences the incidence of infection and the age at which it is acquired. Although women in lower socioeconomic groups are only about twice as likely as other women to have been infected, they are at least three times more likely to transmit infection to their newborn infants. Such increased risk is not due to an increased rate of primary infection during pregnancy ($\sim$5–6 per 1000); rather, it is the result of recurrent maternal infection (Stagno et al., 1982).

195

Excretion and Transmission of Cytomegalovirus During Pregnancy and at Birth

Cervical and urinary excretion of CMV has been monitored in pregnant women in various parts of the world. All studies confirm the high frequency of infection; depending on the population studied, maternal virus excretion ranges from 11 to 28% (Alexander, 1967; Montgomery et al., 1972; Reynolds et al., 1973). Sites of excretion include the cervix, genital tract, urinary tract, oropharynx, and breast. Virus shedding is episodic and rarely persistent, but the percentage of gravidas excreting virus increases steadily throughout pregnancy (see Table 8-2). Although it had previously been assumed that the lower rates seen in the first trimester reflected the usual prevalence of excretion in the female population at large, it has now been demonstrated that the prevalence of genital tract infection in women *at term* most closely matches that found in nongravid females (Reynolds et al., 1973; Stagno et al., 1975; Knox et al., 1979). Consequently, it is now believed that the physiologic changes that accompany the first two trimesters of pregnancy have a suppressive effect that disappears in the last trimester when the rate of virus shedding returns to that seen in the nongravid population.

Cervical excretion of virus may reflect primary infection in the mother, but is about nine times more likely to represent reactivation of latent virus (Stagno et al., 1982). Although transmission and serious congenital disease is much more likely to occur as a result of primary infection, recent observations indicate that recurrent infections in the mother are associated with fetal infection more frequently than had been appreciated in the past. Studies by Stagno and co-workers have documented congenital infection in the offspring of 0.5–1.5% of women who were known to be seropositive before conception

Table 8-2. Rate of Isolation of CMV from Cultures of the Uterine Cervix or Vagina at Different Stages of Pregnancy

	Trimester					
	First		*Second*		*Third*	
Reference	No. Tested	% Positive	No. Tested	% Positive	No Tested	% Positive
Numazaki et al. (1970)	30	0	62	9.6	61	27.8
Montgomery et al. (1972)	43	2	83	7	49	12
Reynolds et al. (1973)	76	1.3	241	6.6	261	13.4

Source: Adapted from Alford et al. (1980).

(Stagno et al., 1982). Similar data comparing the relative risks of congenital CMV infection in a low-income group are outlined in Table 8-3. Additional evidence that congenital infection may occur in infants of antibody-positive mothers comes from studies of women who have delivered more than one affected baby in successive pregnancies (Embil et al., 1970; Stagno et al., 1973). Analysis of the DNA of viruses isolated from several such cases proved that the second infection can result from reactivation of the mother's endogenous strain or from reinfection with a new strain.

In the case of primary infection, transmission of CMV to the fetus occurs as a result of maternal viremia or transplacental passage of infected leukocytes. The route by which virus reaches the fetus in the case of reactivated infection, which is less likely to be accompanied by viremia, has not been established. In this instance, some investigators have suggested that transplacental transit of infected white blood cells or direct spread from the glandular-rich endometrium may be the mechanisms involved.

Transmission of CMV at the time of birth or in the early postpartum period occurs much more frequently than does infection in utero. Most babies so affected begin to excrete CMV at two to six weeks of age. There is marked variability in the rate of perinatal infection. For example, in Helsinki, Finland, 24% of infants are infected by three months of age, compared to a rate of less than 5% in Manchester, England (Collaborative Study, 1970; Granström et al., 1977). The rate in the United States lies midway between those two figures. The highest infection rate occurs in Japan, where 60% of babies are excreting virus by one year of age. In all cases, the major source of

Table 8-3. Rate of Congenital CMV Infection in a Low-Income Population in Relationship to Recurrent Maternal Infection

	No. infants infected [a]	*Percentage infected*
Incidence in general infant population	31 (1412)	2.2
Incidence with recurrent maternal infection		
Mother known to be previously seropositive	8 (457)	1.8
Mother known to have excreted CMV previously	1 (58)	1.7
Mother known to have transmitted CMV in previous pregnancy	1 (26)	3.8

[a] Total number of infants in each group shown in parentheses.

Source: Adapted from Alford et al. (1980).

virus for the neonate is the mother. In addition to an infected genital tract, breast milk appears to be the next most common source of postnatal infection. On average, 18% of seroimmune women shed virus into breast milk or at some other site; and about half of the infants exposed to breast milk virus become infected (Alford et al., 1980). Furthermore, it has been shown that women who have previously delivered a congenitally infected infant are much more likely to be excretors than those who have not. This suggests that there are significant host factors that regulate the extent to which viral activation and excretion occur.

Sequelae of Intrauterine CMV Infection

Despite the high incidence of natally or postnatally acquired CMV infection, in the vast majority of instances the result is asymptomatic infection without apparent long-term sequelae. At birth, 1–3% of all infants are excreting CMV; more than 90% of such congenitally infected infants are asymptomatic. The rest may present clinical manifestations similar to those of congenital rubella. Typical features, which may exist alone or in combination, include intrauterine growth retardation, hepatosplenomegaly, jaundice, petechiae or purpura, microcephaly, chorioretinitis, and cerebral calcifications. Infants with the full-blown syndrome either die, or they survive with profound mental impairment. In the large group of infants who are asymptomatic at birth, damage to the auditory nerve is the most serious sequela (Reynolds et al., 1974; Stagno et al., 1977b). Infection of the auditory mechanism is progressive, and loss of hearing may not become apparent until three to five years of age. It is now estimated that about 7–15% of infected infants who survive the neonatal period without symptoms develop deafness or other late-appearing subtle defects, such as minimal brain dysfunction (Hanshaw et al., 1976). Because 1–3% of all pregnancies will result in the birth of an infant *congenitally* infected with CMV, and approximately 20% of such infants sustain some damage, then in the United States at least 0.2% of all livebirths, or approximately 7000 infants, are affected annually by intrauterine CMV infection.

HERPES SIMPLEX INFECTIONS

Herpes simplex virus exists in two forms, type 1 and type 2, which can be distinguished antigenically, biochemically, and biologically. They are also characterized by different primary sites of attack and modes of transmission. Herpes simplex virus type 1 infects most individuals before five years of age; it may induce gingivostomatitis, encephalitis, or eye infections, but at least 90% of primary infections are asymptomatic. In contrast, HSV type 2 is transmitted venereally and is responsible for most cases of herpes genitalis. Following the primary infection, HSV type 1 generally remains latent in the trigeminal ganglia, and HSV type 2 in the sacral ganglia. At present, 10–25% of genital herpes simplex infections are caused by HSV type 1. This number has been increasing of late and may reflect an increase in orogenital sex. Herpes genitalis is of greatest concern to the practicing obstetrician and pediatrician when infection, either primary or recurrent, occurs during pregnancy, especially around the time of delivery.

Rates of Maternal Genital Herpes Infection and Infection in the Newborn

Antibodies resulting from infection with HSV type 2 are present in 10–70% of women, depending on sexual activity and socioeconomic class (Nahmias et al., 1970; Rawls et al., 1971). In the United States as a whole, the frequency of genital herpes among pregnant women is about 5–10 per 1000. In women of lower socioeconomic status, genital excretion of HSV type 2 occurs more frequently than in private obstetric patients (Ng et al., 1970; Naib et al., 1973). However, there is evidence that the number and rate of consultations with private physicians for genital herpes simplex infection has increased markedly in the United States, from 29,560 in 1966 to 260,890 in 1979 (Centers for Disease Control, 1982).

Despite these high rates of maternal infection and excretion, the number of infants born each year with clinically apparent infections due to HSV are far fewer than one would predict. Studies among low socioeconomic groups in New York and in Atlanta, Georgia, where 80–90% of women are seropositive for HSV type 2, indicate that recognizable congenital HSV infections occur in only about 1 of 7500 deliveries (Nahmias et al., 1970a). In the United States as a whole, the number of reported cases is approximately 120 per year; this is equivalent to 1 in 27,000 livebirths. These discrepancies can only be explained in two ways: Either the risk of neonatal herpes from maternal genital disease is less than expected, or the frequency of unreported, unrecognized, or asymptomatic neonatal infection is far greater than previously suspected.

Maternal Excretion and Transmission

The infant can acquire HSV infection in one of three ways: (1) in utero, presumably in the course of primary infection in the mother, (2) at the time of birth, by exposure to secretions in the maternal genital tract, and (3) postpartum, following exposure to the mother,

other family members, hospital personnel, or other infected neonates, any of whom may be actively excreting HSV type 1 or type 2.

By far the most important source of infection for the fetus is the contaminated genital tract of the mother, although this can be definitely documented in only half the neonatal cases. The major explanation for the difficulty in confirming the source of infection is that most mothers who transmit virus to their babies have asymptomatic infections. Approximately 40–70% have had no symptoms of genital disease at any time during their pregnancies, or have nonspecific abnormal findings that do not suggest herpes to either the physician or the patient (Whitley et al., 1980). In some instances, infected women have no complaints even though their obstetricians find genital vesicles or ulcers in the course of routine care.

Genital excretion, confirmed by culture or cytology, occurs three to seven times more frequently in pregnant women than in nonpregnant women, and the duration of viral excretion accompanying each episode may be longer during pregnancy (Bolognese et al., 1976; Nahmias et al., 1971). Also, the rate of excretion tends to be higher in the last trimester than during the first two, as in CMV infection.

Primary rather than recurrent infection, and active genital shedding of virus at the time of delivery are significant risk factors for the infant. On the basis of the results of one study, when maternal infection is present after 32 weeks gestation the overall risk of neonatal herpes infection is about 10%; when the virus is present at delivery, the risk increases to approximately 40% (Nahmias et al., 1971). Results of another study suggest that the risks associated with vaginal delivery following late gestational infection are lower (Grossman et al., 1981).

There is strong circumstantial evidence that HSV can, in rare instances, cause congenital infection by the transplacental route. There is a threefold greater risk of abortion in women who experience genital infection in the first half of pregnancy when compared with the rate in the general obstetric population, and the risk appears to be higher when the infection is a primary one (Naib et al., 1970; Nahmias et al., 1971). In a few instances virus has been isolated from abortus material, and in one case the fetal membranes were found to contain intranuclear inclusions. Some infants have had herpetic skin lesions at birth in the absence of premature rupture of the membranes, suggesting an ascending route of virus spread. Also, a few infants have been born with a distinctive array of congenital malformations; all have had laboratory evidence of HSV infection at birth, and genital HSV infection during pregnancy was confirmed in their mothers (Shaffer, 1965; South et al., 1969; Florman et al., 1973; Montgomery et al., 1973).

200

Type 2 HSV infections acquired in the early postnatal period have also been described in about 24 infants. Half were acquired from the mother; the rest were apparently acquired from hospital employees or family.

Characteristics of the Maternal and Neonatal Populations Infected with Herpes Simplex Virus

Data collected by members of the Collaborative Antiviral Study Group have helped define the characteristics of mothers and babies infected with herpes simplex virus (Whitley et al., 1980). Of 56 mothers delivering HSV-infected newborns, the majority were white and young, having a mean age of 21 years; eight individuals were between 12 and 17 years of age, and more than half were married. Prior spontaneous abortion had occurred in 21%. The prevalence of other venereal diseases was 11%. Of mothers giving birth to infected babies, 70% were asymptomatic at the time of delivery. However, about 75% of the women in this group had a history of recurrent HSV infections in the past, and 12.5% reported recurrent penile lesions in their sexual partners.

Among the infected neonates, 46% were born prematurely and 23% had birthweights less than 1800 g (Whitley et al., 1980). These findings further support prior observations and implicate HSV as a cause of premature labor, but the pathogenesis of this relationship is not understood. Even among the premature newborns, 31% had uncomplicated nursery courses until the onset of HSV infection, and 67% of the term infants were well in the nursery and had already been discharged when evidence of infection appeared. Transmission, long-term survival, and morbidity were not influenced in any way by the presence of transplacentally acquired antibody to herpes simplex virus.

Managing the Pregnant Woman Infected with Herpes Simplex Virus

The risk of birth defects in infants born to mothers who experience a primary or recurrent infection during the first half of pregnancy is not precisely known, but it is considered to be far too low to consider interruption of the pregnancy.

Current recommendations are that women with a history of genital HSV infection as well as those who have active lesions within two months of delivery should be followed serially with viral cultures or Papanicolaou smears during the last four to six weeks of pregnancy (Visintine et al., 1978). If cultures are positive within a week of

201

delivery, most obstetricians elect to deliver the baby by cesarian section. This course is based on evidence that the principal source of infection for the newborn infant is exposure to virus present in the birth canal. Because disseminated or central nervous system infection in the newborn is relatively rare, and the majority of infants born to mothers with infection are clinically normal, the actual benefits of cesarian section have been difficult to evaluate by prospective study. However, retrospective analysis of the outcome of pregnancies in which the mother was culture-positive at term is shown in Table 8-4. Although the numbers are relatively small, abdominal delivery appears to be a successful tactic (Grossman et al., 1981; Nahmias et al., 1971). There are, however, rare instances in which cesarian section appears not to have been preventive; it is possible that infection may have ascended through microscopic tears in the fetal membranes in these instances.

The newest of the antiviral chemotherapeutic agents, acycloguanosine (Acyclovir), has recently been licensed in the United States as a topical preparation for the treatment of *initial* genital HSV infections. In such cases it has provided symptomatic relief and has reduced the duration of virus shedding by a few days. Acyclovir has no effect on the number or the severity of recurrent infections. Furthermore, strains of HSV resistant to Acyclovir have already been recovered from patients. The number of such resistant isolates will probably increase with more widespread use of the drug. Whether the parenteral or oral forms of the drug will be found safe for use during pregnancy and effective in reducing shedding during recurrent infection is not yet known.

Table 8-4. Risk of Neonatal Herpes Infection in Infants of Mothers with Culture-Proven Genital Infection at Term

Type of delivery	No. infants infected (no. cases)[a]	
	Premature	Full-term[b]
Vaginal	5 (29)	4 (14)
Cesarian section		
Within four hours of membrane rupture	0 (2)	0 (15)
After longer than four hours of membrane rupture	2 (2)	2 (8)

[a] Within one week before delivery.
[b] 36–44 weeks gestation.
Sources: Compiled from Grossman et al. (1981); and Nahmias et al. (1971). Note: *None* of the infants studied by Grossman, et al. became infected.

HEPATITIS B

Hepatitis B is the most extensively studied of the viruses that cause acute and sometimes chronic infection of the liver. Little is known about maternal and neonatal infections with hepatitis A or the non A–non B group of viruses, because serologic and culture techniques for these agents are limited to only a few highly specialized laboratories. In contrast, a veritable explosion of information has accumulated during the past few years regarding hepatitis B. This is primarily the result of seroepidemiologic studies that have been based on well-understood virus antigen–antibody systems: surface antigen (HBs Ag), core antigen (HBc Ag), and e-antigen. Serologic techniques are widely available and have been applied in studies of hepatitis B in the pregnant woman and her offspring. The tests most commonly performed are for HBs Ag and anti-HBs; infectivity is correlated with the presence of HBs Ag in the blood, particularly if e-antigen is also detected.

Prevalence of HBs Antigenemia

In the United States, between 0.1 and 0.3% of individuals are HBs Ag-positive; the highest prevalence is among the indigent, male homosexuals, multiply transfused patients, and drug addicts (Czaja, 1979). In Asia the rates are very much higher, especially among the Taiwanese, where they are around 15% (Stevens et al., 1975). The prevalence of anti-HBs in the United States and western Europe is about 11% (Czaja, 1979). The presence of this antibody indicates that the individual has had infection in the past and is no longer infectious.

The prevalence of HBs Ag in the blood of pregnant women ranges from 0.1 to 16% and reflects the prevalence of antigen carriage in the general ethnic community from which the woman originates (Anderson et al., 1975; Okada et al., 1976; Beasley et al., 1977). Family members of known antigen-positive individuals are ten times more likely to have HBs Ag or anti-HBs in their blood than control families in the same ethnic group. This attests to the frequency of virus transmission among members of the same household. Vertical transmission from mother to infant is considered to be a major source of infection.

Transmission of Infection from Mother to Infant

Antigen-positive mothers, or mothers with acute hepatitis, may transmit hepatitis B to their infants in utero, at the time of birth, or postnatally. Although the rates of premature birth, low birthweight, and neonatal death are somewhat higher in the presence of maternal HBs Ag, there is no evidence for an association between maternal infection and congenital malformation. The usual age at which antigenemia can be detected in infants born to chronic carrier mothers is 8–16 weeks (Derso et al., 1978; Dupuy et al., 1978; Mollica et al., 1979). This temporal pattern is considered to be most compatible with exposure occurring during birth, as a result of contamination by vaginal secretions and maternal blood.

Five studies have specifically addressed the issue of transmission and outcome in mothers who have had acute hepatitis B during pregnancy (Schweitzer et al., 1972, 1973, 1973a; Cossart, 1974; Gerety and Schweitzer, 1977). In one, 56 mother–infant pairs were examined; the mothers had become ill during pregnancy or within six months after delivery. Transmission occurred in nearly 50% of the pairs (Schweitzer et al., 1972). The results of these studies indicate that the risk of neonatal infection appears to be greatest (67–76%) when maternal infection occurs in the third trimester or soon after delivery; when acute hepatitis occurs in the first half of pregnancy the risk is only 10%. Infants born to mothers with acute infection usually become antigen-positive at an earlier age (four to eight weeks) than those who acquire infection perinatally. Although most such infants remain asymptomatic, they may have abnormalities in liver biochemistries. Many maintain HBs Ag in their blood for as long as two years without developing antibody, and some have abnormal hepatic histology on biopsy. Follow-up studies have not yet been conducted over a sufficient period of time to indicate whether the incidence of chronic hepatitis, hepatocellular carcinoma, or immune complex disease in childhood or early adult years are late sequelae.

The risks associated with maternal carriage of HBs Ag have been extensively studied. Hepatitis B surface antigen is vertically transmitted to a large proportion (40–70%) of Japanese and Taiwanese infants born to asymptomatic chronic carrier mothers. The rates are generally lower in the United States and in parts of western Europe (0–36%); however, in several areas they have ranged from 67–86%, even in the presence of low endemicity of the chronic carrier state (Schweitzer et al., 1973a; Okada et al., 1975; Stevens et al., 1975; Gerety and Schweitzer, 1977). There is suggestive evidence that under such circumstances the affected infants remain HBs Ag-positive for only short periods—less than three months—whereas in Japan and Taiwan they are likely to develop persistent antigenemia unaccompanied by overt signs of hepatic disease (Dupuy et al., 1978). Such chronically infected children form the pool from which vertical transmission occurs in the next generation.

Examination of cord blood for the presence of HBs Ag as a means of identifying infected neonates is not a helpful procedure. The cord blood may be falsely positive because of contamination with maternal blood, or it may be negative, because the first exposure often occurs at the time of birth.

Although postpartum transmission is known to occur by the parenteral (blood transfusions) and oropharyngeal routes (breast milk, other maternal secretions), it is not likely that these are important sources as compared to infection at the time of birth.

The accumulated evidence thus points to the association of high rates of transmission of hepatitis B infection with (1) Asian origin, (2) maternal acute hepatitis in the third trimester or in the months immediately postpartum, (3) higher maternal titers of HBs Ag, and (4) presence of e-antigen in maternal serum.

Management of Infection in the Newborn and Prevention with Vaccine

Both immune serum globulin (ISG) and hepatitis B immune globulin (HBIG) are available for prophylaxis of infection in the neonate. Prophylaxis is recommended for infants born to mothers with acute hepatitis in the third trimester and for babies of antigen-positive mothers. Neither ISG nor HBIG is effective in altering the course of already established infection, but HBIG has been shown to be effective in preventing the carrier state in infants of antigenemic mothers (Stevens et al., 1982).

An inactivated hepatitis B vaccine was licensed in the United States in 1981. It is recommended for immunization of infants, children, and adults who are considered to be at increased risk of contracting hepatitis B infection. It has not been studied adequately in pregnant women and nursing mothers, and it is unlikely that such studies will be done. However, because of the demonstrated safety, immunogenicity, and protective efficacy of the vaccine, and because inactivated vaccine does not cause viremia, Krugman suggests that pregnant women should not be denied protection if they are at risk, especially if they live or work in areas where hepatitis is endemic (Krugman, 1982).

RUBELLA

The importance of rubella (German measles) rests almost entirely on the remarkable teratogenicity of the virus, first noted by Gregg, an Australian ophthalmologist, in 1941. It was not until 1962 that the virus was first isolated in tissue culture; yet in 1969, after the short span of only seven years, several effective vaccines had already been developed and licensed. Their use has had a profound impact on the incidence of the disease, which has declined sharply. Yet obstetricians are still confronted with problems related to possible exposure or infection of pregnant women, and inadvertent vaccination during pregnancy.

Rubella exists worldwide and remains an endemic infection in tropical and semitropical areas. Until 1969, epidemics in the United States occurred in 6- to 9-year cycles, with extremely large outbreaks every 10–20 years, the last in 1964. In that year some 450,000 cases were reported, and 20,000 infants were subsequently born with the congenital rubella syndrome. The reported cases of rubella reflect only a fraction of the actual incidence, however, for as with other mild illnesses, underreporting is the rule. Furthermore, the clinical features—fever, rash, and lymphadenopathy—are not highly specific, and cases often go undiagnosed. In addition, approximately two of every three infections are completely asymptomatic.

Before widespread use of rubella vaccine, the disease was commonest among schoolchildren 5–9 years old, but many susceptible adolescents and young adults were also infected. Serologic surveys indicated that as a result of continuous circulation of the virus in the United States and similar countries, approximately 85% of individuals had been infected and were immune by age 15–19, and close to 100% by 35–40 years of age. In developing countries an immunity rate of >90% is achieved much earlier—by age <5–10 years (Horstmann, 1982).

Transmission of rubella is from person to person, presumably via airborne-droplet infection. The period of communicability is from approximately seven days before to five days after onset, but is maximal around the time of appearance of the rash. The most characteristic clinical finding is tender enlargement of posterior auricular and posterior cervical lymph nodes. The rash is maculopapular and is always present on the face, a helpful diagnostic point.

Congenital Rubella

Much of what is known about the epidemiology and pathogenesis of congenital rubella resulted from extensive laboratory investigations during the 1964 epidemic. Tests on abortuses and on newborn infants revealed that there are several possible outcomes when the disease occurs during pregnancy: The fetus may escape infection completely; it may be inapparently infected and suffer no pathologic consequences; or there may be mild to severe single or multiorgan involvement. Both clinically apparent and totally inapparent maternal infection can result in transmission to the fetus.

The risk of fetal damage is greatest when the disease occurs during the first trimester of pregnancy, especially the period of organogenesis, between the fourth and eighth weeks (Cooper and Krugman, 1967; Peckham, 1972). However, infection in the several weeks before conception as well as in the fourth or even fifth months of gestation also carries some risk, particularly for hearing impairment (Hardy et al., 1969; Vejtorp and Mansa, 1980). No cases of congenital rubella have been reported when maternal infection occurred after the twentieth week.

Transmission to the fetus occurs as a result of maternal viremia, which lasts for approximately one week before onset and may seed many fetal tissues. Inflammatory foci regularly develop in the placenta, and occasionally infected cells of the chorionic villi break off and act as emboli (Tondüry and Smith, 1966). The mechanism by which rubella virus induces pathologic changes in the fetus is not well understood. The virus is not a lytic one and therefore does not destroy infected cells but sets up a chronic infection that persists throughout fetal life. The immune response is different from that in postnatally acquired infection. Rubella-specific IgM antibody appears between 16 and 20 weeks of gestation, is present at birth, and continues to rise over the first few months of life (Alford, 1976). Fetal IgG antibodies develop concomitantly and persist, whereas the passively acquired maternal IgG gradually declines in the months following birth. The presence of IgM in cord blood is diagnostic of intrauterine infection, but its absence does not rule out rubella (Alford, 1971).

Despite the presence of specific antibody, newborn infants excrete large amounts of virus from the throat and other sites, and are a source of contagion to susceptibles exposed to them. Virus shedding continues for many months—by approximately 60% of infants at 1–4 months, 30% at 5–8 months, and 5–10% at 9–12 months (Cooper and Krugman, 1967). The agent has been recovered from a cataract removed at three years of age. Auditory nerve deafness and brain damage may be the result of persistent replication of virus in early life (Cooper, 1975; Gumpel, 1972).

The most prominent clinical features of congenital rubella are intrauterine growth retardation, cataract(s), patent ductus arteriosus or other cardiac anomalies, and hearing impairment, which—along with psychomotor retardation—does not usually become apparent until after one to two years of age. Many other abnormalities may also be present, including hepatosplenomegaly, jaundice, thrombocytopenic purpura, and radiolucencies of the long bones; involvement of virtually every organ and tissue has been reported at one time or another (Alford, 1976). Mortality in severely involved infants is high, particularly during the first year of life.

Diagnosis of the congenital disease can often be made on the basis of clinical findings, but laboratory confirmation may be required to differentiate rubella from other congenital infections such as CMV and toxoplasmosis. Virus isolation is slow and difficult; serologic diagnosis is therefore more commonly used (Alford, 1976). The presence of specific IgM in the infant's serum indicates intrauterine infection. If no IgM is detected, it is necessary to examine the serum from *both* newborn infant and mother for antibody; the titers will be similar. The test should be repeated after four to six months, at which time the mother's titer will remain essentially unchanged; in the absence of fetal infection, the infant's antibody level will have declined or disappeared as a result of loss of maternal antibody, but if in utero infection occurred, the titer will remain elevated and may have increased.

Rubella in the Vaccine Era

VACCINATION PROGRAMS

The main objective of all rubella immunization programs is to prevent the congential disease. Two different vaccination policies exist. In the United States, vaccine is recommended for all prepubertal children; at present it is given chiefly to infants 12–15 months old as part of routine immunization. The aim of this policy is to provide herd immunity of a high degree, thereby interrupting the circulation of wild virus and its subsequent transmission to women of childbearing age. In addition, vaccination is recommended for adolescent girls and young adult females, provided they are not pregnant and understand the necessity for birth control measures for the ensuing three months. Prenatal screening for immunity is part of good obstetric practice, and those identified as seronegative can then be immunized in the immediate postpartum period. In the United Kingdom and in some European countries a more select policy exists. Vaccination is recommended primarily for young adolescent girls 13–14 years old and for adult women who are considered to be at "high risk," such as teachers, nurses, and other health personnel.

INADVERTENT VACCINATION DURING PREGNANCY

Despite the strong contraindication to vaccination during pregnancy, there have been many instances in which it has occurred inadvertently. Because of this possibility it is desirable to determine the immune status of postpubertal women prior to vaccine administration, or at least to obtain a serum specimen for subsequent testing should the individual prove to have been pregnant when immunized. If a susceptible pregnant woman is infected by the vaccine virus, the fetus is at risk of developing a chronic infection (Larson et al., 1971; Fleet et al., 1974). The Centers for Disease Control have collected information on 343 such women, 145 of whom elected to terminate the pregnancy; rubella virus was recovered from the abortuses of 6 of 28 (21%) as late as 20 weeks after vaccination (Modlin et al., 1976). Among the 84 susceptibles who chose to carry the pregnancy to term, all delivered infants who appeared normal at birth (Centers for Disease Control, 1980), but 3 of the 30 infants tested had experienced intrauterine infection as evidenced by the presence of rubella-specific IgM, and elevated hemagglutination inhibitor antibody levels persisting at six months of age in several others (Hayden et al., 1980). There is therefore some risk to the fetus as a result of maternal infection with vaccine virus, but this is clearly very low, probably under 5%, in contrast to the approximately 20% with congenital anomalies apparent at birth following natural infection.

Control of Rubella in the United States

The number of cases of rubella reported annually has dropped from approximately 50,000 in 1970 to 4000 in 1980 (Preblud et al., 1980). There appears to have been a concomitant decline in the congenital disease, but because of the late onset of signs in some cases, reporting is often delayed and incomplete. No major epidemics have occurred since 1964, and the cyclic behavior of the disease has been interrupted. However, throughout the 1970s localized outbreaks continued, and a new pattern of age distribution of cases appeared. Rubella ceased being a disease of schoolchildren, and instead of reported cases were in individuals over 15 years old, largely students in high schools and universities, and military recruits (Klock and Rachelefsky, 1973; Preblud et al., 1980). This behavior reflected results of serologic surveys that indicated that the percentage of susceptibles over 15 years of age has not changed significantly since 1969 despite extensive use of the vaccine (Centers for Disease Control, 1976; Horstmann, 1982a). Hospital-based outbreaks involving physicians have been of particular concern (Polk et al., 1980). As a result many hospitals now require antibody testing and immunization of all seronegative personnel, male and female.

Beginning in 1980 and continuing in 1981, the annual incidence of rubella declined further to an all-time low, with sharp reduction in the number of cases in those over 15 and also in young age groups

(Centers for Disease Control, 1980). This pattern is probably a result of intensified efforts to immunize adolescents and young adults and to improve vaccination rates among children. Many states now require proof of vaccination (or a history of the disease) for school entry, a measure that has resulted in considerably higher immunization rates in the childhood population.

In terms of the importance of these changes in the prevention of congenital rubella, a major factor will be the degree to which wild virus continues to circulate in future years. Despite marked decline, it is unlikely that such circulation will completely disappear. On exposure, reinfection is known to occur at a higher rate in individuals with vaccine-induced immunity than in those who experienced natural infection (Horstmann et al., 1970). The crucial question is whether or not viremia will accompany reinfection during pregnancy in young women immunized long before, in infancy. This likelihood should now be less probable, because the only vaccine currently in use in the United States is the more immunogenic RA27/3 strain (Meruvax II), which has been widely available in Europe for many years. It is more effective than earlier vaccines in inducing neutralizing antibodies (which are thought to be the protective ones), it produces higher titers and a wider spectrum of antibody responses than other strains, and it has the added virtue of inducing local secretory antibody in the nasopharynx, the first line of defense (Plotkin et al., 1973). The widespread use of this vaccine should provide a more sturdy and long-lived protective immunity and result in further improvement in the control of rubella in the United States.

REFERENCES

Alexander, E.R. (1967). Maternal and neonatal infection with cytomegalovirus in Taiwan. *Pediatr. Res. 1*, 210 (abstract).

Alford, C.A. (1971). Immunoglobulin determinations in the diagnosis of fetal infection. *Ped. Clin. North Am. 18*, 99–113.

—— (1976). Rubella. In *Infectious diseases of the fetus and newborns*, edited by J. Remington and J. Klein. Philadelphia: W.B. Saunders, pp. 71–106.

——, Stagno, S., Pass, R.F. (1980). Natural history of perinatal cytomegaloviral infection. In *Perinatal infections*, Ciba Foundation Symposium 77, Amsterdam, Oxford, New York: Excerpta Medica, pp. 125–149.

Anderson, K.E., Stevens, C.E., and Tsuei, J.J., (1975). Hepatitis B antigen in infants born to mothers with chronic hepatitis B antigenemia in Taiwan. *Am. J. Dis. Child. 129*, 1389–1392.

Beasley, R.P., Trepo, C., Stevens, C.E., and Szmuness, W. (1977). The e antigen and vertical transmission of hepatitis B surface antigen. *Am. J. Epidemiol. 105*, 94–98.

Bolognese, R.J., Corson, S.L., Fuccillo, D.A., Traub, R., Moder, F., and Sever, J.L. (1976). Herpesvirus hominis type II infections in asymptomatic pregnant women. *Obstet. Gynecol. 48*, 507–510.

Centers for Disease Control (1976). *Rubella surveillance. July 1973–December 1975*. U.S. Public Health Service.

Centers for Disease Control (1980). *Rubella surveillance. Jan. 1976–Dec. 1978*. U.S. Public Health Service.

Centers for Disease Control (1982). Genital herpes infection—United States, 1966–1979. *Morbidity Mortality Weekly Rep. 31*, 137.

Collaborative Study (1970). Cytomegalovirus infection in the northwest of England: A report on a two-year study. *Arch. Dis. Child. 45*, 513–522.

Cooper, L.Z. (1975). Congenital rubella in the United States. In *Symposium on infections of the fetus and newborn infant*, edited by S. Krugman and A.A. Gershon. New York: Alan R. Liss, pp. 1–22.

—— and Krugman, S. (1967). Clinical manifestations of postnatal and congenital rubella. *Arch. Ophthalmol. 77*, 434–439.

Cossart, Y.E. (1974). Acquisition of hepatitis B antigen in the newborn period. *Postgrad. Med. J. 50*, 334–337.

Czaja, A.J. (1979). Serologic markers of hepatitis A and B in acute and chronic liver disease. *Mayo Clin. Proc. 54*, 721–732.

Derso, A., Boxall, E.H., Tarlow, M.J., and Flewett, T.H. (1978). Transmission of Hbs Ag from mother to infant in four ethnic groups. *Br. Med. J. 1*, 949–952.

Driscoll, S.G. (1969). Histopathology of gestational rubella. *Am. J. Dis. Child. 118*, 49–53.

Dupuy, J.M., Giraud, P., Dupuy, C., Drouet, J., and Hoofnagle, J. (1978). Hepatitis B in children. II. Study of children born to chronic HBs Ag carrier mothers. *J. Pediatr. 92*, 200–204.

Embil, J., Ozere, R., and Haldane E. (1970). Congenital cytomegalovirus infection in two siblings from consecutive pregnancies. *J. Pediatr. 77*, 417.

Feldman, R.A. (1969). Cytomegalovirus infection during pregnancy. *Am. J. Dis. Child. 117*, 517–521.

Fleet, W.J., Jr., Benz, E.W., Jr., and Karzon, D.T. (1974). Fetal consequences of maternal rubella immunization. *J.A.M.A. 227*, 621–627.

Florman, A.L., Gershon, A.A., Blackett, P.R., and Nahmias, A.J. (1973). Intrauterine infection with herpes simplex virus. *J.A.M.A. 225*, 129–132.

Gerety, R.J. and Schweitzer, I.L. (1977). Viral hepatitis type B during pregnancy, the neonatal period, and infancy. *J. Pediatr. 90*, 368–374.

Glasgow, L.A. and Overall, J.C. (1977). Viral and protozoal perinatal infections of the fetus and newborn. In *Neonatal-perinatal medicine, diseases of the fetus and infant*, edited by R.E. Behrman. St. Louis: C.V. Mosby.

Granström, M.L., Leinikki, P., Santavuori, P., and Pettay, O. (1977). Perinatal cytomegalovirus infection in man. *Arch. Dis. Child. 52*, 354–359.

Gregg, N. McA. (1941). Congenital cataract following German measles in the mother. *Trans. Opthalmol. Soc. Aust. 3*, 35.

Grossman, J.H., Wallen, W.C., and Sever, J. (1981). Management of genital herpes simplex virus infection during pregnancy. *Obstet. Gynecol. 58*, 1–4.

Gumpel, S.M. (1972). Clinical and social status of patients with congenital rubella. *Arch. Dis. Child. 47*, 330–337.

Hanshaw, J.B., Scheiner, A.P., Moxley, A.W., Gaev, L., Abel, V., and Scheiner, B. (1976). School failure and deafness after "silent" congenital cytomegalovirus infection. *N. Engl. J. Med. 295*, 468–470.

Hardy, J.B., Azarowicz, E.N., Mannini, A., Medearis, D.M., and Cooke, R.E. (1961). The effect of Asian influenza on the outcome of pregnancy. *Am. J. Public Health 51*, 1182–1188.

———, McCracken, G.H., Gilkeson, M.R., and Sever, J.L. (1969). Adverse fetal outcome following maternal rubella after the first trimester of pregnancy. *J.A.M.A. 207*, 2414–2420.

Hayden, G.F., Hermann, K.L., Buimovici-Klein, E. Weiss, K.E., Nieburg, P.I., and Mitchell, J.E. (1980). Subclinical congenital rubella infection associated with maternal rubella vaccination in early pregnancy. *J. Pediatr. 96*, 869–872.

Hildebrandt, R.J., Sever, J.L., Margileth, A.M., and Callagan, D.A. (1967). Cytomegalovirus in the normal pregnant woman. *Am. J. Obstet. Gynecol. 98*, 1125–1128.

Horstmann, D.M. (1982). Rubella. In *Viral infections of humans. Epidemiology and control* (2nd ed.), edited by A.S. Evans. New York: Plenum.

——— (1982a). Rubella. *Clin. Obstet. Gynecol. 25*, 585–597.

———, Banatvala, J.E., Riordan, J.T., Payne, M.C., Whittemore, R., Opton, E.M., and Florey, C. (1965). Maternal rubella and the rubella syndrome in infants. *Am. J. Dis. Child. 110*, 408–415.

———, Liebhaber, H., LeBouvier, G., Rosenberg, D.A., and Halstead, S.B. (1970). Rubella: Reinfection of vaccinated and naturally immune persons exposed in an epidemic. *N. Engl. J. Med. 283*, 771–778.

Huang, E-S., Alford, C.A., Reynolds, D.W., Stagno, S., and Pass, R.F. (1980). Molecular epidemiology of cytomegalovirus infections in women and their infants. *N. Engl. J. Med. 303*, 958–962.

Jespersen, C.S., Littauer, J., and Sagild, U. (1977). Measles as a cause of fetal defects: A retrospective study of ten measles epidemics in Greenland. *Acta Paediatr. Scand. 66*, 367–372.

Klein, J.O., Remington, J.S., and Marcy, S.M. (1976). An introduction to infections of the fetus and newborn infant. In *Infectious diseases of the fetus and newborn infant*, edited by J.S. Remington and J.O. Klein. Philadelphia: W.B. Saunders, pp. 1–32.

Klock, L.E. and Rachelefsky, G.S. (1973). Failure of rubella herd immunity during an epidemic. *N. Engl. J. Med. 288*, 69–72.

Knox, G.E., Pass, R.F., Reynolds, D.W., Stagno, S., and Alford C.A. (1979). Comparative prevalence of subclinical cytomegalovirus and herpes simplex virus infections in the genital and urinary tracts of low-income, urban women. *J. Infect. Dis. 140*, 419–422.

Krech, U., Jung, M., and Jung, F. (1971). *Cytomegalovirus infections of man*. Basel: S. Karger, pp. 1–5.

Krugman, S. (1982). The newly licensed hepatitis B vaccine: Characteristics and indications for use. *J.A.M.A. 247*, 2012–2015.

Lang, D.J. (1975). The epidemiology of cytomegalovirus infections: Interpretation of recent observations. In *Infections of the fetus and newborn infant*, edited by S. Krugman and A.A. Gershan. New York: Alan R. Liss, pp. 35–45.

Larson, H.E., Parkman, P.D., Davis, W.J., Hopps, H.E., and Meyer, H.M., Jr. (1971). Inadvertent rubella virus vaccination during pregnancy. *N. Engl. J. Med. 284*, 870–873.

Li, F.P. and Hanshaw, J.B. (1967). Cytomegalovirus infection among migrant children. *Am. J. Epidemiol. 86*, 137–141.

Modlin, J.F., Hermann, K., Brandling-Bennett, A.D., Eddins, D.L., and Hayden, G.F. (1976). Risk of congenital abnormality after inadvertent rubella vaccination of pregnant women. *N. Engl. J. Med. 294*, 972–974.

Mollica, F., Musumeci, S., Rugolo, S., and Mattina, T. (1979). A prospective study of 18 infants of chronic HBs Ag mothers. *Arch. Dis. Child. 54*, 750–754.

Montgomery, J.R., Flanders, R.W., and Yow, M. (1973). Congenital herpesvirus infection with possibly related anomalies. *Am. J. Dis. Child. 126*, 364–366.

Montgomery, R., Youngblood, L., and Medearis, D. (1972). Recovery of cytomegalovirus from the cervix in pregnancy. *Pediatrics 49*, 524–531.

Nahmias A.J., Josey, W.E., Naib, Z.M., Luce, C.F., and Griest, B.A. (1970). Antibodies to herpesvirus hominis types 1 and 2 in humans. II. Women with cervical cancer. *Am. J. Epidemiol. 91*, 547–552.

——, Alford, C.A., and Korones, S.B. (1970a). Infection of the newborn with herpesvirus hominis. *Adv. Pediatr. 17*, 185–226.

—— and Duffey, C. (1970). Antibodies to herpesvirus hominis types 1 and 2 in humans. I. Patients with genital herpetic infections. *Am. J. Epidemiol. 91*, 539–546.

——, ——, ——, Freeman, M.G., Fernandez, R.J., and Wheeler, J.H. (1971). Perinatal risk associated with maternal genital herpes simplex virus infection. *Am. J. Obstet. Gynecol. 110*, 825–837.

Naib, Z.M., Nahmias, A.J., Josey, W.E., Facog, M.D., and Wheeler, J.H. (1970). Association of maternal genital herpetic infection with spontaneous abortion. *Obstet. Gynecol. 35*, 260–263.

——, ——, ——, and Zaki, S.A. (1973). Relation of cytohistopathology of genital herpesvirus infection to cervical anaplasia. *Cancer Res. 33*, 1452–1463.

Ng, A.B.P., Reagen, J.W., and Yen, S.S.C. (1970). Herpes genitalis—clinical and cytopathologic experience with 256 patients. *Obstet. Gynecol. 36*, 645–651.

Numazaki, Y., Yano, N., Morizuka, T., Takai, S., and Ishida, N. (1970). Primary infection with human cytomegalovirus: Virus isolation from healthy infants and pregnant women. *Am. J. Epidemiol. 91*, 410–417.

Okada, K., Kamiyama, I., Inomata, M., Imai, M., Miyakawa, Y., and Mayumi, M. (1976). e Antigen and anti-e in the serum of asymptomatic carrier mothers as indicators of positive and negative transmission of hepatitis B to their infants. *N. Engl. J. Med. 294*, 746–749.

————, Yamada, T., Miyakawa, Y., and Miyakawa, M. (1975). Hepatitis B surface antigen in the serum of infants after delivery from asymptomatic carrier mothers. *J. Pediatr. 87*, 360–363.

Peckham, C.S. (1972). Clinical and laboratory study of children exposed in utero to maternal rubella. *Arch. Dis. Child. 47*, 571–577.

Plotkin, S.A. (1975). Routes of fetal infection and mechanisms of fetal damage. *Am. J. Dis. Child. 129*, 444–449.

————, Farquhar, J.D., and Ogra, P.L. (1973). Immunologic properties of RA 27/3 rubella vaccine: A comparison with strains presently licensed in the United States. *J.A.M.A. 225*, 585–590.

Polk, B.F., White, J.A., DeGirolami, P.C., and Modlin, J.F. (1980). An outbreak of rubella among hospital personnel. *N. Engl. J. Med. 303*, 541–545.

Preblud, S.R., Serdula, M.K., Frank, J.A., Jr., and Hinman, A.R. (1980). Current status of rubella in the United States, 1969–79. *J. Infect. Dis. 142*, 776–779.

Punyagupta, S., Olson, L.C., Harinasuta, Akarawong, K., and Varawidhya, W. (1973). The epidemiology of hepatitis B antigen in a high prevalence area. *Am. J. Epidemiol. 97*, 349–354.

Rawls, W.E., Gardner, H.L., Flanders, R.W., Lowry, S.P., Kaufman, R.H., and Melnick, J.L. (1971). Genital herpes in two social groups. *Am. J. Obstet. Gynecol. 110*, 682–689.

Reynolds, D.W., Stagno, S., Hosty, T.S., Tiller, M., and Alford, C.A. (1973). Maternal cytomegalovirus excretion and perinatal infection. *N. Engl. J. Med. 289*, 1–5.

————, ————, Stubb, K.G., Dahle, A.J., Livingston, M., Saxon, S.S., and Alford, C.A. (1974). Inapparent congenital cytomegalovirus infection with elevated cord IgM levels. *N. Engl. J. Med. 290*, 291–296.

Schweitzer, I.L., Dunn, A.E.G., Peters, R.L., and Spears, R.L. (1973a). Viral hepatitis B in neonates and infants. *Am. J. Med. 55*, 762–771.

————, Moseley, J.W., Ashcavai, M., Edwards, V.M., and Overby, L.B. (1973). Factors influencing neonatal infection by hepatitis B virus. *Gastroenterology 65*, 277–283.

————, Wing, A., McPeak, C., and Spears, R.L. (1972). Hepatitis and hepatitis-associated antigen in 56 mother-infant pairs. *J.A.M.A. 220*, 1092–1095.

Shaffer, A.J. (1965). *Diseases of the newborn* (2nd ed.). Philadelphia: W.B. Saunders, p. 733.

Siegel, M. and Fuerst, H.T. (1966). Low birth weight and maternal virus diseases: A prospective study of rubella, measles, mumps, chickenpox, and hepatitis. *J.A.M.A. 197*, 88.

South, M.A., Tompkins, W.A.F., Morris, C.R., and Rawls, W.E. (1969). Congenital malformation of the central nervous system associated in the genital type (type 3) herpesvirus. *J. Pediatr. 75*, 13–18.

Stagno, S., Pass, R.F., Dworsky, M.E., Henderson, R.E., Moore, E.G., Walton, P.D., and Alford, C.A. (1982). Congenital cytomegalovirus infection: The relative importance of primary and recurrent maternal infection. *N. Engl. J. Med. 306*, 945–949.

——, Reynolds, D.W., Amos, C.S., Dahle, A.J., McCollister, F.P., Mohindra, I., Ermocilla, R., and Alford, C.A. (1977a). Auditory and visual defects resulting from symptomatic and subclinical congenital and toxoplasma infections. *Pediatrics 59*, 669–678.

——, ——, Huang, E-S., Thames, S.D., Smith, R.J., and Alford, C.A. (1977b). Congenital cytomegalovirus infection: Occurrence in an immune population. *N. Engl. J. Med. 296*, 1254–1258.

——, ——, Lakeman, A. Charamella, L.J., and Alford, C.A. (1973). Congenital cytomegalovirus infection: Consecutive occurrence due to viruses with similar antigenic compositions. *Pediatrics 52*, 788–794.

——, ——, Tsiantos, A., Fuccillo, D.A., Smith, R., Tiller, M., and Alford, C.A. (1975). Cervical cytomegalovirus excretion in pregnant and nonpregnant women: Suppression in early gestation. *J. Infect. Dis. 131*, 522–527.

Stevens, C., Beasley, R., Szmuness, W. et al. (1982). Efficacy of hepatitis B immune globulin in prevention of perinatally transmitted hepatitis B: Results of a second clinical trial in Taiwan. In *Viral hepatitis*, edited by W. Szmuness, H. Alter, and J. Maynard, Philadelphia: Franklin Institute Press.

——, ——, Tsui, J., and Lee, W.-C. (1975). Vertical transmission of hepatitis B antigen in Taiwan. *N. Engl. J. Med. 292*, 771–774.

Tondüry, G. and Smith, D.W. (1966). Fetal rubella pathology. *J. Pediatr. 68*, 867–879.

Vejtorp, M. and Mansa, B. (1980). Rubella IgM antibodies in sera from infants born after maternal rubella later than the 12th week of pregnancy. *Scand. J. Infect. Dis. 12*, 1–5.

Visintine, A., Nahmias, A.J., and Josey, W.E. (1978). Genital herpes. *Perinatal Care 2*, 32.

Wentworth, B.B. and Alexander, E.R. (1971). Seroepidemiology of infections due to members of the herpesvirus group. *Am. J. Epidemiol. 94*, 496–507.

Whitley, R.J., Nahmias, A.J., Visitine, A.M., Fleming, C.L., and Alford, C.A. (1980). The natural history of herpes simplex virus infection of mother and newborn. *Pediatrics 66*, 489–494.

9

Behavioral Teratology

Brenda Eskenazi

The high proportion of children suffering from such developmental disorders as mental retardation, learning disabilities, and hyperactivity has raised concern about their etiology. Some investigators (e.g., Weiss and Spyker, 1974; Buelke-Sam and Kimmel, 1979) have considered perinatal exposure to toxic agents, whether pharmacologic or environmental in origin, as potential causes of developmental behavior disorders. During the 1970s the field of behavioral teratology gained considerable momentum.

Whereas relatively high doses of a neurotoxin may result in structural malformation of the central nervous system (CNS), it is often assumed that lower doses of the same agent may produce subtler malformations evident only in behavioral deficits. Thus behavioral deficits may be the earliest sign of neurotoxicity, frequently occurring before the underlying neurochemical or morphologic defects are apparent (Butcher et al., 1975; Spyker, 1975; Rodier, 1976).

Whether a teratogen affects the development of the nervous system depends not only on the particular affinity of the toxin but also on the stage of fetal development when the agent is introduced. Wilson (1973) proposed that the embryo is not very susceptible to teratogenesis during the early stages of fetal development (the prediffer-entiation period, Days 1–6), because insult to the embryo at this time would most probably have a lethal effect. Maximum susceptibility to teratogenesis occurs during differentiation and early organogenesis. Teratogens introduced at this time to the developing nervous system can result in gross defects of the CNS (e.g., anencephaly). As organogenesis approaches completion at around eight weeks of gestation, the risk of gross morphologic damage or lethal effects of a toxin diminishes.

Neuronal multiplication is most rapid during the tenth to the eighteenth week of gestation, whereas neuronal migration begins around the seventh week and continues into the third trimester (Sidman and Rakic, 1973). By the middle of gestation, most neuronal regions possess the adult number of cells (Dobbing, 1974); however, cell multiplication in the forebrain continues into the second postnatal year (Dobbing and Sands, 1973). Although by midgestation, multiplication of glial and neuronal cells may be nearly complete in many areas of the brain, dendritic arborization, synaptogenesis, and myelinization have just begun. Differentiation and arborization of dendrites in the cerebral cortex occur most rapidly during the eighteenth to thirty-third weeks. Most growth of dendritic trees takes place within the first six months after birth (Purpura, 1974). Between 8 and 18 weeks of gestation, synapses are present above and below the cortical plate, but they are not found within the cortical plate until 23 weeks; the number of synapses increases progressively with age (Molliver et al., 1973). Myelinization of neurons starts during gestation but continues until adolescence.

When low doses of teratogens cause behavioral deficits, they probably do so by interfering with neuronal migration, dendritic differentiation, synaptogenesis, or myelinization. Purpura (1974) proposed that disturbances in synaptic function or dendritic growth could produce "a wide spectrum of disorders ranging from mild learning disabilities to profound mental deficiency" (p. 26). For example, Purpura (1974a) found a paucity of dendritic spines in profoundly retarded children. Toxic agents may cause dysgenesis of dendritic spines and may also interfere with establishment of synaptic connections by disrupting the synthesis, release, or reuptake of neurotransmitters.

Thus, unlike most other organ systems, the nervous system continues to develop until adolescence, remaining vulnerable to potential teratogens for a relatively long period of time. In utero exposure to teratogens may be exacerbated by early postnatal exposures—for example, through breast milk, through the ambient environment, even through contaminants on workclothes brought home by a parent. Although maternal ingestion or exposure was traditionally considered the only route of contamination of the fetus, recent studies suggest that toxic agents in semen could also affect progeny (see Joffe, 1979, for review).

This chapter will examine the literature on pharmacologic and environmental agents that adversely affect neurobehavioral development. Agents that potentially cause congenital CNS malformations but are not known to have adverse effect on behavioral development, such as vinyl chloride (Edmonds et al., 1978), fall outside the scope of

217

this chapter. When reviewing the literature, it is important to bear in mind that research in behavioral teratology is fraught with difficulties and limitations. For instance, there exist the usual problems in definition of exposure (e.g., multiple exposures, dose, timing; see Chapter 18). More significantly, behavioral deficits caused by toxic agents can be too subtle to be uncovered by routine neurologic examination; instead, detailed neurodevelopmental evaluation is necessary (see Chapter 20). Neurobehavioral tests must be both sensitive and valid, and variables—for example, maternal socioeconomic status (SES) or nutrition—that could alter behavioral development and confound the interpretation of the effects of the exposure must be controlled.

MICROENVIRONMENTAL AGENTS

Alcohol

Adverse effects of alcohol on the fetus were suspected in biblical times (Judges 13:7), yet not until recently has a syndrome been described. In 1968, Lemoine and colleagues in France observed in offspring of alcoholics a constellation of deficits including retarded growth, psychomotor disturbances, and peculiar facies. Five years later, in the United States, Jones, Smith, and co-workers (1973) described a similar cluster of characteristics and labeled it the fetal alcohol syndrome (FAS).

The characteristic facial features of FAS include short palpebral fissures, indistinct philtrum, short upturned nose with a low nasal bridge, narrow upper lip, small chin, and flat midface. Other frequently associated features include ptosis, aberrant palmar creases, heart murmurs usually due to atrial septal defects, and posterior rotation of the ears. Children with FAS often show growth deficiencies in weight and height (below 3rd percentile) (Eckardt et al., 1981) that are directly related to the amount of alcohol consumed by the mother particularly in late pregnancy (Little, 1977). Even with adequate caloric intake the infants do not catch up in growth (Jones et al., 1973). Children with FAS often are microcephalic (Hanson et al., 1976; Streissguth et al., 1978; Majewski, 1981).

Mental Retardation. Approximately 85% of children with signs of FAS show mild to moderate retardation (average IQ between 65 and 80). Because the prevalence of FAS is estimated at 1 per 750 births, alcohol is one of the most common *known* causes of mental retardation (Streissguth et al., 1980).

Streissguth et al. (1978) found the degree of mental deficiency in 20 cases of FAS (IQs ranging broadly from 15 to 109) was related to the severity of the dysmorphic features: Children independently judged to have the most severe cases of FAS had an average IQ of 55; those with mild cases had an average IQ of 82. Although few longitudinal studies exist, there is little evidence that the IQs of children with FAS improve over time (Jones et al., 1974; Streissguth et al., 1978a, 1981; Iosub et al., 1981).

Children of alcoholic women do not necessarily manifest the craniofacial features of FAS, but nevertheless may be at risk for low intelligence. This finding has been confirmed cross-culturally, in France (Lemoine et al., 1968), the Soviet Union (Shurygin, 1974), and Sweden (Olegård et al., 1979) (see Abel 1981; Streissguth, 1978, for review). In the United States, 23 offspring of chronic alcoholic women who participated in the Collaborative Perinatal Project were compared in mortality and CNS function to offspring of nondrinkers (Jones et al., 1974). Of the 23, 17% of offspring of alcoholics died in the first week (compared to 2% for controls). Among survivors, 44% had IQs of 79 or below at age seven (compared to 11% for controls). Mental retardation was the most frequent problem noted in these offspring, and was usually accompanied by diminished head size.

Hyperactivity and Irritability. Hyperirritability with hyperacusis in infants, and hyperactivity in children are frequently reported components of FAS (Clarren and Smith, 1978; Streissguth et al., 1980a). Irritability and tremors in infants may be symptoms of withdrawal from ethanol and are frequently observed in conjunction with spontaneous tonic–clonic seizures, opisthotonus, and abdominal distension (Pierog et al., 1977). In some cases, tremors may last beyond the first four weeks and therefore may not be the result of alcohol withdrawal (Jones and Smith, 1973; Havlicek and Childaeva, 1976).

Streissguth and co-workers (1978) reported that many of the children with FAS were described by caretakers as "always on the go"; others were described as fidgety with short attention spans. Shaywitz and associates (1980) found that 15 FAS children of normal intelligence were hyperactive, impulsive, and had short attention spans. Some children with FAS repetitively self-stimulate by head-rolling and head-banging, and by rocking (Jones et al., 1973). Children without signs of FAS but whose mothers were moderate drinkers were found at four years of age to be less attentive, less compliant with parental commands, and more fidgety at meals than children of occasional or nondrinkers (Landesman-Dwyer et al., 1981).

Other Motor Findings. Children with FAS frequently have immature motor behavior associated with spasticity (Olegård et al., 1979), weak grasp, and poor eye–hand coordination (Jones et al., 1973). Hypotonia is also described in children with FAS (Streissguth et al.,

219

1980a); degree of hypotonia is dose-related to maternal alcohol intake in newborns who do not have FAS (Ouellette and Rosett, 1976). However, one study that compared offspring of alcohol-exposed mothers (mild, moderate, and heavy users) to those of unexposed mothers found no difference in the psychomotor developmental milestones of three-year-olds (Mau, 1980).

Sleep Disturbances.   Alcohol exposure in utero has sometimes been associated with sleep problems in infants. Streissguth et al. (1978) reported that sleep disturbances were rare in 20 FAS children. However, children not diagnosed as having FAS but whose mothers were heavy drinkers have been reported to sleep less, to have a greater frequency of wakening during sleep, and to be more restless than children whose mothers drank less than once per month (Rosett et al., 1979).

Havlicek and Childaeva (1976) observed pathologic slow-wave EEG patterns in 15 children of alcoholic mothers as long as four to six weeks after birth. The abnormal EEG patterns were characterized by hypersynchrony in all stages of sleep, especially during periods with prominent delta frequencies (for related findings see Havlicek et al., 1977; Sander et al., 1977). Newborns (some with FAS) of alcoholic mothers have abnormal visual and somatosensory evoked responses (Olegård et al., 1979).

Disturbances in sleep may have grave repercussions in the quality of the parent–child interaction, a relationship that is already tenuous when the mother is alcoholic.

Other Neurobehavioral Disorders.   Children with FAS show lags in language acquisition (Shaywitz et al., 1981) and retardation in reading, arithmetic, and spelling. In a retrospective study, Shaywitz et al. (1980) found that 15 of 87 children of normal intelligence who were referred to a learning disabilities clinic for scholastic failure and hyperactivity had mothers with a history of alcoholism at the time of pregnancy.

Social Drinkers.   There is growing evidence that offspring of women who drink during pregnancy, but are not considered alcoholics, also display disorders in behavior. After controlling for caffeine and nicotine use, Landesman-Dwyer et al. (1978) found that infants of "moderately heavy social drinkers" compared to infants of nondrinkers had significantly more body tremors, atypical head positions, higher activity levels, more hand–face contacts, and spent more time with their eyes open. Some of these behaviors evidenced a dose–response relationship. Other behavioral findings in newborns of "social drinkers" include decreased habituation to repetitive stimuli (Streissguth et al., 1977), weak sucking pressure (Martin et al., 1979), and slow operant learning (Martin et al., 1977). In an ongoing prospective study of 462 eight-month-old infants, mental and motor development on the Bayley Scales was related to maternal alcohol use when nicotine and caffeine use was controlled (Streissguth et al., 1980).

Pathology. There is little evidence to suggest that either vitamin deficiency or malnutrition (both common in alcoholics) is responsible for FAS (Jones and Smith, 1973; Ouellette and Rosett, 1976; see Henderson et al., 1981, for review). Structural abnormalities in brains of infants with FAS are not typical of the neuropathology associated with malnutrition. Neuropathology in infants exposed in utero to alcohol includes aberrant neuronal and glial cell migration, hydrocephalus (Clarren et al., 1978; Majewski, 1981), agenesis of the corpus callosum, relative agyria, and microencephaly (Jones and Smith, 1973).

Comment. Many reports that examine the relationship between maternal alcohol use and infant behavior have failed to control other variables that could confound the association. For example, use of caffeine, nicotine, and licit or illict drugs may be higher in alcoholic women (Sokol et al., 1980). Alcoholic women tend to come from low socioeconomic groups where prenatal nutrition and medical care are often poor. They also tend to have more complications during pregnancy (Kaminski et al., 1978; Sokol et al., 1980). Many offspring of alcoholic women are raised in foster homes, where care may be different from that in natural homes (see Streissguth, 1976). Streissguth et al. (1979) found that children both of alcoholic women and of women who were recovered alcoholics had significantly lower IQs than children of nondrinking women. This result suggests that alcohol may also have an indirect effect. Thus there remains a need for additional studies that control confounding variables before conclusions can be made about the effects of alcohol on neurobehavioral development. Still other studies are necessary to determine the lowest dose associated with behavioral deficits and to examine the effects of "binge" drinking.

Smoking

Since the early investigations of Simpson (1957) and Lowe (1959), maternal cigarette smoking has been consistently associated with retardation in intrauterine growth. Offspring of smoking mothers tend, on average, to weigh about 200 g less than the offspring of nonsmokers (Meredith, 1975), with the extent of weight reduction varying positively with dose (see Landesman-Dwyer and Emanuel, 1979; Abel, 1980, for review). Smoking during pregnancy also has been related to increased prenatal and neonatal mortality (e.g., Butler and Alberman, 1969; Naeye et al., 1976), as well as increased risk of congenital malformations (Fedrick et al., 1971), including anencephaly (Naeye, 1978) and other malformations of the nervous system (Heinonen et al., 1977).

Evidence suggests that cigarette smoke is also a behavioral teratogen. Newborns of mothers who smoked and drank alcohol during pregnancy performed significantly worse than controls in operant conditioning of head-turning and sucking (Martin et al., 1977). Landesman-Dwyer et al. (1978) found that offspring of the heaviest drinking and smoking women yawned and sneezed more often, indicated less alert behavior, and showed frequent atypical head orientation to the left. These effects were greater than predicted on the basis of alcohol and nicotine exposure alone.

Garn et al. (1980), after excluding infants born before 38 weeks' gestation, found that the probability of a low Bayley test score in eight-month-old infants increased 50% with heavy maternal cigarette use. However, Streissguth et al. (1980), who used a more precise measure of nicotine exposure and controlled for alcohol and caffeine exposure as well as gestational age, failed to find a significant relationship of *nicotine* and Bayley scores.

Only a few studies have looked at long-term effects of maternal cigarette smoking on cognitive development and achievement. Hardy and Mellits (1972) studied cognitive development and achievement in offspring of 143 inner-city women drawn from the Collaborative Perinatal Project. Children of mothers who smoked at least ten cigarettes per day were compared to children of 143 nonsmokers matched for gender, race, date of delivery, and maternal age and education; 55 of these pairs were also matched on birthweight. Neither at age four nor at age seven did the offspring of smoking women differ from offspring of nonsmokers on IQ (however, both groups scored below the national mean). In addition, there were no significant differences in the 7 year old offspring of smokers and nonsmokers in reading and arithmetic (Wide Range Achievement Test), vocal association subtest for abstract language usage, Bender–Gestalt, or Goodenough–Harris Draw-a-Person Test. The only significant difference was on the spelling subtest of the Wide Range Achievement Test, where children born to nonsmokers did better.

222

In 1973, Butler and Goldstein reported on the seventh- and eleventh-year follow-up of 12,000 of the 17,000 children who participated in the British National Child Development Study. After controlling for social class and for maternal age and height, Butler and Goldstein found that the 7-year-old children of mothers who smoked after the fourth month of pregnancy (see Butler et al., 1972, for justification) lagged behind children of nonsmokers by 1.0 cm in height and by four months in their average reading level. These decrements were small compared to effects of other factors such as the number of children in the home. At 11 years the children were also evaluated on a general ability test and on a mathematics test. Children of smokers lagged significantly behind children of nonsmokers by three months in general ability, four months in reading, five months in mathematics, and 1.0 cm in height. The adverse effects of smoking in pregnancy on height and reading attainment had not widened between ages 7 and 11. There was also some evidence of a dose–response relationship.

In a prospective study of 319 $6\frac{1}{2}$-year-old children, Dunn et al. (1977) also found a small but significant decrement in cognitive performance, as measured by WISC IQ, associated with maternal smoking. However, when social class was controlled, differences in IQ were no longer statistically significant. Children of smokers were almost twice as frequently diagnosed as having "minimal cerebral dysfunction" (a term that Dunn and co-workers do not define); they also had abnormal EEGs almost twice as often. On average, children of smoking mothers had lower grade placement, and male offspring of smokers were rated by teachers as significantly more misbehaved; these analyses did not control social class.

Three additional studies suggest that maternal smoking is associated with such behavioral problems in offspring as hyperactivity. In a case-control study, Denson et al. (1975) reported that mothers of 20 methylphenidate-sensitive hyperactive children were more than twice as likely to have smoked during pregnancy than mothers of dyslexic children and mothers of normal controls matched for social class and gender. Nichols (1977) found a positive association between number of cigarettes smoked by the mother during pregnancy and hyperactivity in her child. In a prospective study (Landesman-Dwyer et al., 1981), 128 white middle-class women who smoked during pregnancy but who did not drink or who drank occasionally, rated their four-year-old child as more willing to approach strangers and novel situations, and to persevere (sustain involvement with a single activity). They also perceived their children to be more active than children of mothers who did not smoke or drink. However, this result was not confirmed on the mother's ratings of the child on the Werry, Weiss, and Peters Activity Scale or on naturalistic observation by the experimenter, who was blind to the child's exposure.

Mechanism and Pathology.   Although there are several contaminants in cigarette smoke, a major one is carbon monoxide (Garvey and Longo, 1978). Infants exposed to carbon monoxide through sources other than cigarette smoke develop neurologic sequelae including mental retardation (Desclaux et al., 1951), microcephalus (Brander, 1940), and retarded psychomotor development (Zourbas, 1947; see Longo, 1970, for review). Cerebral anoxia during pregnancy, labor, or delivery results in similar sequelae.

Mothers who smoke tend to have larger placentas than do non-smoking mothers, while their infants are smaller; these effects are also found in fetal hypoxia due to high altitude. Christianson (1979) suggested that fetal growth may be decelerated via an adaptive mechanism to reduce the fetus's oxygen demand. Small-for-gestational-age infants born to smoking mothers do not demonstrate the relative sparing of head-growth retardation that is seen in other small-for-gestational-age infants (Persson et al., 1978). Hence infants born to smoking mothers may have fewer brain cells or at least retarded brain development.

Comment.   Women who smoke are more likely to drink coffee and alcohol (Yerushalmy, 1971); yet few studies of effects of smoking have controlled these exposures. The observed effects may be due to the characteristics of the smoker rather than of the smoking (Yerushalmy, 1972). Social class, which is controlled for in only some of the studies, may confound the results. Furthermore, cognitive development is shaped by a host of environmental factors such as parental behavior patterns, which themselves may be related to smoking (Dunn et al., 1977).

Most of these studies have not separated out the independent effects of low birthweight and smoking. Low birthweight is associated with poor neurodevelopmental outcome (Lipper et al., 1981). Thus the behavioral effects of smoking on the offspring may be the secondary result of low birthweight and its effects on behavior rather than of smoking per se (Dunn et al., 1977).

So far, the evidence suggests that maternal smoking may be associated with decrements in intelligence and academic achievement, and with behavioral problems. However, the decrements are so small that large sample sizes are required to detect differences (Hardy and Mellits, 1972; Butler and Goldstein, 1973).

Caffeine

There are few studies on the teratogenic effects of caffeine in humans. Maternal coffee drinking has been associated with low birthweight (Mau and Netter, 1974), reproductive loss (Weathersbee et al., 1977; Weathersbee and Lodge, 1979), and sometimes with congenital malformations (Heinonen et al., 1977; Van den Berg, 1977; Borlée et al., 1978). Only one study to date has related caffeine use during pregnancy to subsequent development of the infant (Streissguth et al., 1980). When maternal alcohol and nicotine use, gestational age, maternal education, and parity were controlled, no significant relationship appeared between maternal caffeine use and the infant's mental and psychomotor development as assessed by the Bayley Scale at eight months.

PHARMACEUTICAL AGENTS: ILLICIT AND LICIT

Narcotics

Over 75% of neonates exposed in utero to heroin or methadone display withdrawal symptoms (Hill and Desmond, 1963; Rosen and Johnson, 1982). Similar symptoms of neonatal withdrawal have been associated with maternal use of codeine (Mangurten and Benwara, 1980), pentazocine (Kopelman, 1975; Preis et al., 1977), glutethimide (Reveri et al., 1977), hydroxyzine (Prenner, 1977), barbiturates (see later sections), and tranquilizers (see on Tranquilizers section) including ethchlorvynol (Rumack and Walravens, 1973), diazepam (Mazzi, 1977; Rementería and Bhatt, 1977), and chlordiazepoxide (Athinarayanan et al., 1976).

At birth the addicted neonate may appear normal. Most studies (Strauss et al., 1974; Rosen and Johnson, 1982), but not all (Ostrea and Chavez, 1979), report that the Apgar scores of addicted neonates do not differ from those of neonates of nonaddicted mothers. However, addicted neonates reportedly have lower birthweights and may be small for gestational age (Vargas et al., 1975; Ostrea and Chavez, 1979; Wilson et al., 1981). Head circumference tends to be below the 10th percentile (Vargas et al., 1975; Chasnoff et al., 1982).

Within 24–72 hours after birth, the addicted neonate may develop the classic symptoms of the narcotic abstinence syndrome (Goodfriend et al., 1956). Starting in the first week of life, methadone-addicted neonates when compared to nonaddicted controls on the Brazelton Neonatal Behavioral Assessment Scale were found to be more active, irritable, tremulous, resistant to cuddling, and difficult to console. They also exhibited more hand-to-mouth movements and motor immaturity (Kaplan et al., 1975; Lodge et al., 1975; Strauss et al., 1975, 1976; Chasnoff et al., 1982). Methadone-addicted neonates showed difficulty in orienting to auditory and visual stimuli as assessed on the Brazelton Scale (Strauss et al., 1975; Chasnoff et al., 1982) and in habituating to visual stimuli (Soule et al., 1973; Lessen-Firestone et al., 1974). Methadone exposure in utero was dose-related to a decrease in sucking rate (Kaplan et al., 1975).

Although most studies examine methadone-addicted neonates, most narcotic-addicted neonates show similar deficits when compared to nonaddicted controls or to neonates of polydrug users (e.g., phenobarbital, diazepam; Chasnoff et al., 1982). One exception (Lodge et al., 1975) was the higher level of activity noted in methadone-addicted neonates compared to heroin-addicted neonates.

As many as one-third of the methadone-addicted infants have abnormal ocular findings such as strabismus, nystagmus, and ocular torticollis (Chavez et al., 1979; Rosen and Johnson, 1982). Lodge et al. (1975) observed that at one month of age, methadone-addicted and methadone/heroin-addicted infants, when compared to controls, had more eye coordination problems; heroin-addicted infants were comparable to controls.

Follow-up evaluation of narcotic-addicted infants are reported in a few investigations. Wilson et al. (1973) found that three to six months after birth, addicted infants continued to be restless, agitated, colicky, tremulous, and hyperacusic. Tremors and irritability, however, had decreased in severity. Hyperphagia, hyperacusis, and hypertonicity were the most prolonged symptoms.

After one year of age, as many as 20% of addicted infants still demonstrated disturbances of activity level or attention span that were associated with sleep disorders and temper tantrums, but no differences were observed between methadone- or heroin-addicted infants and controls in irritability, tremulousness, and consolability (Wilson et al., 1981). One-year-old addicted infants showed considerable delays in developmental milestones such as sitting up. They also showed poorer fine motor coordination (Wilson et al., 1981; Rosen and Johnson, 1982). Muscle tone remained increased in heroin-addicted but not methadone-addicted infants (Wilson et al., 1981). At 18 months, there was little language development, and tone and coordination problems persisted (Rosen and Johnson, 1982).

Performance of heroin- and methadone-addicted infants on the Bayley Scales provides additional evidence of the infants' impaired psychomotor development (Strauss et al., 1976; Wilson et al., 1981; Rosen and Johnson, 1982). Psychomotor and mental development of addicted infants up to 18 months fell within normal limits. However, when compared to nonaddicted controls (even when matched for obstetric complications, gestational age, birthweight, Apgar score, and sex; Rosen and Johnson, 1982), addicted infants have poorer psychomotor development; this discrepancy becomes more pronounced as the children get older (Strauss et al., 1976; Rosen and Johnson, 1982). The psychomotor scores of methadone-addicted one-year-olds were even lower than scores of heroin-addicted infants (Wilson et al., 1981).

Comment. Results of these studies imply that even as long as two years after birth, addicted infants suffer sequelae of in utero exposure to narcotics. It seems that these effects are restricted more to motor than to mental development, and that methadone exposure may result in slightly more profound deficits than does heroin exposure. Defects in motor development include poor fine motor coordination, oculomotor defects, and hyperkinesis. Follow-up studies beyond two years of age are needed.

Whether the observed effects are caused directly by the narcotics or related to other characteristics of the mother is unclear. Addicted mothers are often in poor health and malnourished, and they often abuse other drugs as well. Usually the mother is a single parent, and the paternal drug history, which may also affect the infant's development, is unknown (Strauss et al., 1976). Although most studies have controlled for differences in SES, race, or maternal age, few studies have controlled for alcohol use, smoking, birthweight, or gestational age.

Marijuana

In utero exposure to marijuana has been consistently reported to have adverse affects on the neurobehavioral development of rats (Borgen et al., 1973; Abel, 1979; Kawash et al., 1980). Although one study found that almost 20% of women smoked marijuana during pregnancy (Fried, 1980), the effects of exposure in humans have not been clarified. Two investigations have examined the neurobehavioral effects of in utero exposure to marijuana (Abrams, 1979; Fried, 1980) in humans, but their results are contradictory and are based on small sample sizes of slightly different ages.

Offspring of 12 irregular users of marijuana (one joint per week), 1 moderate user (two to five joints per week), and 10 heavy users (more than five joints per week) were evaluated on the Brazelton Neonatal Assessment Scale, 60–80 hours after birth (Fried, 1980), and compared with 66 offspring of mothers who did not smoke marijuana. Significantly more infants exposed to marijuana failed to habituate to a repeated visual stimulus. Although alcohol and nicotine use was significantly associated with marijuana use in a previous study of this sample (Fried et al., 1980), these variables were not controlled in the analysis of habituation rates. Infants whose mothers smoked marijuana were significantly more likely to startle easily or to have tremors independent of alcohol and nicotine exposure. Over one-third of the babies born to regular users emitted shrill cries similar to those described in infants withdrawing from narcotics.

Abrams (1979) compared 12 infants of mothers who smoked marijuana with 12 infants of nonmarijuana smokers. The two groups were matched for age, SES, and other drug use, but not for tobacco or alcohol use. In sharp contrast to Fried (1980), Abrams reported that the marijuana-exposed infants scored significantly *better* on the Bayley Motor Scale at 1 and 12 weeks. Additionally, these infants had *better* scores in eye movement pursuit of visual stimuli, alertness, lability of sleep–wake states, and motor coordination assessed on the Brazelton Neonatal Assessment Scale at one and six weeks. Clearly, these studies need replication.

Amphetamines

Prenatal injection in mice of D-amphetamine sulfate alters levels of brain catecholamines and increases activity levels (Zemp and Middaugh, 1975). In humans, 86% of one-year-old children of women who abused amphetamines (one-third of them had also abused alcohol) had normal fine and gross motor development; 80% were judged free of emotional disturbance (Billing et al., 1980). However, infants whose mothers remained addicted throughout pregnancy and who were raised by foster parents were slow in their early development and showed marked apathy throughout the first six months of life.

Antipsychotics

Neuroleptic drugs such as penfluridol and haloperidol (Engel et al., 1973), and psychotropic drugs such as prochlorperazine, fenfluramine, and propoxyphene (Vorhees et al., 1979), have adverse effects on locomotor development of rodents. Two offspring of women given combinations of phenothiazine derivatives (chlorpromazine, thioridazine, and hydrochlorothiazide) during pregnancy developed extrapyramidal-type motor disturbances (Hill et al., 1966). These motor signs, which persisted for six months in one infant and ten months in the more severe case, included nystagmus, tremors, hypertonia, posturing of the hands, and flapping of the arms and hands. Other studies on phenothiazines have failed to associate poor development (Ayd, 1964) or lower IQ (Slone et al., 1977) with prenatal exposure.

228

Anticonvulsants

DIPHENYLHYDANTOIN (DILANTIN)

Infants of epileptic mothers may be at risk for congenital malformations. Dysmorphic facial features have been described in infants exposed in utero to hydantoins (Meadow, 1968; Hill et al., 1974; Hanson and Smith, 1975). These features include short nose with broad bridge and inner epicanthal folds, hypertelorism, ptosis, strabismus, wide mouth, and neck webbing (Hanson, 1976). In addition to craniofacial anomalies, in utero exposure to hydantoin is related to an increased prevalence of congenital heart anomalies, limb defects, cleft lip and palate (Speidel and Meadow, 1972; Hill et al., 1974), and growth deficiencies including small head circumference (Hanson and Smith, 1975).

Some reports indicating a higher incidence of mental retardation in infants exposed to hydantoins are case studies without comparison populations. Hanson and Smith (1975) found that 4 out of 5 cases of fetal hydantoin syndrome had mental deficiency, and all were microcephalic. Annegers et al. (1974) reported that among 76 children of epileptic women taking anticonvulsant medication and followed for at least five years, 3 were severely retarded and warranted institutionalization. It is not clear which anticonvulsant medications these children's mothers were taking. In a study of 35 children exposed to hydantoins in utero, 4 were diagnosed as having fetal hydantoin syndrome, and in 11 others mental deficiency was the most serious single feature (Hanson and Smith, 1976).

A number of controlled studies have also reported an increased incidence of mental retardation in infants exposed in utero to hydantoins. Some investigations conducted formal follow-up testing of these children. In a retrospective survey of 427 pregnancies of 186 epileptic women (Speidel and Meadow, 1972), mental subnormality occurred in 1.5% of offspring compared with 0.2% in controls. Some of the epileptic women were taking anticonvulsants other than hydantoin, and not all were using medication.

Hanson et al. (1976a) found that the 104 hydantoin-exposed infants drawn from the Collaborative Perinatal Project had significantly lower IQs at seven years, and smaller head circumference at birth than children (pair-matched for SES, age, race, and institution of birth) whose mothers were not epileptic and who did not take hydantoin medications. Six of the eleven children who showed the clear pattern of fetal hydantoin syndrome had IQs between 31 and 84.

Hill et al. (1974) performed follow-up evaluations of 28 children exposed to anticonvulsive agents and 165 children not exposed to these agents. At 18 months, 5 of 11 exposed infants but only 3 of 36 controls (significantly fewer) had developmental quotients less than 90. Moreover, at 21 months, developmental quotients were significantly lower for 7 anticonvulsant-exposed infants as compared to 27 controls.

Another study based on infants participating in the Collaborative Perinatal Project (Shapiro et al., 1976) found mental and motor scores at eight months, and IQ at four years, to be nonsignificantly lower among children born to epileptic mothers taking either phenobarbital or phenytoin than children of mothers who were not epileptic. Because the performance of children of mothers taking phenobarbital was not different from those taking phenytoin, the authors concluded there was no evidence that phenytoin caused mental deficiency; the association of mental deficiency and phenytoin found in previous investigations could be due to use of a nonepileptic comparison group (see Comment below).

Comment. A question that has been repeatedly addressed is whether the observed physical anomalies and mental retardation are specifically due to the effects of hydantoin medications, or rather due to a direct or even genetic effect of maternal epilepsy (Hill, 1976; Bruni and Willmore, 1979). Hill (1976) suggests that if the effects are drug-induced they may be the residue of "long-term deficiency states or impaired metabolism imposed on the female because of long-term (10 to 20 years) drug ingestion" (p. 925). Although a genetic component may in part explain the observed defects, hydantoin has not been ruled out as a cause. The incidence of congenital anomalies in offspring of untreated epileptic mothers and of epileptic fathers is intermediate between offspring of medicated epileptic mothers and normal controls (Speidel and Meadow, 1972; Monson et al., 1973; Shapiro et al., 1976). That infants born to epileptic mothers not exposed to hydantoin have malformation rates similar to those of unmedicated nonepileptic control populations strongly suggests that epilepsy per se is not responsible for teratogenesis (Hill, 1973; Monson et al., 1973).

Trimethadione. Trimethadione, a drug prescribed for petit mal seizures, has been associated with a configuration of malformations including malformed and low-set ears, palatal anomalies (cleft or high-arched), teeth irregularities, cardiac anomalies, and V-shaped eyebrows (German et al., 1970; Zackai et al., 1975; Feldman et al., 1977). About half of children exposed in utero to trimethadione or related drugs (e.g., paramethadione) were mentally retarded, 62%

were speech-impaired, 40% were visually impaired, and 25% suffered hearing loss (Feldman et al., 1977).

Infants whose mothers took barbiturates during pregnancy may show withdrawal symptoms similar to infants addicted to narcotics. Whether mothers were addicted to barbiturates or had them prescribed for anxiety or epilepsy, their infants showed the same symptomatology.

Barbiturate-addicted infants are initially hyperactive and tremulous (Bleyer and Marshall, 1972). They cry constantly and have difficulty sleeping. Later, they may show symptoms of hyperphagia, hyperacusis, sweating, episodic irritability, and prolonged crying (Desmond et al., 1972). Unlike narcotic-exposed infants, these infants are usually full-sized. They also have Apgar scores within normal limits (Desmond et al., 1972). The age at onset of hyperexcitability may be later than in opiate addiction, but the duration of symptoms is similar to that for narcotics and may last six months (see Barbiturates Section under Obstetric Medications).

So far, the only suggestion that early exposure to barbiturates may have long-term behavioral effects has come from studies evaluating offspring of patients on anticonvulsants (see Dilantin effects), and from studies of infants who received phenobarbital to prevent recurrent febrile seizures (Wolf and Forsythe, 1978; Camfield et al., 1979; Wolf et al., 1981). Follow-up studies are needed of infants exposed in utero to barbiturates.

Thalidomide

Thalidomide, a sedative drug widely prescribed to pregnant women in Europe in the 1960s, typically caused congenital deformities of the limbs, ears, eyes, and viscera (Ministry of Health, 1964). At first, the central nervous system was rarely thought to be involved. However, follow-up studies of thalidomide children have suggested that CNS function may be affected.

Illingworth (1966) initially hypothesized that thalidomide children may be below normal intelligence. The investigation of Gouin-Décarie (1969) supported the hypothesis by finding that one-third of 33 Canadian children exposed to thalidomide (aged $1\frac{1}{2}$ to $3\frac{1}{2}$ years) had borderline or mentally defective IQs. McFie and Robertson (1973) found that 4 of 56 thalidomide-exposed children, aged 7 to 10 years, had subnormal IQs, this proportion being higher than expected from a random sample of the population; however, the mean IQ of the group was within the normal range. McFie and Robertson (1973) also found a much higher percentage of the children than expected showed left-sided lateral preference, a finding also described by Smithells (1970). The mean reading and spelling grade levels of the thalidomide-exposed children were below that grade expected by chronologic age or IQ. However, Pringle and Fiddes (1970) who studied children with limb deformities (three-quarters were thalidomide-exposed), failed to confirm that these children were poorer readers.

Thalidomide children may also suffer from other neurobehavioral defects. Stephenson (1976) observed that 7 of 408 thalidomide children had epileptic seizures between birth and 9 years of age, and 5 had epilepsy at the time of study (13- and 14-year-olds). These numbers are six to eight times the prevalence rates expected; the annual incidence in the first 7 years of life for the thalidomide children was five times the figure for the general population. Abnormalities on EEG has been noted previously in association with thalidomide exposure (Horstmann, 1966).

Betamethasone

Betamethasone, a drug given to mothers in preterm labor for prevention of respiratory distress in the offspring, has detrimental effects on myelinization and cellular development of the CNS in animals (Gumbinas et al., 1973; Weichsel, 1974). However, a four-year followup study of 177 children treated prenatally with betamethasone (MacArthur et al., 1981) indicates that these children were comparable to normal controls in developmental motor milestones, speech development, social maturity, IQ, and visual perceptual skills.

Hormones

The fetus may be exposed to exogenous sex hormones when, for example, the mother receives them for prevention of miscarriage, for antitumor therapy, during a pregnancy test, or when oral contraceptives are taken inadvertently after conception. Sex hormones have been associated with a wide variety of adverse effects on the fetus (see Schardein, 1980, for review). These effects, which depend on dose, timing, and type of steroid, include masculinization (pseudohermaphroditism) of female genitalia, usually with androgens or with progestins (e.g., Ehrhardt and Money, 1967), and feminization of male offspring with DES, progesterone, and estrogens (e.g., Kaplan, 1959; Heinonen et al., 1977; Lorber et al., 1979).

Some evidence suggests that progesterones exert a feminizing effect on behavior of the male offspring. For example, Yalom et al. (1973) found that 16- to 17-year-old males born of diabetic or toxemic mothers who had taken DES and progesterone were less aggressive, less athletic, and had decreased heterosexual experiences and overall masculine interests. However, Meyer-Bahlberg et al. (1977) could not confirm these results in a younger sample of 13 males (average age of 11) drawn from the Collaborative Perinatal Project. Boys exposed in utero to medroxyprogesterone acetate (Provera-MPA) did not differ from 40 controls (matched for age, sex, SES, and history of maternal vaginal bleeding) in IQ, athletic skills, sex of playmates, gender preference, areas of energy expenditure, toy preference, or interest in marriage or children.

Prenatal progesterone effects also have been examined in females. Zussman et al. (1975) found that 16- to 19-year-old girls exposed to progesterone in utero were less likely to report having been a "tomboy" during childhood, were less active in play and sports, and were more concerned about clothes and hairstyles. Ehrhardt et al. (1977) confirmed these findings.

Exogenous sex hormones also have been thought to cause an "embryo fetal exogenous sex steroid exposure syndrome" (EFESSES). This syndrome is characterized by such craniofacial anomalies as facial elongation, obtuse chin, primary telecanthus, downward-slanting palpebral fissures, broad nose bridge, and pouting lower lip (Lorber et al., 1979). Many cases had sacral defects and were growth-retarded; hypospadias was common in males. Six out of nine cases were severely mentally retarded.

Clomiphene, which is not a hormone itself but is used to enhance fertility, has been suspected of being associated with increased risk of anencephaly in the offspring (Schardein, 1980). Gonadotropin therapy, employed for induction of ovulation, is not associated with increased malformations in the liveborn, or with retarded physical or psychomotor development (Caspi et al., 1976). Abnormalities in offspring whose mothers used hormones or fertility drugs may be related to underlying infertility rather than to the treatment (Schardein, 1980).

Obstetric Medications

Numerous studies have examined the effects of obstetric medications on neonatal behavior, although few investigations followed the neonate beyond the first month of life (for more complete reviews see Dubowitz, 1975; Scanlon, 1981). In many of the investigations cited, the comparison groups comprised small samples of infants who received multiple agents during delivery, thereby complicating the interpretation of the specific effects of a given agent (see Aleksandrowicz and Aleksandrowicz, 1974). The present chapter includes only those investigations where specific drug effects can be identified.

Analgesia. The most commonly used analgesic agent is meperidine (Demerol) given intravenously. In the first week of life, neonates exposed to meperidine (often in conjunction with other medications) were more immature on motor function (Standley et al., 1974), less active (Horowitz et al., 1977), more difficult to console and cuddle, and were drowsier (Brackbill et al., 1974), less alert (Hodgkinson et al., 1978b), less responsive to voices, sounds, and lights, and habituated more slowly (Brackbill et al., 1974; Hodgkinson et al., 1978, 1978b). Meperidine-exposed neonates exhibited weaker sucking and diminished primitive reflexes (Hodgkinson et al., 1978b). Most of these deficits were observed in the first three days of life. At four months of age, infants of mothers who received analgesics (usually meperidine) showed less habituation to visual stimuli (Friedman et al., 1978). Because few studies have examined the behavior of meperidine-exposed infants after the first week, the time course of recovery is unknown.

Epidural Anesthesia. Epidural anesthesia is performed by injecting local anesthetics such as bupivacaine, mepivacaine, lidocaine, or chloroprocaine into the epidural space, usually of the lumbar area. All epidural anesthetics are present in the blood of the newborn after delivery, mepivacaine having the longest half-life (nine hours) and chloroprocaine the shortest (43 seconds) (Ralston and Shnider, 1978). The amount of bupivacaine that crosses the placenta is about one-half that of mepivacaine or lidocaine (Hodgkinson et al., 1975).

Neonates born after epidural block with lidocaine or mepivacaine tend to be "floppy but alert," that is, their muscle strength and tone are decreased for at least the first 12 hours of life (Scanlon et al., 1974; Scanlon, 1976; Tronick et al., 1976). They show weak primitive reflexes (Moro's and rooting) and, in some studies, slow habituation to pinprick (Scanlon et al., 1974). During the first ten days of life, muscle tone slowly improves, although by Day 10 the infants still are less active and display poorer hand-to-mouth movements than infants exposed to minimal levels of obstetric medications (Tronick et al., 1976). Infants delivered by cesarean section under lidocaine epidural anesthesia were more hypotonic and, even at three days old, showed weaker sucking, rooting, and palmar grasp reflexes than infants delivered by cesarean under general anesthesia (thiopental) (Palahniuk et al., 1977; Hollman et al., 1978).

Immediately after delivery, infants born under bupivacaine epidural anesthesia were less responsive to the human voice. However, subsequent assessment on the Brazelton Scale failed to reveal differences between infants delivered under bupivacaine and nonmedicated controls (Lieberman et al., 1979). Thus, bupivacaine-exposed neonates did not show the decrease in muscle tone and strength noted in infants delivered under lidocaine or mepivacaine (Scanlon, 1976).

Paracervical or Pudendal Nerve Block. Local anesthetics administered by these techniques cross the placental barrier. The overall behavior, as assessed by Scanlon's Early Neonatal Neurobehavioral Test (Scanlon et al., 1974), on infants born under lidocaine pudendal anesthesia, was inferior to that of infants delivered under chloroprocaine epidural anesthesia (Hodgkinson et al., 1978b). Infants delivered under paracervical block (bupivacaine or lidocaine) habituated more slowly to pinprick and to light than infants delivered with no anesthesia (Nesheim et al., 1979).

There exist a number of case reports of neonates who suffered mepivacaine intoxication following paracervical or pudendal blocks during labor (Guillozet, 1975; Hillman et al., 1979). Neurologic examinations revealed decreased spontaneous movement, hypotonia, abnormalities of pupil or oculomotor reflexes, and hyperreflexia. Tonic–clonic seizures began in the first day of life, although all patients were seizure-free by age $4\frac{1}{2}$. One child, perhaps the worst case of intoxication (Guillozet, 1975), exhibited considerable motor and language delays.

Spinal and General Anesthesia. Spinal anesthesia is performed by injecting a local anesthetic, such as tetracaine, into the cerebrospinal fluid, usually in the lumbar region. Because the amount of anesthetic used in spinal block is minimal, little crosses the placental barrier (Hodgkinson et al., 1975). Thiopental, a rapid-acting barbiturate that crosses the placenta within one minute, and ketamine, a phencyclidine, are the general anesthetic agents most frequently used in the United States. Two-day old neonates delivered by cesarean section under general anesthesia were more alert, had better muscle tone, sucking, and primitive reflexes than neonates delivered by cesarean section under spinal anesthesia or pudendal block. Ketamine anesthesia resulted in more alert infants than did thiopental anesthesia (Hodgkinson et al., 1978a).

Barbiturates (see section on Anticonvulsants). Because of their rapid transplacental passage and selective storage in the immature brain, barbiturates (e.g., secobarbital) have a deep depressant effect on the neonate; hence they are rarely used in present-day obstetrics. Barbiturates adversely affect feeding in the first few days of life by reducing the infant's sucking rate and amount of milk consumption (Kron et al., 1966) and by decreasing the neonate's responsivity to breast-feeding (Brazelton, 1961).

Tranquilizers. Diazepam (Valium) is used in pregnancy for the management of preeclampsia and eclampsia, and during delivery as a tranquilizer. Cree et al. (1973) observed that of 32 infants exposed to diazepam, 10 had low Apgar scores and required tracheal intubation; 13 were hypotonic, often with depressed reflexes (lasting 36–72 hours after birth); 9 were hypothermic within the first 12 hours; and 12 were reluctant to suck and required tube-feeding for up to three days. These effects were particularly pronounced in infants whose mothers received more than 30 mg of diazepam within 15 hours of delivery. There are apparently no follow-up studies on neurobehavioral development in infants exposed to diazepam in utero or during delivery. However, follow-up of infants exposed to two other tranquilizers, meprobamate (Miltown) and chlordiazepoxide (Librium), have suggested that mental and motor development at eight months, and IQ at four years, are not different from nonexposed controls (Hartz et al., 1975).

Oxytocin. Children delivered after exposure to oxytocin, used either to induce labor or as part of a challenge test, did not show abnormalities on the Brazelton Neonatal Behavioral Scale during Day 1 or 3 (Scanlon et al., 1978), on developmental milestones (Friedman et al., 1979), on intelligence even when assessed at age five (Niswander et al., 1966; McBride et al., 1977), or on fine and gross motor coordination (Niswander et al., 1966; McBride et al., 1977). There is limited evidence that seizures were more common in infants born after induction of labor with oxytocin (Niswander et al., 1966; Ghosh, 1975).

Comment. Most anesthetic and analgesic agents cross the placenta. The impact of obstetric medication on the fetus depends on how much medication crosses the placenta, its dose, and the stage of delivery at which it is given. Only a few reports provide information about the pharmacokinetics of the anesthetic or analgesic agent such as the amount of medication in the neonate's blood (although even this is an imprecise measure of exposure; Scanlon, 1981). To date, only one investigator (Brackbill, 1977) has attempted to correlate long-term (up to seven years) behaviorial change with obstetric medication; how-

236

ever, no conclusive information has been published, and unpublished reports have engendered much controversy (see Kolata, 1979; Scanlon, 1981).

ENVIRONMENTAL AGENTS

Methyl Mercury

In 1952, Engleson and Herner described cerebral palsy-like symptoms and mental retardation in an infant exposed in utero to methyl mercury. Subsequently, two major disasters resulted in fetal methyl mercury poisoning; one accident occurred in Minamata Bay, Japan around 1953, and the other in Iraq in 1971.

In Minamata, mercury was discharged into local waters as an effluent of a plant producing acetylaldehyde. Microorganisms in the bay methylated the mercury, the methylated mercury was ingested by the fish, and the contaminated fish entered the food chain, poisoning more than 800 persons and 40 infants in utero. The Iraqi outbreak of methyl mercury poisoning, which resulted in hospital admissions of more than 6000 persons with at least 80 cases poisoned in utero, was caused by accidental ingestion of seed grain treated with a methyl mercury fungicide (see Bakir et al., 1973). Unlike the exposure at Minamata Bay, which was severe, prolonged, and continuous, the exposure in Iraq was of higher doses for a shorter period of time (September–December 1971). Also, because Iraqi infants were breast-fed and Japanese infants were not, exposure in Iraqi infants continued into the early postnatal period. Differences in exposure may account for slight discrepancies in the effects of these two accidents.

In general, methyl mercury had a much worse effect on the fetus than on the mother (Marsh et al., 1981). Although the majority of mothers showed few or mild toxic signs, their newborns were severely affected (Amin-Zaki et al., 1974). Infants exposed in utero had higher blood mercury levels after birth than their mothers (Amin-Zaki et al., 1974); furthermore, as infants they may excrete mercury less rapidly than adults (Weiss and Doherty, 1975).

Congenital malformations were rare in Iraq and Minamata (Weiss and Doherty, 1975). Mild to moderate microcephaly was reported in 5 cases (of 26 affected infants) in Japan (Murakami, 1972), and 3 cases (of 15) in Iraq (Amin-Zaki et al., 1974). Malocclusion ($N = 14$), skull deformities ($N = 11$), and strabismus ($N = 13$) were noted among 26 fetal Minamata victims (Murakami, 1972). Although the incidence of these defects appears elevated, the incidence in the unexposed population in these countries is not known.

237

Symptoms reported in the Minamata infants included cerebral palsy-like symptoms, lethargy, failure to follow visual stimuli, uncoordinated sucking or swallowing, and convulsions. Many were emaciated (Reuhl and Chang, 1979). In Iraq, 10 of 32 infants exposed to methyl mercury had signs of cerebral palsy, and 14 showed hyperreflexia. Cerebral palsy-like symptoms were associated with the highest mercury concentrations in mother's hair and with exposure in the third trimester (Amin-Zaki et al., 1979). Psychomotor retardation was dose-related to fetal exposure of methyl mercury (Marsh et al., 1980). Unlike the Minamata infants, the Iraqi infants were irritable ($N = 14$), had exaggerated reactions to noise, and cried excessively. Eight tended to smile, laugh, or cry without provocation, and eight were blind or had impaired vision (Amin-Zaki et al., 1979). Bakir et al. (1980) noted that four infants had impaired hearing and four had severely affected "mental power." Hearing deficits and blindness were not observed in Minamata cases, although constriction of visual fields was noted in some cases as they grew older (Harada, 1976; Reuhl and Chang, 1979).

Other neurologic symptoms became apparent as the Japanese children grew older. These defects included marked incoordination with both spastic and flaccid paralysis and ataxia, delayed motor and language developmental milestones, dysarthria, and involuntary movements. Mental retardation (IQ 75 or less) was noted in all 23 cases in Japan (Harada, 1977). During 15 years of follow-up of the Minamata cases, motor function improved in mild cases; but even in these cases, deficits in intelligence remained unimproved (Harada, 1978). Ataxia and speech disturbances persisted in almost all Japanese cases, and abnormal EEG was observed in two-thirds of them (Harada et al., 1971; see Kojima and Fujita, 1973).

Harada (1976) reported that 29% of children in Minamata born between 1955 and 1958 were mentally retarded, a percentage significantly higher than in age-matched control populations. Sensory disturbances and clumsiness in movement of fingers and other motor dysfunctions were seen in the mentally retarded children of Minamata. These results suggest that more children than initially observed were exposed to the adverse effects of methyl mercury in utero or during their early postnatal lives.

Thirty-two infants exposed in utero in Iraq were examined over a five-year period (Amin-Zaki et al., 1979). Of the 14 children who initially had symptoms, 5 who had cerebral palsy died, and of the 18 exposed children who were initially symptomless, 4 died. Most of the remaining children had histories of motor, speech, or mental developmental delay, and neurologic signs such as Babinski and hyperreflexia.

Pathology. Autopsy examinations of the brains of two Iraqi cases (Choi et al., 1978) and two Japanese cases (Matsumoto et al., 1964) have been reported. The exposure and disease course differed in the four cases. In the two Japanese cases, both profoundly retarded, autopsy revealed general brain atrophy, with hypoplasia of the cortex, especially of the granular cell layer in the calcarine and central gyri and in the corpus callosum. Abnormalities were noted in cytoarchitecture. In the two Iraqi cases, Choi et al. (1978) found abnormalities in migration of neurons in cerebral and cerebellar cortices, and in cytoarchitecture.

Lead

Lead is ubiquitous in the environment; children can be exposed to lead in drinking water, in air contaminated by automobile exhaust or lead smelter fumes, or by pica, especially through eating leaded paint chips (see Rutter, 1980, for review).

It is well known that large doses of lead exposure in children can result in encephalopathy. However, even relatively low levels of lead exposure have been associated with lower IQs (Perino and Ernhardt 1974; Landrigan et al., 1975), poorer academic skills (Pihl and Parkes, 1977), increased motor activity (Baloh et al., 1975; Needleman et al., 1979), and hyperactivity (David et al., 1972; Gittelman and Eskenazi, 1983).

Most studies are based on school-age children, so that no estimates can be provided of effects of in utero exposure. However, a retrospective study (Beattie et al., 1975; Moore et al., 1977) of 77 mentally retarded children aged two to six years found higher water lead levels in homes where the infants' mothers lived during pregnancy than in homes of mothers of nonretarded infants matched for social class. In a subsample of these children, lead concentrations were measured retrospectively using the heel blood samples used to evaluate phenylketonuria in the first two weeks of life. Concentrations were higher in the mentally retarded children.

Wibberley et al. (1977) found an excess of lead in the placentas of infants who failed to survive the neonatal period. Palmisano et al. (1969) reported an infant intoxicated by lead when her mother ingested "moonshine" (untaxed whiskey) during pregnancy. The infant exhibited hypertonus, tremulousness, and hyperreflexia. These symptoms may have resulted from exposure to alcohol as well as lead.

Although lead is one of the best-known and most researched neurotoxins, almost no studies have followed the behavioral development of infants with high lead levels at birth or with parents who had high lead exposures. (See Bridbord, 1978, for occupational lead exposure in women.) Such studies would provide further information about whether lead plays an etiologic role in behavioral disorders or whether increased lead burden is a consequence of lead ingestion by children who already have behavioral disorders (e.g., pica).

Solvents

In a case-control study of children with CNS malformations, Holmberg (1979) observed that significantly more case mothers had been exposed to at least 1 of 14 different organic solvents in the workplace. However, potential confounders such as SES, age, and parity were not controlled (Shiekh, 1979).

Fetal solvent syndrome had been described in an infant of a woman who severely abused solvents (toluene) and also drank about one six-pack of beer a week (Toutant and Lippman, 1979). The infant had craniofacial features similar to those described for FAS children, was below the 10th percentile in height, weight, and head circumference, and showed poor sucking reflex and jerky, uncoordinated movements. Epidemiologic studies are needed to clarify whether this syndrome results from solvent exposure, alcohol exposure, or the combined effects of both.

Halogenated Aromatic Hydrocarbons

In 1973, polybrominated biphenyl (PBB), a fire retardant, was accidently confused with cattle feed and entered the food chain in Michigan. Children were exposed to PBB in utero, and postnatally in cow's and mother's milk. These compounds are fat-soluble and, consequently were excreted in large quantities in mothers' milk (Finberg, 1977). In a study by Weil et al. (1981), children exposed to PBB did not differ from a control group on the McCarthy Developmental Scales. However, within the exposed group, a significant negative relationship appeared between body burden of PBB and performance on four of the five subscales of the McCarthy. More PBB-exposed children were reported by their parents to be excessively clumsy, but this was not confirmed on neurologic examination.

In 1968, as a result of contamination of rice oil with polychlorinated biphenyl (Kuratsune et al., 1972), more than 300 people developed a skin disease similar to chloracne; 11 liveborn infants and 2 stillborns had been exposed in utero (Yamaguchi et al., 1971). Although the typical symptoms of congenitally exposed children included stained skin and nails, eye discharge, and jaundice, 12 of 13 infants were also small by national standards and 4 were small for gestational age. Thus

240

far no evidence exists of physical or mental retardation in these children (Yamaguchi et al., 1971; Kuratsune et al., 1972).

CONCLUSIONS

Review of the behavioral teratology literature indicates that in just over a decade many behavioral teratogens have been uncovered. Nevertheless, what has been discovered so far probably represents only a fraction of the behavioral teratogens that exist.

In spite of major advances in this field, many questions remain unanswered: Why are some fetuses more susceptible than others to behavioral teratogenic effects? How do variables such as SES, prenatal nutrition, and gender contribute to this susceptibility? Which behavioral teratogens exert their effects directly on the fetus and which indirectly—for example, by reducing birthweight? At what point in gestation is the introduction of an agent most likely to result in postnatal behavioral disorder? What pathologies underlie these behavioral changes? What are the most sensitive tools to assess them? Clearly, follow-up studies of the long-range effects of in utero exposures must be conducted in order to clarify the role that early exposures play in the etiology of developmental disorders of behavior.

REFERENCES

Abel, E.L. (1979). Behavioral teratology of marijuana extracts in rats. *Neurobehav. Toxocol. Teratol. 1*, 235–247.

———— (1980). Smoking during pregnancy: A review of effects on growth and development of offspring. *Hum. Biol. 52*, 593–625.

———— (1981). Behavioral teratology of alcohol. *Psychol. Bull. 90*, 564–581.

Abrams, J.H. (1979). Developmental assessment of human infants through 12 weeks of age following chronic prenatal exposure to marijuana. *Diss. Abs. Int. 39*, 3495-B.

Aleksandrowicz, M.K. and Aleksandrowicz, D.R. (1974). Obstetrical pain-relieving drugs as predictors of infant behavior variability. *Child Dev. 45*, 935–945.

Amin-Zaki, L., Elhassani, S., Majeed, M.A., Clarkson T.W., Doherty R.A., and Greenwood, M. (1974). Intra-uterine methylmercury poisoning in Iraq. *Pediatrics 54*, 587–595.

————, Majeed, M.A., Elhassani, S.B., Clarkson, T.W., Greenwood, M.R., and Doherty, R.A. (1979). Prenatal methylmercury poisoning. Clinical observation over five years. *Am. J. Dis. Child. 133*, 172–177.

Annegers, J.F., Elveback, L.R., Hauser, W.A., and Kurland, L.T. (1974). Do anticonvulsants have a teratogenic effect? *Arch. Neurol. 31*, 364–373.

Athinarayanan, P., Pierog, S.H., Nigam, S.K., and Glass, L. (1976). Chlordiazepoxide withdrawal in the neonate. *Am. J. Obstet. Gynecol. 124*,
212–213.

Ayd, F.J. (1964). Children born to mothers treated with chlorpromazine
during pregnancy. *Clin. Med. 71*, 1758–1763.

Bakir, F., Damluji, S.F., Amin-Zaki, L., Murtadha, M., Khalidi, A., Al-Rawi,
N.Y., Tikriti, S., Dhahir, H.I., Clarkson, T.W., Smith, J.C., and Doherty,
R.A. (1973). Methylmercury poisoning in Iraq. An interuniversity report.
Science 181, 230–241.

———, Rustam, H., Tikriti, S., Al-Damluji, S.F., and Shihristani, H. (1980).
Clinical and epidemiological aspects of methylmercury poisoning. *Postgrad. Med. J. 56*, 1–10.

Baloh, R., Sturm, R., Green, B., and Gleser, G. (1975). Neuropsychological
effects of chronic asymptomatic increased lead absorption. A controlled
study. *Arch. Neurol. 32*, 326–330.

Beattie, A.D., Moore, M.R., Goldberg, A., Finlayson, M.J.W., Graham, J.F.,
Mackie, E.M., Main, J.C., McLaren, D.A., Murdoch, R.M., and Stewart,
G.T. (1975). Role of chronic low-level lead exposure in the aetiology of
mental retardation. *Lancet 1*, 589–592.

Billing, L., Eriksson, M., Larsson, G., and Zetterström, R. (1980). Ampheta-
mine addiction and pregnancy. III. One year follow-up of the children.
Psychosocial and pediatric aspects. *Acta Paediatr. Scand. 69*, 675–680.

Bleyer, W.A. and Marshall, R.E. (1972). Barbiturate withdrawal syndrome in
a passively addicted infant. *J.A.M.A. 221*, 185–186.

Borgen, L.A., Davis, W.M., and Pace, H.B. (1973). Effects of prenatal Δ⁹THC
on the development of rat offspring. *Pharmacol. Biochem. Behav. 1*,
203–206.

Borlée, I., Lechat, M.F., Bouckaert, A., and Misson, C. (1978). Le café,
facteur de risque pendant la grossesse? *Louvain Méd. 97*, 279–284.

Brackbill, Y. (1977). Long-term effects of obstetrical anesthesia on infant
autonomic function. *Dev. Neurobiol. 10*, 529–535.

———, Kane, J., Manniello, R.L., and Abramson, D. (1974). Obstetric
premedication and infant outcome. *Am. J. Obstet. Gynecol. 118*, 377–384.

Brander, T. (1940). Microcephalus und Tetraplegie bei einem Kinde nach
Kohlen monoxydvergiftung der Mutter während der Schwangerschaft.
Acta Paediatr. (Suppl.) 28, 123–132.

Brazelton, T.B. (1961). Psychophysiologic reactions in the neonate. II. Effect
of maternal medication. *J. Pediatr. 58*, 513–518.

Bridbord, K. (1978). Occupational lead exposure and women. *Prev. Med. 7*,
311–321.

Bruni, J. and Willmore, L.J. (1979). Epilepsy and pregnancy. *Can. J. Neurol.
Sci 6*, 345–349.

Buelke-Sam, J. and Kimmel, C.A. (1979). Development and standardization
of screening methods for behavioral teratology. *Teratology 20*, 17–30.

Butcher, R.E., Hawver, K., Burbacher, T., and Scott, W. (1975). Behavioral
effects from antenatal exposure to teratogens. In *Aberrant development
in infancy: Human and animal studies*, edited by N.R. Ellis. Hillside,
N.J.: Lawrence Erlbaum Associates.

Butler, N.R. and Alberman, E.D. (1969). *Perinatal problems. The second report of the 1958 British Perinatal Mortality Survey.* Edinburgh and London: E. and S. Livingstone, pp. 47–71.

—— and Goldstein, H. (1973). Smoking in pregnancy and subsequent child development. *Br. Med. J. 4,* 573–575.

——, ——, and Ross, E.M. (1972). Cigarette smoking in pregnancy: Its influence on birth weight and perinatal mortality. *Br. Med. J. 2,* 127–130.

Camfield, C.S., Chaplin, S., Doyle, A-B., Shapiro, S.H., Cummings, C., and Camfield, P.R. (1979). Side effects of phenobarbital in toddlers; behavioral and cognitive aspects. *J. Pediatr. 95,* 361–365.

Caspi, E., Ronen, J., Schreyer, P., and Goldberg, M.D. (1976). The outcome of pregnancy after gonadotrophin therapy. *Br. J. Obstet. Gynaecol. 83,* 967–973.

Chasnoff, I.J., Hatcher, R., and Burns, W.J. (1982). Polydrug- and methadone-addicted newborns: A continuum of impairment. *Pediatrics 70,* 210–213.

Chavez, C.J., Ostrea, E.M., Stryker, J.C., and Strauss, M.E. (1979). Ocular abnormalities in infants as sequelae of prenatal drug addiction. *Pediatr. Res. 13,* 367.

Choi, B.H., Lapham, L.W., Amin-Zaki, L., and Saleem, T. (1978). Abnormal neuronal migration, deranged cerebral cortical organization and diffuse white matter astrocytosis of human fetal brain: A major effect of methylmercury in utero. *J. Neuropathol. Exp. Neurol. 37,* 719–733.

Christianson, R.E. (1979). Gross differences observed in the placentas of smokers and nonsmokers. *Am. J. Epidemiol. 110,* 178–187.

Clarren, S.K., Alvord, E.C., Sumi, S.M., Streissguth, A.P., and Smith, D.W. (1978). Brain malformations related to prenatal exposure to ethanol. *J. Pediatr. 92,* 64–67.

—— and Smith, D.W. (1978). The fetal alcohol syndrome. *N. Engl. J. Med. 298,* 1063–1067.

Cree, J.E., Meyer, J., and Harley, D.M. (1973). Diazepam in labour: Its metabolism and effect on the clinical condition and thermogenesis of the newborn. *Br. Med. J. 4,* 251–255.

David, O., Clark, J., and Voeller, K. (1972). Lead and hyperactivity. *Lancet 2,* 900–903.

Denson, R., Nanson, J.L., and McWatters, M.A. (1975). Hyperkinesis and maternal smoking. *Can. Psychiatr. Assoc. J. 20,* 183–187.

Desclaux, P., Soulairac, A., and Morlon, C. (1951). Intoxication oxycarbonée au cours d'une gestation (cinquième mois), arriération mentale consécutive. *Arch. Fr. Pediatr. 8,* 316–318.

Desmond, M.M., Schwanecke, R.P., Wilson, G.S., Yasunaga, S., and Burgdorff, I. (1972). Maternal barbiturate utilization and neonatal withdrawal symptomatology. *J. Pediatr. 80,* 190–197.

Dobbing, J. (1974). Human brain development and its vulnerability. *Mead Johnson Symp. Perinat. Dev. Med. 6,* 3–12.

—— and Sands, J. (1973). The quantitative growth and development of the human brain. *Arch. Dis. Child. 48,* 757–767.

Dubowitz, V. (1975). Neurological fragility in the newborn: Influence of medication in labour. *Br. J. Anaesth. 47*, 1005–1010.

Dunn, H.G., McBurney, A.K., Ingram, S., and Hunter, C.M. (1977). Maternal cigarette smoking during pregnancy and the child's subsequent development: II. Neurological and intellectual maturation to the age of $6\frac{1}{2}$ years. *Can. J. Public Health 68*, 43–50.

Eckardt, M.J., Harford, T.C., Kaelber, C.T., Parker, E.S., Rosenthal, L.S., Ryback, R.S., Salmoiraghi, G.C., Vanderveen, E., and Warren, K.R. (1981). Health hazards associated with alcohol consumption. *J.A.M.A. 246*, 648–666.

Edmonds, L.D., Anderson, C.E., Flynt, J.W., and James, L.M. (1978). Congenital central nervous system malformations and vinyl chloride monomer exposure: A community study. *Teratology 17*, 137–142.

Ehrhardt, A.A., Grisanti, G.C., and Meyer-Bahlburg, H.F.L. (1977). Prenatal exposure to medroxyprogesterone acetate (MPA) in girls. *Psychoneuroendocrinology 2*, 391–398.

———— and Money, J. (1967). Progestin-induced hermaphroditism: I.Q. and psychosexual identity in a study of 10 girls. *J. Sex Res. 3*, 83–100.

Engel, J., Ahlenius, S., Brown, R., and Lundborg, P. (1973). Behavioural effects in offspring of nursing mothers. *Proc. Eur. Soc. Study of Drug Toxicity 15*, 20–24.

Engleson, G. and Herner, T. (1952). Alkylmercury poisoning. *Acta Paediatr. Scand. 41*, 289–294.

Fedrick, J., Alberman, E.D., and Goldstein, H. (1971). Possible teratogenic effect of cigarette smoking. *Nature 231*, 529–530.

Feldman, G.L., Weaver, D.D., and Lovrien, E.W. (1977). The fetal trimethadione syndrome. *Am. J. Dis. Child. 131*, 1389–1392.

Finberg, L. (1977). PBBs: The ladies' milk is not for burning. *J. Pediatr. 90*, 511–512.

Fried, P.A. (1980). Marihuana use by pregnant women: Neurobehavioral effects in neonates. *Drug Alcohol Depend. 6*, 415–424.

————, Watkinson, B., Grant, A., and Knights, R.M. (1980). Changing patterns of soft drug use prior to and during pregnancy: A prospective study. *Drug Alcohol Depend. 6*, 323–343.

Friedman, E.A., Sachtleben, M.R., and Wallace, A.K. (1979). Infant outcome following labor induction. *Am. J. Obstet. Gynecol. 133*, 718–722.

Friedman, S.L., Caron, A.J., Brackbill, Y., and Caron, R.F. (1978). Obstetric medication and visual processing in 4- and 5-month old infants. *Merrill-Palmer Q. 24*, 111–128.

Garn, S.M., Petzold, A.S., Ridella, S.A., and Johnson, M. (1980). Effect of smoking during pregnancy on Apgar and Bayley scores. *Lancet 2*, 912–913.

Garvey, D.J. and Longo, L.D. (1978). Chronic low level maternal carbon monoxide exposure and fetal growth and development. *Biol. Reprod. 19*, 8–14.

German, J., Ehlers, K.H., Kowal, A., DeGeorge, F.V., Engle, M.A., and Passarge, E. (1970). Possible teratogenicity of trimethadione and paramethadione. *Lancet 2*, 261–262.

Ghosh, A. (1975). Oxytocic agents and neonatal morbidity. *Lancet 1*, 453.

Gittelman, R. and Eskenazi, B. (1983). Lead and hyperactivity revisited: An investigation of non-disadvantaged children. *Arch. Gen. Psychiatry 40*, 827–833.

Goodfriend, M.J., Shey, I.A., and Klein, M.D. (1956). The effects of maternal narcotic addiction on the newborn. *Am. J. Obstet. Gynecol. 71*, 29–36.

Gouin-Décarie, T. (1969). A study of the mental and emotional development of the thalidomide child. In *Determinants of infant behavior*, edited by Methuen. London: B.M. Foss.

Guillozet, N. (1975). The risks of paracervical anesthesia: Intoxication and neurological injury of the newborn. *Pediatrics 55*, 533–536.

Gumbinas, M., Oda, M., and Huttenlocher, P. (1973). The effects of cortico-steroids on myelination of the developing rat brain. *Biol. Neonate 22*, 355–366.

Hanson, J.W. (1976). Fetal hydantoin syndrome. *Teratology 13*, 185–188.

———, Jones, K.L., and Smith, D.W. (1976). Fetal alcohol syndrome. Experience with 41 patients. *J.A.M.A. 235*, 1458–1460.

———, Myrianthopoulos, N.C., Sedgwick-Harvey, M.A., and Smith, D.W. (1976a). Risks to the offspring of women treated with hydantoin anticonvulsants, with emphasis on the fetal hydantoin syndrome. *J. Pediatr. 89*, 662–668.

——— and Smith, D.W. (1975). The fetal hydantoin syndrome. *J. Pediatr. 87*, 285–290.

——— and ——— (1976). Fetal hydantoin syndrome. *Lancet 1*, 692.

Harada M. (1976). Intrauterine poisoning, clinical and epidemiological studies and significance of the problem. *Bull. Instit. Constitutional Med.*, Kumamoto University (Suppl. 25), 1–60. Cited by Harada 1978.

——— (1977). Study on methylmercury concentration in the umbilical cords of the inhabitants born in the Minamata area. *Brain Dev. 9*, 79–84.

——— (1978). Congenital Minamata disease: Intrauterine methylmercury poisoning. *Teratology 18*, 285–288.

———, Moriyama H., and Nonaka M. (1971). Investigation on babies of Minamata disease at the later period. *Jpn. J. Clin. Exp. Med. 48*, 1431–1440 (Jap). Cited by Kojima and Fujita (1973).

Hardy, J.B. and Mellits, E.D. (1972). Does maternal smoking during pregnancy have a long-term effect on the child? *Lancet 2*, 1332–1336.

Hartz, S.C., Heinonen, O.P., Shapiro, S., Siskind, V., and Slone, D. (1975). Antenatal exposure to meprobamate and chlordiazepoxide in relation to malformations, mental development, and childhood mortality. *N. Engl. J. Med. 292*, 726–728.

Havlicek, V. and Childaeva, R. (1976). E.E.G. component of fetal alcohol syndrome. *Lancet 2*, 477.

———, ———, and Chernick, V. (1977). E.E.G. frequency spectrum characteristics of sleep states of alcoholic mothers. *Neuropaediatrie 8*, 360–373.

Heinonen, O.P., Slone, D., and Shapiro, S. (1977). *Birth defects and drugs in pregnancy*. Littleton, Mass.: Publishing Sciences Group.

Henderson, G.I., Patwardhan, R.V., Hoyuma, A.M., and Schenker, S. (1981). Fetal alcohol syndrome: Overview of pathogenesis. *Neurobehav. Toxicol. Teratol. 3*, 73–80.

Hill, R.M. (1973). Teratogenesis and antiepileptic drugs. *N. Engl. J. Med. 289*, 1089–1090.

—— (1976). Fetal malformations and antiepileptic drugs. *Am. J. Dis. Child. 130*, 923–925.

—— and Desmond, M.M. (1963). Management of the narcotic withdrawal syndrome in the neonate. *Pediatr. Clin. North Am. 10*, 67–87.

——, ——, and Kay, J.L. (1966). Extrapyramidal dysfunction in an infant of a schizophrenic mother. *J. Pediatr. 69*, 589–595.

——, Verniaud, W.M., Horning, M.G., McCulley, L.B., and Morgan, N.F. (1974). Infants exposed in utero to antiepileptic drugs. A prospective study. *Am. J. Dis. Child. 127*, 645–653.

Hillman, L.S., Hillman, R.E., and Dodson, W.E. (1979). Diagnosis, treatment, and follow-up of neonatal mepivacaine intoxication secondary to para-cervical and pudendal blocks during labor. *J. Pediatr. 95*, 472–477.

Hodgkinson, R., Bhatt, M., Grewal, G., and Marx, G.F. (1978). Neonatal neurobehavior in the first 48 hours of life: Effect of the administration of meperidine with and without naloxone in the mother. *Pediatrics 62*, 294–298.

——, ——, Kim, S.S., Grewal, G., and Marx, G.F. (1978a). Neonatal neurobehavioral tests following cesarean section under general and spinal anesthesia. *Am. J. Obstet. Gynecol. 132*, 670–673.

——, ——, and Wang, C.N. (1978b). Double-blind comparison of the neurobehavior of neonates following the administration of different doses of meperidine to the mother. *Can. Anaesth. Soc. J. 25*, 405–411.

——, Marx, G.F., and Kaiser, J.H. (1975). Local regional anesthesia during childbirth and newborn behavior. *Science 189*, 571–572.

Hollman, A.I., Jouppila, R., Koivisto, M., Maatta, L., Pihlajaniemi, R., Puuka, M., and Rantakyla, P. (1978). Neurologic activity of infants following anesthesia for cesarean section. *Anesthesiology 48*, 350–356.

Holmberg, P.C. (1979). Central-nervous-system defects in children born to mothers exposed to organic solvents during pregnancy. *Lancet 2*, 177–179.

Horowitz, F.D., Ashton, J., Culp, R., and Gaddis, E. (1977). The effects of obstetrical medication on the behavior of Israeli newborn infants and some comparisons with Uruguayan and American infants. *Child Dev. 48*, 1607–1623.

Horstmann, W. (1966). Hinweise auf zentral-nervöse Schäden im Rahmen der Thalidomid-Embryopathie. *Z. Kinderheilkd. 96*, 291. Cited by Stephenson (1976).

Illingworth, R.S. (1966). *Development of the infant and young child, normal and abnormal* (3rd ed.). Edinburgh: E. and S. Livingstone.

Iosub, S., Fuchs, M., Bingol, N., Stone, R.K., and Gromisch, D.S. (1981). Long-term follow-up of three siblings with fetal alcohol syndrome. *Alcohol Clin. Exp. Res. 5*, 523–527.

Joffe, J.M. (1979). Influence of drug exposure of the father on perinatal outcome. *Clin. Perinatol. 6*, 21–36.

Jones, K.L. and Smith, D.W. (1973). Recognition of the fetal alcohol syndrome in early infancy. *Lancet 2*, 999–1001.

————, ————, Streissguth, A.P., and Myrianthopoulos, N.C. (1974). Outcome in offspring of chronic alcoholic women. *Lancet 1*, 1076–1078.

————, ————, Ulleland, C.N., and Streissguth, A.P. (1973). Pattern of malformation in offspring of chronic alcoholic mothers. *Lancet 1*, 1267–1271.

Kaminski, M., Rumeau, C., and Schwartz, D. (1978). Alcohol consumption in pregnant women and the outcome of pregnancy. *Alcohol Clin. Exp. Res.* 2, 155–163.

Kaplan, N.M. (1959). Male pseudohermaphrodism. Report of a case, with observations on pathogenesis. *N. Engl. J. Med. 261*, 641–644.

Kaplan, S.L., Kron, R.E., Litt, M., Finnegan, L.P., and Phoenix, M.D. (1975). Correlations between scores on the Brazelton Neonatal Assessment Scale, measures of newborn sucking behavior, and birthweight in infants born to narcotic addicted mothers. In *Aberrant development in infancy: Human and animal studies*, edited by N.R. Ellis. Hillsdale, N.J.: Lawrence Erlbaum Associates.

Kawash, G.F., Yeung, D.L., and Berg, S.D. (1980). Effects of administration of cannabis resin during pregnancy on emotionality and learning in rats' offspring. *Percept. Mot. Skills 50*, 359–365.

Kojima, K. and Fujita, M. (1973). Summary of recent studies in Japan on methyl mercury poisoning. *Toxicology 1*, 43–62.

Kolata, G. (1979). Scientists attack report that obstetrical medications endanger children. *Science 204*, 391–392.

Kopelman, A.E. (1975). Fetal addiction to pentazocine. *Pediatrics 55*, 888.

Kron, R.E., Stein, M.S., and Goddard, K.E. (1966). Newborn sucking behavior affected by obstetrical sedation. *Pediatrics 37*, 1012–1016.

Kuratsune, M., Yoshimura, T., Matsuzaka, J., and Yamaguchi, A. (1972). Epidemiologic study on Yusho, a poisoning caused by ingestion of rice oil contaminated with a commercial brand of polychlorinated biphenyls. *Environ. Health Perspect 1*, 119–128.

Landesman-Dwyer, S. and Emanuel, I. (1979). Smoking during pregnancy. *Teratology 19*, 119–125.

————, Keller, L.S., and Streissguth, A.P. (1978). Naturalistic observations of newborns: Effects of maternal alcohol intake. *Alcohol Clin. Exp. Res.* 2, 171–177.

————, Ragozin, A.S., and Little, R.E. (1981). Behavioral correlates of prenatal alcohol exposure: A four-year follow-up study. *Neurobehav. Toxicol. Teratol. 3*, 187–193.

Landrigan, P.J., Whitworth, R.H., Baloh, R.W., Staehling, N.W., Barthel, W.F., and Rosenblum, B.F. (1975). Neuropsychological dysfunction in children with chronic low-level lead absorption. *Lancet 1*, 708–712.

Lemoine, P., Harrousseau, H., Borteyru, J.P., and Menuet, J. (1968). Les enfants de parents alcooliques. Anomalies observeés. A propos de 127 cas. *Ouest Méd. 25*, 477–482.

Lessen-Firestone, J.K., Strauss, M.E., Starr, R.H., and Ostrea, E.H. (1974). *Behavioral characteristics of methadone-addicted neonates*, Tech. Rep. No. 02–74, Spencer Foundation. Detroit: Wayne State University. Cited by Lodge et al. (1975).

Lieberman, B.A., Rosenblatt, D.B., Belsey, E., Packer, M., Redshaw, M., Mills, M., Caldwell, J., Notarianni, L., Smith, R.L., Williams, M., and Beard, R.W. (1979). The effects of maternally administered pethidine or epidural bupivacaine on the fetus and newborn. *Br. J. Obstet. Gynaecol. 86*, 598–606.

Lipper, E., Lee, K., Gartner, L.M., and Grellong, B. (1981). Determinants of neurobehavioral outcome in low-birth-weight infants. *Pediatrics 67*, 502–505.

Little, R. (1977). Alcohol consumption during pregnancy and decreased birthweight. *Am. J. Public Health 67*, 1154–1156.

Lodge, A., Marcus, M.M., and Ramer, C.M. (1975). Behavioral and electrophysiological characteristics of the addicted neonate. *Addict. Dis. 2*, 235–255.

Longo, L.D. (1970). Carbon monoxide in the pregnant mother and fetus and its exchange across the placenta. *Ann. N.Y. Acad. Sci. 174*, 313–341.

Lorber, C.A., Cassidy, S.B., and Engel, E. (1979). Is there an embryo-fetal exogenous sex steroid exposure syndrome (EFESSES)? *Fertil. Steril. 31*, 21–24.

Lowe, C.R. (1959). Effect of mothers' smoking habits on birthweight of their children. *Br. Med. J. 2*, 673–676.

MacArthur, B.A., Howie, R.N., Dezoete, J.A., and Elkins, J. (1981). Cognitive and psychosocial development of 4-year old children whose mothers were treated antenatally with betamethasone. *Pediatrics 68*, 638–643.

Majewski, F. (1981). Alcohol embryopathy: Some facts and speculations about pathogenesis. *Neurobehav. Toxicol. Teratol. 3*, 129–144.

Mangurten, H.H. and Benawra, R. (1980). Neonatal codeine withdrawal in infants of nonaddicted mothers. *Pediatrics 65*, 159–160.

Marsh, D.O., Myers, G.J., Clarkson, T.W., Amin-Zaki, L., Tikriti, S., and Majeed, M.A. (1980). Fetal methylmercury poisoning: Clinical and toxicological data on 29 cases. *Ann. Neurol. 7*, 348–353.

——, ——, ——, ——, ——, ——, and Dabbagh, A.R. (1981). Dose-response relationship of human fetal exposure to methylmercury. *Clin. Toxicol. 18*, 1311–1318.

Martin, D.C., Martin, J.C., Streissguth, A.P., and Lund, C.A. (1979). Sucking frequency and amplitude in newborns as a function of maternal drinking and smoking. In *Currents in alcoholism.* Vol. 5, *Biomedical issues and clinical effects of alcoholism*, edited by M. Galanter. New York: Grune and Stratton.

Martin, J., Martin, D.C., Lund, C.A., and Streissguth, A.P. (1977). Maternal alcohol ingestion and cigarette smoking and their effects on newborn conditioning. *Alcohol Clin. Exp. Res. 1*, 243–247.

Matsumoto, H., Koya, G., and Takeuchi, T. (1964). Fetal Minamata disease. A neuropathological study of two cases of intrauterine intoxication by a methyl mercury compound. *J. Neuropathol. Exp. Neurol. 24*, 563–574.

Mau, G. (1980). Moderate alcohol consumption during pregnancy and child development. *Eur. J. Paediatr. 133*, 233–237.

——, and Netter, P. (1974). Kaffee- und Alkaholkonsum-Risikofaktoren in der Schwangerschaft? *Geburtshilfe Frauenheilkd. 34*, 1018–1022.

Mazzi, E. (1977). Possible neonatal diazepam withdrawal: A case report. *Am. J. Obstet. Gynecol. 129*, 586–587.

McBride, W.G., Lyle, J.G., Black, B., Brown, C., and Thomas, D.B. (1977). A study of five year old children born after elective induction of labour. *Med. J. Aust. 2*, 456–459.

McFie, J. and Robertson, J. (1973). Psychological test results of children with thalidomide deformities. *Dev. Med. Child Neurol. 15*, 719–727.

Meadow, S.R. (1968). Anticonvulsant drugs and congenital abnormalities. *Lancet 2*, 1296.

Meredith, H.V. (1975). Relation between tobacco smoking of pregnant women and body size of their progeny: A compilation and synthesis of published studies. *Hum. Biol. 47*, 451–472.

Meyer-Bahlburg, H.F.L., Grisanti, G.C., and Ehrhardt, A.A (1977). Prenatal effects of sex hormones on human male behavior: Medroxyprogesterone acetate (MPA). *Psychoneuroendocrinology 2*, 383–400.

Ministry of Health (1964). *Deformities caused by thalidomide.* London: Her Majesty's Stationery Office.

Molliver, M.E., Kostović, I., and Van der Loos, H. (1973). The development of synapses in cerebral cortex of the human fetus. *Brain Res. 50*, 403–407.

Monson, R.R., Rosenberg, L., Hartz, S.C., Shapiro, S., Heinonen, O.P., and Slone, D. (1973). Diphenylhydantoin and selected congenital malformations. *N. Engl. J. Med. 289*, 1049–1052.

Moore, H.R., Meredith, P.A., and Goldberg, A. (1977). A retrospective analysis of blood-lead in mentally retarded children. *Lancet 1*, 717–719.

Murakami, U. (1972). The effect of organic mercury on intrauterine life. *Adv. Exp. Med. Biol. 27*, 301–336.

Naeye, R.L. (1978). Relationship of cigarette smoking to congenital anomalies and perinatal death. *Am. J. Pathol. 90*, 289–293.

———, Ladis, B., and Drage, J.S. (1976). Sudden infant death syndrome: A prospective study. *Am. J. Dis. Child. 130*, 1207–1210.

Needleman, H.L., Gunnoe, C., Leviton, A., Reed, R., Peresie, H., Maher, C., and Barrett, P. (1979). Deficits in psychologic and classroom performance of children with elevated dentine lead levels. *N. Engl. J. Med. 300*, 689–694.

Nesheim, B.I., Lindbaek, E., Storm-Mathisen, I., and Jenssen, H. (1979). Neurobehavioral response of infants after paracervical block during labor. *Acta Obstet. Gynaecol. Scand. 58*, 41–44.

Nichols, P.L. (1977). *Minimal brain dysfunctions: Association with perinatal complications.* Paper presented at the Society for Research in Child Development. Cited by Landesman-Dwyer and Emanuel (1979).

Niswander, K.R., Turoff, B.B., and Romans, J. (1966). Developmental status of children delivered through elective induction of labour. *Obstet. Gynecol. 27*, 15–20.

Olegård, R., Sabel, K.-G., Aronsson, M., Sandin, B., Johansson, P.R., Carlsson, C., Kyllerman, M., Iverson, K., and Hrbek, A. (1979). Effects on the child of alcohol abuse during pregnancy. *Acta Paediatr. Scand. (Suppl.) 275*, 112–121.

Ostrea, E.M. and Chavez, C.J. (1979). Perinatal problems (excluding neonatal withdrawal) in maternal drug addiction: A study of 830 cases. *J. Pediatr.* 94, 292–295.

Ouellette, E.M. and Rosett, H.L. (1976). A pilot prospective study of the fetal alcohol syndrome at the Boston City Hospital. Part II: The infants. *Ann. N.Y. Acad. Sci.* 273, 123–129.

Palahniuk, R.J., Scatliff, J., Biehl, D., Wiebe, H., and Sankaran, K. (1977). Maternal and neonatal effects of methoxyflurane nitrous oxide and lumbar epidural anaesthesia for Caesarean section. *Can. Anaesth. Soc. J.* 24, 586–596.

Palmisano, P.A., Sneed, R.C., and Cassady, G. (1969). Untaxed whiskey and fetal lead exposure. *J. Pediatr.* 75, 869–872.

Perino, J. and Ernhardt, C.B. (1974). The relation of subclinical lead level to cognitive and sensorimotor impairment in black preschoolers. *J. Learning Disabil.* 7, 26–30.

Persson, P., Grennert, L., Gennser, G., and Kullander, S. (1978). A study of smoking and pregnancy with special reference to fetal growth. *Acta Obstet. Gynaecol. Scand. (Suppl.)* 78, 33–39.

Pierog, S., Chandavasu, O., and Wexler, I. (1977). Withdrawal symptoms in infants with the fetal alcohol syndrome. *J. Pediatr.* 90, 630–633.

Pihl, R.O. and Parkes, M. (1977). Hair element content in learning disabled children. *Science* 198, 204–206.

Preis, O., Choi, S.J., and Rudolph, N. (1977). Pentazocine withdrawal syndrome in the newborn infant. *Am. J. Obstet. Gynecol.* 127, 205–206.

Prenner, B.M. (1977). Neonatal withdrawal syndrome associated with hydroxyzine hydrochloride. *Am. J. Dis. Child.* 131, 529–530.

Pringle, M.L.K. and Fiddes, D.O. (1970). *The challenge of thalidomide.* London: Longmans.

Purpura, D.P. (1974). Neuronal migration and dendritic differentiation: Normal and aberrant development of human cerebral cortex. *Mead Johnson Symp. Perinat. Dev. Med.* 6, 13–27.

——— (1974a). Dendritic spine dysgenesis and mental retardation. *Science* 184, 1126–1128.

Ralston, D.H. and Shnider, S.M. (1978). The fetal and neonatal effects of regional anesthesia in obstetrics. *Anesthesiology* 48, 34–64.

Rementería, J.L. and Bhatt, K. (1977). Withdrawal symptoms in neonates from intrauterine exposure to diazepam. *J. Pediatr.* 90, 123–126.

Reuhl, K.R. and Chang, L.W. (1979). Effects of methylmercury on the development of the nervous system: A review. *Neurotoxicology 1*, 21–55.

Reveri, M., Pyati, S.P., and Pildes, R.S. (1977). Neonatal withdrawal symptoms associated with glutethimide (Doriden) addiction in the mother during pregnancy. *Clin. Pediatr.* 16, 424–425.

Rodier, P. (1976). Critical periods for behavioral anomalies in mice. *Environ. Health Perspect.* 18, 79–83.

Rosen, T.S. and Johnson, H.L. (1982). Children of methadone-maintained mothers: Follow-up to 18 months of age. *J. Pediatr.* 101, 192–196.

Rosett, H.L., Snyder, P., Sander, L.W., Lee, A., Cook, P., Weiner, L., and Gould, J. (1979). Effects of maternal drinking on neonate state regulation. *Dev. Med. Child Neurol.* 21, 464–473.

Rumack, B.H. and Walravens, P.A. (1973). Neonatal withdrawal following maternal ingestion of ethchlorvynol (Placidyl). *Pediatrics 52*, 714–716.

Rutter, M. (1980). Raised lead levels and impaired cognitive/behavioural functioning: A review of the evidence. *Dev. Med. Child Neurol. (Suppl.) 22*, 1–26.

Sander, L.W., Snyder, P.A., Rosett, H.L., Lee, A., Gould, J.B., and Ouellette, E. (1977). Effects of alcohol intake during pregnancy on newborn state regulation: A progress report. *Alcohol Clin. Exp. Res 1*, 233–241.

Scanlon, J.W. (1976). Effects of local anesthetics administered to parturient women on the neurological and behavioral performance of newborn children. *Bull. N.Y. Acad. Med. 52*, 231–240.

—— (1981). Effects of obstetric anesthesia and analgesia on the newborn: A select, annotated bibliography for the clinician. *Clin. Obstet. Gynecol. 24*, 649–670.

——, Brown, W.V., Weiss, J.B., and Alper, M.H. (1974). Neurobehavioral responses of newborn infants after maternal epidural anesthesia. *Anesthesiology 40*, 121–128.

——, Ostheimer, G.W., Lurie, A.O., Brown, W.V., Weiss, J.B., and Alper, M.H. (1976). Neurobehavioral responses and drug concentrations in newborns after maternal epidural anesthesia with bupivacaine. *Anesthesiology 45*, 400–405.

——, Suzuki, K., Shea, E., and Tronick, E. (1978). Clinical and neurobehavioral effects of repeated intrauterine exposure to oxytocin: A prospective study. *Am. J. Obstet. Gynecol. 132*, 294–296.

Schardein, J.L. (1980). Congenital abnormalities and hormones during pregnancy: A clinical review. *Teratology 22*, 251–270.

Shapiro, S., Hartz, S.C., Siskind, V., Mitchell, A.A., Slone, D., Rosenberg, L., Monson, R.R., Heinonen, O.P., Idanpaan-Heikkila, J., Haro, S., and Saxén, L. (1976). Anticonvulsants and parental epilepsy in the development of birth defects. *Lancet 1*, 272–275.

Shaywitz, S.E., Caparulo, B.K., and Hodgson, E.S. (1981). Developmental language disability as a consequence of prenatal exposure to ethanol. *Pediatrics 68*, 850–855.

——, Cohen, D.J., and Shaywitz, B.A. (1980). Behavior and learning difficulties in children of normal intelligence born to alcoholic mothers. *J. Pediatr. 96*, 978–982.

Sheikh, K. (1979). Teratogenic effects of organic solvents. *Lancet 2*, 963.

Shurygin, G.I. (1974). Characteristics of the mental development of children of alcoholic mothers (Russian). *Pediatriia 11*, 71–73.

Sidman, R.L. and Rakic, P. (1973). Neuronal migration, with special reference to developing human brain: A review. *Brain Res. 62*, 1–35.

Simpson, W.J. (1957). A preliminary report of cigarette smoking and the incidence of prematurity. *Am. J. Obstet. Gynecol. 73*, 808–815.

Slone, D., Siskind, V., Heinonen, O.P., Monson, R.R., Kaufman, D.W., and Shapiro, S. (1977). Antenatal exposure to the phenothiazines in relation to congenital malformations, perinatal mortality rate, birth weight, and intelligence quotient score. *Am. J. Obstet. Gynecol. 128*, 486–488.

Smithells, R.W. (1970). Hand and foot preference in thalidomide children. *Arch. Dis. Child.* 45, 274.

Sokol, R.J., Miller, S.I., and Reed, G. (1980). Alcohol abuse during pregnancy: An epidemiologic study. *Alcohol Clin. Exp. Res.* 4, 135–145.

Soule, B., Standley, K., Copans, S., and Davis, M. (1973). *Clinical implications of the Brazelton Scale.* Paper presented at the annual meeting of the Society for Research in Child Development. Cited by Lodge et al. (1975).

Speidel, B.D. and Meadow, S.R. (1972). Maternal epilepsy and abnormalities of the fetus and newborn. *Lancet 2*, 839–843.

Spyker, J.M. (1975). Assessing the impact of low level chemicals on development: Behavioral and latent effects. *Fed. Proc. 34*, 1835–1844.

Standley, K., Soule, A.B., Copans, S.A., and Duchowny, M.S. (1974). Local-regional anesthesia during childbirth: Effect on newborn behaviors. *Science 186*, 634–635.

Stephenson, J.B.P. (1976). Epilepsy: A neurological complication of thalidomide embryopathy. *Dev. Med. Child Neurol. 18*, 189–197.

Strauss, M.E., Andresko, M., Stryker, J.C., Wardell, J.N., and Dunkel, L.D. (1974). Methadone maintenance during pregnancy: Pregnancy, birth, and neonate characteristics. *Am. J. Obstet. Gynecol. 120*, 895–900.

———, Lessen-Firestone, J.K., Starr, R.H., and Ostrea, E.M. (1975). Behavior of narcotic-addicted newborns. *Child Dev. 46*, 887–893.

———, Starr, R.H., Ostrea, E.M., Chavez, C.J., and Stryker, J.C. (1976). Behavioral concomitants of prenatal addiction to narcotics. *J. Pediatr. 89*, 842–846.

Streissguth, A.P. (1976). Maternal alcoholism and the outcome of pregnancy: A review of the fetal alcohol syndrome. In *Alcoholism problems in women and children*, edited by M. Greenblatt and M.A. Schuckit. New York: Grune and Stratton.

———, Barr H.M., Martin D.C., and Herman, C.S. (1980). Effects of maternal alcohol, nicotine, and caffeine use during pregnancy on infant mental and motor development at eight months. *Alcohol Clin. Exp. Res. 4*, 152–164.

———, Herman C.S., and Smith, D.W. (1978). Intelligence, behavior, and dysmorphogenesis in the fetal alcohol syndrome: A report on 20 patients. *J. Pediatr. 92*, 363–367.

———, ———, and ——— (1978a). Stability of intelligence in the fetal alcohol syndrome: A preliminary report. *Alcohol Clin. Exp. Res. 2*, 165–170.

Streissguth, A.P. (1978). Fetal alcohol syndrome: An epidemiologic perspective. *Am. J. Epidemiol. 107*, 467–478.

———, Landesman-Dwyer, S., Martin, J.C., and Smith, D.W. (1980a). Teratogenic effects of alcohol in humans and laboratory animals. *Science 209*, 353–361.

———, Little, R.E., Herman, C., and Woodell, S. (1979). IQ in children of recovered alcoholic mothers compared with maternal controls. *Alcohol Clin. Exp. Res. 3*, 197.

———, Martin, D.C., and Barr, H.M. (1977). *Neonatal Brazelton assessment and relationship to maternal alcohol intake.* Paper presented at American Psychological Association meeting. Cited by Streissguth et al. (1980).

———, ———, Martin, J.C., and Barr, H.M. (1981). The Seattle longitudinal prospective study on alcohol and pregnancy. *Neurobehav. Toxicol. Teratol. 3*, 223–233.

Toutant, C. and Lippmann, S. (1979). Fetal solvents syndrome. *Lancet 1*, 1356.

Tronick, E., Wise, S., Als, H., Adamson, L., Scanlon, J.W., and Brazelton, T.B. (1976). Regional obstetric anesthesia and newborn behavior: Effect over the first ten days of life. *Pediatrics 58*, 94–100.

van den Berg, J. (1977). Epidemiologic observations of prematurity: Effects of tobacco, coffee, and alcohol. In *Epidemiology of prematurity*, edited by D.M. Reed and F.J. Stanley. Baltimore, Md.: Urban and Schwarzenberg, 157–176.

Vargas, G.C., Pildes, R.S., Vidyasagar, D., and Keith, L.G. (1975). Effect of maternal heroin addiction on 67 liveborn neonates. *Clin. Pediatr. 14*, 751–757.

Vorhees, C.V., Brunner, R.L., and Butcher, R.E. (1979). Psychotropic drugs as behavioral teratogens. *Science 205*, 1220–1225.

Weathersbee, P.S. and Lodge, J.R. (1979). Alcohol, caffeine, and nicotine as factors in pregnancy. *Postgrad. Med. 66*, 165–169.

———, Olsen, L.K., and Lodge, J.R. (1977). Caffeine and pregnancy. A retrospective survey. *Postgrad. Med. 62*, 64–69.

Weichsel, M.E. (1974). Glucocorticoid effect upon thymidine kinase in the developing cerebellum. *Pediatr. Res. 8*, 843.

Weil, W.B., Spencer, M., Benjamin, D., and Seagull, E. (1981). The effect of polybrominated biphenyl on infants and young children. *J. Pediatr. 98*, 47–51.

Weiss, B. and Doherty, R.A. (1975). Methylmercury poisoning. *Teratology 12*, 311–314.

——— and Spyker, J.M. (1974). Behavioral implications of prenatal and early postnatal exposure to chemical pollutants. *Pediatrics 53*, 851–859.

Wibberley, D.G., Khera, A.K., Edwards, J.H., and Rushton, D.I. (1977). Lead levels in human placentae from normal and malformed births. *J. Med. Genet. 14*, 339–345.

Wilson, G.S., Desmond, M.M., and Verniaud, W.M. (1973). Early development of infants of heroin-addicted mothers. *Am. J. Dis. Child. 126*, 457–462.

———, ———, and Wait, R.B. (1981). Follow-up of methadone-treated and untreated narcotic-dependent women and their infants: Health, developmental, and social implications. *J. Pediatr. 98*, 716–722.

Wilson, J.G. (1973). *Environment and birth defects.* New York: Academic Press.

Wolf, S.M. and Forsythe, A. (1978). Behavior disturbance, phenobarbital, and febrile seizures. *Pediatrics 61*, 728–731.

———, ———, Stunden, A.A., Friedman, R., and Diamond, H. (1981). Long-term effect of phenobarbital on cognitive function in children with febrile convulsions. *Pediatrics 68*, 820–823.

Yalom, I.D., Green, R., and Fish, N. (1973). Prenatal exposure to female hormones. Effect on psychosexual development in boys. *Arch. Gen. Psychiatry 28*, 554–561.

Yamaguchi, A., Yoshimura, T., and Kuratsune, M. (1971). A survey on pregnant women having consumed rice oil contaminated with chloro-biphenyls and their babies. *Fukuoka Igaku Zasshi 62*, 112–117.

Yerushalmy, J. (1971). The relationship of parents' cigarette smoking to outcome of pregnancy—implications as to the problem of inferring causation from observed associations. *Am. J. Epidemiol. 93*, 443–456.

———— (1972). Infants with low birth weight born before their mothers started to smoke cigarettes. *Am J. Obstet. Gynecol. 112*, 277–284.

Zackai, E.H., Mellman, W.J., Neiderer, B., and Hanson, J.W. (1975). The fetal trimethadione syndrome. *J. Pediatr. 87*, 280–284.

Zemp, J.W. and Middaugh, L.D. (1975). Some effects of prenatal exposure to D-amphetamine sulfate and phenobarbital on development neuro-chemistry and on behavior. *Addict. Dis. 2*, 307–331.

Zourbas, J. (1947). Encéphalopathie congénitale avec troubles du tonus neuro-musculaire vraisemblement consécutive à une intoxication par l' oxyde de carbone. *Arch. Fr. Pediatr. 4*, 513–515.

Zussman, J.V., Zussman, P.P., and Dalton, K. (1975). *Postpubertal effects of prenatal administration of progesterone*. Paper presented at meeting of the Society for Research in Child Development. Cited by Ehrhardt et al. (1977).

10

Infertility: Prevalence, Etiology, and Natural History

Mark A. Belsey

The importance of infertility as a health and a social problem can be judged from several perspectives. Infertile couples often require detailed, sophisticated, and costly clinical and laboratory examinations stretched out over a period of months. Prospects for the diagnosis of a treatable condition are variable but rarely good. In addition, adoptable children have become less available with the wider accessibility of effective contraceptive methods, the option of induced abortion, and the increasing tendency for single mothers to keep their babies. In developing countries, where the traditional emphasis of a woman's role is often defined in terms of her fertility, involuntary infertility represents a social stigma that is usually, and frequently unfairly, borne by the woman. Failure to bear children is an accepted basis for divorce in many cultures. When couples with involuntary infertility are either inadequately or insufficiently counseled, or fail to adjust, marital stress and instability may result.

In some developing countries infertility consumes a large proportion of reproductive health service resources. In such areas it is not unusual to find that as many as one-third of either family planning or gynecologic consultations relate to complaints of infertility. The routine management of an infertile couple may require repeated visits and procedures. In one report, the average number of clinic consultations for infertility was seven per couple, and over 20% of the couples had between 11 and 40 consultation visits (Collado Martinez, 1977).

DEFINITIONS

The lack of an adequate definition of infertility has led to some confusion, particularly between clinicians and epidemiologists on the one hand, and demographers on the other. Infertility, sometimes referred to as infecundity, sterility, or physiologic infertility, is defined by demographers as the incapacity "of a man, woman or couple to participate in reproduction (i.e. the production of a live child)" (United Nations Dept. of Economic and Social Affairs, 1958). The inability to conceive or to impregnate, and the inability to carry a conceptus to a livebirth, reflect different processes and etiologies, with distinct implications for their amelioration or prevention.

The working definitions that relate to couples and are relevant to defining infertility in epidemiologic terms were set out by a World Health Organization (1975) Scientific Group on the Epidemiology of Infertility as follows:

a. *Primary infertility*: The woman has never conceived despite cohabitation and exposure to pregnancy* for a period of two years.

b. *Secondary infertility*: The woman has previously conceived, but is subsequently unable to conceive, despite cohabitation and exposure to pregnancy for a period of two years; if the woman has breast-fed a previous infant then exposure to pregnancy should be calculated from the end of the period of lactational amenorrhoea.

c. *Pregnancy wastage*: The woman is able to conceive, but unable to produce a live birth. Loss of pregnancy during the first 28 weeks is referred to as early and intermediate fetal death, or abortion, and may be spontaneous or induced. Beyond 28 weeks of gestation and up to term, such losses are referred to as late fetal deaths, or stillbirths.

d. *Child mortality*: All deaths of children born alive up to their fifth birthday. (Perinatal mortality, i.e. stillbirth plus all deaths of offspring within the first week after birth, may be recorded separately. In some cultures, however, the early neonatal deaths may be perceived as stillbirths and hence be difficult to elicit.)

e. *"Unproven infertility" or "unproven fertility"* refers to problems sometimes perceived by individuals or couples as infertility or included as infertility in demographic surveys, whereas in fact, the woman is virtually not at risk of conception. The problem may be biological, such as among lactating women who are anovulatory, or couples practising contraception; or circumstantial, when there is the absence of cohabitation or coitus (e.g. women whose consort is temporarily away).

---

* The Scientific Group, after reviewing the subject, concluded that "exposure to pregnancy" is difficult to define and standardize except in the context of specific local conditions.

PREVALENCE

Primary Infertility

In the absence of specific epidemiologic studies on the prevalence of infertility, the estimates of the magnitude of the problem are often imprecise, being based either on demographic data or on health service statistics. The difficulty in using these sources of data for assessing the magnitude is illustrated in Figs. 10-1 and 10-2a to c. Figure 10-1 represents the universe of couples in which the woman is of reproductive age. Demographic data, as shown in Fig. 10-2a, provide only estimates of primary infertility but they rarely differentiate among involuntary infertility, voluntary infertility, and unknown fertility. Hospital or clinic-based data (Fig. 10-2b) do not indicate the prevalence of the problem unless there is ascertainment of all affected couples in *all* services providing infertility care and unless the vast majority of couples suffering from involuntary infertility avail themselves of the services. However, such health service–based data do provide important information on the current demands for infertility services.

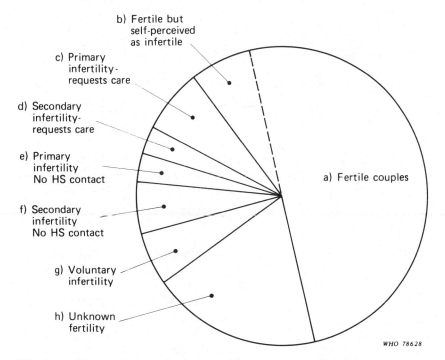

Fig. 10-1. The universe of couples with the woman of reproductive age.

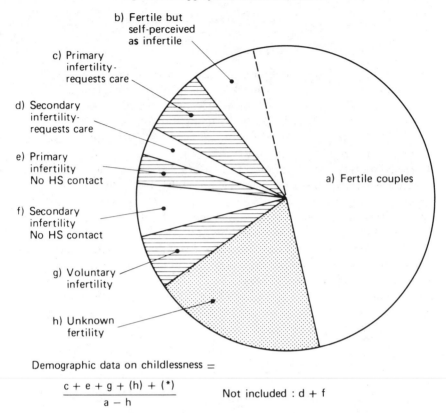

b) Fertile but
self-perceived
as infertile

c) Primary
infertility-
requests care

d) Secondary
infertility-
requests care

e) Primary
infertility
No HS contact

f) Secondary
infertility
No HS contact

g) Voluntary
infertility

h) Unknown
fertility

a) Fertile couples

Demographic data on childlessness =

$$\frac{c + e + g + (h) + (*)}{a - h}$$ Not included : d + f

*women with no children due to abortion and child loss   *WHO 78629*

Fig. 10-2a.   Demographic data on childlessness as an indicator of infertility.

Estimating the prevalence of infertility involves identifying couples who have primary or secondary infertility, regardless of whether they have requested care from the health services (Fig. 10-2c). Such prevalence data would be obtainable from community-based surveys of a population sample; however, this would not provide information on etiology.

Accepting the limitation of the available information, it still provides the basis for some speculation on the epidemiology of infertility in different parts of the world.

There exists a base rate or "core" of infertility representing the biologic variation of human populations with respect to chromosomal, congenital, and endocrinologic abnormalities affecting both men and women. To these base rates might also be added the occurrence of certain acquired disorders present to a greater or lesser degree in

258

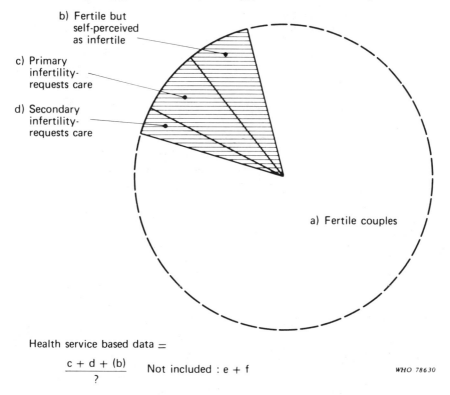

b) Fertile but
self-perceived
as infertile

c) Primary
infertility-
requests care

d) Secondary
infertility-
requests care

a) Fertile couples

Health service based data =

$$\frac{c + d + (b)}{?}$$ Not included : e + f

WHO 78630

Fig. 10-2b. Health service-based data as an indicator of infertility.

most communities, such as fallopian tubal occlusion following pelvic inflammatory disease or postpartum sepsis, the sequelae of mumps orchitis in adult men, and occupational exposures to chemicals such as 1,2-dibromo-3-chloropropane. When the occurrence of certain of these acquired conditions reaches epidemic proportions, or when there appears to be an unusual clustering of cases among certain population groups or occupations, then infertility becomes a major public health problem.

Infertility is a problem that takes on different dimensions in different parts of the world. There are wide variations in the prevalence rate of infertility, depending on the underlying cause, variations in the response of the couple and society, and variations in the diagnostic and therapeutic facilities. We can examine infertility from several different perspectives: (a) that of countries where rates are high or quite low, (b) that of developed or developing countries with their respective differences in resources for diagnosis and treatment, and (c) that of social and cultural responses to the problem.

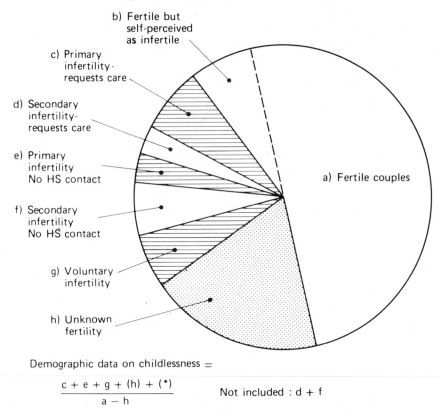

b) Fertile but self-perceived as infertile

c) Primary infertility - requests care

d) Secondary infertility - requests care

e) Primary infertility No HS contact

f) Secondary infertility No HS contact

g) Voluntary infertility

h) Unknown fertility

a) Fertile couples

Demographic data on childlessness =

$$\frac{c + e + g + (h) + (*)}{a - h}$$

Not included : d + f

*women with no children due to abortion and child loss

WHO 78629

Fig. 10-2c. The prevalence rate of infertility.

With respect to the prevalence rate of involuntary infertility, text-books on human reproduction and on infertility generally give this value as 10% (Behrman and Kistner, 1975). A reassessment of the census data from Canada, analysis of data from the World Fertility Survey, and data from other censuses and other studies do not substantiate a "core" rate of infertility of 10%. Instead, there appears to be wide variation in the rates of the different indices of infertility, as noted in Table 10-1.

The indices of primary infertility vary, from a low of 1.0 and 1.5% (never pregnant) for married women of 35 to 39 years of age in Thailand (World Fertility Survey, 1977) and Korea (Korean Institute for Family Planning, 1971), respectively, to a high of 13 and 23% for similar women in urban areas of Colombia (Estrada et al., 1972) and one rural area of New Guinea (Ring and Scragg, 1973), respectively (Table 10-1). The higher levels of either childlessness or nulliparity in the urban areas, as represented by Canada and Colombia (Table 10-1), suggest that either voluntary infertility is higher in the urban areas, or certain of the "acquired" causes of infertility, such as pelvic inflammatory disease, are more common in these areas.

In recent years the phenomenon of voluntary infertility appears to be emerging in some developed countries and within particular social groups. Thus, for example, data from Rumania illustrate the possibility that voluntary infertility and social factors play a significant part in the apparently high level of infertility (Muresan et al., 1969). The data also illustrate the variations within countries between social groups. Childlessness among women married five to nine years is over 20% among intellectuals, but not even 5% among farming families. The possibility of "true" biologic variation in infertility between population groups is yet to be tested.

In the developing countries, particularly Africa, there appear to be even wider variations in infertility from country to country, and within countries from region to region and between tribal groups. The prevalence of childlessness among married women who have completed their reproductive years varies from a low of 1.0% to a high of 42.5% for different districts in the Sudan (Sudan, Population Census Office, 1958, and Fig. 10-3). Similar wide ranges in childlessness are noted in other areas of Africa (Table 10-2).

Failure to bear children is an accepted basis for divorce in many cultures: Whether it represents cause or effect, in some developing countries in Africa there is a higher rate of childlessness among divorced women.

Secondary Infertility

Community-based data on the prevalence of secondary infertility do not exist, although some indirect indicators can be obtained from fertility surveys. One possible indicator of secondary infertility would be the frequency of women who have borne only one child after some 10–19 years of marriage. Voluntary infertility confounds any interpretation of such data, as do such factors as postpartum sexual abstinence, breast-feeding customs, adaptation and acceptance by a secondarily infertile couple to their infertile state, and long-term separation of husband and wife.

Some inferences on secondary infertility might be made from an examination of data from countries characterized by traditional cultures where the norms for average family size are well above two children. For example, in the World Fertility Survey conducted in Pakistan and Thailand among women 35–39 years of age and married for 10 to 19 years, 4.0 and 5.1%, respectively, had only one child ever

Table 10-1. Indices of Infertility in Various Countries

Country	Never pregnant (%)	Nulliparous (%)	No children ever born (%)	Only one child ever born (%)	Childless (%)
Zambia (Central Statistical Office, 1975)					
Women 35–39, eight provinces		6–24			
Colombia (Estrada et al., 1972)					
Married women 35–39					
Urban		13			
Rural		7			
Korea (Korean Institute for Family Planning, 1971)					
Married women 35–39					
Seoul	1	1			
Other urban	2	3			
Rural	1	1			
Thailand (World Fertility Survey, 1977)					
Ever married women 35–39	1.5				
Women married 10–19 years			1.5	5.1	
Pakistan (World Fertility Survey, 1976)					
Ever married women 35–39	4.0				
Women married 10–19 years			4.0	4.0	
Canada (Ussing et al., 1972)					
Married women 35–39		7.0			
Denmark (Veevers, 1972)					
Women aged 30–44 whose first marriage was at age 15–19					
Urban					4.4
Rural nonfarm					2.9
Rural farm					2.5
New Guinea (Ring and Scragg, 1973)					
Women 35–39					
Buka		2	2	6.4	
New Ireland		22.8	22.8	9.6	

Fiji (World Fertility Survey, 1976a)			
Fijian women married			
5–9 years		8	12
10–14 years		7	7
15–19 years		6	7
Indian women married			
5–9 years		5	12
10–14 years		3	5
15–19 years		2	2
Rumania (Muresan et al., 1969)			
Women married 5–9 years		4.8	39.6
Collective farmers		14.6	48.0
Workers		20.6	58.9
Intellectuals			
Malaysia (World Fertility Survey, 1974)			
Currently married women age 35–39	1.9		
Women currently married for 10–14 years		2.7	3.5
Women currently married for 15–19 years		0.7	2.5
Nepal (World Fertility Survey, 1976b)			
Women ever married age 35–39 years	3.1		
Women currently married age 35–39 years	2.4		
Women currently married 10–14 years		5.6	9.5
Women currently married for 15–19 years		3.9	5.1
Dominican Republic (Encuesta Nacional de Fecundidad			
Informe General, 1976)			
Women ever married age 35–39 years	2.6		
Women currently married age 35–39 years	2.7		
Women currently married for 10–14 years		3.7	4.9
Women currently married for 15–19 years		2.3	2.7

263

Table 10-2. Indices of Infertility and General Fertility in Central and West Africa

Country and/or region	Population in 1000s	General fertility rate (No. births/ 1000 women aged 15–44 years)	Crude livebirth rate per 1000 population	Percentage of childless women aged 25–29 years	Percentage of childless women aged 50+ years
Cameroon					
West	1,025	196	49.8	7.0	6.7
Southeast	1,185		36.4	28	23
North	1,395		41.0	21	15
Central African Empire	1,021	157	48	25.2	13.6
Banda	318	122	40.6		
Nzakara	30	48	20.0		
Baya	294	194	54.6		
Center region	240	125	41.0	34.7	15.0
West region	643	187	53	19.4	10.4
River region	134	101	36	36.3	19.0
Gabon	440	116	35	34	31.9
Wolen N'tem	78	122	37		31.2
Ogoone Lolo	37	80	25		46.2
Nyange	37	170	52		17.8
Upper Volta	4,440	194	49.6	7.2	6
Niger	2,600	232	50.55	12.8	5.2
Mali (Toureg)	76	209	52	26	15
Senegal	3,049	178	43.3	12	5.6

Sudan	10,262		51.7		9.6
Bahr el Ghazal	991		84.6		4.2
Blue Nile	2,070		45.7		8.4
Darfur	1,329		41.8		7.3
Equatoria	904		54.1		21.2
Kassala	941		42.6		13.5
Khartoum	505		40.7		9.7
Kordofan	1,762		50.0		9.9
Northern	873		43.0		7.8
Upper Nile	889		69.3		2.3
Zaire	21,800	171	42.7	22.1	17.6
Kwango	466	203	48.1	6.8	3.4
S. Kivu	831	211	52.3	7.1	4.6
Equateur	302	133	33.7	39.1	40.0
Tshuapa	395	113	30.5	44.1	33.0
Stanleyville	635	123	34.0	34.4	23.3
Bas-Vele	468	64	19.1	50.7	37.3
Haut-Velo	589	83	23.2	46.2	36.9
Nanie-Ma	447	129	34.3	27.9	23.5
Congo[a]		145	41.1	17	15

[a] Excludes Brazzaville and Pointe Noire.

Source: Belsey, M.A. (1976).

265

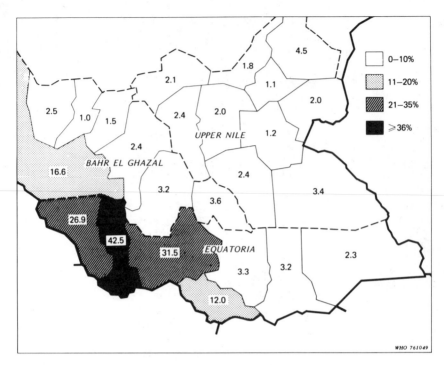

Fig. 10-3. Percentage childlessness among women completing reproductive age in the districts of three southern Sudan provinces.
Source: Besley, M.A. (1976).

born (the comparable figures for no children ever born were 4.0 and 1.5%) (World Fertility Survey, 1976, 1977). For two areas of New Guinea the comparable figures of "presumed secondary infertility" were 6.4 and 9.6% (Ring and Scragg, 1973). Although voluntary infertility or lack of exposure to pregnancy could account for a portion of the women with only one pregnancy during 10–19 years of marriage, it seems reasonable to assume that a large proportion of these women probably represent cases of secondary infertility in these countries. In contrast, the high percentage (40–60%) of one-child families among women married 5–9 years in Rumania (Muresan et al., 1969) contrasts with the much lower figure (12%) for Fiji women (World Fertility Survey, 1976a), suggesting a high level of voluntary infertility in the former.

The use of data on "one child ever born" during a defined duration of marriage or by a certain age excludes from the estimate secondary infertility following subsequent pregnancies. However, with increasing parity it is almost impossible to separate out voluntary infertility from demographic data. Furthermore, of the women with only one child within a defined duration, a variable proportion will not have been exposed to pregnancy during that interval or may have experienced a series of spontaneous or induced abortions, thus not meeting the above-cited definitions of infertility.

PRIMARY VERSUS SECONDARY INFERTILITY

Examination of the proportion of couples suffering from primary versus secondary infertility may in some circumstances provide some suggestions as to the etiology of infertility in that particular setting. Variation in the rates of primary and secondary infertility reflect differences in the pattern of underlying causes. Health service statistics may not provide an accurate reflection of the proportion of primary versus secondary infertility. In the published reports on large series of cases from 13 countries there was no instance of the rate of secondary infertility being greater than primary infertility among those presenting themselves to the clinic. These clinic-based data generally suggest a predominance of primary infertility, affecting from 53 to 87% of couples seeking assistance (Table 10-3).

In contrast to the impression derived from clinical data, the impression from the various demographic indices from several developing countries might suggest that secondary infertility was as frequent as if not more frequent than primary infertility. So, for example, in Malaysia among women currently married 15–19 years, 0.7% have never borne a child whereas 2.5% have borne only one child (World Fertility Survey, 1974). The corresponding figures for Nepal are 3.9 and 5.1% (World Fertility Survey, 1976b), and for the Dominican Republic 2.3 and 2.7% (Encuesta Nacional de Fecundidad Informe General, 1976). Unfortunately, no data are available from clinical sources corresponding to the data from the demographic sources. However, on the basis of these crude comparisons it would not be unreasonable to hypothesize that secondary infertility would tend to be "underrepresented" in hospital and clinic data. Couples who have already had at least one or more children may be more likely to accept a situation where they subsequently have difficulty in conceiving, whereas couples suffering from primary infertility may be more likely to seek medical attention. In cultures where numerous pressures exerted on the woman to become pregnant soon after marriage, consultation may be sought for even short delays in conception, sometimes resulting in overestimates of the prevalence of primary infertility by inclusion of fertile couples who perceive themselves to be infertile.

Table 10-3. Clinical Patterns of Infertility Based on Infertility Clinics (%)

Reference and country	Years of observation	No. of couples	Source	Primary	Secondary
Dor et al. (1977) Israel	1958–73	665	One physician	65.5	34.5
Nakamura (1975) Brazil	1951–71	1000	One clinic of one hospital	58.3	41.7
Ratnam et al. (1976) Singapore	1970–74	709	University Ob/Gyn Dept.	75.5	24.5
Gargoucha et al. (1976) Tunisia Le Kef	1972–74	114	Regional hospital Clinic and MCH clinic	52.7	47.3
Newton et al. (1974) London	1970–72	872	University clinic		
Cambell et al. (1974) New Guinea	1972	118	Regional hospital	62.7	26.3
Chatfield et al. (1970) Kenya	n.s.[b]	200	Gynecology outpatient dept., national hospital	58.0	42.0
Baeyertz (1976) New Zealand	1958–66	307	Private patients, one physician	53.4	46.6
Anderson (1968) Denmark[a]	1959–62	183	Hospital clinic	74.9	25.1
Čočev (1972) Bulgaria	1965–69	744	Couples seeking diagnosis and treatment in a district	62.9	37.1
Raymont (1969) Canada[a]	10 years	500	Infertility center, one hospital	68.2	31.8
Cox (1975) Australia	1964–73	900	Referrals to University dept.		
Gunaratne (1979) Sri Lanka	1976–77	393	University infertility clinic	86.8	13.2
Insler et al. (1981) Israel	1975–79	583	Sole infertility clinic serving 238,000 population	72.9	27.1

[a] Categories >100% because multiple factors were present in some couples.

[b] n.s., not stated.

[c] An additional 14.7% had unilateral tube involvement.

[d] 10.5% described as congenital malformations.

[e] Endometriosis.

[f] Tuberculosis.

[g] Normal.

[h] 6.5% both male and female and 14.1% apparently normal.

[i] Sperm count <20 million/ml.

In the extreme situations where the levels of infertility are high and predominantly either primary or secondary, it may be possible to hypothesize a single underlying mechanism or cause. Thus, for example, in the southern Sudan (Belsey, 1976), although high levels of infertility are noted in one district (Pibor), the pattern is almost exclusively one of secondary infertility, which suggests a major role

Tubal	Disturbed ovulation	Cervix/ uterine	Other	Unknown	Total female	Male factor	Azoo- spermia	Oligo- spermia
16.2	33.4	5.1	1.2	16.1	72.1	27.9	11.8	16.1
34.9	10.9	18.4	8.5		72.1	27.9		
11.7	22.5	5.8	14.7[e]	22.1		23.1		
40.4[c]		21.1[d]	5.3[f]					
18.0	27.0	7–9					25	
86.4							6.9	16.9[i]
56.1	2.0		2.0[f]			Not done	—	—
							6.3	25.0
36.1 (10.0)	29.5	48.0		6.0[g]			5.5	41.0
76.7	12.4	3.2	4.2	3.5[g]			9.8	31.1 (of 414 men)
32.2	16.9	25.6	26.2		76.4	26.2	4.7	21.5
11.0	42.9		8.9	17.6[g]		19.7		
15.3	16.2	16.6			44.3[h]	41.6	13.7	
— (6.7)	49.1	— (6.7)	0.7	1.4		30.2		

for postpartum factors such as sepsis (Fig. 10-4). In another area in the southern Sudan (Zande East), the problem appears to be predominantly one of primary infertility, suggesting etiologic factors operating before or at the time of puberty, affecting ovulation, the patency of the fallopian tube, or spermatogenesis.

The need for precise information on the prevalence of infertility is of obvious importance to governments in their efforts to develop diagnostic, preventive, and therapeutic services.

Several years ago a strategy for epidemiologic research on infertility was developed by a group of experts. Although specifically oriented to the problem of infertility in developing countries, with particular reference to Africa, the approach may also be relevant to other countries, both developed and developing. The report of

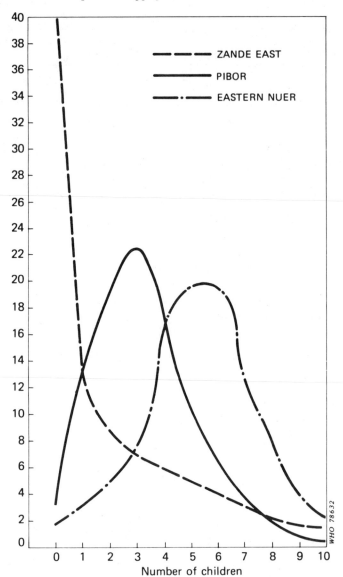

Fig. 10-4. Percentage distribution by number of children of women past childbearing age, three districts in the Sudan.

this group of experts outlined a strategy for defining the magnitude and the causes of infertility in any community based on the use of epidemiologic techniques (World Health Organization, 1975, and Fig. 10-5). Three or more levels of investigation were set out: (1) compilation and analysis of existing information, including demographic

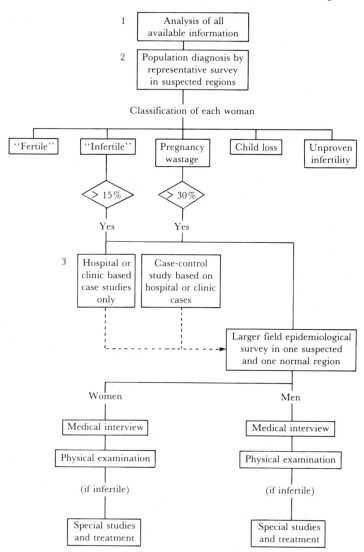

Fig. 10-5. The sequence of, and alternative approaches to, research on the magnitude, distribution, and causes of infertility and pregnancy wastage. *Source:* Modified from W.H.O. (1975).

data and hospital and clinical records, (2) population diagnosis based on representative surveys, and (3) clinicoepidemiologic studies.

The World Health Organization (1975) Scientific Group noted the need to differentiate among the categories of conditions that might be perceived to be infertility. Although both infections and endocrinologic disorders may underlie pregnancy wastage, the infectious

Table 10-4. Information Required for Community-Based Epidemiologic Studies of Infertility

a. Identifying data: name, age, residence, ethnic group

b. Marital status: duration of current union; whether divorced/widowed/separated—duration

c. Current situation: pregnant, breast-feeding—duration; amenorrhea—duration

d. Most recent pregnancy: date, outcome of pregnancy (abortion, stillbirth, or livebirth); for livebirths, whether child is alive or dead

e. Total number of livebirths, total number of children living now

f. Husband: name, age, whether he has other wives, and whether they have had children by him

g. Cohabitation status: whether husband is at home; whether couple is having intercourse, and how frequently

h. Contraceptive practice: type and duration since last pregnancy

Source: World Health Organization (1975).

agents and endocrinologic mechanisms causing spontaneous abortion are both quite distinct from the factors associated with infertility. Furthermore, the prevention, therapy, and prognosis of pregnancy wastage are also quite distinct from infertility.

A group of experts from several countries comprising a WHO Task Force on Infertility have developed and undertaken preliminary testing of a simplified questionnaire to be used in the categorization of both the level and the nature of the problem perceived to be infertility in different communities. The items of information to be collected are set out in Table 10-4 and permit classification of couples according to primary and secondary infertility, pregnancy wastage, child loss, and fertility and unknown fertility status.

As recommended by the WHO Scientific Group, married or cohabiting couples in which the woman is 20–29 years of age should be used as the indicator group for whether a problem of infertility does or does not exist in a community. Application of this system in Nigeria has shown it to be useful in estimating the level of primary and secondary infertility, but there may be a tendency to underreport pregnancy wastage and child loss.

DIAGNOSTIC AND ETIOLOGIC CATEGORIES OF INFERTILITY

A discussion of the epidemiology of infertility should describe the persons affected as well as the broad etiologic categories and factors contributing to the overall problem of infertility; it should not concern itself with details on the mechanisms by which infertility occurs, or with diagnostic or therapeutic procedures to be used.

A cursory comparison of the pattern of categories of infertility used by clinicians suggests a wide variation among countries (Table 10-3). The validity of such comparisons between countries is tenuous at best. First, most clinical reports represent an ill-defined and incomplete population, being composed of self-selected couples or couples referred from other clinics because of the expertise or interest of the center. Thus, for example, the high rate of ovulatory disturbances in the series of Cox (1975) in Table 10-3 represents the selective referral of cases for specific therapy. Second, variation between centers may also be attributable to differences in diagnostic techniques and the definition of abnormal results. The greater sensitivity and specificity of hysterosalpingography and laparoscopy over tubal insufflation has been described. The interpretation of semen examinations, particularly sperm counts characterized as oligospermic, is subject to a wide variation in the technique for collecting and counting, as well as their interpretation. Recently, WHO has published a manual for the standard examination of human semen and semen–cervical mucus interaction in order to provide a basis of comparability among clinical and research workers (Belsey et al., 1980).

Further difficulties arise in assessing the importance of different categories of infertility, because the patients seen in a single facility represent an unknown and not necessarily representative sample of the universe of infertile couples.

In one report, where one health facility was the only source of care for infertility and the population served was well defined both geographically and in social characteristics, the sociocultural profile of those requesting infertility care differed from the population in general (Insler et al., 1981). The authors interpreted this observation as reflecting differences in health care utilization patterns by different sociocultural groups. They could equally reflect differences in infertility rates by the same groups.

Despite the limitations in comparing data from different countries, it would still appear worthwhile to examine the available data on diagnostic categories of couples seen at infertility clinics in different parts of the world. Certain common patterns emerge, yet at the same time there are some obvious differences not entirely attributable to case or clinic selection bias. Excluding African countries characterized by high levels of infertility, and where data on males is often lacking, male factors associated with either azoospermia or oligospermia are implicated in about 20 to 30% of the couples seen in infertility clinics, with the exception of one report from Sri Lanka (Gunaratne, 1979; Table 10-3).

The greatest variation in the patterns of diagnosis occur in women. As noted previously, these differences may be partially due to variations in diagnostic techniques and procedures or in the interpretation of results. However, the differences may also be due to true differences in the epidemiology of infertility in these countries. Tubal factors, as the underlying cause of infertility, range from 12 to 86% of infertile couples seen at a particular facility in different countries (Table 10-3).

With the advent of drugs and hormones that are effective in the induction of ovulation, establishing the relative importance of ovulatory problems in the epidemiology of infertility becomes more important for those responsible for the organization and provision of health care, because such problems require specialized facilities for laboratory diagnosis and treatment. Thus, whereas the high proportion of ovulatory problems seen by Cox (1975) may be attributed to a selective case bias, the equally high proportion seen by Insler et al. (1981) appears to be more representative of the population served by the health facility.

Among the reports from the large series of cases from 13 countries (Table 10-3) are a large number of couples in whom no organic pathology can be found. These rates vary from 1.4 to 27% in different reports. Because this latter group has the highest rate of successful conceptions and deliveries among all classes of infertile couples, it is possible that either psychologic factors or ignorance have been important in the etiology of infertility. However some centers may have a high proportion of couples without an etiologic diagnosis because lack of facilities render complete diagnostic examinations impossible.

ETIOLOGY OF INFERTILITY

Often cited as evidence for the importance of psychologic factors underlying infertility in some couples is the clinical observation that a large proportion of couples, often lacking an obviously organic cause of infertility, conceive during the course of diagnostic studies. Thus, for example, 10.8% of the pregnancies occurring in the series of Insler et al. (1981) were considered spontaneous and unrelated to any therapy or procedure. Also cited as similar evidence is the occurrence of postadoption conception. In neither case are there much more than anecdotal data, whereas those few controlled studies that do exist fail to confirm that there is a significant increase in conceptions among apparently normal infertile couples, either at the time of adoption or as long as two years thereafter (Tyler et al., 1960; Weir and Weir, 1966).

Table 10-5. Fertility Rates and Mean Delay in Conception by Age at Marriage

Age at marriage (years)	Fertility Rates per 1000 women	Mean conception delay in months
12–15	90	13.4
16	93	11.7
17	128	10.4
18	121	9.2
19	151	8.7
20	180	7.2
21	209	6.4
22	226	6.4
23	203	6.0
24	276	5.3
25	214	6.4
26	180	8.9

Source: Gain cited by Behrman and Kistner (1975).

The role of ignorance may be more important than generally recognized. Of the studies cited in Table 10-3, only one noted it as a specific cause or contributing factor (Raymont et al., 1969). Age and frequency of sexual intercourse are both interrelated and related to fertility, although not always fully appreciated by both couples and physicians. Thus, there appears to be an age of optimum fecundity as shown in data on age at marriage, fecundity, and mean conception delay in Table 10-5. Frequency of intercourse affects fertility, as shown in Table 10-6. Finally, the timing of intercourse will obviously affect fertility. Studies on the knowledge of the reproductive cycle among even college-educated women demonstrate the high levels of ignorance and misinformation. In one study, 40% of the women

Table 10-6. Conceptions in Less than Six Months for Various Rates of Intercourse

Average frequency of intercourse per week	Number of cases	Conceptions in under six months (%)
<1 time	24	16.7
1 but <2	109	32.1
2 but <3	123	46.3
3 but <4	100	51.0
≥4 times	72	83.3

Source: MacLeod, J. and Gold, R.Z., cited by Behrman and Kistner (1975).

thought that ovulation took place during menstruation. Under such circumstances it is not surprising that at least 50% of the "normal" infertile couples conceive while under care of the infertility clinics.

Although the proportion of total cases attributable to tubal occlusion varies widely, it remains one of the major causes of infertility in nearly all clinical settings. Presumably tubal obstruction, whether complete or partial, is a consequence of infection, either sexually transmitted or following pregnancy or abortion. In either case, when sequelae of genital infection in either the woman or the man are presumed to be the basis of the infertility, it is often impossible to identify the causative organism or even the sequence of events leading to the infertility. The interval between genital tract infection and the complaint of infertility is often several years. Furthermore, we are increasingly becoming aware of the significant occurrence of asymptomatic carriers and mildly symptomatic cases of *Neisseria gonorrhoeae* among both men and women. Repeated episodes of pelvic inflammatory disease are more often associated with microorganisms other than *N. gonorrhoeae* (Eschenbach et al., 1975), although the initiating infection may still be with *N. gonorrhoeae*.

To establish an infectious disease agent as the source of a significant factor in the etiology of infertility, where the levels of infertility are high, requires the use of epidemiologic data to demonstrate an association between the indicators of infertility and the particular infectious disease or its indicators. Thus, Griffith (1963–64), using data from different provinces in Uganda, demonstrated the correlation of the crude birthrate and general fertility rates with the rates of gonorrhea isolates and with urethral stricture. Similar uses of epidemiologic data have shown the association of mumps orchitis and male infertility (Table 10-7), and also that, although syphilis in its early stages results in pregnancy wastage, late stages have less effect; indeed, excellent results may be anticipated if the condition is treated in pregnancy (Table 10-8).

The epidemiologic importance of postpubertal mumps in male infertility is suggested in at least one report. Gunaratne (1979), reporting from Sri Lanka, found a history of postpubertal mumps in 84 men among a consecutive series of 393 infertile couples. Of these men, 19 had atrophic testes and 7 had small testes; 13 were azoospermic and 23 oligospermic.

The recent development and refinement of serologic techniques for identifying previous infections with *Neisseria gonorrhoeae* and *Chlamydia trachomatis* has contributed to establishing the relative importance of these agents in infertility.

N. gonorrhoeae is a well-known cause of pelvic inflammatory disease and subsequent infertility. However, nongonococcal infec-

Table 10-7. Marriage Rate and Fertility Orchitis and Control Patients

	Men with bilateral orchitis		Control cases	
	No.	%	No.	%
Total number	98	100	98	100
Married men	68	69.4	85	86.7
Fertile men	47	48	81	82.7
Fertile married men	46	67.6	80	94.1
Conceptions				
Total	112	—	205	—
Per man	1.1	—	2.1	—
Per married man	1.6	—	2.4	—
Per married fertile man	2.4	—	2.5	—
Average duration of marriage (years)	12.5	—	13.6	—

Source: Belsey, M.A. (1976).

Table 10-8. Effect of Syphilis on the Outcome of Pregnancy Compared with the Results of Nonsyphilitic Pregnancies

Pregnancy outcome	Nonsyphilitic		Untreated early syphilis		Untreated late syphilis		Syphilis treated during pregnancy	
	No.	%	No.	%	No.	%	No.	%
Normal full-term living infant	8,897	85.3	40	18.2	61	74.4	435	94.0
Living syphilitic infant	—	—	90	40.9	2	2.4	5	1.1
Premature,[a] nonsyphilitic	930	9.0	5	2.3	2	2.4	2	0.4
Neonatal death								
Full-term infant	49	0.5	4	1.8	1	1.2	1	0.2
Premature infant[a]	177	1.7	26	11.8	6	7.4	4	0.9
Stillborn								
At full term	57	0.5	40	18.2	10	12.2	11	2.3
Premature[a]	213	2.1	15	6.8	0	0	5	1.1
Total	10,323		220		82		463	

[a] Defined as ≤2.27 kg at birth.
Source: Belsey, M.A. (1976).

tions are being implicated more often in the etiology of acute pelvic inflammatory disease and tubal occlusion. Reports from the United States (Eschenbach et al., 1975) and Sweden (Weström, 1975) indicate that, despite extensive diagnostic studies, *N. gonorrhoeae* is shown to be the cause of salpingitis in less than half the patients with pelvic inflammatory disease. A previous delivery, abortion, or curettage has been associated with about 20% of such cases.

Bacteroides fragilis, C. trachomatis, and possibly cytomegalovirus, *Ureaplasma urealyticum*, and other organisms have recently been associated with nongonococcal salpingitis (Henry-Suchet et al., 1980). Furthermore, nongonococcal salpingitis, despite early and prolonged therapy, has been associated with an even higher rate of tubal occlusion (16.6%) than that following gonococcal infection (5.5%), presumably because of the greater resistance of a mixed group of organisms to antibiotics more specific to *N. gonorrhoeae*. Similar differences in the sequelae of gonococcal and nongonococcal salpingitis have been noted by Falk (1965). The role of these other infections as causes of infertility in men has not been evaluated.

The role of occupational, environmental, and drug exposures in the etiology of infertility has become of greater concern with the accumulation of reports on the association of male infertility with such pesticides as 1,2-dibromo-3-chloropropane (Whorton et al., 1977) and drugs such as sulfasalazine (Levi et al., 1979). The increasing dependence of developed and developing societies on herbicides, pesticides, and other chemical agents also increases the need for health and epidemiologic surveillance for the adverse consequences of exposure to these agents. In a recent report, a group of men working in a pesticide factory became increasingly aware that few of them had recently fathered a child, although they were in their late twenties and early thirties (Whorton et al., 1977). On detailed clinical epidemiologic investigation of the men who had worked three or more years in the factory, none had sperm counts above 1 million and most were azoospermic. The presumed etiologic agent resulting in infertility, 1,2-dibromo-3-chloropropane, has been shown previously to be toxic to the testes of rats, guinea pigs, and rabbits. Other chemical agents may also be implicated in infertility.

Occupational exposure to lead is associated with a significant increase in the percentage of spermatozoa with morphologic defects, with low sperm density, and with poor motility (Lancranjan et al., 1975). Recently it has been suggested that drug exposure in utero may have an effect on subsequent fertility. Testicular cysts and testicular hypoplasia has been noted to be over four times as common (31.5 versus 7.9%) in a group of males exposed in utero to diethylstilbestrol (DES) as compared with a group receiving a placebocontrol (Gill et al., 1979). Using the sperm penetration assay (zona-free hamster eggs), Stenchever et al. (1981) have shown that the majority of men exposed in utero to DES have an impaired test as compared to a group not exposed to DES. A group of men known to be fertile were shown to have no impairment of the sperm penetration assay.

CONCLUSION

In order to describe the epidemiology of infertility, the need for standardized procedures and definitions is obvious. Such standardization also assists health service planners in developing the appropriate diagnostic and therapeutic services for a country. In addition, the establishment of baseline data on the prevalence and categories of infertility in different communities facilitates further investigation of the underlying etiology using epidemiologic techniques and provides for public health authorities a means by which infertility can be monitored in a community. Unusual increases in overall rates or categories can be investigated and presumably prevented, as in the case of toxic chemical or other environmental exposures.

Infertility is an important health problem in many countries, sometimes reaching levels high enough to have significant impact on the health services and to cause concern because of the social and economic consequences. Infertility levels, underlying causes, and contributing factors clearly vary from one country to another and even from one locale to another. Such variation underlines the importance and need for a precise clinical and epidemiologic definition of the problem in any particular country.

REFERENCES

Anderson, A.J.B., Kristoffersen, K., Salazar, B., and Ramos, E. (1968). Infertilitet: Resultater og problemer i et tre års hospitalsmateriale. *Ugeskrift fur Laeger 130*, 633–639.

Baeyertz, J.D. (1967). A review of 307 cases of infertility. *Australian and New Zealand Journal of Obstetrics and Gynaecology 7*, 204–217.

Behrman, S.J. and Kistner, R.W. (1975). *Progress in Infertility*, 2nd edition, Boston: Little, Brown & Co.

Belsey, M.A. (1976). The epidemiology of infertility: a review with particular reference to sub-Saharan Africa. *Bull. WHO 54*, 319–341.

———, Eliasson, R., Gallegos, A.J., Moghissi, K.S., Paulsen, C.A., and Prasad, M.R.N. (1980). *Laboratory manual for the examination of human semen and semen–cervical mucus interaction*. Based on consultations held within the WHO Special Programme of Research, Development and Research Training in Human Reproduction. Singapore, Press Concern.

Campbell, G.R. and Roberts-Thomson, K. (1974). Infertility in the Highlands. *Papua New Guinea Med. J. 17*(4), 347–353.

Central Statistical Office (1975). *Inter-regional variations in fertility in Zambia.* Population Monographs No. 2, Republic of Zambia.

Chatfield, W.R., Suter, P.E.N., Bremner, A.D., Edwards, E., and McAdam, J.H. (1970). The investigation and management of infertility in East Africa: a prospective study of 200 cases. *East Afr. Med. J. 47*, 212–216.

Čočev, D. (1972). Results of studies and treatment of sterility in families in Blagoengrade district during a period of five years. *Akush. Ginekol. (Sofia) 11*, 133–141.

Collado Martinez, H. (1977). Estudio de 350 parejas esteriles en el Instituto Materno Infantil Carit, *Revista Medical del Hospital General de Mexico 40*, 45–53.

Cox, L.W. (1975). Infertility: a comprehensive programme. *Br. J. Obstet. Gynaecol. 82*, 2–6.

Dor, J., Homburg, R., and Rabau, E. (1977). An evaluation of etiologic factors and therapy in 665 infertile couples. *Fertility and Sterility 28*, 718–722.

Encuesta Nacional de Fecundidad Informe General (1976) Santo Domingo, Consejo nacional de Poblacions y Familia, Republica Dominicana.

Eschenbach, D.A., Buchanan, T.M., Pollock, H.M., Forsyth, P.S., Alexander, E.R., Lin, J.S., Wang, S.P., Wentworth, B.B., McCormack, W.M., and Holmes, K.K. (1975). Polymicrobial etiology of acute pelvic inflammatory disease. *N. Engl. J. Med. 293*, 166–171.

Estrada, A. et al. (1972). *Resultados Generales: Encuesta Nacional de Fecundidad*, Publication No. 1. Bogota. Associacion Colombiana de Facultades de Medicina, Division de Medicina Social y Poblacion.

Falk, V. (1965). Treatment of acute non-tuberculous salpingitis with antibiotics alone and in combination with glucocorticoids. *Acta Obstet. Gynecol. Scand. 44*(Suppl. 6), 1–118.

Gargoucha, E., Ryjik, V., and Maximov, G. (1976). Certain causes de Stérilité Féminine dans la région du Kef (Tunisie). *La Tunisie Médicale 54*(6), 833–836.

Gill, W.B., Schumacher, G.F.B., Bibbo, M., Strauss, F.H., and Schoenberg, H.W. (1979). Association of diethylstilbestrol exposure *in utero* with cryptorchidism, testicular hypoplasia and semen abnormalities. *J. Urol. 122*, 36–39.

Griffith, H.B. (1963–64) Gonorrhea and fertility in Uganda. *Eugen. Rev. 55*, 103–108.

Gunaratne, M. (1979). The epidemiology of infertility: a selected clinic study. *Ceylon Med. J. 24*, 36–42.

Henry-Suchet, I., Catalan, F., Loffredo, V., Ferfaty, D., Siboulet A., Perol, Y., Sanson, M.J., DeBache, C., Pigeau, F., Coppin, R., DeBrux, J., and Poynard, T. (1980). Microbiology of specimens obtained by laparoscopy from controls and from patients with pelvic inflammatory disease or infertility with total obstruction: *Chlamydia trachomatis* and *Ureaplasma urealyticum. Am. J. Obstet. Gynecol. 138*, 1022–1025.

Insler, V., Potashnik, G., and Glassner, M. (1981). Some epidemiological aspects of fertility evaluation. In: *Advances in Diagnosis and Treatment of Infertility*, edited by V. Insler and G. Bettendof. North-Holland: Elsevier, 165–177.

Korean Institute for Family Planning (1971). *Fertility-Abortion Survey*. Seoul.

Lancranjan, I., Popescu, H.I., Găvănescu, O., Klepsch, I., and Serbănescu, M. (1975). Reproductive ability of workmen occupationally exposed to lead. *Arch. Environ. Health 30*, 396–401.

Levi, A.J., Fisher, A.M., Hughes, L., and Hendry W.F. (1979). Male infertility due to sulphasalazine, *Lancet 2*, 276–278.

Muresan, P. et al. (1969). Recherches medico-sociales sur la fertilité de la population feminine de la Republique socialiste de Roumanie: Enquête expérimentale 1967–1968. *Santé publique (Bucarest) 12*, 131–140.

Nakamura, M.S., Porto, R.L., Jr., and Mueller, F. (1975). Etiologia da esterilidade conjugal no Departamento de Ginecologia da Facultade de Medicina da Universidade de Sao Paula. *Reproduction 2*, 39–44.

Newton, J., Craig, S., and Joyce, D. (1974). The changing pattern of a comprehensive infertility clinic. *J. Biosoc. Sci. 6*, 477–482.

Ratnam, S.S., Chew, P.C., and Tsakok, M. (1976). Experience of a comprehensive infertility clinic in the Department of Obstetrics and Gynaecology, University of Singapore. *Singapore Med. J. 17*, 157–159.

Raymont, A., Arronet, G.H., and Arrata, W.S.M. (1969). Review of 500 cases of infertility. *Intern. J. fertility 14*, 141–153.

Ring, A. and Scragg, R. (1973). A demographic and social study of fertility in rural New Guinea. *J. Biosoc. Sci. 5*, 89–121.

Stenchever, M.A., Williamson, R.A., Leonard, J., Karp, L.E., Ley, B., Shy, K., and Smith, D. (1981). Possible relationship between *in utero* diethylstilbestrol and male infertility. *Am. J. Obstet. Gynecol. 140*, 186–193.

Sudan, Population Census Office (1958). *The first population census of Sudan, 1955/56*. Khartoum, Ministry of Social Affairs.

Tyler, E.T., Bonapart, J., and Grant, J. (1960). Occurrence of pregnancy following adoption. *Fertility and Sterility 11*, 581–589.

United Nations Department of Economic and Social Affairs (1958). *Multilingual Demographic Dictionary*. New York (Population Studies No. 29).

Ussing, Jytte and Brunn-Schmidt (1972). Nogle resultatet fra fertilitetsundersögelsen. Studie 22, Kobenhaven.

Veevers, J.E. (1972). Declining childlessness and age at marriage: a test of a hypothesis. *Social Biology 19*, 285–288.

Weir, W.C. and Weir, D.R. (1966). Adoption and subsequent conceptions. *Fertility and Sterility 17*, 283–288.

Weström, L. (1975). Effect of acute pelvic inflammatory disease on fertility. *Am. J. Obstet. Gynecol. 121*, 707–713.

Whorton, D. Krauss, R.M., Marshall, S., and Milby, T.H. (1977). Infertility in male pesticide workers, *Lancet 2*, 1259–1261.

World Fertility Survey (1974). Malaysian Fertility and Family Survey. First

Country Report, Department of Statistics, Kuala Lumpur National Family Planning Board, Malaysia, K.L.

World Fertility Survey (1976). *Pakistan Fertility Survey*, 1st Report. Islamabad, Population Planning Council of Pakistan.

World Fertility Survey (1976a). *Fiji Fertility Survey 1974, Principal Report.* Bureau of Statistics, Suva, Fiji.

World Fertility Survey (1976b). First Report His Majesty's Government Health Ministry Nepal Family Planning and Maternal and Child Health Project, Kathmandu.

World Fertility Survey (1977). *The Survey of Fertility in Thailand: Country Report*, Report No. 1, Institute of Population Studies. Bangkok Chulalongkorn University and Population Survey Division, National Statistical Office.

World Health Organization (1975) Technical Report Series, No. 582. The Epidemiology of Infertility: Report of a WHO Scientific Group.

11

Unwanted Pregnancy

Lorraine V. Klerman and James F. Jekel

The first step in determining the epidemiology of any condition is to establish rigorous criteria for its occurrence. This task is particularly difficult when the condition is unwanted pregnancy.

THE CONCEPT OF AN UNWANTED PREGNANCY

Rosen (1982) has noted the existence of a historical trend in definitions of unwanted pregnancy. Formerly, motherhood was expected of married women. All pregnancies within marriage were therefore defined as wanted and all outside of marriage as unwanted. The widespread availability of abortion, however, has made it possible to decide that even a marital pregnancy is unwanted because abortions provide a way to prevent an unwanted pregnancy from becoming an unwanted birth. Also, major changes in societal attitudes and behavior toward births outside of marriage for adult women, and similar changes in parental attitudes and behavior toward adolescent pregnancies, have made it possible for a nonmarital pregnancy to be considered wanted.

Many researchers have struggled with the problems of defining unwanted pregnancies. As early as 1959, Lehfeldt described the ambivalence often experienced by women even before conception. He discussed a condition he called "willful exposure to unwanted pregnancy." The subject was explored in great depth by Pohlman and Pohlman (1969), who suggested many factors that should be considered before a pregnancy was labeled as unwanted: Several family members may be involved and their opinions may differ;

feelings about a particular pregnancy or about childbearing in general may change over time; some children may be wanted, but not all; children may be wanted of a particular sex or age only; children may be wanted for unhealthy reasons; and an individual may be in conflict, that is, both want and not want a pregnancy or child, and this ambivalence may be experienced at both the conscious and unconscious levels. The authors warn:

> [These problems in defining wantedness] should serve as a caution to researchers not to take their classification categories of "wanted" or "unwanted" too seriously. Such labels are usually based on respondents' answers to one or two questions and these answers do not support all the meanings a researcher sometimes wishes to load onto his concept. The researcher's clear dichotomy may hide very hazy parent feelings (pp. 181–182).

The report of the Commission on Population Growth and the American Future (Westoff and Parke, 1972) contained two chapters on unwanted pregnancies. David (1972), in his discussion of the costs and alternatives, defined an unwanted pregnancy as one "unintended and consciously unwanted at the time of conception." His definition of an unwanted child as "the product of an unwanted pregnancy" is questionable. He focused on number of failures (having more children than wanted) rather than on timing failures (having children at the wrong time) and on prospective judgment (before conception) rather than afterthoughts. In the same volume Ryder and Westoff (1972) reviewed the operational definitions and findings of the 1965 and 1970 National Fertility Studies. The principal source of information on unwanted births in those surveys of ever-married women was the question, "Did you yourself want a child but not until *later* or did you really want *no more* children?"

Hass (1974) critiqued American fertility studies and their measures of wantedness. She suggested that the measurement tools were inadequate, particularly in their insensitivity to timing failures; that conceptualizations were too narrow, focusing on conscious feelings only and almost exclusively the woman's; and that surveys depended on recall and did not allow for changes over time. Her own fertility decision-making model had three stages—preconception, pregnancy, and postnatal—and included factors such as perceived susceptibility to conception, couple communication, and attitudes toward conception, pregnancy, and childbearing.

Miller (1974) specifically studied the relationship between the intendedness of conception and the wantedness of pregnancy. Unfortunately, his findings, based on a study of 221 women and 379 conceptions, were limited to predominantly white, married, middle-class women and thus may not be generalizable to other groups. Nevertheless the concepts are important. He distinguished between "those psychological states occurring prior to conception which reflect the individual's orientation toward the possibility of conception occurring, and those psychological states occurring after conception which reflect how the individual feels about the pregnancy or child" (p. 396). This distinction is essentially the difference between the intentions of an individual (or couple) with respect to conception and feelings of wantedness for the pregnancy or child after conception. Miller was also able to develop an "intendedness" scale based on contraceptive use, and a "wantedness" scale based on the feelings of the female and her partner toward the pregnancy. As would be expected, almost all consciously intended conceptions led to fully wanted pregnancies. Less obviously, but of considerable potential significance, "conceptions resulting from inadequate contraception or from contraceptive accidents fell evenly across the full range of wantedness." Miller concluded that there exists a "wantedness reserve," that is, that less than fully intended conceptions may lead to fully wanted pregnancies. In his study, the proportion of fully *intended* pregnancies (45%) was lower than the proportion of fully *wanted* pregnancies (60%). He preceived this difference as "an adaptive reserve which enables [the population] to mobilize positive feelings and respond to its subintended (less than fully intended) conceptions with an increase in wantedness feelings" (p. 404). Miller also found that the "wantedness reserve" differed in magnitude depending on the time in a woman's marriage and reproductive cycle. It was lower immediately after marriage and the birth of a child, and higher from 6 to 9 months after a marriage and 12–15 months after the birth of a child. An important conclusion from this research is that the levels of intendedness of a conception should not be equated with the levels of wantedness of the children produced.

The extensive literature on this subject indicates that a simple definition of unwanted pregnancy is impossible. At a minimum, the epidemiologist must consider what is being measured, how quantitatively it is to be measured, and the time of the questions with reference to conception and birth. For example, is pregnancy the subject, or are all conceptions to be studied, including those terminating in abortion? Alternatively, is the analysis to be limited to those that end in a livebirth? In this latter case is it unwanted pregnancies that are being studied, or unwanted livebirths? Many unwanted pregnancies lead to the birth of children who are loved and nurtured despite the initial unwantedness of the pregnancy. Also, are conceptions, pregnancies, or births to be studied in terms of their wanted, intended, or planned status? How should one classify mistimed conceptions?

Quantitatively, the epidemiologist must decide whether these variables are to be treated dichotomously or in a scale or score, as Miller (1974), Sears et al. (1957), and Bracken et al. (1978) have attempted.

The time dimension is crucial, both in terms of when the question is *asked* (e.g., prior to conception, during pregnancy, or after birth) and in terms of the *reference* period (i.e., what time period is referred to in the question). Recall errors are very likely.

The answer to a question about an unwanted pregnancy is also subject to variation depending on circumstances under which the question is asked. Because pregnancies are socially rewarded under some conditions and socially disapproved under others, interview or questionnaire factors are important. Answers given in the welfare office may differ from those given to a physician or to an interviewer at home. An adolescent or an unmarried woman may be reluctant to admit that a pregnancy was deliberate. In contrast, a married woman may feel awkward stating that her pregnancy was unwanted. The sex and race of the interviewer may also affect responses. Moreover, the answer may certainly vary depending on whether the woman, her male partner, or some other significant individual is asked the question. Family circumstances at the time of the questioning may result in unintentional or intentional falsification of response. For example, a woman burdened with a child handicapped from birth, or with children no longer receiving support from a father, may believe that her pregnancy was unwanted, even though if she had been asked at the time she was pregnant she would have stated that the pregnancy was wanted.

Finally, estimates may err in either direction. Because of embarrassment, denial, or repression, a woman or her partner may say a conception, pregnancy, or child was wanted when it was not. This is probably more likely with an adult than an adolescent. Alternatively, a woman may say a conception, pregnancy, or child was unwanted when it was, because she believes this is the expected or culturally correct answer, particularly if the birth is outside of marriage or the mother is an adolescent.

Because of these problems as well as the many others cited in the literature, a definitive epidemiology of unwanted pregnancy is probably impossible. What can be expected, however, is greater precision and comparability over time in the definition of terms and a broad sampling of women including the never or not yet pregnant, as well as those who have been pregnant or given birth.

FEDERAL ESTIMATES OF UNWANTEDNESS

Two major data collection programs of the National Center for Health Statistics ask questions about the wantedness of pregnancies and births: the National Survey of Family Growth and the National Natality Survey.

National Survey of Family Growth

In 1973 and again in 1976, the National Survey of Family Growth (NSFG) conducted national surveys of fertility based on household interviews (Munson, 1977; Eckard, 1980). Respondents included women between the ages of 15 and 44 who were currently married or previously married, or who had never married but had natural children presently living in the household. Thus, never-married women who had no natural children living with them were not sampled, nor were any females under age 15 or over age 44.

Among the questions asked were a series on wantedness. The authors describe this sequence, which was the same in both surveys, as follows:

> For women reporting that contraceptive use was stopped prior to conception or that no contraceptive method was used in the interval preceding conception (which begins with the end of the preceding pregnancy, if there is one), the question on wantedness was phrased as follows: "Was the reason you (were not/stopped) using any method because, you, yourself, wanted to become pregnant?" If the woman answered negatively, she was asked two further questions, which were also asked of all other respondents. These questions are: "At the time you became pregnant (THIS INTERVAL), did you, yourself, actually want to have a(nother) baby at some time?" and "As you recall, is that how you felt before you became pregnant, or did you come to feel that way later?" A subsequent question for those who did not know or care whether or not they wanted to have "a(nother)" baby was:
> "It is sometimes difficult to recall these things, but as you look back to just before that pregnancy began, would you say you probably wanted a(nother) baby sometime or probably not?" (Eckard, 1980, p. 9)

A pregnancy was defined as wanted if the woman reported that:

a. contraception was not used in the interval or was stopped prior to conception *because* the woman wanted to become pregnant;

287

  b. she wanted to have "a(nother)" baby at some time and felt that way *before* becoming pregnant;

  c. she reported that she probably wanted "a(nother)" baby at some time. (Eckard, 1980, p. 10)

A pregnancy was defined as "unwanted" if the woman reported that she did not want, or probably did not want, to have a baby at some time and felt that way before becoming pregnant. All other pregnancies were termed "undetermined." These included those that women came to want sometime after conception, those that came to be unwanted sometime after conception, and those for which feelings at time of conception could not be reported.

It should be noted that although the reports of these surveys are titled "Wanted and Unwanted Births" the wantedness status refers to the pregnancy resulting in the birth. Also, the questions focus on the woman's feeling in the period before the pregnancy in order to determine her desire for a child rather than her feelings during pregnancy or toward the child once it is born, and probably reflect intention, as recalled at a later date. Thus, the results should probably be reported in terms of intended and unintended conceptions. This summary, however, will follow the language of the reports, that is, unwanted births.

The 1973 survey, based on almost 10,000 interviews, reported that 79.7% of the births in the women surveyed were wanted, 13.1% unwanted, and 7.3% undetermined. Unwantedness varied significantly with age, race, parity, education, family income, religion, desired family size, marital status, and contraceptive sterilization (Munson, 1977). The 1976 survey was based on almost 9000 interviews. The comparative figures were 79.9% wanted, 12.0% unwanted, and 7.1% undetermined. In this survey, however, the undetermined group was further divided: 5.3% wanted after conception, 1.6% unwanted after conception, and 1.2% unknown. Total unwantedness, defined as unwanted at conception plus unwantedness after conception, varied significantly with age: Older mothers had the highest rates (16.0% for those aged 35–39 and 17.8% for those aged 40–44), followed by women 30–34 years of age (12.2%) and teenagers (11.4%). Almost 30% of black births were unwanted at or after conception as compared to 10.6% of white births. Unwantedness increased with parity, with 5% or less of first and second births being unwanted and over 13% of subsequent births.

Analyses of other variables were limited to unwantedness at conception only. They showed that unwantedness decreased with the education of the woman and her husband, and with income. It was higher among women working full-time and unemployed at the time than among those working part-time or not in the labor force. Unwantedness was highest among respondents who claimed no religion (16.1%), followed by Protestants (13.1%), Catholics (9.6%), Jews (5.2%), and others (5.1%). It decreased with increases in desired family size. Those never married had the highest percentage of unwanted pregnancies (27.2%), followed by those with one or more previous marriages (15.1%) and those with no previous marriages (10.8%). Hispanic origin, geographic origin, and previous fetal loss were not significantly associated with unwantedness (Eckard, 1980).

Anderson (1981) analyzed the 1973 and 1976 NSFG to determine trends in the planning status of marital births. He concluded that the proportion of births within marriage that were unwanted fell from 12 to 9% between the two studies. Although these declines were experienced by most groups in the population, distinct differences still existed, for example, between Catholics and non-Catholics and between Hispanics and non-Hispanics, probably caused by underlying differences in fertility preferences. There were also variations among women of different income levels, possibly related to their ability to control their fertility. Poor and black women remained more likely to have unwanted births than women in other groups. Utilizing other techniques to analyze the 1976 NSFG, Westoff (1981) also described a significant decline in unwanted fertility, although there were differences among sub-groups, with black women having the highest proportion of unwanted births.

National Natality Survey

The data from the National Natality Survey (NNS) provide more biased estimates of the frequency of unwanted pregnancies than the NSFG data because they exclude pregnancies that terminate in illegitimate births and abortions, both of which are the most likely to be unwanted. The NNS, however, may provide a more accurate picture than the NSFG of wantedness prior to conception among women delivering, because information is sought from women who gave birth within the year whereas the NSFG asks about all pregnancies, regardless of how many years have passed. Women may not recall accurately their feelings prior to a pregnancy in the distant past.

In 1968, 1969, 1972, and 1980 the NNS conducted followback surveys of samples of legitimate livebirths that had occurred during those years. Data were obtained by mailed questionnaire with a follow-up by phone or personal interview for mothers who did not respond or whose responses were largely incomplete. In 1968 and 1969 the sampling fraction was 1 in 1000 for white births and 1 in 500 for all other births. In 1972 it was 1 in 500 for all births. The response rate from the 3595 mothers selected in 1968 was 88.9%; it was 84.8% from 3666 mothers in 1969 and 71.5% from 5689 mothers in 1972 (Weller, 1976; Weller and Heuser, 1978).

The 1968 and 1969 surveys included the following questions on wantedness:

> "Just before you became pregnant with your new baby, did you want to become pregnant?"

Possible answers were "Yes," "No, wanted a baby, but did not want to become pregnant yet," and "No, did not want a baby."

In 1972 the wording was changed to the following:

> "Thinking back, just before you became pregnant with your new baby, did you want to become pregnant at that time?"

Possible responses were "I wanted this pregnancy *at an earlier time*, as well as at that time," "I wanted to become pregnant *at that time*," "I did not want to become pregnant at that time, but I wanted another child *sometime in the future*," and "I did not want to become pregnant at that time, or at any time in the future" (Weller and Heuser, 1978, p. 3). For comparative purposes, the first two answers on the 1972 instrument were considered the equivalent of "yes" in the 1968 and 1969 ones. Births wanted at a later time (third answer) were referred to as "timing failures." "Unwanted" refers only to a birth that was not wanted at all. As in the case of the NSFG, the question probably was responded to in terms of the intendedness of the conception, but because only women who gave birth to a live infant were sampled, the data analyses are worded in terms of births; that wording is followed in this summary.

The rate of unwanted births declined during the period covered by the three surveys. It was 12.7% in 1968, 11.5% in 1969, and 8.2% in 1972. The 1973 data for the NSFG indicate that 13.1% of all births were unwanted. The difference between surveys suggests the bias introduced by eliminating illegitimate births.

The 1972 NNS found that unwanted legitimate births were highest among women 35 years of age and over (32.9%) and lowest (less than 5%) in all age groups under 25, except 18- and 19-year-olds (5.7%). Unwanted births were more frequent among nonwhites (9.5%) than whites (8.1%), but the decline in unwantedness was more striking among nonwhites than whites, reducing the differences in the two groups. Unwanted births increased with parity, with less than 5% of first and second births and over 15% of subsequent births being unwanted. Unwantedness decreased with the years of school com-

290

pleted by the mother, except that women who had 1–3 years of education past high school had a higher percentage of unwantedness than women who had completed high school only. It decreased with the number of years of school completed by the father, except that men who had 16 or more years of education had a higher percentage of unwantedness than did men with 13–15 years of education. Unwantedness increased with increasing annual income, except in the under-$2000 category, where the percentage of unwantedness was as high as for groups with much higher income. Women who expected no more children were much more likely than women who expected more children to state that their last child was unwanted. This suggests timing failures rather than unwanted births for those wanting more children at some time. Over half (53.4%) of the first births that were probably premaritally conceived were wanted later, and less than 1% were unwanted.

WANTEDNESS OF BIRTHS TO TEENAGERS

It is generally believed that the overwhelming percentage of pregnancies among teenagers are unwanted, particularly if they are unmarried. To some extent this belief results from society's attitudes toward pregnancy outside of marriage, adolescent sexuality, and adolescent childrearing; that is, all pregnancies among unmarried females should be unwanted, and teenagers are too immature to be sexually active and to rear a child successfully.

Johns Hopkins Surveys of Young Women

This belief has been supported by the three nationwide surveys of 15- to 19-year-old women conducted by Johns Hopkins University (Zelnik and Kantner, (1980) in 1971, 1976, and 1979. The question on wantedness was asked the same way in each survey and was part of the pregnancy history. It dealt with pregnancy intention at the time of conception. For each pregnancy, the respondent was asked, "Did you want to become pregnant the (1st, 2nd, 3rd, 4th) time?" (Kantner, 1981). Among 15- to 19-year-old women who had ever experienced a premarital first pregnancy and either were unmarried at the time the pregnancy was resolved or were pregnant and unmarried at the time of the survey, the percentage of unwanted pregnancies was 75.8% in 1971, 75.4% in 1976, and 82.0% in 1979. Further analyses are difficult, however, because of the small sample sizes.

The Johns Hopkins data are particularly important because they have been used as the basis for two influential reports on the

291

wantedness of births to teenagers: one by the federal government's Centers for Disease Control (CDC) in 1978 and the other by the Alan Guttmacher Institute (AGI) in 1981.

Centers for Disease Control Estimates

In a report entitled "Unintended Teenage Childbearing," the Family Planning Evaluation Division of CDC (CDC, 1978) estimated that 273,000 unintended births occurred among teenage women 15–19 years old during 1974. This represented approximately 46% of all births to this age group. This estimate was obtained by applying the Hopkins 1971 survey percentages of births to married and single teenagers that were unintended (Zelnik and Kantner, 1974) to state data on the number of births by race and marital status, and calculating an estimated intended fertility rate for each state for 1974. Subtracting this rate from the actual fertility rate gave an estimate of the unintended fertility rate. Multiplying the unintended fertility rate by the number of females aged 15–19 in each state provided an estimate of the number of unintended births.

The CDC estimated that 63% of births to black teenagers were unintended as compared to 38% of those to whites. White teenagers, however, had a higher absolute number of unintended births (161,668 as compared to 104,340). Unintended fertility rates for females aged 15–19 ranged from 12.8% in Massachusetts to 53.4% in Mississippi (CDC, 1978a).

These data excluded pregnancies ending in induced abortion and thus underestimated the rate and number of unwanted conceptions. The reliability of the CDC estimates, however, is heavily dependent on both the accuracy and transferability of the findings of the Hopkins studies to the 1974 U.S. population and on the accuracy of the fertility data for this age group.

Alan Guttmacher Institute Estimates

In 1976 the AGI stated that "nearly two-thirds of all adolescent pregnancies and one-half of births are not intended" (p. 16). The sources were the 1971 Hopkins data adjusted for nonresponse, and unpublished data from the 1972 National Natality Survey.

In 1981 the AGI issued an updated monograph stating that "eight in ten premarital teenage pregnancies and two-thirds of premarital teenage births are unintended" (p. 16). The AGI estimated that 86% of pregnancies among unwed teenagers were unintended and 51% among the married. For births, the figures were 66% unintended among the unmarried and 48% unintended among the married. The variation by age was 65% unintended pregnancies among 18- and 19-year-olds, 87% among 15- to 17-year-olds, and virtually all unintended among those under 15. By race, 82% of pregnancies and 70% of births were unintended among blacks, and 71% of pregnancies and 49% of births among whites.

The 1981 AGI estimates of pregnancy intentions are unique in that they are based on estimates of actual abortions and miscarriages as well as on questionnaire responses (Dryfoos and Bourque-Scholl, 1981). Data sources included the natality statistics of the National Center for Health Statistics, abortion data from CDC and AGI's own surveys, unpublished calculations of the 1976 NSFG, and the 1971 and 1976 Hopkins surveys. (For a more recent analysis of the pregnancy intentions of adolescents and older women using similar data sources, see Dryfoos, 1982 and Ory, Forrest, and Lincoln, 1983, pp. 14, 15.)

Philadelphia Studies

All the studies of teenage pregnancy previously cited are based at least partly on questions asked the already pregnant or parenting adolescent. A more valid estimate of the wantedness of teenage pregnancy might be obtained by asking nonpregnant adolescents for their perceptions of the costs and benefits of pregnancy and parenthood in the adolescent years. According to Luker (1975), if those who perceived more costs than benefits became pregnant before age 20, presumably that pregnancy would be unwanted as well as unplanned; but if those who perceived more benefits than costs became pregnant, the pregnancy would be wanted, although possibly un planned. (For a criticism of Luker's theories see Crosbie and Bitte, 1982.) Of course, it is probable that costs and benefits are not fixed or related to enduring personality characteristics, but rather that they fluctuate with circumstances such as current sexual partner, relations with parents and peers, and school performance (Rosen et al., 1979; Klerman et al., 1982).

A series of studies in Philadelphia have provided some information about the attitudes of the nonpregnant. The first (Freeman et al., 1980) was a report on unmarried black urban youth, 13–18 years of age, of both sexes. Only 35% of the respondents felt that having a child now would make life "worse" or "ruined." Twenty-two percent said it would make life no different or better, and 43% did not know how a child would affect their lives. There were no significant differences between male and female respondents. Thus, only slightly over one-third of the respondents would state definitively that pregnancy would be unwanted. These attitudes were confirmed by the answer to a subsequent question, which indicated that if the female respondents or the female partners of the male respondents became pregnant within the next month, 15% would be happy with the pregnancy and 31% would be upset but believed that having a baby would "work out."

A second report (Freeman et al., 1982) resulted from a study of black never-pregnant females aged 17 or younger enrolled in a family planning clinic designed for teenagers. Only 22% wanted their first baby before age 20. In answer to another question, 22% thought a pregnancy in the next year would make their life situation better or no different; to this latter group should probably be added the 38% who did not know what effect the pregnancy would have. Thus, only the remaining 40% who said pregnancy would make their situation worse, could be said definitely not to want pregnancy. At one-year follow-up, 47% of this latter group stated they always used a contraceptive, as compared to 22% of the "situation better/no different" and 31% of the "do not know" groups.

A third study (Freeman, 1982) was of black unmarried 14- to 17-year-olds divided into those who delivered a first pregnancy, aborted a first pregnancy, and were never pregnant but were enrolled in a family planning clinic. Respondents were asked to indicate on three scales their feelings when they "just knew they were pregnant" (for deliverers and aborters) and "if they became pregnant during the next year" (for the never pregnant). The three scales were "very unhappy–very happy," "very unwanted–very wanted," and "very unplanned–very planned." Of the never-pregnant group, 78% said a pregnancy would be unplanned and an additional 10% gave ambivalent answers. When asked about happiness, however, only 64% said they would be unhappy and an additional 16% were ambivalent. A pregnancy would be unwanted by 62%, and 14% were ambivalent. The deliverers and aborters felt similarly about the planning status of their pregnancies.

Other Studies

Other studies of low-income, mostly black teenage populations have also inquired about the wantedness of their pregnancies. Furstenberg (1976) noted that the adolescents and their parents were astonished to learn of the pregnancy and that a feeling of despair accompanied this reaction. But one in five of the adolescents reported "kind of good" or "sort of happy" responses to the pregnancies, and another fifth reported mixed feelings or indicated that they had not been affected much one way or the other.

Some of these women expressed a fatalistic resignation to their pregnancies, and many reacted by asserting that everyone can make one mistake. A number of the adolescents with mixed reactions said that they looked forward to having a child, at the same time admitting that they were not really ready to be parents and that the child was going to interfere with their goals. Three-fifths of the expectant mothers stated their first reactions in unambivalently negative terms, and an even larger proportion (75%) said they wished they had not become pregnant. (Furstenberg, 1976, p. 53)

Furstenberg also notes that almost all responses to the pregnancy became more positive as the pregnancy advanced.

In a study of primiparous adolescent mothers 18 years of age and younger, Zuckerman (1980) found that only 10% were upset about being pregnant—a percentage similar to that of older women. In another study of adolescent, mostly black 12- to 19-year-olds in prenatal clinics, Ryan and Sweeney (1980) reported that 30% of pregnancies were intentional but an additional 33% were unintentional but wanted. Less than 10% of the total sample felt that their pregnancies caused any family problems, and 76% said their parents felt happy or "OK" about the situation. A study of very young adolescent mothers (12- to 15-year-olds) by the Child Welfare League of America (Miller, 1981) reported on the initial reaction of these young women to the discovery of their pregnancy. Negative reactions were felt by 80% , 4% reacted with disbelief, and 16% had positive feelings about being pregnant.

The range of unwantedness in studies of adolescents undoubtedly reflects differences in samples, in pregnancy status when asked, and in the questions themselves. Nevertheless, it seems likely that many teenage births, although unintended, are not unwanted. Many of the pregnancies that are truly unwanted terminate in abortions. If the adolescent chooses to carry her pregnancy to term, it seems possible that her feelings and those of her sexual partner may be positive or ambivalent. As the Select Panel for the Promotion of Child Health (1981) noted in the section of its report devoted to education on human sexuality,

A variety of emotional factors appear to be involved in teenage pregnancies including a desire for love and acceptance, for "proof" of maturity, for status with peers. Adolescents are seldom aware of the adverse impact early birth will have on their own future education and income, or of the expense and strain inherent in childrearing (p. 122).

Henderson (1980) was able to document this problem by showing differences in the perceptions of the consequences of school-age pregnancy and motherhood among the young mothers themselves, their parents, and school personnel. The mothers and their parents mentioned a limited number of consequences, which were generally short-term, immediate, and nonsevere. School personnel, however, listed numerous long-term and severe consequences.

IMPLICATIONS FOR PROGRAMS AND POLICIES

While the planned alternatives to childrearing (induced abortion and adoption) are themselves stressful, the birth of an unwanted child is probably more so and may result in emotional strain on the mother, child abuse and neglect, and family problems (David and Matejeck, 1981; Furstenberg, 1976; McAnarney, 1983, Ch. 10–16). Consequently, society should put considerable resources into the prevention of unwanted pregnancies and births. A more complete epidemiology of these phenomena would make it easier to decide what strategies would be most effective. Epidemiologic studies should help pinpoint groups who are particularly at risk for unwanted pregnancies and births, and for whom better contraceptive methods, greater access to these methods, and more family planning education are particularly needed. The U.S. National Committee on Vital and Health Statistics has made several recommendations regarding the measurement of desired and actual births (National Center for Health Statistics, 1978, pp. 13–14):

1. Data on the number and timing of births that occur to the various birth cohorts and the extent to which these are wanted should continue to be collected in the National Survey of Family Growth and the National Natality Followback Survey.
2. The National Natality Followback Survey should collect at regular intervals, perhaps biennially, information on the mothers' marital and pregnancy histories.
3. Data on unwanted pregnancies and their outcomes should be collected in the National Survey of Family Growth from all never-married as well as all ever-married women.[1]
4. Longitudinal panel data should be collected in which family size desires and expectations (among numerous variables) are measured at successive intervals, beginning soon after marriage. In addition to permitting studies of the stability of desires and expectations, this would allow an estimation of the effects of number and timing failures on subsequent family size desires and expectations.

[1] Cycle III of the NSFG, conducted in 1982–1983, includes all women in the childbearing years, regardless of marital status.

5. Data on unplanned births should be collected from husbands as well as wives.
6. Data should be collected which allow a determination of the extent to which preferences and/or strategies of timing and spacing of births exist, to what extent these are stable, and whether timing failures produce changes in the overall plans.
7. Longitudinal studies are needed in which the personal, social, and health characteristics of children reported as wanted are compared with children reported as unwanted by parents with matching socioeconomic and personality characteristics.

Programmatic efforts, however, should not wait on study results. Evidence already available points to the need for improved contraceptive devices, particularly for adolescents who are worried about the pill, should not use the IUD, and dislike barrier methods. Greater availability of family planning facilities and more education about contraception are also high-priority needs, both for adolescents (Forrest et al., 1981) and for older women (Dryfoos, 1982).

The sizeable proportion of unintended pregnancies that lead to wanted children suggests that additional strategies may be needed, especially among adolescents. The prevention of unintended pregnancies in this group will require educational and employment policies that provide young men and women with sources of gratification, enhancement of self-esteem, creativity, and independence other than pregnancy and parenthood.

CONCLUSION

The epidemiologic study of unwanted pregnancies and births is still relatively unsophisticated. More thought needs to be given to sample selection, definitions, questionnaire design, and ways to overcome respondent bias. More comprehensive, in-depth information will enable federal and state governments to develop programs to assist those who know they do not want to become pregnant, or to make others pregnant. Still needed is information that will help those who are uncertain about their desire to become parents make the best decisions for their circumstances.

REFERENCES

Alan Guttmacher Institute (1976). *11 million teenagers: What can be done about the epidemic of adolescent pregnancies in the United States.* New York: Planned Parenthood Federation of America.

———— (1981). *Teenage pregnancy: The problem that hasn't gone away*. New York: Alan Guttmacher Institute.

Anderson, J.E. (1981). Planning status of marital births, 1975–1976. *Fam. Plann. Perspect. 13*(2), 62–70.

Bracken, M.B., Klerman, L.V., and Bracken, M. (1978). Abortion, adoption, or motherhood: An empirical study of decision-making during pregnancy. *Am. J. Obstet. Gynecol. 130*(3), 251–262.

Centers for Disease Control (1978). Unintended teenage childbearing, United States, 1974. *Morbidity Mortality Weekly Rep. 27*(16), 131–132.

———— (1978a). *Teenage fertility in the United States: 1960–1970, 1974, regional and state variation and excess fertility*. Washington, D.C.: U.S. Government Printing Office.

Crosbie, P.V. and Bitte, D. (1982). A test of Luker's theory of contraceptive risk-taking. *Stud. Fam. Plann. 13*(3), 67–68.

David, H.P. (1972). Unwanted pregnancies: Costs and alternatives. In *Demographic and social aspects of population growth*, edited by C.F. Westoff, and R. Parke, Jr. Washington, D.C.: U.S. Government Printing Office, pp. 439–466.

———— and Matejcek, Z. (1981). Children born to women denied abortion: An update. *Fam. Plann. Perspect. 13*(1), 32–34.

Dryfoos, J.C. (1982). Contraceptive use, pregnancy intentions and pregnancy outcomes among U.S. women. *Fam. Plann. Perspect. 14*(2), 81–94.

———— and Bourque-Scholl (1981). *Factbook on teenage pregnancy*. New York: Alan Guttmacher Institute. Eckard, E. (1980). Wanted and unwanted births reported by mothers 15–44 years of age: United States, 1976. *Advance Data from Vital and Health Statistics 56*, 1–10.

Forrest, J.D., Hermalin, A.I., and Henshaw, S.K. (1981). The impact of family planning clinic programs on adolescent pregnancy. *Fam. Plann. Perspect. 13*(3), 199–216.

Freeman, E.W. (1982). Personal communication.

————, Rickles, K., Huggins, G.R., Mudd, E.H., Garcia, C.R., and Dickens, H.O. (1980). Adolescent contraceptive use: Comparison of male and female attitudes and information. *Am. J. Public Health 70*(8), 790–797.

————, ————, Mudd, E.B.H., and Huggins, G.R. (1982). Never-pregnant adolescents and family planning programs: Contraception, continuation, and pregnancy risk. *Am. J. Public Health 72*(8), 815–822.

Furstenberg, F.F., Jr. (1976). *Unplanned parenthood—the social consequences of teenage childbearing*. New York: The Free Press.

Hass, P.H. (1974). Wanted and unwanted pregnancies: A fertility decision-making model. *J. Soc. Issues 30*(4), 125–165.

Henderson, G.H. (1980). Consequences of school-age pregnancy and motherhood. *Fam. Relations 29*, 185–190.

Kantner, J.F. (1981). Personal communication.

Klerman, L.V., Bracken, M.B., Jekel, J.F., and Bracken, M. (1982). The delivery–abortion decision among adolescents. In *Pregnancy in adolescence—needs, problems, and management*, edited by I.R. Stuart and C.F. Wells. New York: Van Nostrand Reinhold, pp. 219–235.

Lehfeldt, H. (1959). Willful exposure to unwanted pregnancy (WEUP). *Am. J. Obstet. Gynecol. 78*(3), 661–665.

Luker, K. (1975). *Taking chances: Abortion and the decision not to contracept.* Berkeley: University of California Press.

McAnarney, E.R., editor. (1983). *Premature adolescent pregnancy and parenthood.* New York: Grune and Stratton.

Miller, S. (1981). *Children as parents: A progress report on a study of childbearing and childrearing among 12–15 year olds.* New York: Child Welfare League of America, Inc.

Miller, W.B. (1974). Relationship between the intendedness of conception and the wantedness of pregnancy. *J. Nerv. Ment. Dis. 159*(4), 396–406.

Munson, M.L. (1977). Wanted and unwanted births reported by mothers 15–44 years of age: United States, 1973. *Advance Data from Vital and Health Statistics 9,* 1–11.

National Center for Health Statistics (1978). *Statistics needed for national policies related to fertility.* A report of the U.S. National Committee on Vital and Health Statistics. Hyattsville, Md.: U.S. Department of Health, Education and Welfare.

Ory, H.W., Forrest, J.D., and Lincoln, R. (1983). *Making choices: Evaluating the health risks and benefits of birth control methods.* New York: Alan Guttmacher Institute.

Pohlman, E. and Pohlman, J.M. (1969). *The psychology of birth planning.* Cambridge, Mass.: Schenkman.

Rosen, R.H. (1982). Pregnancy resolution decisions: A review and appraisal of research. In *The childbearing decision—fertility attitudes and behavior,* edited by G.L. Fox. Beverly Hills, Calif: Sage Publications.

————, Ager, J.W., and Martindale, L.J. (1979). Contraception, abortion, and self-concept. *J. Popul. 2,* 118–139.

Ryan, G.M. and Sweeney, P.J. (1980). Attitudes of adolescents toward pregnancy and contraception. *Am. J. Obstet. Gynecol. 137*(3), 358–366.

Ryder, N.B. and Westoff, C.F. (1972). Wanted and unwanted fertility in the United States: 1965 and 1970. In *Demographic and social aspects of population growth,* edited by C.F. Westoff and R. Parke, Jr. Washington, D.C.: U.S. Government Printing Office, pp. 466–503.

Sears, R.R., Maccoby, E.E., and Levin, H. (1957). *Patterns of child rearing.* Evanston, Ill.: Row, Peterson.

Select Panel for the Promotion of Child Health (1981). *Better health for our children.* Vol. 1, *Major findings and recommendations.* Washington, D.C.: U.S. Department of Health and Human Services, Publication No. 79-55071.

Weller, R.H. (1976). Number and timing failures among legitimate births in the United States: 1968, 1969, and 1972. *Fam. Plann. Perspect. 8*(3), 111–116.

———— and Heuser, R.L. (1978). Wanted and unwanted childbearing in the United States: 1968, 1969, and 1972 national natality surveys. *Vital Health Stat. (21),* No. 32. Hyattsville, Md.: National Center for Health Statistics, Publication No. 78-1918.

Westoff, C.F. (1981). The decline in unwanted fertility, 1971–1976. *Fam. Plann. Perspect. 13*(2), 70–72.

Westoff, C.F. and Parke, R., Jr., editors (1972). *Demographic and social aspects of population growth*, Vol. 1. Research reports of the Commission on Population Growth and the American Future. Washington, D.C.: U.S. Government Printing Office.

Zelnik, M. and Kantner, J.F. (1974). The resolution of teenage first pregnancies. *Fam. Plann. Perspect. 6*(2), 74–80.

————— and ————— (1980). Sexual activity, contraceptive use and pregnancy among metropolitan-area teenagers: 1971–1979. *Fam. Plann. Perspect. 12*, 230–237.

Zuckerman, B. (1980). Personal communication.

12

Induced Abortion

Willard Cates, Jr.

To survey the epidemiology of induced abortion is a multifaceted venture that enters the territory of the behavioral scientist, the public health practitioner, the political analyst, the clinician, the demographer, and the statistician. Because induced abortion concerns a woman's choice about her pregnancy, it reflects personal decision-making behavior. Because these choices involve differences in safety, induced abortion has a public health impact. Because the issue has become highly political, it influences public policy formation. As it involves operative intervention into a pregnancy, induced abortion is a surgical procedure. Finally, induced abortion directly influences the outcome of the current pregnancy and may influence the outcome of future pregnancies; therefore, it affects demographic measures.

Induced abortion concerns many individuals. In 1978, over 50 million women of reproductive age lived in the United States, 60% of whom were estimated to be sexually active and fertile (Table 12-1). Approximately 5.6 million pregnancies occurred in this population, 3.1 million of which were unintended. Nearly half of these unintended pregnancies were terminated by legally induced abortion, accounting for 1.4 million procedures in the United States in 1978 (Henshaw et al., 1981).

The remainder of this chapter will expand on the topics mentioned above. The focus will be on knowledge gained through studies conducted primarily in the United States. Data of varying quality pertaining to induced abortion are available from other countries (Tietze, 1981), and they correlate with many of the trends found in the United States.

The author thanks David A. Grimes, M.D. and Gail D. Carpenter for their constructive input to this chapter.

Table 12-1. Women at Risk of Pregnancy and
Estimated Pregnancy Outcomes, United States, 1978

Characteristic	Number
Women aged 15–44	51,033,000
Fertile, sexually active women aged 15–44	31,460,000
Total pregnancies	5,610,000
Intended—total	2,515,000
Livebirths	2,096,000
Spontaneous abortions	419,000
Unintended—total	3,095,000
Livebirths	1,287,000
Legal abortions	1,410,000
Spontaneous abortions	398,000

Source: Henshaw et al. (1981), Table I-1.

PERSONAL DECISION MAKING

A woman faced with an unplanned pregnancy has two basic choices:
She can end the pregnancy by induced abortion or continue it to
term. If she chooses pregnancy termination and if legal abortion is
available, she can obtain induced abortion from a physician; if legal
abortion is not available, she can seek an illegal induced abortion
from an unlicensed practitioner or else self-induce her abortion.
Regardless of these choices, she may suffer a spontaneous abortion
before her intended outcome occurs.

Women Obtaining Legal Abortions

In the United States, most women who obtain legal abortions are
young, white, unmarried, childless, and obtain their abortions close
to home (Table 12-2). In 1978, about 31% of the women obtaining abortions were teenagers, 35% were aged 20–24, and 34% were
25 or over; 69% were white; 77% were unmarried. These distributions generally reflect the characteristics of women with unintended
pregnancy (Henshaw et al., 1981). Over 90% of women obtaining
abortions in the United States in 1978 did so in their own state of
residence (Centers for Disease Control, 1980). As abortion services
became more widely available after 1973, fewer women had to travel
long distances to obtain them.

The distribution of women who obtain abortions, however, does not
reflect the likelihood of choosing induced abortion if a woman becomes
pregnant. Rather, adding denominators of estimated pregnancies

Table 12-2. Number and Percentage Distribution of Legal Abortions and Percentage of Pregnancies Terminated by Legal Abortion, United States, 1978

Characteristic	Number	(%)	*Pregnancies terminated by abortion (%)*
Total	1,409,600	(100.0)	29.4
Age			
<20	433,900	(30.8)	38.2
20–24	489,410	(34.7)	29.5
25–29	265,990	(18.9)	21.4
30–34	134,280	(9.5)	23.4
35–39	65,350	(4.6)	36.8
>40	20,670	(1.5)	50.8
Race			
White	969,410	(68.8)	26.3
Black and other	440,190	(31.2)	39.9
Marital status			
Married	330,630	(23.5)	10.5
Unmarried	1,078,970	(76.5)	66.2

Source: Henshaw et al. (1981), Tables II-2 and II-3.

to the above distribution revealed different patterns (Table 12-2). Women at both ends of the reproductive age spectrum were more likely to terminate pregnancies by legal abortion than women aged 25–34. This indicates women in the middle reproductive years are more likely to plan their pregnancies and to carry them to term. Nearly 40% of pregnancies in women of black and other races were terminated by legal abortion, compared to about 25% of those to white women. Finally, unmarried women were more than six times more likely to terminate pregnancies by legal abortion as married women. This large difference between married and unmarried women does not take into account those women who conceived premaritally and subsequently gave birth while married. This situation would tend to shift livebirths from the unmarried to the married category, thereby decreasing the denominator for unmarried women to a greater degree than for married women because of the large number of livebirths for the latter.

Psychosocial Correlates

Whereas these epidemiologic measures indicate which general characteristics are correlated with a woman's obtaining an induced abortion, each decision is unique; the specific circumstances surrounding a particular pregnancy are the most important factors affecting a woman's decision to abort (Bracken et al., 1978; Smetana and Adler, 1979). Many women have already made informed decisions about reproductive behavior before becoming pregnant (Luker, 1975); they have weighed contraception against pregnancy. Once pregnant, a new set of values applies (Smetana and Adler, 1979), and feelings of anxiety and depression increase (Freeman, 1978). The decision to abort is rarely taken lightly; nearly nine in ten women report conflicting emotions (Bracken et al., 1974; Freeman, 1978).

Ambivalence about the pregnancy is apparently not associated with major psychologic sequelae (David et al., 1981; Doan and Quigley, 1981). Rather, data indicate that the woman's own perceived ability to cope with her emotions is an important factor affecting her postabortion mental state (Bracken et al., 1974). In this regard, parental support is important to younger women in their coping; for older women, their partner's support is most important.

Repeat Abortions

A woman's decision to terminate one pregnancy is associated with her decision about others (Bracken and Kasl, 1975; Tietze, 1978). Women who have undergone a previous induced abortion have threefold higher abortion rates than those obtaining abortions for the first time (Tietze, 1978). Several factors explain this difference: (1) Women who have already had one abortion are generally in their prime reproductive years; (2) they are demonstrably sexually active; (3) they are of proven fecundity; (4) they are willing to accept induced abortion as a way of preventing an unplanned birth; and (5) they have demonstrated their ability to overcome barriers that may deter other women from obtaining abortion services.

The increasing number and rate of repeat abortions in the United States occurring after abortion became legalized have raised public concern (Lake, 1980). From 1974 to 1978, the number of repeat abortions more than tripled, accounting for more than half the total increase in the number of induced abortions during this interval (Centers for Disease Control, 1980). These trends have been cited as evidence that legalization of abortion leads to deteriorating contraceptive practice.

The data indicate that the primary reason for the increase in repeat abortions was an increase in the "population at risk"—that is, as the number of women undergoing abortion for the first time increases, the number at risk of a repeat abortion also increases (Tietze and Jain, 1978). Between 1970 and 1978, the number of women having their first legal abortion, and thus at risk of repeat legal abortion, increased more than 30-fold (Centers for Disease Control, 1980; Tietze, 1981).

PUBLIC HEALTH IMPACT

A pregnant woman is at increased risk of death as the pregnancy progresses no matter what her choice of outcomes. The risks associated with pregnancy and childbirth are usually acceptable to a woman if her pregnancy is wanted; however, they are less acceptable if the pregnancy is unwanted. Of the options available to a woman with an unintended pregnancy, legally induced abortion is safer for her than either illegally induced abortion or continuing the pregnancy to term. The increasing availability of legal induced abortion has had a marked positive public health impact on women of reproductive age.

Legal Versus Illegal Abortion

Before 1969, the best estimates of the annual rate of induced abortion in the United States ranged widely, between 200,000 and 1.2 million (Calderone, 1958; Abernathy et al., 1970). Nearly all these abortions were illegally induced, which caused sizeable numbers of deaths and complications among American women of reproductive age. For example, in 1965, 235 deaths, or 20% of all deaths related to pregnancy and childbirth, were attributed to abortion (National Center for Health Statistics, 1968). After 1969, the number of reported legal abortions increased from approximately 22,000 to over 1.4 million in 1978 (Centers for Disease Control, 1980; Henshaw et al., 1981). Initially, the increase in legal abortions was accompanied by a progressive decline in the estimated number of illegal abortions. Thus, most of the initial increase in legal abortions went largely to replace illegal abortions (Tietze, 1973; Cates and Rochat, 1976; Tietze and Bongaarts, 1976) and did not dramatically influence birth trends.

This shift from illegal to legal abortion has directly affected overall abortion mortality (Fig. 12-1). In 1965, total abortion mortality began to decline faster than other pregnancy-related causes, probably because more effective contraceptive methods led to fewer unwanted pregnancies, which in turn led to fewer attempted illegal abortions (Westoff, 1972). In 1970, total abortion mortality declined even more rapidly and continued at an accelerated pace through 1976. This accelerated decline further implies that legal abortions primarily replaced illegal abortions, because if they had substituted for term

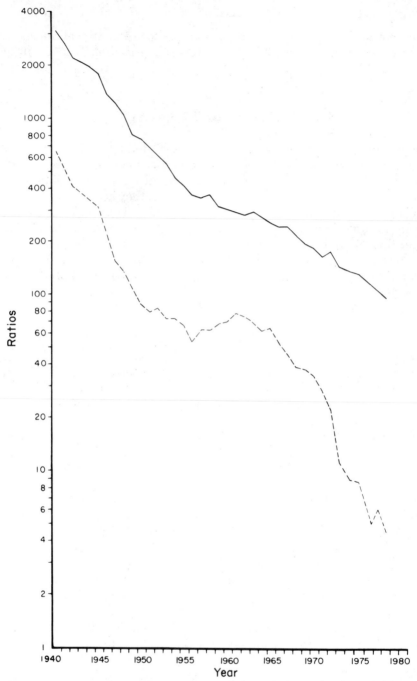

Fig. 12-1. Maternal mortality ratios, excluding abortion deaths (solid line; equal to total maternal deaths minus abortion deaths), and abortion mortality ratios (broken line; deaths per 1 million livebirths), United States, 1940–1978. From U.S. Vital Statistics, Final Mortality Statistics, National Center for Health Statistics.

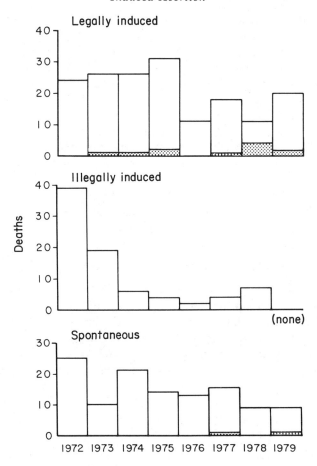

Fig. 12-2. Abortion-related deaths by category (excluding unknown category) and year (1979 data are provisional). Shaded areas, ectopic pregnancy—related to abortion.

births, abortion mortality would have increased relative to maternal mortality.

The categorization of abortion-related deaths into one of three categories—legally induced, illegally induced, and spontaneous—further underscores these trends (Fig. 12-2). In 1972, 90 abortion-related deaths occurred; by 1979, the number had declined to less than one third this number (Centers for Disease Control, 1981a). Through 1976, nearly all of this decline occurred in the illegally induced category, where the number of deaths decreased from 39 in 1972 to 2 in 1976. The reduction in illegal abortion mortality had a

307

distinct temporal association with the increasing availability of legal abortion (Gates et al., 1978).

Morbidity trends for abortion in recent years parallel those of mortality. Studies performed at national, state, and local levels show that hospitalization of women with complications resulting from abortion has decreased. Estimates based on the Hospital Discharge Survey from 1970 to 1977 show a general decline in hospital discharges for women with diagnoses relating to other than legal abortion and its complications; the greatest part of this decline occurred in 1973, immediately after the Supreme Court decisions (Bracken et al., 1982). In addition, individual hospitals on both the East and West coasts of the United States, have shown similar declines (Goldstein and Stewart, 1972; Seward et al., 1973; Lanman et al., 1974; Kahan et al., 1975).

Legal Abortion Versus Childbearing

Legally induced abortion is safer for the pregnant woman than childbearing (Cates and Tietze, 1978; Cates et al., 1979b). Between 1972 and 1978, the risk of dying from terminating a pregnancy by legal abortion before 15 weeks' gestation was one seventh that of continuing the pregnancy to term (Fig. 12-3). Adjusting the death-to-case rates for age, race, and preexisting conditions further increases the

Fig. 12-3. Death-to-case rates for legal abortion by weeks of gestation, compared with birth-related mortality rate, United States, 1972–1978.

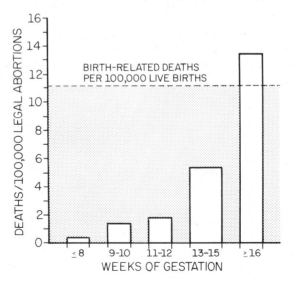

relative safety of induced abortion compared to childbearing (Cates and Tietze, 1978).

The relative risk of a woman's suffering serious complications if she elects to continue rather than abort her pregnancy is even greater than her risk of dying. For example, between 15 and 20% of term births are delivered by cesarean section (Placek and Taffel, 1980), whereas less than 1 in 500 abortion procedures performed in the first trimester results in unintended surgery (Cates et al., 1979b). Thus, the public health gains in mortality and morbidity for pregnant women have occurred primarily because legal abortion is proportionally safer than the alternative outcomes available to a pregnant woman.

PUBLIC POLICY IMPACT

More than any other surgical issue in the United States, abortion is a persistent focus for political action. The media have raised abortion to a level of importance that is not supported by its relatively low ranking as an issue of concern to most Americans (Traugott and Vinovskis, 1980). Political actions concerning legal abortion services have primarily involved two issues: (1) the possible limitation of public funds for legal abortions (Cates, 1981) and (2) regulating the conditions under which abortions could be performed (Cates et al., 1979a). Monitoring the health impact of these public policies has contributed to the legal and judicial decisions on abortion.

Abortion Funding

The Hyde Amendment, which restricted federal funds for abortion, was passed by Congress in 1976 and went into effect in 1977. The year before its implementation, approximately one fourth (295,000) of the abortions in the United States were obtained by low-income women through Medicaid. During the following two years, the number of federally funded abortions averaged 3000 per year, only 1% of the previous figure. The amendment therefore effectively stopped federally funded abortions.

However, several states continued to fund abortions using state revenues (Gold, 1980); approximately 85% of the low-income women likely to seek abortion were still covered by state funds. Thus, for the nation as a whole, more than nine in ten low-income women obtained a legal abortion despite the Hyde Amendment (Fig. 12-4). Seventy percent of these abortions were financed by state revenues, the rest by other sources of funds, including personal finances, reduced provider fees, and private contributions. About 7% of the low-income

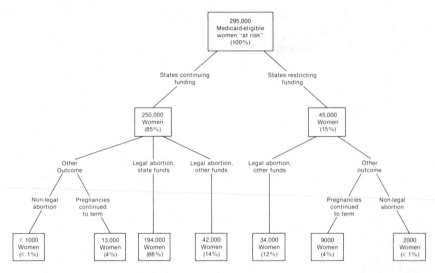

Fig. 12-4. Estimated Medicaid-eligible women at risk of restricted federal funds for abortion, by state funding status and projected outcome of pregnancy, United States, August 1977–February 1980. Estimates of state funding status from the Alan Guttmacher Institute, based on fiscal years 1977 and 1978 survey of states and monthly monitoring of state funding status. Estimates of projected outcome of pregnancy from the Centers for Disease Control, based on studies in restricted states and on national surveillance on abortion morbidity and mortality.

women continued their pregnancies to term, whereas only an estimated 1% resorted to illegal abortion (Cates, 1981).

However, there was a real difference in outcome between states that funded abortions and those that did not. In the former, 94% of the women "at risk" had abortions; only 5% carried their pregnancy to term. In the states restricting funding, 4% carried their pregnancies to term. Thus, it appears that a total funding cutoff would cause approximately one in five women to carry a pregnancy to term that might otherwise have been aborted.

Abortion Regulations

Legislation has been introduced in the United States at local, state, and national levels to regulate abortion services (Cates et al., 1979a). The alleged purpose of this legislation is to provide more comprehensive information for women considering pregnancy termination and to guard the health of women who choose abortion by providing safer conditions for the procedure. The regulations gen-

310

erally contain five provisions affecting delivery of abortion services: (1) the content of information provided in the preoperative counseling session, (2) a waiting period between obtaining informed consent for the procedure and its being performed, (3) parental notification if the pregnant woman is under 18 years of age and unmarried, (4) proscription of the use of agents with adverse effects on the fetus *in utero*, and (5) a requirement that all abortions after 12 weeks gestation be performed in hospitals.

Available epidemiologic data raise questions whether the regulations will achieve their stated goals. For example, laws that require the woman to be informed only of the risks of pregnancy termination without consideration of the risks of pregnancy continuation do not accurately represent all factors necessary in her giving an "informed consent" (Miller, 1980). Waiting periods have been shown to increase both the risks (Cates et al., 1977) and costs (Lupfer and Silber, 1981) of the abortion procedure, without substantially deterring the woman from terminating her pregnancy.

The actual effect of parental notification requirements has not been investigated. Parents are usually important influences on pregnancy decision making for the pregnant adolescent (Bracken et al., 1974). Responses to a national survey of abortion providers indicated that over half of teenagers younger than 18 obtaining abortions told their parents before the procedure (Torres et al., 1980). The younger the woman, the more likely her parents were to know and to suggest the abortion in the first place. Yet one fourth of teenagers obtaining legal abortion stated they would not do so if parental notification were required (Torres et al., 1980), preferring either to have an illegal abortion or to continue the pregnancy to term. Legislation to forbid particular abortion methods such as hypertonic saline instillation, or to require that all second-trimester abortion procedures be performed in hospitals, would increase the risks to the patient (Grimes et al., 1977; Cates and Grimes, 1981).

Although neither of the two main approaches to regulate abortion services has greatly affected the number of procedures performed, they have made legal abortion more difficult to obtain. Current efforts in Congress to restrict abortion services altogether would have a different impact. If legal abortion were no longer available, data presented above indicate that most women desiring to terminate unwanted pregnancies will do so regardless of its legal status (Cates and Rochat, 1976). Thus, indeed abortion per se will not be eliminated by restrictive legislation; rather, most women will still obtain abortion, albeit under less safe conditions. This will lead to a predictable increase in illness and death among women of reproductive age—the magnitude of which is uncertain.

311

Table 12-3. Categories and Variables Affecting Risk of Abortion Complications

Category	Variable
Patient's demographic profile	Age
	Race
	Gravidity
	Parity
	Socioeconomic status
Patient's medical risk factors	Preexisting conditions
	Gestational age
	Position of the uterus
Operator's skill	Level of training
	Previous abortion experience
	Innate ability
Type of anesthesia	None
	Local
	General
	Regional
	Combination
Type of dilatation	None
	Metal
	Plastic
	Laminaria-single
	Laminaria-multiple
	Chemical
	Vibrator
Amount of dilatation	As recorded in millimeters
Type of instrumentation	Uterine sound
	Flexible suction curette
	Rigid suction curette
	Sharp curette
	Ring forceps

Source: Cates and Grimes (1981).

INDUCED ABORTION AS A SURGICAL PROCEDURE

Induced abortion may be the most frequently performed operation in the world, with annual estimates ranging from 30 to 50 million, most of which are illegally induced (Tietze, 1981). About 2 million legally induced abortions are reported, nearly three fourths from the United States. Because of public interest in the issue and the large number of procedures performed, much has been learned regarding the epidemiology of abortion techniques. This has directly affected clinical practice. Also, epidemiologic expertise gained through studying

Category	Variable
	Intrauterine catheter
	Combination
	Postevacuation sharp curette
Size of instrumentation	As recorded in millimeters
Length of operative procedure	As recorded in minutes or hours
Type of abortifacient	Saline
	Prostaglandin
	Urea
	Oxytocin
	Combination
Type of facility and/or service	Hospital inpatient
	Hospital outpatient
	Type of hospital
	Freestanding clinic
	Physician's office
Use of prophylactic antibiotics	No
	Yes
	Type of antibiotic
Concurrent sterilization	Laparoscopic cauterization
	Laparoscopic clip
	Minilaparotomy with ligation
	Abdominal laparotomy with ligation
	Vaginal approach with ligation
	Hysterectomy
Postabortion contraception	None
	IUD inserted after uterine evacuation
	Oral contraceptives initiated
	Barrier methods

legal abortion as a surgical procedure has been used to investigate risk factors with other operations as well (Centers for Disease Control, 1981b).

Variations in Procedure

The term "induced abortion" is used generically to describe many permutations of operative procedures (Table 12-3); each variation can independently influence abortion morbidity. Factors related to the technical aspects of the procedure include type of anesthesia, method of dilatation, extent of dilatation, and mode of instrumentation and abortifacient used.

313

Other factors, not directly related to the abortion procedure itself, also affect the risk of complications (Table 12-3). Such variables as the woman's demographic characteristics, the woman's medical risk status, the type of facility in which the procedure is performed, concurrent sterilization, use of prophylactic antibiotics, and the type of postabortion contraception may independently influence the incidence and spectrum of abortion morbidity.

Physician's Skill

An important technical factor affecting the results of any surgical procedure, including induced abortion, is the skill of the physician. Unfortunately, valid criteria to measure a physician's skill have not been resolved by the different studies of abortion morbidity. Three variables probably have an influence on the skill of the physician: level of operative training, experience of the physician, and innate operative ability. Regarding training, the largest multicenter prospective study of abortion complications, the Joint Program for the Study of Abortion (JPSA/CDC), found no significant difference between major complication rates for abortions performed by residents and interns versus those performed by attending staff (Cates et al., 1979b). With respect to experience, no consistent pattern was found in Chicago between the number of procedures a physician had performed and the physician's complication rate compared to that of colleagues with either more or less experience (Bozorgi, 1977). In Yugoslavia, Andolsek (1974) found physicians performing between 100 and 300 abortions over the two-year study interval had lower complication rates than those who performed fewer than 100 or more than 300 procedures; she suggests that overscheduling may contribute to the higher complications rates among physicians doing the most procedures.

The innate ability of the physician is even more difficult to assess. In Chicago and Yugoslavia, some physicians with similar training and experience had different complication rates even though using identical protocols (Andolsek, 1974; Bozorgi, 1977). In St. Louis, some clinicians had higher rates of perforation despite having a background similar to that of other colleagues (Freiman and Wulff, 1977).

Gestational Age

The most important nontechnical risk factor is gestational age. The risk of abortion morbidity increases continually with advancing gestational age (Fig. 12-5). The two largest studies have documented that the seven- to eight-week gestational age interval has the lowest

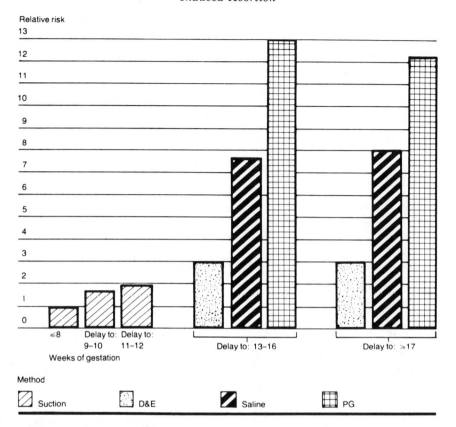

Relative risk

Method

Suction   D&E   Saline   PG

Fig. 12-5. Relative risk of major abortion-related morbidity due to length of gestation and choice of method, compared with risk associated with suction at ≤8 weeks gestation. From Cates et al. (1977).

major complication rate; the complication rate at six weeks or earlier was slightly higher (Tietze and Lewit, 1972; Cates et al., 1979b). After eight weeks gestation, the risk of major complications appears to rise approximately 15–30% for each week of delay (Fig. 12-5). In the JPSA/CDC study (Cates et al., 1977), a two-week delay at eight weeks gestation increases the relative risk of major complications at a faster rate than a two-week delay at ten weeks gestation (Table 12-4).

Therefore, existing data support two important conclusions regarding gestational age. First, early abortions are safer than later abortions. As a corollary, delays of any sort—whether administrative, medical, or social—increase the risk of complications. Second, there exists no gestational age threshold beyond which complication rates increase exponentially. Instead, complication rates increase linearly with advancing gestation during the first two trimesters.

315

Table 12-4. Total and Major Complications per 100 Women, by Gestation, Procedure, and Sterilization, for Total Patients and for Patients with Follow-up (FU), United States, 1971–1975

Gestation (weeks), procedure, and sterilization	Total complications		Major complications	
	Total patients	Patients with FU	Total patients	Patients with FU
All patients				
6 or less	7.2	10.3	0.4	0.6
7–8	4.7	6.6	0.3	0.4
9–10	5.6	7.7	0.4	0.6
11–12	8.2	9.9	0.8	1.0
13–14	17.0	18.1	1.4	1.6
15–16	33.1	36.2	1.9	2.1
17–20	39.9	47.4	2.2	2.5
21 or more	36.1	47.5	2.3	2.9
All gestations	12.3	14.9	0.8	1.0
Patients without pre-existing complications or concurrent sterilization				
6 or less	7.2	10.3	0.2	0.3
7–8	4.4	6.1	0.2	0.3
9–10	5.3	7.3	0.4	0.5
11–12	7.7	9.1	0.6	0.8
13–14	16.4	17.0	1.0	1.1
15–16	33.1	35.7	1.4	1.5
17–20	39.7	46.7	1.9	2.3
21 or more	34.6	45.2	1.7	2.2
All gestations	12.1	14.5	0.7	0.8
Procedure[a]				
Suction curettage[b,c]	4.7	6.5	0.3	0.4
D&E[c,d]	5.5	6.7	0.6	0.6

[a] Without preexisting complications.
[b] At 12 weeks gestation or earlier.
[c] Without tubal sterilization.
[d] Dilatation and evacuation at 13 weeks gestation or later.

Abortion Procedure

Legally induced abortion is a remarkably safe surgical procedure. Overall, about 12% of women undergoing legal abortions sustain a complication of any type, whereas fewer than 1% develop a major complication (Table 12-4). The JPSA/CDC (Cates and Grimes, 1981) indicates that the risk of complications, both total and major, are lower if women with preexisting medical conditions or concurrent sterilization are excluded from analysis. In contrast, if only women

Gestation (weeks), procedure, and sterilization	Total complications		Major complications	
	Total patients	Patients with FU	Total patients	Patients with FU
Saline[c,e]	38.0	47.0	1.7	2.1
Prostaglandin[c,e]	53.1	54.5	2.8	2.6
Hysterotomy[f]	47.0	48.1	13.9	15.2
Hysterectomy	49.5	48.8	13.4	13.4
Suction curettage[a,c]				
6 or less	6.0	9.2	0.2	0.3
7–8	4.0	5.7	0.2	0.3
9–10	4.7	6.6	0.3	0.4
11–12	5.2	6.5	0.4	0.6
D&E[a,c,d]				
13–16	5.6	6.8	0.6	0.7
17 or more	4.8	5.3	0.5	0.5
Saline [a,c,e]				
13–16	42.1	50.9	1.7	1.7
17 or more	36.3	45.4	1.7	2.2
Prostaglandin[a,c,e]				
13–16	55.0	55.5	2.8	2.1
17 or more	51.9	53.9	2.8	3.0
Tubal sterilization[a,b,g]				
Not done	4.7	6.5	0.3	0.4
By laparotomy	22.6	24.5	3.2	3.1
By laparoscopy	7.6	8.5	0.8	1.2

[e] Intraamniotic instillation.
[f] With tubal sterilization.
[g] Aborted by suction curettage.
Source: Cates and Grimes (1981).

with follow-up information are included in the analysis, these rates necessarily increase slightly.

Besides operator skill and gestational age, the choice of abortion method is also a major determinant of abortion complications. In the United States, five main abortion procedures have been used: suction curettage, dilatation and evacuation (D&E), intraamniotic saline instillation, intraamniotic prostaglandin $F_{2\alpha}$ ($PGF_{2\alpha}$) instillation, and hysterotomy/hysterectomy (Centers for Disease Control, 1980). In general, suction curettage is the safest available method of abortion.

Dilatation and evacuation at ≥13 weeks' gestation has higher complication rates than suction abortion at ≤12 weeks but lower rates than instillation methods using either saline or ($PGF_{2\alpha}$). Finally, hysterotomy and/or hysterectomy have major complication rates so high that these procedures cannot be considered appropriate as primary means of abortion in the United States except in unique situations.

Trends in Complications and Deaths

In the United States, the increasing availability of legal abortion has been associated with changes in the distribution of all three risk factors, which together has improved the safety of legally induced abortion during the 1970s (Grimes and Cates, 1979). An increasing percentage of training programs in obstetrics and gynecology are teaching abortion techniques, along with other ambulatory surgical procedures (Lindheim and Cotterill, 1978). Abortions are being performed at progressively earlier gestational ages (Centers for Disease Control, 1980). In 1970, nearly one in four legal abortions was performed at gestational ages of 13 weeks or later; by 1978, less than one in ten abortions was performed this late in pregnancy. Finally, the increasing use of suction rather than sharp curettage, and D&E rather than instillation procedures, has influenced the safety of legal abortion. Between 1970 and 1978, the death-to-case rate for legal abortion declined from 6.2 per 100,000 abortions to 0.9, an 85% decline (Centers for Disease Control, 1980).

DEMOGRAPHIC IMPACT

Induced abortion has a potential demographic impact in two ways: (1) its effect on the outcome of the current pregnancy and (2) its effect on the outcome of future pregnancies. To the extent that an induced abortion prevents the occurrence of a spontaneous abortion, a stillbirth, or a livebirth during the *same pregnancy*, the absolute number of these events would be reciprocally related to the number of abortions. To the extent that induced abortion influences the outcome of *subsequent pregnancies*, the incidence of any adverse outcomes would change in a direction determined by whether the association with induced abortion is harmful or protective. Finally, whether the induced abortion was performed legally or illegally may have a different impact on *both* currrent and subsequent pregnancy outcomes; thus the relative ratio between these two categories of induced abortion must also be considered in projecting demographic impact.

Current Pregnancy

In the first half of the 1970s most legal abortions in the United States terminated pregnancies that would have resulted in illegally induced abortions (p. 305); yet, because some women were deterred from illegal abortion and instead continued unwanted pregnancies to term, the increasing availability of legal abortion contributed to a decline in unintended births. In the early 1970s, legalization of abortion has been temporally associated with decreases in out-of-wedlock births in New York City (Pakter et al., 1973), California (Sklar and Berkov, 1973), Oregon (Quick, 1978), and the United States as a whole (Sklar and Berkov, 1974). Teenage birthrates were particularly influenced. State-to-state variation in teenage childbearing patterns shows a significant correlation with the abortion:livebirth ratio (Bauman et al., 1977; Brann, 1979).

Induced abortion may also influence the reported incidence of other perinatal outcomes in three ways. First, some clandestine abortions were erroneously categorized as spontaneous abortions and resulted in liveborn but nonviable infants (Glasss et al., 1974); although the same phenomenon occasionally occurs with legal abortion, current abortion techniques make this less likely (Cates and Grimes, 1981). Second, women generally at highest risk of adverse perinatal events—the youngest, oldest, and those with lowest income—have the highest legal abortion: livebirth ratios (Henshaw et al., 1981); legalization of abortion may have allowed these women to terminate unintended high-risk pregnancies voluntarily. Third, selective abortion of planned pregnancies with known congenital anomalies determined through prenatal diagnostic techniques would reduce the number of infants born with these conditions.

Most investigators have found a temporal association between the increase in legal abortion and decreasing neonatal mortality (Pakter et al., 1973; Garfinkel et al., 1975; Quick, 1978; Wallace, 1978). However, further, more sophisticated analytic approaches to determining the etiologic role of legal abortion in this decline have led to differing conclusions (Bauman and Anderson, 1980; Grossman and Jacobovitz, 1981).

Subsequent Pregnancy

The demographic influence of induced abortion on a woman's future pregnancies is likewise an unsettled issue (Bracken, 1978; Hogue, 1978; Cates, 1979). Some studies have demonstrated that women with prior induced abortions, especially previous multiple abortions, have an increased risk of such adverse events as spontaneous abortions, preterm deliveries, low-birthweight infants, and pregnancy complications. Others have found no such association.

The issue is particularly difficult to study because of inherent methodologic problems. Because long-term morbidity after legal abortion often requires many years before any effect is seen, and because the possible adverse sequelae are relatively rare occurrences, studies to detect late complications must be rigorously designed to avoid possible bias. Because of these difficulties, no single investigation can form the basis for establishing a causal relationship. Rather, each study should be considered separately for its strengths and weaknesses.

The best data currently available do not permit a firm conclusion as to whether one induced abortion per se, or even multiple abortions, produces increased risks of adverse reproductive outcomes in subsequent desired pregnancies. Those studies that demonstrate significant associations have primarily implicated the particular type of abortion procedure—especially sharp curettage (Harlap et al., 1979; World Health Organization, 1979). Because variations in abortion technique produce different short-term complications, they might also be expected to have a differential influence on late sequelae. Perhaps the manner and extent of dilatation is the most important factor in the induced abortion procedure, influencing future pregnancies.

CONCLUSION

Induced abortion influences many parameters of reproductive health and perinatal epidemiology. It offers women faced with unintended pregnancies an option other than childbearing. The choice to terminate a pregnancy, though hardly an easy decision, can be made less traumatic if legal and social barriers are reduced. If induced abortion can be performed within the limits of the law, it is a remarkably safe surgical procedure. The availability of legally induced abortion has had a dramatic public health impact in most countries by reducing deaths and complications to women of reproductive age.

The effect of induced abortion on other perinatal measures is more difficult to document. Whereas it directly affects the outcome of a woman's current pregnancy, induced abortion may also have a lingering influence on her subsequent pregnancies. Future research should focus on (1) factors influencing the dilemma of resolving unintended pregnancy, (2) the impact of policies limiting the availability of legally induced abortion, (3) techniques for reducing morbidity and mortality of the abortion procedure, and (4) analyses addressing the question of the late effects of induced abortion.

REFERENCES

Abernathy, J.R., Greenberg, B.G., and Horvitz, D.G. (1970). Estimates of induced abortion in urban North Carolina. *Demography 7*, 19–29.

Andolsek, L. (1974). *The Ljubljana Abortion Study, 1971–1973*. National Institute of Health, Center for Population Research, Bethesda, Md., pp. 15–16.

Bauman, K.E. and Anderson, A.E. (1980). Legal abortions and trends in fetal and infant mortality rates in the United States. *Am. J. Obstet. Gynecol. 136*, 194–202.

———, ———, Freeman, J.L., and Koch, G.G. (1977). Legal abortions, subsidized family planning services, and the U.S. "birth dearth." *Soc. Biol. 24*, 183–191.

Bracken, M.B. (1978). Induced abortion as a risk factor for perinatal complications: A review. *Yale J. Biol. Med. 51*, 539–548.

———, Freeman, D.H., and Hellenbrand, K. (1982). Hospitalization for legal induced and other abortions in the United States 1970–1977. *Am. J. Public Health 72*, 30–37.

———, Hachamovitch, M., and Grossman, G. (1974). The decision to abort and psychological sequelae. *J. Nerv. Ment. Dis. 158*, 154–162.

——— and Kasl, S.V. (1975). First and repeat abortions: A study of decision-making and delay. *J. Biosoc. Sci. 7*, 473–491.

———, Klerman, L.V., and Bracken, M. (1978). Abortion, adoption or motherhood: An empirical study of decision-making during pregnancy. *Am. J. Obstet. Gynecol. 130*, 251–262.

Brann, E.A. (1979). A multivariate analysis of interstate variation in fertility of teenage girls. *Am. J. Public Health 69*, 661–666.

Bozorgi, N. (1977). Statistical analysis of first-trimester pregnancy terminations in an ambulatorysurgical center. *Am. J. Obstet. Gynecol. 127*, 763–768.

Calderone, M.S. (1958). *Abortion in the United States*. New York: P.B. Hoeber.

Cates, W. Jr. (1979). Late effects of induced abortion: Hypothesis or knowledge? *J. Reprod. Med. 22*, 207–212.

——— (1981). The Hyde Amendment in action: How did the restriction of federal funds for abortion affect low-income women? *J.A.M.A. 246*, 1109–1112.

———, Gold, J., and Selik, R.M. (1979a). Regulation of abortion services: For better or worse? *N. Engl. J. Med. 301*, 720–723.

——— and Grimes, D.A. (1981). Deaths from second-trimester abortion by dilatation and evacuation: Causes, prevention, facilities. *Obstet. Gynecol. 58*, 401–408.

——— and ——— (1981). Morbidity and mortality of abortion in the United States. In *Abortion and sterilization: Medical and social aspects*, edited by J.E. Hodgson. London: Academic Press, pp. 155–180.

——— and Rochat, R.W. (1976). Illegal abortion in the United States, 1972–1974. *Fam. Plann. Perspect. 8*, 86–92.

———, ———, Grimes, D.A., and Tyler, C.W. Jr. (1978). Legalized abortion:

Effect on national trends of maternal and abortion-related mortality (1940–1976). *Am. J. Obstet. Gynecol. 132,* 211–214.

———, Schulz, K.F., Grimes, D.A., and Tyler, C.W. Jr (1977). The effect of delay and choice of method on the risk of abortion morbidity. *Fam. Plann. Perspect. 9,* 266–273.

———, ———, ———, and ——— (1979b). Short-term complications of uterine evacuation techniques for abortions at 12 weeks gestation or earlier. In *Pregnancy termination: Procedures, safety and new developments,* edited by G.I. Zatuchni, J.J. Sciarra, and J.J. Speidel. Hagerstown, Md: Harper & Row, pp. 127–135.

——— and Tietze, C. (1978). Standardized mortality rates associated with legal abortion: United States, 1972–1975. *Fam. Plann. Perspect. 10,* 109–112.

Centers for Disease Control (1980). *Abortion surveillance, 1978.* Atlanta, Ga.: Centers for Disease Control.

——— (1981a). Abortion. In *MMWR Annual Summary, 1980.* Atlanta, Ga.: Centers for Disease Control, pp. 103–104.

——— (1981b). *Sterilization surveillance, 1976–1978.* Atlanta, Ga.: Centers for Disease Control.

David, H.P., Rasmussen, N. Jr., and Holst, E. (1981). Postpartum and postabortion psychotic reactions. *Fam. Plann. Perspect. 13,* 88–92.

Doane, B.K. and Quigley, B.G. (1981). Psychiatric aspects of therapeutic abortion. *Can. Med. Assoc. J. 125,* 427–432.

Freeman, E.W. (1978). Abortion: Subjective attitudes and feelings. *Fam. Plann. Perspect. 10,* 150–155.

Freiman, S.M. and Wulff, G.J.L. (1977). Management of uterine perforation following elective abortion. *Obstet. Gynecol. 50,* 647–650.

Garfinkel, J., Chabot, M.J., and Pratt, M.W. (1975). Infant, maternal, and childhood mortality in the U.S.: 1968–1973. Rockville, Md.: U.S. Department of Health, Education and Welfare.

Glass, L., Evans, H.E., Swartz, D.P., Rajegowda, B.K., and LeBlanc, W. (1974). Effects of legalized abortion on neonatal mortality and obstetrical morbidity at Harlem Hospital Center. *Am. J. Public Health 64,* 717–718.

Gold, R.B. (1980). After the Hyde Amendment: Public funding for abortion in FY 1978. *Fam. Plann. Perspect. 12,* 131–134.

Goldstein, P. and Stewart, G. (1972). Trends in therapeutic abortion in San Francisco. *Am. J. Public Health 62,* 695–699.

Grimes, D.A. and Cates, W. Jr. (1979). Complications from legally induced abortion: A review. *Obstet. Gynecol. Surv. 13,* 177–191.

———, Schulz, K.F., Cates, W. Jr., and Tyler, C.W. Jr. (1977), Midtrimester abortion dilatation and evacuation: A safe and practical alternative. *N. Engl. J. Med. 296,* 1141–1145.

Grossman, M. and Jacobowitz, S. (1981). Variations in infant mortality rates among counties of the United States: The roles of public policies and programs. *Demography 18,* 695–713.

Harlap, S., Shiono, P., Ramcharan, S., Berendes, H., and Pellegrin, F. (1979). A prospective study of spontaneous fetal losses after induced abortions. *N. Engl. J. Med. 301,* 677–681.

Henshaw, S.K., Forrest, J.D., Sullivan, E., and Tietze, C. (1981). *Abortion 1977–1979: Need and services in the United States, each state and metropolitan area.* New York: Alan Guttmacher, pp. 1–13.

Hogue, C.J.R. (1978). Review of postulated fertility complications subsequent to pregnancy termination. In *Risks, benefits, and controversies in fertility control,* edited by J.J. Sciarra, G.I. Zatuchni, and J.J. Speidel. Hagerstown, Md.: Harper & Row, pp. 356–367.

Kahan, R.S., Baker, L.D., and Freeman, M.G. (1975). The effect of legalized abortion on morbidity resulting from criminal abortion. *Am. J. Obstet. Gynecol. 121,* 114–116.

Lake, A. (1980). The abortion repeaters. *McCall's,* September 1980, pp. 58–62.

Lanman, J.T., Kohl, S.G., and Bedel, J.H. (1974). Changes in pregnancy outcome after liberalization of the New York State abortion law. *Am. J. Obstet. Gynecol. 118,* 485–492.

Lindheim, B.L. and Cotterill, M.A. (1978). Training in induced abortion by obstetrics and gynecology residency programs. *Fam. Plann. Perspect. 10,* 24–28.

Luker, K. (1975). *Taking chances: Abortion and the decision not to contracept.* Berkeley: University of California Press.

Lupfer, M. and Silber, B.G. (1981). How patients view mandatory waiting periods for abortion. *Fam. Plann. Perspect. 13,* 75–79.

Miller, L.J. (1980). Informed consent: I. *J.A.M.A. 244,* 2100–2103.

National Center for Health Statistics (1968). *Final mortality statistics—1965.* Washington, D.C.: U.S. Government Printing Office.

Pakter, J., O'Hare, D., Nelson, F., and Svigir, M. (1973). Two years' experience in New York City with the liberalized abortion law—progress and problems. *Am. J. Public Health 63,* 524–535.

Placek, T.J. and Taffel, S.M. (1980). Trends in cesarean section rates for the United States, 1970–78. *Public Health Rep. 95,* 540–548.

Quick, J.D. (1978). Liberalized abortion in Oregon: Effects on fertility, prematurity, fetal death, and infant death. *Am. J. Public Health 68,* 1003–1008.

Seward, P.N., Ballard, C.A., and Ulene, A.L. (1973). The effect of legal abortion on the rate of septic abortion at a large county hospital. *Am. J. Obstet. Gynecol. 115,* 335–338.

Sklar, J. and Berkov, B. (1973). The effects of legal abortion on legitimate and illegitimate birth rates: The California experience. *Stud. Fam. Plann. 4,* 381–392.

———— and ———— (1974). Abortion illegitimacy and the American birth rate. *Science 185,* 909–915.

Smetana, J.G. and Adler, N.E. (1979). Decision-making regarding abortion: A value × expectancy analysis. *J. Population 2,* 338–357.

Tietze, C. (1973). Two years' experience with a liberal abortion law: Its impact on fertility trends in New York City. *Fam. Plann. Perspect. 5,* 36–41.

———— (1978). Repeat abortion—why more? *Fam. Plann. Perspect. 10,* 286–288.

—— (1981). *Induced abortion; A world review, 1981.* New York: The Population Council.

—— and Bongaarts, J. (1976). The demographic effect of induced abortion. *Obstet. Gynecol. Surv. 31,* 699–709.

—— and Jain, A.K. (1978). The mathematics of repeat abortion: Explaining the increase. *Stud. Fam. Plann. 9,* 294–299.

—— and Lewit, S. (1972). Joint Program for the Study of Abortion (JPSA): Early medical complications of legal abortion. *Stud. Fam. Plann. 3,* 98–122.

Torres, A., Forrest, J.D., and Eisman, S. (1980). Telling parents: Clinic policies and adolescents' use of family planning and abortion services. *Fam. Plann. Perspect. 12,* 284–292.

Traugott, M.W. and Vinovskis, M.A. (1980). Abortion and the 1978 Congressional elections. *Fam. Plann. Perspect. 12,* 238–246.

Wallace, H.M. (1978). Status of infant and perinatal morbidity and mortality: A review of the literature. *Public Health Rep. 93,* 386–393.

Westoff, C.F. (1972). The modernization of United States contraceptive practice. *Fam. Plann. Perspect. 4,* 9–12.

World Health Organization Task Force on the Sequelae of Abortion (1979). Gestation, birth weight, and spontaneous abortion in pregnancy after induced abortion. *Lancet 1,* 142–145.

13

Hydatidiform Mole

Kenji Hayashi and Michael B. Bracken

Hydatidiform mole (HM), a condition in which there is partial or complete conversion of the chorionic villi into grapelike vesicles, has attracted the interest of endocrinologists, immunologists, and, more recently, geneticists as a result of its variety of biological characteristics. A number of descriptive epidemiologic studies have been done, but few etiologic ones have been published to date.

Hydatidiform mole itself is considered benign although it has been identified as the commonest precursor of choriocarcinoma, one of the most malignant forms of cancer. A review of the literature indicates that 40–80% of choriocarcinomas were preceded by HM (Marquez-Monter et al., 1968; Matalon and Modan, 1972). Conversely, 11.6% of HM subsequently developed into malignancy (Takeuchi, 1978).

In HM patients, painless vaginal bleeding, usually beyond ten weeks of conception, is almost universally present, ranging from spotting to profuse haemorrhage. The uterus is large for the stage of pregnancy, and toxemia prior to 20 weeks and absent fetal parts and heart tones are among major clinical signs (Becker and Avioli, 1977). In addition, it should be noted that 8–10% of HM patients show signs of hyperthyroidism arising from production of thyrotropin by the trophoblast (Goldstein et al., 1979).

With the advent of methotrexate in 1956 and actinomycin D in 1962, the cure rates of choriocarcinoma have markedly improved, even in patients with metastatic lesions (Hertz, 1967). Because many patients are of childbearing age and hope to become pregnant again, a potential problem concerns the long-lasting side effects of chemotherapy. At present, then, attention needs be focused on primary prevention. In addition to indicating possible avenues for lowering the incidence of HM, etiologic studies may also provide some new insight into other basic issues such as mechanisms of maintenance of normal pregnancy especially in terms of histocompatibility between mother and fetus, the etiology of cancer, the origin of some congenital malformations, and the etiology of some spontaneous abortions.

CLINICAL CHARACTERISTICS OF HYDATIDIFORM MOLE

Morphologically, HM typically fits into two major categories: complete (or classic) and partial. Complete HM is a conceptus that lacks an intact fetus and shows gross, cystlike swelling of its chorionic villi due to the accumulation of fluid within the mesenchymal core. Partial moles show some of the same histologic picture as complete moles but coexist with a normal, separate conceptus. In addition, Hertig and Edmonds (1940) suggested an intermediate subtype, the transitional mole, as an early stage of complete mole, which preserves an ovisac that does not contain a fetus.

Because hydatidiform mole, invasive mole (choriocarcinoma destruens), and choriocarcinoma all originate from the trophoblast, they have been defined as trophoblastic neoplasms. However, whether each is an independent entity or whether they reflect different phases of a continuous spectrum of the same disease process is still controversial. From the former viewpoint, HM is regarded as an atypical missed abortion and invasive mole or choriocarcinoma as a secondary malignant transformation of HM (Hertig and Edmonds, 1940). The spectrum theory expounded by Park (1959) is based on observation of the clinical course and the patient's response to chemotherapy. It provides an analogy to the development of cervical cancer from dysplasia, carcinoma in situ, and invasive carcinoma, and led to the application of primary chemotherapy to trophoblastic malignancy, although this treatment has been critically reviewed (Hammond et al., 1973).

EPIDEMIOLOGY OF HYDATIDIFORM MOLE

Geographic Distribution

There are wide variations in reports on the incidence of HM throughout the world, ranging from 1 in 120 deliveries in Taiwan to 1 in 1000–2000 deliveries in the United States (Table 13-1). In countries where many births occur in the home, hospital-based studies tend to inflate the incidence artificially. Pregnancies are used as the denominator in some studies, but deliveries are used in others. Because all

Table 13-1. Incidence of Hydatidiform Mole Reported in Previous Studies[a]

Region	Incidence Per 1000 deliveries	Incidence Per 1000 pregnancies	References
United States			
Boston	0.48	—	Hertig and Edmond (1940)
Jersey City, N.J.	0.76	—	Chesley et al. (1946)
Philadelphia	0.67	—	Stroup (1956)
New York City	—	0.50	Douglas (1957)
New Orleans	0.45	—	Reiner and Dougherty (1960)
Hawaii	—	0.75	McCorriston (1968)
Rhode Island	—	0.63	Yen and MacMahon (1968)
Los Angeles	0.90	—	Westerhout et al. (1969)
New York	—	0.74	Muellar and Lapp (1969)
Rochester, N.Y.	—	0.58	Slocum and Lund (1969)
United States	—	1.08	Hayashi et al. (1982)
Latin America			
Mexico	—	0.46	Marquez-Monter et al. (1968)
Mexico	1.97	1.63	MacGregor et al. (1969)
Venezuela	—	0.92	Agüero et al. (1973)
Paraguay	—	0.23	Rolon and Lopez (1977)
Asian countries			
Philippines	5.0	—	Acosta-Sison (1959)
Japan	4.4	—	Hasegawa et al. (1960)
Japan (Wakayama)	2.55	1.92	Sasaki et al. (1979)
Taiwan	8.3	—	Wei and Ouyang (1963)
Hongkong	4.1	—	Chun et al. (1964)
Malaysia	1.5	—	Ong et al. (1978)
Israel	0.9	—	Matalon and Modan (1972)
Iran	—	3.2	Javey and Sajadi (1978)
Africa			
Uganda	1.03	—	Leighton (1973)
Nigeria	4.88	—	Ogunbode (1978)
Scandinavia			
Norway	0.77	—	Kolstad and Hognestad (1965)
Sweden	0.71	0.64	Ringertz (1970)
Australia			
Sydney	—	1.2	Coppelstone (1958)

[a] None of the studies listed classifies hydatidiform moles by completeness.

products of conception have the potential for developing into HM, it is also advisable to include induced abortions in the denominator with other pregnancy outcomes. However, many investigators have been unable to do so because the earlier illegal status of induced abortion precluded reliable data collection. Although it is uncertain how much variation is due to methodologic irregularities, marked differences in incidence among countries are widely accepted. The true incidence seems to be much higher in Asian countries and Central America than in the United States and Scandinavian countries. Hayashi et al. (1982) have recently provided national estimates of the incidence of HM per 1000 pregnancies for the years of 1970–1977 in the United States. The overall eight-year rate was 1.1 per 1000 pregnancies or one case of HM for every 923 pregnancies.

Most regional reports in the United States are from the East Coast, and their incidence rates are quite similar (Table 13-1). Hayashi et al. (1982) also studied regional differences in incidence in the United States. Within the nine census regions, rates were lowest in New England, Middle Atlantic, and East South Central, and highest in the Mountain and West South Central regions (Fig. 13-1).

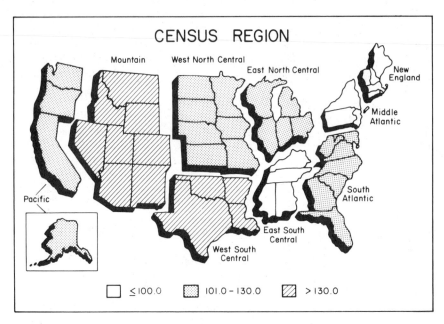

Fig. 13-1. Incidence of hydatidiform mole in the United States by census region adjusted by race per 100,000 pregnancies.
Source: Hayashi et al. (1982).

Incidence by Race

The differences in HM incidence among countries lead us to expect some discrepancy in incidence by race. In Hawaii, a polyracial community, the Japanese account for 54% of all trophoblastic disease compared with only 14% for Caucasians, although the populations of both groups are almost equal (McCorriston, 1968). Another report from Singapore, also a polyracial region, showed little difference in incidence among Malaysian, Chinese, and Indian races, but all had higher rates than whites (Teoh et al., 1971).

The incidence in the black population in the United States has rarely been studied. Yen and MacMahon (1968) suggested that blacks had a higher incidence than whites, but Westerhout et al. (1969) found the reverse. Hayashi et al. (1982) reported the rate in blacks to be about half that in whites. A study in Nigeria showed a relatively high incidence (Ogunbode, 1978), but a report from Uganda indicated an incidence for blacks in between that of whites and Orientals (Leighton, 1973).

Among Caucasians, Scandinavians seem to be relatively low in incidence and Latin groups much higher, although the literature is far from convincing on this point.

Parental Age Distribution and Parity

Most studies on incidence by maternal age confirm the same general pattern: a remarkably high rate of HM in women over 34 years old and another, somewhat less elevated, high rate in women under 20 years old as compared to women in the age group 20–34. In the national U.S. data (Hayashi et al., 1982), these age relationships were consistent in both whites and blacks (Fig. 13-2). In contrast, paternal age has rarely been studied but was not significant in one investigation (Yen and MacMahon, 1968), whereas the difference between maternal and paternal ages was not a factor in another (Sasaki et al., 1979).

Parity does not appear to be associated with occurrence of HM when maternal age is taken into account (Yen and MacMahon, 1968). However, many investigators have not made this type of adjustment, and further study of the independent effects of parity is needed.

Time Trends in Incidence

Acosta-Sison (1959) reported that the incidence of HM was 7.9 per 1000 deliveries in the Philippines during the years before 1945 when the Japanese military forces occupied the Islands, and gradually

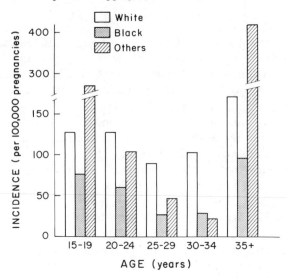

Fig. 13-2. Incidence of hydatidiform mole by maternal age and race. *Source*: Hayashi et al. (1982).

decreased thereafter. In the three-year period 1955–1957, the rate was 5.0 per 1000. This observation led Acosta-Sison to suggest that malnutrition contributed to the occurrence of HM. Yen and MacMahon's report (1968) from Rhode Island showed an increasing HM rate from 1930 to 1964, interrupted by a remarkable drop between 1940 and 1949. Matalon and Modan (1972) reported that the incidence of HM in Israel increased linearly from 1950 through 1965, a trend that was primarily due to a rise in incidence in the over-40 and teenage groups. At a New York City hospital, HM increased eight fold from 1957–1959 to 1966–1968 in young women, an observation prompting the suggestion that the disease might be transmitted by sexual contact (Slocumb and Lund, 1969). Hayashi et al. (1982) observed an increase in the United States from 1970 through 1975 followed by a slight drop in the 1976–1977 period. The increases were observed in all age groups except women 30–34.

It is unclear whether the increase observed in the incidence of HM is a true finding or an artifact due to changes in referral patterns or diagnostic criteria. There has been no significant change in the method of diagnosing HM in the United States during the last decade. However, the increasing availability of induced abortion may artificially increase the incidence of HM, because women with HM diagnosed at abortion may be referred to hospital for treatment whereas normal aborted pregnancies are less likely to enter national statistical records. If this is the case, the greater number of induced abortions in recent years may account for some of the increase observed in HM, especially in younger women.

HYPOTHESES ON THE ETIOLOGY OF HM

Geographic and time-related variation in the incidence of HM suggests that environmental factors play a role in the development of the disease. However, racial differences in incidence within a single community and the remarkable age distribution of HM imply that genetic factors are at play.

The major etiologic factors proposed for HM are discussed below.

Malnutrition and Low Socioeconomic Status

The hypothesis that malnutrition increases the risk for HM has been elaborated since the 1960s. The initial report came from the Philippines where Acosta-Sison (1959) observed a high incidence of trophoblastic disease among poor pregnant women, not infrequently complicated with pulmonary tuberculosis. Their staple food was rice, and their diet was deficient in proteins. Douglas (1959) did not find a high incidence in a New York City hospital, where the study population was drawn from the lowest socioeconomic groups in the city; however, the diet of these patients was much better than that in Asian countries during the same period. Race was not considered. Several studies refute the nutrition hypothesis. McCorriston (1968) reported that although the Japanese in Hawaii enjoy a high standard of living, they have higher incidence rates of HM than whites, albeit lower than those in Japan. In Alaska, native Alaskans have a high incidence of HM despite what was considered adequate protein intake (Martin 1978). MacGregor et al. (1969) could not find any different nutritional patterns in Mexico between HM patients and a control group. In the United States, the East South Central region had the lowest average per capita income in 1975 and also the lowest incidence of HM. Moreover, when all the states were ranked on incidence of HM and on per capita income, there was no meaningful association (Hayashi et al., 1982). At present, therefore, malnutrition and low socioeconomic status do not appear to be important risk factors for HM.

Infection

The possible involvement of a virus in the etiology of HM has been suggested in at least two reports (Marquez-Monter and Benitez-Gurrola, 1966; Arora, 1967) because of the abnormal morphology of the trophoblast cells, which resemble human kidney cells infected with SV40 virus. Some types of congenital anomalies, such as the rubella syndrome, are known to be induced by viruses (see Chapter 8), but in HM the evidence is too scarce to be conclusive.

Consanguinity

The trophoblastic tumor, like normal fetal parts, has been regarded as a form of natural homograft, because it carries paternal genetic traits that differ antigenically from those of the mother. Although a mother is usually capable of detecting an ordinary homograft from her child, the fetus and placenta are effectively shielded from the maternal immune system. Similarly, successful growth of HM is likely to be immunologically protected. From this perspective, it has been hypothesized that members of a relatively inbred community would tolerate a higher proportion of trophoblastic growth because of reduced differences in histocompatibility genes between both parents (Iliya et al., 1967).

Some efforts have been made to examine the incidence of trophoblastic disease in a community where endogamous marriage is prevalent. In the Near East, Iliya et al. (1967) reported a higher incidence of choriocarcinoma in rural and nomadic communities where consanguinity is common. Martin (1978) suspected that the isolation of native Alaskan villages might contribute to the relatively high incidence of HM in Eskimo women, and Miller and Barnhardt (1975) suggested that mixed marriage reduces the frequency of HM among Japanese women in Okinawa. In this latter study, Japanese couples had a three times higher incidence of HM than that of Japanese women married to American servicemen. Although it is unclear whether consanguinity could be directly related to the occurrence of HM, this possibility cannot be ruled out.

Blood Type as a Risk Factor

Parental blood type may be related to the risk of having choriocarcinoma. Bagshaw and Rawlines (1971) reported that group A women married to group O men had the highest risk, whereas group A women married to group A men had the lowest. Spontaneous regression of histologically malignant trophoblastic disease, after evacuation of HM, occurs most commonly in women mated to men of the same ABO phenotype.

Dawood and Teoh (1971) compared the ABO blood group distribution in patients with trophoblastic disease to that in the normal Singapore population. They found no significant shift in the ABO blood group distribution in HM patients but a higher incidence in group A and a lower incidence in group B among the patients with choriocarcinoma regardless of race.

In association with blood type studies, human leukocyte antigen (HLA) has also been examined, but most studies have been unsuccessful in relating HLA to the development of HM (Lewis and Terasaki, 1971; Rudolph and Thomas, 1971).

Blood type is rarely detected in human trophoblast, except type A, which can be found only in early gestation (Gross, 1966). Moreover, it is well known that normal cells lose their original antigenic character when they develop into malignant forms. Thus there is still considerable doubt as to whether blood type is a risk factor for HM.

Missed Abortion Theory

Hertig and Edmonds (1940) studied a number of cases of spontaneous termination of pregnancy and noted that hydatidiform degeneration (small swelling cyst of less than 2 mm diameter) was extremely common in pathologic ova in which the embryo was absent or showed evidence of having ceased to develop at a very early stage. From this observation they concluded that although most pathologic ova resulted in abortion by 10 to 12 gestational weeks, debris retained in the uterus might develop into classic moles typically found later in gestation. Takeuchi (1978) confirmed the pathologic findings and accepted the missed abortion theory, while at the same time introducing an immunological concept to explain how potential HM is retained in the uterus. In view of recent findings that almost all hydatidiform moles are genetically female (see below), he suggested that the female trophoblast is antigenically much more likely to be compatible with, rather than rejected by, the maternal host. Most recent genetic studies, which indicate that HM originates at fertilization, seem to conflict with the missed abortion theory (Holland and Hreshchyshyn, 1967; Kaji and Ohama, 1977; Jacobs et al., 1978; Wake et al., 1978; Lawler et al., 1979).

Genetic Etiology

Recent genetic studies have produced a major advance in our understanding of the etiology of HM. In 1977, Vassilakos et al. published evidence that HM consists of two distinct entities—"complete" and "partial"—that can be distinguished by morphologic and cytogenetic criteria.

Complete HM never contains an embryo, umbilical cord, or amniotic membranes and has abnormal chorionic villi. Its chromosomes are typically 46XX, or sex chromatin positive if karyotyping cannot be performed. *Partial HM* contains embryo, umbilical cord, amniotic membranes, and normal chorionic villi. Chromosomes in the partial mole usually include triploidies, although trisomies and tetraploidies are also found.

In the same year Kaji and Ohama (1977), who had studied the inheritance of molar chromosomes, reported that complete moles were androgenetic in origin, receiving all their chromosomes (including both X chromosomes) from the father. The ovum that develops into a complete mole, therefore, is under the influence of a spermatozoan nucleus. These studies have been confirmed in Hawaii (Jacobs et al., 1978), Japan (Wake et al., 1978), and England (Lawler et al., 1979).

INTERPRETATION OF RECENT GENETIC FINDINGS

Because the complete mole always has an androgenetic, 46XX karyotype, three methods of fertilization are possible. First, fertilizaton may be caused by two sperms (dispermy). This seems a highly improbable mechanism, however, because many heterozygous paternal chromosomes would need to become homozygous in the mole. Second, fertilization may be by a diploid sperm resulting from failure of the second meiotic division of spermatogenesis. Because several genetic foci known to be heterozygous in the father were all found to be homozygous in the mole, this is also an unlikely process (Lawler et al., 1979). The third and at present most likely possibility, is fertilization by a normal haploid sperm whose nuclear material parthenogenetically divides in the ovum. From this process one would expect as many YY as XX zygoids to be formed, the YY cells being more likely to be lost during early cleavage.

By contrast, genetic studies of partial moles indicate that there is a maternal contribution to the karyotype. Thus, dispermy or failure of the first paternal meiotic division may play an etiologic role (Vassilakos et al., 1977). Problems in late meiosis of the ova's nucleus may also lead to the development of partial HM, particularly trisomies. The majority of partial moles are triploid, however, and appear to be of dispermic origin (Szulman et al., 1981; Lawler et al., 1982).

FUTURE GENETIC EPIDEMIOLOGIC STUDIES

The new genetic studies of HM indicate that a revision of our understanding of the epidemiology of HM is called for. If HM does actually represent two discrete disease entities, then the risk factors for each need to be elucidated. This is extremely important, because complete moles frequently show marked hyperplasia and anaplasia of the trophoblast with a high risk of trophoblastic neoplasia, choriocarcinoma, and metastases. The partial mole, however, is probably not associated with chorioadenoma destruens or choriocarcinoma (Vassilakos et al., 1977).

Future epidemiologic investigation must include detailed genetic analysis to classify each type of mole under study. Additionally, genetic studies of both parents are necessary. Examination of other possible risk factors such as occupation or environmental exposures for both parents will probably also be revealing. Epidemiologic studies of the occurrence and distribution of diploid spermatozoa and defective ova might also provide useful insights into the etiology of HM.

There is only one epidemiologic study in the literature that classifies moles, by chromosome analysis and histopathology, as being complete or partial (Jacobs et al., 1982). Forty complete and 88 partial moles were studied in Hawaii. Increased incidence of HM in women under 20 was found only for complete moles when compared to a control group of spontaneous abortions. Filipino women had an excess of complete but not partial moles, whereas Japanese and other Orientals in Hawaii did not have elevated rates of either type of mole. Because the majority of Filipinos, unlike the Japanese, were born in their home country, the genetic versus environmental effects could not be isolated in the study. From data provided in the article, we calculated the incidence of complete mole in Hawaii to be 1.44 per 1000 livebirths as compared to 3.17 for partial moles.

Complete moles may be influenced by risk factors similar to incomplete moles, at least in part. Development of ova with absent or inactive nuclei may be associated with maternal age and ethnicity. Production of diploid sperm, however, is an entirely paternal condition subject to both genetic and environmental influences.

Although only one epidemiologic study begins to address these issues, the extant literature has identified risk factors reviewed in this chapter that should be reexamined in future studies. None of the genetic findings precludes a role for environmental influences in the etiology of HM. As documented in other chapters of this volume, genetic mutation, chromosome translocations, and other natural reproductive anomalies are all known to be increased by viral, chemical, and other environmental factors.

REFERENCES

Acosta-Sison, H. (1959). Observation which may indicate the etiology of hydatidiform mole and explain its high incidence in the Philippines and Asiatic countries. *Philippines J. Surg. 14*, 209–297.

Agüero, O., Kizer, S., and Pinedo, G. (1973). Hydatidiform mole in Conception Palacios Maternity Hospital. *Am. J. Obstet. Gynecol. 116*, 1117–1120.

Arora, B. (1967). Infective hepatitis and pregnancy in Bristol. *J. Obstet. Gynaecol. Br. Commonw. 74*, 763–765.

Bagshaw, K.D. and Rawlines, G. (1971). ABO blood groups in trophoblastic neoplasia. *Lancet 1*, 553–556.

Becker, R.L. and Avioli, L.V. (1977). Gestational trophoblastic disease. *Arch. Intern. Med. 137*, 221–225.

Chesley, L.C., Cosgrove, S.A., and Preece, J. (1946). Hydatidiform mole, with special reference to recurrence and associated eclampsia. *Am. J. Obstet. Gynecol. 52*, 331–320.

Chun, D., Braga, C., Chow, C., and Lok, L. (1964) Clinical observations on some aspects of hydatidiform moles. *J. Obstet. Gynaecol. Br. Commonw. 71*, 180–184.

Coppelstone, M. (1958). Hydatidiform mole and its complications. *J. Obstet. Gynaecol. Br. Emp. 65*, 238–252.

Dawood, M.Y. and Teoh, E.S. (1971). ABO blood group in trophoblastic disease. *J. Obstet. Gynaecol. Br. Commonw. 78*, 918–923.

Douglas, G.W. (1957). The diagnosis and management of hydatidiform mole. *Surg. Clin. North Am. 37*, 379–392.

——— (1959). The joint project for study of choriocarcinoma and hydatidiform mole in Asia: Geographic variation in the occurrence of hydatidiform mole and choriocarcinoma, *Ann. N.Y. Acad. Sci. 80*, 195.

Goldstein, D.P., Berkowitz, R.S., and Cohen, S.M. (1979). *The current management of molar pregnancy: Current problems in obstetrics and gynecology*, Vol. 3 (No. 4). Chicago, London: Year Book Medical Publishers.

Gross, S.J. (1966). Human blood group A substance in human endometrium and trophoblast localized by chromatographed rabbit antiserum. *Am. J. Obstet. Gynecol. 95*, 1149–1159.

Hammond, C.B., Borchert, L.G., Tyrey, L., Creasman, W.T, and Parker, R.T. (1973). Treatment of metastatic trophoblastic disease—good and poor prognosis. *Am. J. Obstet. Gynecol. 115*, 451–457.

Hasegawa, T., Kawai, N., and Shintani, S. (1960). Hydatidiform mole and chorioepithelioma as they are in Japan. *Jpn. J. Obstet. Gynecol. 12*, 1875–1887.

Hayashi, K., Bracken, M.B., Freeman, D.H., and Hellenbrand, K. (1982). Hydatidiform mole in the United States (1970–1977): A statistical and theoretical analysis. *Am. J. Epidemiol. 115*, 67–77.

Hertig, A.T. and Edmonds, H.W. (1940). Genesis of hydatidiform mole. *Arch. Pathol. 30*, 260–291.

Hertz, R. (1967). *Choriocarcinoma*, UICC monograph series 3. Berlin: Springer Verlag, pp. 66–71.

Holland, J.F. and Hreshchyshyn, M.M. (1967). Choriocarcinoma. Transactions of a Conference of the International Union against cancer. Berlin-Heidelberg-New York: Springer Verlag.

Iliya, F.A., Williamson, S., and Azar, H.A. (1967). Choriocarcinoma in the

Near East. Consanguinity as a possible etiologic factor. *Cancer 20*, 144–149.

Jacobs, P.A., Hassold, T.J., and Newlands, I.M. (1978). Chromosome constitution of gestational trophoblastic disease. *Lancet 2*, 49.

———, Hunt, P.A., Matsuura, J.S., and Wilson, C.C. (1982). Complete and partial hydatidiform mole in Hawaii: Cytogenetics, morphology and epidemiology. *Br. J. Obstet. Gynecol. 89*, 258–266.

Javey, H. and Sajadi, H. (1978). Hydatidiform mole in southern Iran: A statistical survey of 113 cases. *Int. J. Gynaecol. Obstet. 15*, 390–395.

Kaji, T. and Ohama, K. (1977). Androgenetic origin of hydatidiform mole. *Nature 268*, 633–634.

Kolstad, P. and Hognestad, J. (1965). Trophoblastic tumors in Norway. *Acta Obstet. Gynecol. Scand. 44*, 80–88.

Lawler, S.D., Fisher, R.A., Pickthall, V.J., Povey, S., and Evans, M.W. (1982). Genetic studies on hydatidiform moles. 1. The origin of partial moles. *Cancer Genet. Cytogenet. 5*, 309–320.

———, Pickthall, V.J., Fisher, R.A., Povey, S., Evans, M.W., and Szuiman A.E. (1979). Genetic studies of complete and partial hydatidiform mole. *Lancet 2*, 580.

Leighton, P.C. (1973). Trophoblastic disease in Uganda. *Am. J. Obstet. Gynecol. 117*, 341–344.

Lewis, J.L. and Terasaki, P.L. (1971). HL-A leukocyte antigen studies in women with gestational trophoblastic neoplasms. *Am. J. Obstet. Gynecol. 111*, 547–554.

MacGregor, C., Ontiveros, E.C., Vargas, E.L., and Valenzuela, L.S. (1969). Hydatidiform mole. Analysis of 145 patients. *Obstet. Gynecol. 33*, 343–351.

Marquez-Monter, H. and Benitez-Gurrola, S. (1966). Abnormal trophoblast in tissue culture. *Am. J. Obstet. Gynecol. 94*, 939–941.

———, Vega, G.A., Ridaura, C., and Robeles, M. (1968). Gestational choriocarcinoma in the general hospital of Mexico. *Cancer 22*, 91–98.

Martin, P.M. (1978). High frequency of hydatidiform mole in native Alaskans. *Int. J. Gynaecol. Obstet. 15*, 395–396.

Matalon, M. and Modan, B. (1972). Epidemiologic aspects of hydatidiform mole in Israel. *Am. J. Obstet. Gynecol. 122*, 107–112.

———, Paz, B., Modan, M., and Modan, B. (1972). Malignant trophoblastic disorders. *Am. J. Obstet. Gynecol. 112*, 101–106.

McCorriston, C.C. (1968). Racial incidence of hydatidiform mole. *Am. J. Obstet. Gynecol. 101*, 377–382.

Miller, F.L. and Barnhardt, R.J. (1975). Mixed marriage may offer Asian women protection against hydatidiform mole. *Ob Gyn News 10*, 16.

Muellar, C.W. and Lapp, W.A. (1969). Hydatidiform mole followed by postpartum eclampsia and chorioepithelioma, with recovery. *Am. J. Obstet. Gynecol. 58*, 133–138.

Ogunbode, O. (1978). Benign hydatidiform mole in Ibadan, Nigeria. *Int. J. Gynaecol. Obstet. 15*, 387–396.

Ong, H.C., Lee, P.Y.A., Ng, T.K.F, and Chong, C.H. (1978). Clinical observations of hydatidiform moles in a Malaysian hospital. *Singapore Med. J. 19*, 33–36.

Park, W.W. (1959). In discussion on H.W. Edmonds: Genesis of hydatidiform mole, old and new concepts. *Ann. N.Y. Acad. Sci. 80*, 99–104.

Reiner, I. and Dougherty, C.M. (1960). Clinical and pathologic aspects of hydatidiform mole. *Obstet. Gynecol. 15*, 735–739.

Ringertz, N. (1970). Hydatidiform mole, invasive mole, and choriocarcinoma in Sweden 1958–1965. *Acta Obstet. Gynecol. Scand. 49*, 195–203.

Rolon, P.A. and Lopez, B.H. (1977). Epidemiological aspects of hydatidiform mole in the Republic of Paraguay (South America). *Br. J. Obstet. Gynaecol. 84*, 862–864.

Rudolph, R.H. and Thomas, E.D. (1971). HL-A antigens and choriocarcinoma. *Lancet 2*, 408–409.

Sasaki, K., Yamoto, M., Hata, H., and Nakano, R. (1979). The relationship between maternal aging and the incidence of hydatidiform mole and malignant changes. *Acta Obstet. Gynaecol. Jpn. 31*, 292–296.

Slocumb, J.C. and Lund, C.J. (1969). Incidence of trophoblastic disease: Increased rate in youngest age group. *Am. J. Obstet. Gynecol. 104*, 421–423.

Stroup, P.E. (1956). A study of thirty-eight cases of hydatidiform mole at the Pennsylvania Hospital. *Am. J. Obstet. Gynecol. 72*, 294–303.

Szulman, A.E., Philippe, E., Boué, J.G., and Boué, A. (1981). Human triploidy: Association with partial hydatidiform moles and non-molar conceptuses. *Hum. Pathol. 12*, 1016–1021.

Takeuchi, S. (1978). *Hojokitai No Subete*, Series 20. Nankodo: Tokyo, pp. 98–106.

Teoh, E.S., Dawood, M.Y., and Ratnum, S.S. (1971). Epidemiology of hydatidiform mole in Singapore. *Am. J. Obstet. Gynecol. 110*, 415–420.

Vassilakos, P., Riotton, G., and Kaji, T. (1977). Hydatidiform mole: Two entities. *Am. J. Obstet. Gynecol. 127*, 167–170.

Wake, N., Takagi, N., and Sasaki, M. (1978). Androgenesis as a cause of hydatidiform mole. *J. Natl. Cancer Inst. 60*, 51–53.

Wei, P. and Ouyang, P. (1963). Trophoblastic disease in Taiwan. *Am. J. Obstet. Gynecol. 85*, 844–849.

Westerhout, F.C., Morel, E., and Slate, W. (1969). Observation on 138 molar pregnancies. *Am. J. Obstet. Gynecol. 103*, 56–59.

Yen, S. and MacMahon, B. (1968). Epidemiologic features of trophoblastic disease. *Am. J. Obstet. Gynecol. 101*, 126–132.

14

Sudden Infant Death Syndrome

Donald R. Peterson

Sudden infant death syndrome (SIDS) refers to the sudden death of an infant that is unexpected in relation to its medical history and for which no specific lethal lesion can be identified at autopsy (Peterson, 1980). The rationale for including a chapter on SIDS in a book on perinatal epidemiology rests on the premise that although SIDS occurs almost without exception during the postperinatal period, it shares many epidemiologic attributes with the major causes of death during the perinatal period. Previous reviews have been written from an epidemiologic (Peterson, 1980) and more clinical perspective (Kendeel and Ferris, 1977; Read et al., 1979; Valdes-Dapena, 1980).

Sudden infant death syndrome is synonymous with cot death, crib death, and sudden unexplained infant death. Few, if any, SIDS episodes occur during the first week of life; the frequency peaks during the second and third months, and then it subsides gradually so that 80–90% of the total occur by the age of six months. In 1974 Raring analyzed age distribution patterns from seven published studies in widely separated geographic locations in the United States and elsewhere during the 1960s or before; he concluded that the similarity in patterns was consistent with the hypothesis that SIDS is a "single disease entity" (Raring, 1974).

Figure 14-1 depicts the SIDS age distribution patterns from six subsequent studies conducted in the 1970s in King County, Washington (Peterson et al., 1979), Cook County, Illinois (data provided by Julius Goldberg, Ph.D., Dr.P.H.), upper New York State (Standfast et al., 1979), Auckland, New Zealand (Tonkin, 1974), South Australia (Beal, 1972), and Norway (data provided by Lorentz M. Irgens, M.D.). The composite SIDS pattern closely resembles the one described by Raring. Both closely approximate a log-normal distribution

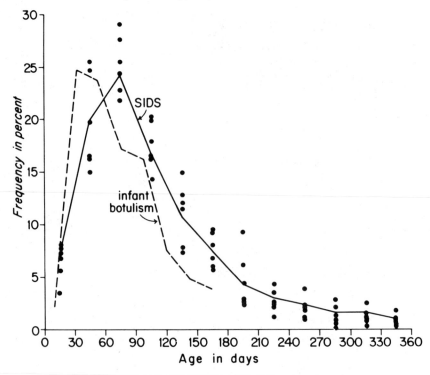

Fig. 14-1. SIDS age distribution compared with infant botulism (see text).

pattern. Using log-normality of the age distribution frequency as a single source criterion, as originally suggested by Sartwell, Armenian and Khoury (1981) concluded that SIDS did not fit their model. The validity of this analytic methodology remains conjectural.

For comparison, Fig. 14-1 also includes the age-at-onset distribution of 186 cases of infant botulism reported worldwide since it was first recognized in 1976 (Arnon et al., 1978). *Clostridium botulinum* organisms and/or toxin have been recorded from approximately 5% of SIDS stool specimens that have been examined. The relationship of the infant botulism age-at-onset distribution to the age-at-death distribution of SIDS shown in Fig. 14-1 is virtually identical to an earlier analysis of approximately half as many infant botulism cases (Arnon et al., 1981).

Although age at onset of respiratory syncytial virus bronchiolitis corresponds closely to the SIDS age distribution, virologic and immunologic studies reveal no consistent associations (Ray and Hebestreit, 1971; Urquhart and Grist, 1972; Ferris et al., 1973; Downham et al., 1975; Cunningham, 1979; Pavri, 1979); furthermore, respiratory syncytial virus bronchiolitis occurs epidemically in contrast to SIDS, which occurs endemically.

From historical records, Read concluded that the age at onset of infantile beriberi (thiamine deficiency) corresponded to the SIDS age distribution (Read, 1978). However, subsequent study failed to implicate thiamine deficiency in the etiology of SIDS (Peterson et al., 1981).

The consistency and uniqueness of the SIDS age distribution pattern strongly favor the contention that most SIDS episodes probably stem from a single etiologic circumstance. Indeed, virtually all epidemiologists who have studied SIDS have either explicitly or implicitly embraced this concept as a working hypothesis. The possibility remains, however, that SIDS episodes are causally heterogeneous.

HISTORICAL NOTE

The following letter, written almost 150 years ago (Fearn, 1834), describes the gross postmortem findings in two instances of sudden infant death in a manner that would credit a contemporary pathologist with respect to both careful observation and insight into probable pathophysiology. Its reproduction here in its entirety not only displays an interesting antique that might otherwise remain hidden from the scientific community, but also clearly documents the occurrence of SIDS in the distant past.

To the Editor of the *Lancet*

Sir,—I have lately been called upon to examine two children, who, without having been previously indisposed, were found dead in bed.

In the first case the child was about six months old and was lying in bed with its mother, who discovered in the middle of the night that it was dead. An inquest was held upon the body, and I was directed, in the absence of anything like testimony as to the cause of its dissolution, to make a postmortem investigation. I should mention that the mother stated positively that the child had not lain near her, and that it was impossible it could have been suffocated, either from its mouth having been applied to any part of her person or to the bed linen.

I found nothing unusual in the cavity of the skull,—no engorgement of the vessels,—no sanguineous or serous effusion. The viscera of the belly were in every respect of healthy appearance, and there was nothing in the stomach to indicate that it had come by its death unfairly. In the chest, however, I found, upon the surface of the thymus gland, numerous spots of extravasated blood, similar spots upon the surface of the lower and back parts of each lung, and many patches of ecchymosis upon the margin of the right ventricle of the heart, and along the course of the trunk of the coronary vein. There was no engorgement, however, of the pulmonary vessels, of the coronaries, or of the vessels of the thymus.

In the second case the child was five months old. It had been pretty well, had been suckled by its mother, and laid in bed upon its side, and in about an hour and a half afterwards was discovered to be dead. There was some frothy matter in and about the mouth, and its hands were firmly clenched. From the position in which it was found it was impossible it could have been smothered.

The appearance exhibited in the autopsy was strikingly the same as in the first case. The contents of the skull and belly were in a perfectly natural condition. The extravasated spots upon the thymus gland were more numerous than in the first case, and those upon the heart and the surface of the lungs were fewer in number. There was about half an ounce of serous fluid in the pericardium.

In these cases one naturally asks,—what was the cause of death? The similarity of the postmortem appearance would lead one to suppose that the cause must in each case have been the same. In the first case I was strongly disposed to think, in spite of the evidence of the mother, that the child must have been destroyed by overlaying it; but after the occurrence of the last case, where, from all the testimony that could be obtained, it seemed impossible that the child could have been suffocated, as it was lying in bed by itself, and was not obstructed in its breathing by the bedclothes, I confess that the opinion I had formed was a good deal shaken, and that I became almost entirely at a loss how to account for death in either. In both cases there seems to have been, from some cause or other, a sudden and violent action of the heart,—and numerous small vessels, from the increased force of its contraction, appear as a consequence to have given way. But so trifling a lesion could hardly, in either instance, be supposed to be of itself sufficient to produce death, and it is with the hope that some of your correspondents who may have seen similar cases, and who may be better able to offer an explanation of the phenomena they present than I am, will take the trouble of enlightening me upon the subject that I am induced to forward you this communication.

At all events the cases may, I think, be considered of some interest, as well in a pathological as a legal point of view. I have the honor to be, Sir, your obliged servant, Saml. W. Fearn, Derby, October 19, 1834.

GEOGRAPHIC DISTRIBUTION

A recent review of SIDS epidemiology includes SIDS incidence data from habitable areas throughout the world ranging from Pt. Barrow, Alaska, to Tasmania, Australia (Peterson, 1980). Despite variability in ascertainment and diagnosis inherent in such data, rates ranged narrowly from 0.6 to 3.0 per 1000 livebirths with northern European countries tending to congregate near the lower end of the distribution.

Significant urban–rural rate differences have not been found (Blok, 1978); within communities, economically depressed neighborhoods tend to exhibit higher SIDS incidence, however. Population density per se apparently does not influence risk appreciably.

CHRONOLOGIC ATTRIBUTES

By and large the scientific community paid little attention to SIDS until, as infant mortality rates declined, it became apparent that SIDS accounted for 40 to 60% of postperinatal mortality (Peterson, 1980). Secular trends of SIDS incidence disclose no evidence of epidemicity, nor have substantial SIDS outbreaks occurred. More SIDS episodes occur during colder than warmer months of the year in both the northern and southern hemispheres. Attempts to explain SIDS seasonality on the basis of exposure to infectious agents have thus far failed.

ECOLOGIC SUMMARY

For the most part, SIDS appears to be a discrete pathophysiologic entity, occurring endemically with seasonal peaks, with roots deeply imbedded in time and broadly dispersed geographically. These features support the inference that the underlying cause or causes of SIDS intrinsically attend the process of human reproduction. Consideration of other epidemiologic attributes of SIDS rests on these fundamental precepts.

Heritability

Evidence from studies of concordance among monozygotic and dizogotic twins and full first cousins of SIDS probands contradicts genetic predisposition along classical Mendelian lines (Peterson et al., 1980). Polygenic inheritance remains a possibility. A preliminary study of HLA phenotypes of 66 parents of 33 SIDS victims disclosed a significant difference when compared with 375 blood donors and unrelated volunteers tested for heterogeneity over all A loci (Tait et al., 1977).

Sudden infant death rates for males consistently exceed those for females by about one and one-half times. Under the Lyon–Barr hypothesis, all autosomal cells in males contain only X chromosomes contributed by the mother, whereas autosomal cells of females exhibit mosaicism—a mixture of cells with X chromosomes of either maternal or paternal derivation. Because of this cellular dimorphism, females may by inherently more resistant to a lethal outcome from a pathophysiologic insult.

Multiple Births

Rates of SIDS for multiple births exceed those for singleton births. Two recent reports indicate that the second twin born of a twin pair is in greater jeopardy of SIDS than the first twin born (Standfast et al., 1980; Getts, 1981).

Repetitions in Families

Repetitions of SIDS within families occur at a rate of about 2% of subsequently born siblings or approximately ten times the empirical risk (Peterson et al., 1980).

Fortunately, SIDS repetitions are rare events in a community. Assuming a repetition rate of 0.02, an overall annual incidence rate of 0.002, and an average family size of two children (an intentionally conservative overestimate), the expected SIDS repetition rate in a population of neonates would be on the order of 2 per 100,000 livebirths ($0.02 \times 0.002 \times 10^5/2$). Thus, repetitions would be encountered seldom, if at all, in most epidemiological studies of SIDS. Available evidence discloses no excess risk among blood relatives of these families. Curiously, siblings of the mothers who experience SIDS repetition, differ significantly from siblings of their spouses as well as from siblings of mothers and fathers without repetitions, in that a significantly higher proportion are not fully related (i.e., half, step, or adopted brothers or sisters). This observation may indicate that mothers who experience SIDS more than once were reared under circumstances that predisposed them to SIDS in later years perhaps on an intergenerational but nongenetic basis.

Maternal Age and Parity

Figure 14-2 illustrates that SIDS rates increase as parity increases and decrease with advancing maternal age. The strength of association with parity diminishes among the older mothers. Figure 14-3, which compares this association for SIDS with other categorical causes of death in infancy after maternal age adjustment, reveals a similar pattern only for respiratory distress syndrome.

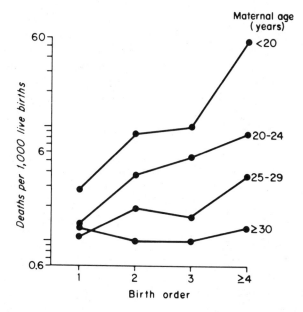

Fig. 14-2. Distribution of SIDS rates per 1000 livebirths by maternal age and birth order, King County, Washington, 1968–1977.

Fig. 14-3. Birth order distribution of SIDS compared with other major components of infant mortality. Rates adjusted for maternal age. King County, Washington, 1968–1977. *Rate irrespective of birth order.

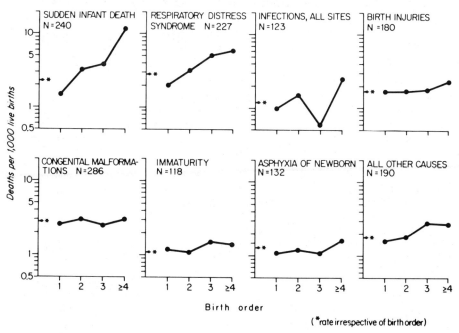

(*rate irrespective of birth order)

Maternal age under 20 at first livebirth or pregnancy has been reported to be the common underlying risk factor for the high rate of SIDS in young mothers as well as older mothers of high parity (Standfast et al., 1980). These authors caution that, with respect to SIDS, any biological or sociological explanation for the association of infant death with early age at first childbirth must be compatible with the relative sparing of the firstborn infant.

Fetal Growth

An inverse association between birthweight and risk of SIDS, which persists after adjustment for maternal age, has been repeatedly documented by epidemiologic studies. Table 14-1 depicts the SIDS birthweight distribution compared with other major mortality components that occur, wholly or in part, during the first week of life. The skewness toward the left of the distribution patterns of all but SIDS strongly suggests that prematurity may be the primary factor responsible. The SIDS pattern, in contrast, appears compatible with intrauterine growth retardation. At birth, infants who later succumb to SIDS have been found to be, on the average, both shorter and lighter than peers who survive infancy (Peterson, 1981). The only SIDS study in which birthweights were adjusted for gestational age supports the view that the inverse association between birthweight and risk of SIDS results from intrauterine growth retardation rather than prematurity per se.

Table 14-1. Major Components of Infant Mortality with Birthweight Distribution (%), King County, Washington, 1969–1977

Infant mortality component	Birthweight class (g)			
	<1500	1500–2000	2001–2500	>2500
Hyaline membrane disease	41.3	28.0	14.7	16.0
Respiratory distress syndrome	65.3	17.3	10.2	7.1
Asphyxia of the newborn	63.2	9.8	5.2	21.8
Immaturity	92.8	3.6	1.4	2.2
Birth injuries	63.6	8.3	6.6	21.5
Congenital malformation	7.4 (5.1)[a]	10.9 (6.2)	13.7 (12.4)	68.0 (76.3)
Infection	22.0 (17.7)	10.6 (8.3)	9.9 (8.8)	57.4 (65.6)
Sudden infant death syndrome	4.4	5.0	15.6	75.1
All other	1.8 (11.0)	11.8 (7.6)	11.3 (11.9)	49.3 (69.5)
All components	0.9	1.6	5.1	92.4

[a] Percentages given in parentheses are restricted to deaths at age ≥7 days.

Postnatal Growth

Anthropomorphic evidence indicates that the growth retardation associated with SIDS that begins *in utero* continues postnatally (Froggatt et al., 1971; Peterson et al., 1973; Naeye et al., 1976b). Cellular hypoplasia at the costrochondral junction in SIDS victims also supports this inference (Sinclair-Smith et al., 1976). Table 14-2 provides a descriptive summary of SIDS growth retardation. These observations belie the long-held notion that SIDS affects perfectly healthy infants.

Behavioral Attributes of the Mother

Cigarette smoking during pregnancy and afterwards has been found to be more common among SIDS mothers than among controls (Steele and Langworth, 1966; Schrauzer et al., 1975; Bergman and Wiesner, 1976; Naeye et al., 1976b), with estimated relative risks of about 2.4. The analogy between the summary description in Table 14-2 and the fetal and postnatal growth retardation that has been known for some time to be associated with maternal smoking may be indicative of some causal relationship either primarily or secondarily; the test of this hypothesis awaits further investigation (Peterson, 1981).

Studies repeatedly reveal that SIDS occurs proportionately more often among mothers who received little or no health supervision during the course of their pregnancies.

Drug-dependent mothers (methadone) also experience inordinately high SIDS risk (Chavez et al., 1979).

Recent reports indicate that subsequent siblings of "abused" probands may be at excess risk of SIDS (Creighton, 1980; Roberts et al., 1980).

Table 14-2. SIDS Growth Pattern Descriptive Summary: Interpretations Based on Mean Values Compared with Live Controls, King County, Washington, 1968–1971

Growth Parameter	Birth	Postnatal life
Weight	Light	Light
Length	Short	Short
Weight:Length	Light for length	Light for length
Ponderal index	Adequately fat	Lean
Weight gain velocity	—	Slow, no catch-up
Length gain velocity	—	Slow, no catch-up

Sociodemographic Attributes of the Mother

The occurrence of SIDS is proportionately more frequent among mothers who are poor, unmarried, relatively uneducated, and of non-Caucasian ethnicity—in the United States especially blacks and native Americans. Incidence of SIDS tends to parallel fertility rate trends. The inverse risk gradient of SIDS associated with advancing maternal age, as previously described, does not result from the mix of maternal age cohorts from cross-sectional analyses of data but accurately reflects an age-dependent relationship.

Reproductive Experience of the Mother

Reproductive histories disclose fewer prior fetal or liveborn deaths among SIDS mothers than among mothers whose infants died from other causes (after adjusting for gravidity). This curious finding thus far defies explanation.

Infertility or spontaneous abortion during the year following SIDS exceeds the expected rate (Mandell and Wolfe, 1975). A shortened interpregnancy interval typically occurs among SIDS mothers who succeed in becoming pregnant.

Disproportionately more SIDS mothers experience abnormal uterine bleeding, abruptio placentae, and placenta previa than mothers of infants who died from other causes (Standfast et al., 1980). However, comparison of SIDS victims with live controls matched for age, sex, race, and maternal gravidity did not corroborate these associations (Arsenault, 1980). Such disparate results illuminate the difficulty inherent in selection of an appropriate comparison group for SIDS victims. Perhaps the most appropriate would be age-matched infants who died suddenly from obvious accidental violence, but these occur too infrequently to provide an adequate number. Investigators have therefore chosen dead or live controls more or less as fancy, fortune, and feasibility dictate. This methodologic issue complicates attempts to assess the significance of many associations that have been addressed by various investigators.

INFANT SUSCEPTIBILITY TO SIDS

The distinctive age distribution pattern described at the beginning of this chapter dramatically defines the period of vulnerability to SIDS and has spawned hypotheses and investigations addressed at virtually every facet of anatomy, physiology, and environment imaginable. These endeavors have not only been complicated but often compromised by the lack of opportunity for antemortem observation and measurement. Nevertheless, considerable useful information has accrued from postmortem studies supplemented by studies in animals, infants surviving a "near-miss" SIDS episode, and siblings of SIDS probands. The mechanism of death remains a mystery despite intensive effort; the common presence of intrathoracic petechiae, as accurately described as "spots of extravasated blood" by Samuel Fearn almost 150 years ago, has not yet been entirely explained. The SIDS victim has understandably been the primary target of investigations seeking to implicate, for example: infection, immunodeficiency, nutritional deficiency, endocrine aberration, and anatomic anomalies but to no avail. Because no definitive anatomic or histologic marker of SIDS exists, even the diagnosis of SIDS rests on exclusion of other recognizable causes of death—a process that depends on the training, experience, and judgment of the examiner. This situation lends an aura of uncertainty to all SIDS research.

Dr. Fearn's early SIDS description implies a silent demise during sleep—an observation confirmed by later accounts that in turn spurred interest in sleep physiology as related to SIDS susceptibility. A recent report concludes that age distribution pattern of SIDS may reflect a developmentally increased susceptibility to hypoxia secondary to hypoventilation (but not necessarily apnea) during periods of quiet sleep (McGinty and Sterman, 1980; Harper et al., 1981).

Evidence of Antemortem Hypoxia in SIDS Victims

A substantial proportion of SIDS cases (approximately 60%) exhibit tissue changes indicative of chronic hypoxia prior to death such as hypertrophy and hyperplasia of pulmonary arterioles, extramedullary hematopoesis, periadrenal brown fat retention, right ventricular hypertrophy, depletion of the adrenal medulla, fat-laden macrophages in the cerebrospinal fluid, and in periventricular areas of the brain, leukomalacia of the periventricular and subcortical white matter of the brain, and morphologic distortions of the carotid body (Naeye, 1973, 1974, 1976; Gadson and Emery, 1976; Naeye et al., 1976a; Valdes-Dapena et al., 1976; Takashima et al., 1978a,b; Cole et al., 1979; Williams et al., 1979).

The Brain Stem in SIDS Victims

In 1976 Naeye identified astroglial cell proliferation in the brain stem of many SIDS victims. Subsequently Takashima et al. (1978a,b) found that astroglial cell proliferation occurred most prominently in the region of the nucleus ambiguous near centers for breathing and heart rate control. More recently, studies of enzymes involved in norepinephrine and epinephrine synthesis in the brain stem indicate hypoactivity of adrenergic neurons in respiratory and cardiac centers (Denoroy et al., 1980). Persistence of reticular dendritic spines in the brain stem of SIDS victims but not that of controls has been interpreted as indicative of a specific lag in the normal maturation of the respiratory control centers (Quattrochi et al., 1978). A recent study reveals a striking reduction in the number of small myelinated fibers in the vagus nerve of SIDS victims, which the authors ascribe to abnormal or delayed development (Sachis et al., 1981).

PATHOGENESIS OF SIDS

Alterations in brain stem structure and function may be either the cause or effect of hypoxia—or, for that matter, a self-perpetuating combination of cause and effect by the development of a positive feedback cycle. Damage to vital centers in the medulla originating during pregnancy that insidiously compounds itself until acute decompensation occurs, would seem to provide a logical explanation of the course of pathogenesis. The SIDS age distribution pattern, which is approximately log-normal, may reflect random distribution in times of acute decompensation, influence of the sleep cycle maturation process, or both in combination. Growth retardation and many of the epidemiologic and clinical descriptors of SIDS accord with this hypothesis. In line with this reasoning, sudden infant deaths might be more aptly termed "subtle" infant deaths.

PREVENTION OF SIDS

Because in this model, the course of pathogenesis, once established, usually proceeds inexorably toward death, successful intervention would depend on identification of factors that initiate the process, perhaps very early in pregnancy. The occurrence of unrecognized maternal infection or nutritional inadequacy during organogenesis has not been explored but perhaps should be despite the obvious difficulties that such efforts would entail. Congenital rubella syndrome and the recently discovered association of subclinical nutritional deficiency in mothers of infants born with neural tube defects serve as precedents for this point of view (Korobkin and Guilleminault, 1978; Laurence et al., 1980).

SOCIETY AND SIDS

Samuel Fearn's nineteenth-century description of SIDS remains valid to this day. Another nineteenth-century figure, the prominent Irish poet and playwright, W.B. Yeats, was similarly prophetic in describing society's reaction to SIDS. In his "Ballad of Moll Magee," an SIDS mother laments her fate and describes her estrangement from her husband and friends (Yeats, 1940). To this day social consequences of SIDS include suspicion on the part of law enforcement personnel, marital disruption, change of residence, and uncertainty with regard to future pregnancies.

CONCLUSION

Sudden infant death syndrome, a medical enigma and a social problem for decades, has been addressed by epidemiologists for only about 20 years. Despite difficulties in applying the epidemiologic approach to this phenomenon, much has been learned of a descriptive nature. The time may now be propitious for analytic studies directed at events or circumstances attending early gestation for clues to the etiology of SIDS.

REFERENCES

Armenian, H.K. and Khoury, M.J. (1981). Age at onset of genetic diseases: An application for Sartwell's model of the distribution of incubation periods. *Am. J. Epidemiol. 113*, 596–605.

Arnon, S.S., Midura, T.F., Damus, K., Wood, R.M., and Chin, J. (1978). Intestinal infection and toxin production by *Clostridium botulinum* as one cause of sudden infant death syndrome. *Lancet 1*, 1273–1276.

Arnon, S.S., Damus, K., and Chin, J. (1981). Infant botulism: epidemiology and relation to sudden infant death syndrome. *Epidemiol. Rev. 3*, 45–66.

Arsenault, P.S. (1980). Maternal and antenatal factors in the risk of sudden infant death syndrome. *Am. J. Epidemiol. 111*, 279–284.

Beal, S. (1972). Sudden infant death syndrome. *Med. J. Aust. 2*, 1223–1229.

Bergman, A.B. and Wiesner, L.A. (1976). Relationship of passive cigarette smoking to sudden infant death syndrome. *Pediatrics 58*, 665–668.

Blok, J.H. (1978). The incidence of sudden infant death syndrome in North Carolina's cities and counties: 1972–1974. *Am. J. Public Health 68*, 367–372.

Chavez, C.J., Ostrea, E.M., Stryker, J.C., and Smialek, Z. (1979). Sudden infant death syndrome among infants of drug dependent mothers. *J. Pediatr. 95*, 407–409.

351

Cole, S., Lindenberg, L.B., Galioto, F.M., Howe, P.E., DeGraff, A.C., Davis, J.M., Lubka, R., and Gross, E.M. (1979). Ultrastructural abnormalities of the carotid body in sudden infant death syndrome. *Pediatrics* 63, 13–17.

Creighton, S. (1980). Deaths from non-accidental injury to children. *Br. Med. J. 281*, 147.

Cunningham, A.S. (1979). Respiratory syncytial virus and sudden infant death (letter to the editor). *N. Engl. J. Med. 300*, 1440–1441.

Denoroy, L., Kopp, N., Gay, N., Bertrand, E., Pujol, J-F., and Gilly, R. (1980). Activities des enzymes de synthese des catecholamines dans des regions du tronc cerebral an cours de la mort subite du nourrisson. *C.R. Acad. Sci. [D] (Paris) 291*, 245–248.

Downham, M.A.P.S., Gardner, P.S., McQuillin, J., and Ferris, J.A.J. (1975). Role of respiratory viruses in childhood mortality. *Br. Med. J. 1*, 235–239.

Fearn, S.W. (1834). Sudden and unexplained death of children (letter to the editor). *Lancet 1*, 246.

Ferris, J.A.J., Aherne, W.A., Locke, W.S., McQuillin, J., and Gardner, P.S. (1973). Sudden and unexpected deaths in infants: Histology and virology. *Br. Med. J. 1*, 439–442.

Froggatt, P., Lynas, M.A., and MacKenzie, G. (1971). Epidemiology of sudden unexpected death in infants ("cot death") in northern Ireland. *Br. J. Prev. Soc. Med. 25*, 119–134.

Gadson, D.R. and Emery, J.L. (1976). Fatty change in the brain in perinatal and unexpected death. *Arch. Dis. Child. 51*, 42.

Getts, A. (1981). SIDS: Increased risk to second born twins (letter to the editor). *Am. J. Public Health 71*, 317–318.

Harper, R.M., Leake, B., Hoffman, H., Walter, D.O., Hoppenbrouwers, T., Hodgman, J., and Sterman, M.B. (1981). Periodicity of sleep states is altered in infants at risk for the sudden infant death. *Science 213*, 1030–1032.

Kendeel, S.R.M. and Ferris, J.A.J. (1977). Sudden infant death syndrome: a review of literature. *J. Forens. Sci. Soc. 17*, 223–255.

Korobkin, R. and Guilleminault, C. (1978). Neurologic abnormalities in near misss for sudden infant death syndrome infants. *Pediatrics 64*, 369–374.

Laurence, K.M., James, N., Miller, M., and Campbell, H. (1980). Increased risk of recurrence of pregnancies complicated by fetal neural tube defects in mothers receiving poor diets and possible benefit of dietary counselling. *Br. Med. J. 281*, 1592–1594.

Mandell, F. and Wolfe, L.C. (1975). Sudden infant death syndrome and subsequent pregnancy. *Pediatrics 56*, 774–776.

McGinty, D.J. and Sterman, M.B. (1980). Sleep physiology hypoxemia, and the sudden infant death syndrome. *Sleep 3*, 361–373.

Naeye, R.L. (1973). Pulmonary arterial abnormalities in the sudden infant death syndrome. *N. Engl. J. Med. 289*, 1167–1170.

——— (1974). Hypoxemia and the sudden infant death syndrome. *Science 186*, 837–838.

——— (1976). Brain stem and adrenal abnormalities in the sudden infant death syndrome. *Am. J. Clin. Pathol. 66*, 526–530.

————, Fisher, R., Ryser, M., and Whalen, P. (1976a). Carotid body in the sudden infant death syndrome. *Science 191*, 567–569.

————, Ladis, B., and Drage, J.S. (1976b). Sudden infant death syndrome: A prospective study. *Am. J. Dis. Child. 130*, 1207–1210.

————, Whalen, P., Ryser, M., and Fisher, R. (1976a). Cardiac and other abnormalities in the sudden infant death syndrome. *Am. J. Pathol. 82*, 1–8.

Pavri, K.M. (1979). Neonatal respiratory syncytial virus infection (letter to the editor). *N. Engl. J. Med. 301*, 332.

Peterson, D.R. (1980). Evolution of the epidemiology of sudden infant death syndrome. *Epidemiol. Rev. 2*, 97–112.

———— (1981). The sudden infant death syndrome: Reassessment of growth retardation in relation to maternal smoking and the hypoxia hypotheses. *Am. J. Epidemiol. 113*, 583–589.

————, Benson, E.A., Fisher, L.D., Chinn, N.M., and Beckwith, J.B. (1973). Postnatal growth and the sudden infant death syndrome. *Am. J. Epidemiol. 99*, 389–394.

————, Chinn, N.M., and Fisher, L.D. (1980). The sudden infant death syndrome: Repetitions in families. *J. Pediatr. 97*, 265–267.

————, Labbe, R.F., van Belle, G., and Chinn, N.M. (1981). Erythrocyte transketolase activity and sudden infant death. *Am. J. Clin. Nutr. 34*, 65–67.

————, van Belle, G., and Chinn, N.M. (1979). Epidemiologic comparisons of the sudden infant death syndrome with other major components of infant mortality. *Am. J. Epidemiol. 110*, 699–707.

Quattrochi, J.J., Baba, N., and Liss, L. (1978). Sudden infant death syndrome (SIDS): Reticular dendritic spines in infants with SIDS. *Soc. Neurol. Sci. Abstr. 4*, 390.

Raring, R.H. (1974). SIDS—A note on age distribution of the syndrome. In *SIDS 1974: Proceedings of the Francis E. Camps International Symposium on Sudden and Unexpected Deaths in Infancy*, edited by R.R. Robinson. Toronto: The Canadian Foundation for the Study of Infant Deaths, pp. 151–156.

Ray, C.G. and Hebestreit, N.M. (1971). Studies of the sudden infant death syndrome in King County, Washington; II. Attempts to demonstrate evidence of viremia. *Pediatrics 48*, 79–82.

Read, D.J.C. (1978). The aetiology of the sudden infant death syndrome: Current ideas on breathing and sleep and possible links to deranged thiamin neurochemistry. *Aust. N.Z. J. Med. 8*, 322–336.

Read, D.J.C., Williams, A.L., Hensley, W., Edwards, M., and Peal, S. (1979). Sudden infant deaths: some current research strategies. *Med. J. Aust. 2*, 236–244.

Roberts, J., Lynch, M.A., and Golding, J. (1980). Postneonatal mortality in children from abusing families. *Br. Med. J. 281*, 102–104.

Sachis, P.N., Armstrong, D.L., Becker, L.E., and Bryan, A.C. (1981). The vagus nerve and sudden infant death syndrome. A morphometric study. *J. Pediatr. 98*, 278–280.

Schrauzer, G.N., Rhead, W.J., and Saltzstein, S.L. (1975). Sudden infant death syndrome: Plasma vitamin E levels and dietary factors. *Ann. Clin. Lab. Sci. 5,* 31–37.

Sinclair-Smith, C., Dinsdale, F., and Emery, J. (1976). Evidence of duration and type of illness in children found unexpectedly dead. *Arch. Dis. Child. 51,* 424–429.

Standfast, S.J., Jereb, S., and Janerich, D.T. (1979). The epidemiology of sudden infant death in upstate New York. *J.A.M.A. 241,* 1121–1124.

——, ——, and —— (1980). The epidemiology of sudden infant death in upstate New York: II. Birth Characteristics. *Am. J. Public Health 70,* 1061–1067.

Steele, R. and Langworth, J.T. (1966). The relationship of antenatal and postnatal factors to sudden unexpected death in infancy. *Can. Med. Assoc. J. 94,* 1165–1171.

Tait, B.D., Williams, A.L., Mathews, J.D., and Cowling, D.C. (1977). HLA and the sudden infant death syndrome. *Monogr. Allergy 11,* 55–59.

Takashima, S., Armstrong, D., Becker, L., and Bryan, C. (1978a). Cerebral hypoperfusion in the sudden infant death syndrome? Brain Stem Gliosis and Vasculature. *Ann. Neurol. 4,* 257–262.

——, ——, ——, and Huber, J. (1978b). Cerebral white matter lesions in sudden infant death syndrome. *Pediatrics 62,* 155–159.

Tonkin, S. (1974). Epidemiology of SIDS in Auckland, New Zealand. In *SIDS 1974: Proceedings of the Francis E. Camps International Symposium on Sudden and Unexpected Deaths in Infancy,* edited by R.R. Robinson. Toronto: The Canadian Foundation for the Study of Infant Deaths, pp. 169–175.

Urquhart, G.E.D. and Grist, N.R. (1972). Virological studies of sudden unexplained infant deaths in Glasgow 1967–70. *J. Clin. Pathol. 25,* 443–446.

Valdes-Dapena, M.A., Gillane, M.M., and Catherman, R. (1976). Brown fat retention in sudden infant death syndrome. *Arch. Pathol. Lab. Med. 100,* 547–549.

Valdes-Dapena, M.A. (1980). Sudden infant death syndrome: a review of the medical literature 1974–1979. *Pediatrics 66,* 597–614.

Williams, A., Vawter, G., and Reid, L. (1979). Increased muscularity of the pulmonary circulation in victims of the sudden infant death syndrome. *Pediatrics 63,* 18–23.

Yeats, W.B. (1940). Collected poems. New York: MacMillan, pp. 26–28. (Originally published in 1906.)

II
Methodological Issues
in Perinatal Epidemiology

15

Sample Size Determination in Comparative Studies

Daniel H. Freeman, Jr.

Most epidemiologists are well trained in formulating a set of objectives to test a hypothesis about the relationship between a risk factor and a disease or other health outcome. They are also skilled in operationalizing these objectives in a field study. When the relevant data have been collected, most investigators can implement an appropriate statistical analysis, often utilizing one or more standard computer packages. One point that seems regularly to lead investigators to seek biostatistical advice is the determination of required sample size. The question investigators pose takes one of three forms:

1. For a given sample size and strength of association, how likely is the study to detect the association?
2. For a given sample size and probability of detection, how small an effect can be detected?
3. For a given detection probability and strength of association, how large a sample is required?

The first two questions presuppose that the data have been collected, because there is an assumed sample size. The third question is more appropriate for planning a study, because its answer will determine, in part, the resources required for implementing the study. For this reason, it is the question most often answered in statistics texts such as those by Colton (1974), Fleiss (1981), and Snedecor and Cochran (1967). The first two questions are, in principle, no more difficult to answer but are less frequently found in statistics texts. The question of minimum detectable associations is addressed for categorical data by Walter (1977). The likehood of detection problem is usually mentioned in developing an answer to the third question.

This chapter will address all three questions with a unified notation. The answers are limited to studies where only two groups are compared. For more complex problems the reader should consult one of the many texts on experimental design, for example, Cochran and Cox (1957) or Cox (1958). For bivariate categorical data where each variable has several levels, an answer to the problem of sample size is discussed by Lachin (1977). A comprehensive discussion of "power analysis" is found in the text by Cohen (1969). The present discussion begins by defining the parameters of study design in statistical language. Using this notation, the problem of comparing a continuous variable across two groups is addressed with three examples. Next a dichotomous variable is examined. In this discussion, prospective and retrospective studies are considered separately. Finally, a limited discussion of sources of preliminary data for study planning is given.

NOTATION AND DEFINITIONS

Statisticians and investigators who use statistics are immediately confronted with two problems. The first is the reduction of measurements to a simple set of numerical statements or summaries. The two most common are the population mean and the population proportion. The former is the arithmetic average of a continuous variable across the members of a population. The latter is the number of members of a population with a particular characteristic divided by the total number of elements in the population. For the moment, either can be represented by the Greek letter θ. When populations are compared, θ is subscripted with the letter i. Using this notation, hypotheses about the populations may be expressed as

$$H_0: \theta_1 - \theta_2 = 0 \qquad \text{versus} \qquad H_1: \theta_1 - \theta_2 \neq 0 \qquad (1)$$

The first hypothesis is usually referred to as the null hypothesis and the second as the alternative hypothesis. After data collection and analysis, the investigator will conclude that the available evidence indicates H_0 is either true or false and, conversely, that H_1 is either false or true.

The statement that H_0 is true or false presents the second problem with which analysts are confronted. If we conclude that H_0 is false, it may be true and we have committed a Type 1 error. The probability that this will occur is the "significance level" of the test and is denoted α. Paralleling this is the conclusion that, given the available evidence, H_0 cannot be rejected. Then there is a probability that H_0 is in fact false. Incorrectly concluding that H_0 is true is a Type 2 error, the probability of which is denoted β. The probability, for a given study design and statistical test, that a false null hypothesis will be rejected is termed the power of the test. This is denoted $1 - \beta$. Finally,

Table 15-1. Probabilities Associated with the Statistical Test of Hypothesis

		True state of affairs	
		$\theta_1 = \theta_2$	$\theta_1 \neq \theta_2$
Statistical test of H_0	Accept	$1 - \alpha$	β
	Reject	α	$1 - \beta$

whether H_0 is rejected or not, it is common practice to construct a confidence interval estimate to characterize the precision of the study estimates. The confidence interval width is determined, in part, by the confidence coefficient: $1 - \alpha$. It should be noted that when the study variable is normally distributed, then the confidence interval will include zero if H_0 has been accepted. This notation is summarized in Table 15-1. The diagonal elements of Table 15-1 ($1 - \alpha$ and $1 - \beta$) are the probabilities of reaching a correct conclusion about H_0. The off-diagonal elements (α and β) are the probabilities of the two types of errors. Clearly, the scientist can specify these in advance of the study. In practice, $\alpha = 0.05$, and the study is designed so as to minimize β.

If θ_1 and θ_2 could be determined exactly, then the possibility of either type of error can be made exceedingly small. This is the common situation in the physical sciences. The medical and social sciences are less fortunate in that most observations on the study variable will differ from the population mean. This variation is summarized in terms of the population's standard deviation σ_i; $i = 1,2$, which in turn determines the variability of our estimates of θ_i:

$$V(\hat{\theta}_i) = \sigma_i^2/n_i \qquad i = 1,2 \tag{2}$$

Here $V(\hat{\theta}_i)$ is the variance associated with the estimate of θ_i, and n_i is the corresponding sample size. The square root of $V(\hat{\theta}_i)$ is the standard error of $\hat{\theta}_i$. In practice, σ_i^2 is estimated from the sample data. Finally, it is usually assumed that $\hat{\theta}_1$ and $\hat{\theta}_2$ are independent or at least uncorrelated. It is evident from eq. (2) that increasing sample size has the effect of generating more precise estimates of the study parameter θ_i, when $\hat{\theta}_i$ is statistically unbiased.

The preceding notation may be used to write out the fundamental equation of sample size determination:

$$c_{1-\beta} = (\theta_1 - \theta_2)\sqrt{\frac{n_1 n_2}{n_2\sigma_{11}^2 + n_1\sigma_{21}^2}} - c_{1-\alpha/2}\sqrt{\frac{n_2\sigma_{10}^2 + n_1\sigma_{20}^2}{n_2\sigma_{11}^2 + n_1\sigma_{21}^2}} \tag{3}$$

Here, $c_{1-\beta}$ and $c_{1-\alpha/2}$ are the $(1 - \beta)100$ and $(1-\frac{\alpha}{2})100$ percentiles of the standard normal distribution or Student's t distribution with $n_1 + n_2 - 2$ degrees of freedom when n_1 and n_2 are small. This formulation applies to "two-tailed" alternative hypotheses when $\theta_1 > \theta_2$. If a "one-tailed" alternative hypothesis is of interest, then $\frac{\alpha}{2}$ is replaced by α. If $\theta_1 < \theta_2$ and a two-tailed alternative is appropriate, then $(\theta_1 - \theta_2)$ is replaced by $(\theta_2 - \theta_1)$. The population variances (σ_{ij}^2) in eq. (3) have a second subscript, so that different variances under the null and alternative hypotheses may be considered. This is particularly important when considering dichotomous variables. When continuous variables are considered it is common practice to assume $\sigma_{10}^2 = \sigma_{20}^2 = \sigma_{11}^2 = \sigma_{21}^2 = \sigma^2$. In this circumstance a considerable simplification in eq. (3) is obtained:

$$c_{1-\beta} = \frac{(\theta_1 - \theta_2)\sqrt{f(1-f)n}}{\sigma} - c_{1-\alpha/2} \qquad (4)$$

where $n = n_1 + n_2$ and $f = n_1/n$. Now it is apparent that $c_{1-\beta}$ increases for larger n values or for greater $(\theta_1 - \theta_2)$ values. Similarly, $c_{1-\beta}$ increases with reductions in either σ or $c_{1-\alpha/2}$. Because $f(1 - f)$ is maximized for $f = \frac{1}{2}$, it follows that $c_{1-\beta}$ is maximized for equal sample sizes. Finally, recall that β is the probability of a Type 2 error, so increasing $c_{1-\beta}$ decreases the probability of a Type 2 error.

The usual practice for sample size determination is to solve eq. (3) or (4) for n. Because the particular solution of interest depends on the study context, we will focus on solutions in specific applications.

CONTINUOUS VARIABLES

Sample Size

Suppose one wished to evaluate a new prophylactic drug treatment for premature infants. One measure of drug efficacy is days of oxygen therapy. The study planner reviews a long case series and finds that among otherwise healthy infants weighing between 1000 and 1700 g, the mean days of oxygenation is ten days, with a standard deviation of ten days. The large standard deviation occurs because many infants have little if any oxygenation, whereas others have quite substantial periods. It is believed that a two-day reduction in oxygenation is required for the drug to be clinically significant as an intervention. The statistical question is, how large a sample is required in order to detect a two-day reduction due to the new drug?

The statistician answers this question by asking (1) how significant is the result to be and (2) how large a risk of failing to detect a difference is the investigator willing to take? These questions correspond to the probabilities of Type 1 and Type 2 errors. The former is usually set at $\alpha = 0.05$, whereas several values of the latter may be considered, for example, $\beta = 0.2, 0.1, 0.05$. Next, the statistician restates the problem in terms of the population parameters and the corresponding hypotheses. Because the outcome is continuous, θ_i is a mean usually denoted by μ_i. In this case, let μ_1 denote the mean days of oxygenation in the control group and μ_2 that of the treated infants. The hypotheses are as follows:

$$H_0: \mu_1 - \mu_2 = 0 \qquad \text{versus} \qquad H_1: \mu_1 - \mu_2 > 0$$

The alternative reflects the investigator's interest in a reduction in oxygenation. All other things being equal, if the drug increases oxygenation it should not be used. The final step is solved in eq. (4) for n:

$$n = \frac{(c_{1-\beta} + c_{1-\alpha/2})^2 \, \sigma^2}{(\mu_1 - \mu_2)^2 \, f(1 - f)} \tag{5}$$

The case series review and ensuing discussion have now provided all of the elements for determining the sample size n. Because a 0.05 significance level and a one-tailed test are desired, $c_{1-0.05} = c_{0.95} = 1.645$. A typical Type 2 error rate is 0.20, so $c_{1-0.20} = c_{0.80} = 0.842$. Next, a two-day shift is claimed to be clinically significant, so $\mu_1 - \mu_2 = 2$. The reported standard deviation for days of oxygenation is ten days, so $\sigma = 10$. Finally the discussion following eq. (4) indicates that equal sample sizes are optimal, so $f = 0.50$. These are now entered into eq. (5):

$$n = \frac{(0.842 + 1.645)^2 (10)^2}{(2)^2 (0.5)(0.5)}$$

$$= 618.5$$

or 310 infants per group. Note that the solution is rounded up to the nearest even integer to permit equal sample sizes.

Minimum Detectable Shift

It is evident from eq. (5) that increasing $1 - \beta$ increases $c_{1-\beta}$ and therefore the sample size. Similarly any shift away from 0.5 in the sample allocation f will also increase the sample size. Finally, σ is largely determined by the study population. It follows that an increase in the detectable difference is the only reasonable method for reducing sample size. Having indicated that at most 50 infants will be available for study, the investigator therefore wishes to know the minimum reduction in days of oxygenation that can be detected for the specified significance and power. This corresponds to the second question on page 357. The answer may be obtained by solving eq. (4) or (5) for $(\mu_1 - \mu_2)$:

$$\mu_1 - \mu_2 = \frac{(c_{1-\beta} + c_{1-\alpha})\sigma}{\sqrt{f(1-f)\,n}} \tag{6}$$

Note that $c_{1-\alpha}$ rather than $c_{1-\alpha/2}$ is used, because a one-tailed alternative is of interest. Using the same study parameters as before and $n = 50$, we obtain:

$$\mu_1 - \mu_2 = \frac{(0.842 + 1.645)(10)}{\sqrt{(0.5)(0.5)(50)}} = \frac{24.87}{\sqrt{12.5}} = 7.03$$

Thus a seven-day reduction in the days of oxygenation can be detected with a significance level $\alpha = 0.05$ and 80% power ($\beta = 0.2$).

Power Calculations

The investigator is somewhat more pleased with this result but would like to probe the question somewhat further. Specifically, an article on the prophylactic use of indomethacin for patent ductus arteriosus in very low birthweight infants is cited (Mahoney et al., 1982). Among a group of 47 infants with weights of under 1700 g who were otherwise healthy, a diagnosis of subclinical patent ductus arteriosus was made based on a murmur. These were allocated at random to a treatment group ($n_1 = 21$) and a placebo group ($n_2 = 26$). A pooled standard deviation of about 25 days was reported. What is the probability that a 14-day reduction in oxygenation would be detected at the usual levels of significance? The answer to this may be obtained from eq. (4):

$$c_{1-\beta} = \frac{14}{25}\sqrt{\frac{21(26)}{47}} - 1.645 = 0.263$$

Here $$f(1-f)n = \left(\frac{n_1}{n}\right)\left(\frac{n_2}{n}\right)n = \frac{n_1 n_2}{n} = \frac{21(26)}{47}$$

Using the standard normal distribution we find $1 - \beta = 0.604$ or $\beta = 0.396$. Thus Mahoney et al. had a 40% chance of failing to detect a two-week reduction in days of oxygenation. In fact, they detected such a reduction. Moreover they isolated the effect to infants weighing under 1000 g.

In summary, for data with continuous outcome variables, eq. (5) can be used to determine sample size, eq. (6) can be used to determine detectable shift, and eq. (4) can be used for power calculations. These all assume some prior estimate of σ is available and the sample sizes ($fn = n_1 > 25$ and $(1 - f)n = n_2 > 25$) are reasonably large. When σ is unknown, the analysis can proceed by specifying $(\mu_1 - \mu_2) = k\sigma$. Then eq. (4) becomes

$$c_{1-\beta} = k\sqrt{f(1 - f)n} - c_{1-\alpha/2} \qquad (7)$$

When fn or $(1 - f)n$ are small, say less than 25, then $c_{1-\alpha/2}$ and $c_{1-\beta}$ may be based on student's t-distribution. Because the degrees of freedom $(n - 2)$ now depend on n, an exact solution is not possible. A method of successive approximations is outlined in Cochran and Cox (1957).

DICHOTOMOUS VARIABLES

Dichotomous study variables occur in many epidemiologic investigations. The variable may be the occurrence or nonoccurrence of a particular disease, the presence or absence of a risk factor, or the recovery or lack of recovery from an illness. In each of these circumstances the comparison of two populations leads the investigator to summarize the data with a fourfold or 2 × 2 table. The study variable is usually assumed to follow a binomial distribution. This means that the population variances are readily available once the probability of the event of interest is specified. As will be seen, this is both an advantage and a disadvantage. A second issue for dichotomous variables is that the design of the study affects the sample size calculation.

Three different designs will be considered. The easiest is the usual experimental design where a treatment group, such as patients receiving a new drug, is compared to a control group. The second design is an observational study, either prospective or cross sectional, where the objective is to determine whether two groups differ with respect to prevalence or incidence when they also differ in their exposure to a suspected risk factor. Finally we will examine the retrospective or case-control study, where one wishes to determine whether a group of diseased patients (cases) differs from a group of controls with respect to some risk factor. The distinction among the three types of studies is in how the investigator creates the comparison groups. This can be by explicit randomization in the experimental study, by an assumed or "natural randomization" of the risk factor in the prospective or cross-sectional study, or by a "natural randomization" of the disease outcome in the case-control study. In the language of sampling, the experimental study is characterized by prior stratification of the population into treated and untreated groups; the prospective and cross-sectional studies are characterized by postsampling stratification into treated or exposed and untreated or unexposed groups; the retrospective study is stratified according to the disease outcome.

The general format for reporting any of these studies is shown in Table 15-2. Here P_i denotes the underlying probability of reporting the study outcome in group i, $i = 1,2$. Let $Q_i = 1 - P_i$, and $\bar{P} = fP_1 + (1 - f)P_2$. The relevant hypotheses are given by

$$H_0: P_1 = P_2 \qquad \text{versus} \qquad H_1: P_1 \neq P_2$$

Using the notation given in the last section, $\theta_i = P_i$. If we assume that the two groups can be modeled by a binomial distribution, then the variances of eq. (3) are given:

$$\sigma_{10}^2 = \sigma_{20}^2 = \bar{P}\bar{Q}$$
$$\sigma_{11}^2 = P_1Q_1 \qquad \sigma_{21}^2 = P_2Q_2 \tag{8}$$

Substituting these values into eq. (3) yields the result:

$$c_{1-\beta} = \frac{(P_1 - P_2)\sqrt{f(1 - f)n} - c_{1-\alpha/2}\sqrt{\bar{P}\bar{Q}}}{\sqrt{(1 - f)P_1Q_1 + fP_2Q_2}} \tag{9}$$

The sample size question is answered by solving eq. (9) for n:

$$n = \frac{[c_{1-\beta}\sqrt{(1 - f)P_1Q_1 + fP_2Q_2} + c_{1-\alpha/2}\sqrt{\bar{P}\bar{Q}}]^2}{f(1 - f)(P_1 - P_2)^2} \tag{10}$$

An advantage of working with dichotomous data, in planning studies, is evident from these two equations. Once P_1 and a clinically interesting shift $P_1 - P_2$ are specified, the required sample size n or the power of test $1 - \beta$ can be readily determined. There is no need to obtain a prior estimate of σ as with continuous data. A disadvantage is that the equations are considerably more complex than their counterparts eqs. (4) and (5). Moreover it is not possible to obtain an exact solution

Table 15-2. Summary Table for a Study of a Dichotomous Variable

Group	Outcome Present	Absent	Total sample
1	P_1	Q_1	$n_1 = fn$
2	P_2	Q_2	$n_2 = (1 - f)n$
Total	$\bar{P}$	$\bar{Q}$	n

for $P_1 - P_2$ in terms of only f, $c_{1-\alpha/2}$, $c_{1-\beta}$, and n. Finally, the application of eqs. (9) and (10) depends on the study design, as is illustrated in the following three examples.

Experimental Studies

An investigator claims that a new antenatal drug will reduce the risk of intraventricular hemorrhage (IVH) among very low birthweight infants (<1500 g) by half. A prior case series indicates the incidence rate of IVH among this group of infants is about 25%. To simplify the discussion we consider babies who remain free of IVH two weeks after delivery as a successful outcome. Thus $P_2 = 0.750$, and the claim is that use of the drug will yield $P_1 = 0.875$. From the earlier discussion it is evident that minimum sample size will be obtained when there are an equal number of treated and control babies, that is, $f = 0.5$. Finally, set $\alpha = 0.05$ and $\beta = 0.10$, so the risks of Type 1 and Type 2 errors are 5 and 10%, respectively. Using standard tables we find $c_{1-\alpha/2} = 1.960$ and $c_{1-\beta} = 1.282$. Finally $\bar{P} = \frac{1}{2}(0.75 + 0.875) = 0.8125$. Inserting these values in eq. (10) yields:

$$n = \frac{[1.282\sqrt{0.5(0.875)(0.125) + 0.5(0.75)(0.25)} + 1.960\sqrt{0.8125(0.1875)}]^2}{(0.875 - 0.75)^2(0.5)(0.5)}$$

$$= 405.74$$

Thus 406 mothers, 203 per group, are required for a test of the new drug.

Prospective and Cross-Sectional Studies

A second common study design in epidemiology is the prospective study. For example, suppose it was hypothesized that prior use of oral contraceptives increases the risk of low birthweight (<2500 g) in subsequent livebirths. One approach would be to indentify women in their first trimester of pregnancy and interview them to determine their contraceptive history. Then the women would be followed until delivery to determine the incidence of low birthweight as well as other possible outcomes. Data from the National Survey of Family Growth could be combined with birth registration data to assist in planning the study. From the former it can be estimated that 32.1% of fecund women are past oral contraceptive users (Mosher, 1981). The incidence of low birthweight among women receiving prenatal care in the first trimester is between 6.4 and 7.0% (Querec, 1978). Finally, it is felt that a relative risk of 2 or greater is clinically interesting. Here relative risk is $R = P_1/P_2$, where P_1 is the incidence rate among former users and P_2 is the incidence rate among nonusers. Unfortunately some algebra is required before eq. (10) can be utilized. Specifically we must solve

$$R = P_1/P_2$$
$$\bar{P} = fP_1 + (1 - f)P_2 \tag{11}$$

for P_1 and P_2. The result, for prospective and cross-sectional studies, is

$$P_1 = R\bar{P}/[1 + f(R - 1)]$$
$$P_2 = P_1/R \tag{12}$$

Using the lesser incidence rate for $\bar{P}$ we obtain

$$P_1 = 2(0.064)/(1 + 0.321(2 - 1)) = 0.097$$
$$P_2 = 0.097/2 = 0.048$$

Assuming $\alpha = 0.05$ and $\beta = 0.10$, we can use eq. (10):

$$n = \frac{(1.282\sqrt{(1 - 0.321)(0.097)(0.903) + (0.321)(0.048)(0.952)} + 1.96\sqrt{(0.064)(0.936)})^2}{(0.321)(1 - 0.321)(0.097 - 0.048)^2}$$

$$n = \frac{(1.282(0.272) + 1.96(0.245))^2}{(0.321)(0.679)(0.048)^2} = 1368.21$$

Hence the investigator will need to include at least 1369 women. The same calculation is appropriate whether a prospective study or a cross-sectional study is proposed, because both will yield appropriate estimates of R. This is not always true of the retrospective study (see also Chapter 16).

Retrospective or Case-Control Designs

The retrospective study is usually characterized by selecting subjects with an outcome of interest (cases) and an appropriate comparison group (controls). The subjects are then studied to determine whether they have been exposed to some risk factor of interest. Unfortunately, the relative risk cannot be estimated directly from such a study. However, if the disease or outcome is rare it may be approximated by the odds ratio:

$$OR = (P_1/Q_1)/(P_2/Q_2) = P_1Q_2/P_2Q_1 \tag{13}$$

Here P_1 and P_2 denote the prevalence of the risk factor in the respective case and control groups. Solving eq. (13) for P_1 yields

$$P_1 = P_2OR/(Q_2 + P_2OR) \tag{14}$$

Because, the disease is rare, it follows that reasonable estimates of P_2 may be obtained from published data. For example, suppose we wish to study the association between congenital malformation in offspring and oral contraception prior to pregnancy. On the basis of the National Survey of Family Growth we would assume $P_2 = 0.321$. Suppose relative risks of at least 2 are of interest; then

$$P_1 = (0.321)(2)/[0.679 + (0.321)(2)] = 0.486$$

Suppose three controls are available for each case; then $f = 0.25$, $1 - f = 0.75$, and

$$\bar{P} = (0.25)(0.486) + (0.75)(0.321) = 0.362$$

Setting $\alpha = 0.05$ and $\beta = 0.10$, we can use eq. (10) and the above results to obtain our sample size:

$$n = \frac{(1.282\sqrt{(0.75)(0.486)(0.514) + (0.25)(0.321)(0.679)} + 1.960\sqrt{(0.362)(0.638)})^2}{(0.25)(0.75)(0.486 - 0.362)^2}$$

$$= \frac{(1.282(0.492) + 1.960(0.481))^2}{0.002883} = 858.8$$

thus 859 observations will be required. Because there are three controls for each case, this translates into 215 cases and 644 controls. An important advantage of this type of study is that the underlying disease incidence does not directly affect the sample size calculation as it did in the experimental, prospective, and cross-sectional study designs.

The discussion for dichotomous data has focused on the computation of sample size. Clearly, if power $(1 - \beta)$ is of interest, eq. (10) can be used directly. However, when we wish to estimate the least significant relative risk that can be detected, the problem is more complex. It requires either a computer solution to eq. (9) or an approximation as discussed by Walter (1977).

CONCLUSIONS

The calculation of sample size is critical both for planning a study and for evaluating completed studies. The preceding discussion has centered around the problem of testing a simple null hypothesis, $H_0: \theta_1 = \theta_2$. It should be evident that the calculations are straightforward although somewhat tedious. The important issue is that some preliminary estimates of the underlying population parameters must be available. Moreover, the investigator must have in mind what constitutes an interesting difference, $\theta_1 - \theta_2$. Finally, it should be kept in mind that these calculations serve as a rough guide rather than an ironclad set of rules.

The usual source of information about the population parameters is the existing literature. This can consist of previously reported estimates of the phenomenon under investigation. The National Health Survey as reported in *Vital and Health Statistics* (the "rainbow series") can provide prevalence estimates for a wide variety of health data. Alternatively, pretests and feasibility studies can provide preliminary estimates about the study parameters. It should be noted that data from such studies can also be used to help the investigators formulate their objectives and hypotheses with greater specificity.

The second question concerns what constitutes an interesting effect. Frequently this can be specified in terms of the population standard deviation. That is, set $\mu_1 - \mu_2 = k\sigma$. As noted in the discussion of continuous data, this leads to a particularly simple equation for the power of the study $(1 - \beta)$. Specifically, if we assume equal allocation ($f = 0.5$), then solving eq. (7) for n yields

$$n = 4(c_{1-\beta} + c_{1-\alpha/2})^2/k^2 \qquad (15)$$

If we set $\alpha = \beta = 0.5$, then $c_{1-\beta} = 1.645$ and $c_{1-\alpha/2} = 1.960$. Hence $n = 51.98/k^2$. This means that 26 individuals per group are required to detect a shift of σ units. Moreover the sample size changes inversely with the square of the "interesting shift." The problem is computationally more complex for dichotomous data but is in principle the same.

The final point concerns the use of these calculations in study planning and evaluation. In practice, more investigations extend beyond the test of a simple hypothesis about two subpopulations. When a truly randomized trial is undertaken and several factors are investigated, then the calculation can be carried out following the methods outlined in Cochran and Cox (1957), Cox (1958), or Cohen (1969). However, for observational studies (cohort, cross-sectional, or case-control designs) the sample distributions are not easily specified a priori, and the standard methods do not apply. In this situation it is still good practice to undertake the sample size calculations for the test of a simple hypothesis. The results can then be inflated on an ad hoc basis to reflect the number of variables that are to be considered in any particular analysis. Of course, this inflation should reflect not just the number of variables but the degrees of freedom associated with the categorical variables used. Moreover, if interactions among the variables are expected, then the sample size inflation should reflect this as well.

In conclusion, sample size calculations are simple and straightforward. They serve as a key ingredient to study planning. If they are incorporated systematically into an investigator's thinking, then studies with little chance of success can be avoided.

REFERENCES

Cochran, W.G. and Cox, G.M. (1957). *Experimental designs*, 2nd Ed. New York: Wiley, pp. 17–29.

Cohen, J. (1969). *Statistical power analysis for the behavioral sciences.* New York: Academic Press.

Colton, T.H. (1974). *Statistics in medicine.* Boston: Little, Brown, pp. 142–146; 168–169.

Cox, D.R. (1958). *Planning of experiments.* New York: Wiley, pp. 154–190.

Fleiss, J.L. (1981). *Statistical methods for rates and proportions*, 2nd Ed. New York: Wiley, pp. 33–49.

Lachin, J.M. (1977). Sample size determinations for r × c comparative trials. *Biometrics 33*, 315–324.

Mahoney, L., Carnero, V., Brett, C., Hayman, M.A., and Clyman, R.I. (1982). Prophylactic indomethacin therapy for patent ductus arteriosus in very low birthweight infants. *N. Engl. J. Med. 309*(9), 506–510.

Mosher, W.D. (1981). Trends in contraceptive practice, United States, 1965–76. *Vital Health Stat. 23*(10), Department of Health and Human Services Publ. No. (PHS) 82-1986.

Querec, L.J. (1978). Characteristics of births. *Vital Health Stat. 21*(30), Department of Health and Human Services Publ. No. (PHS) 78-1908.

Snedecor, G.W. and Cochran, W.G. (1967). *Statistical methods*, 6th Ed. Ames, Iowa: The Iowa State University Press, pp. 111–114, 221–223.

Walter, S.D. (1977). Determination of significant relative risks and optimal sampling procedures in prospective and retrospective comparative studies of various sizes. *Am. J. Epidemiol. 105*(4), 387–397.

16

Strategies for the Analysis of Case-Referent and Cohort Studies

Theodore R. Holford

The purpose of analyzing a set of data is to give a summary that accurately describes the results. In an epidemiologic study of one or more risk factors, a succinct summary can often be provided by giving an appropriate equation or model for which parameters can be estimated. For most diseases this is an empiric process because the state of knowledge is such that a theoretic model cannot be derived. Hence it is not possible to devise a set of formulas that always gives a correct summary of the results. Instead, the data need to be explored in order to discover new relationships or validate known ones. We discuss here a strategy for exploring data whereby one (1) visualizes a relationship, (2) fits a model to the data, and, (3) determines the adequacy of that fit.

The log-linear model provides a flexible analytic method that enables one to consider a variety of possible relationships. A special case of the log-linear model is the linear logistic model, which is sometimes more easily adapted for consideration of particular kinds of association between putative risk factors and disease. An advantage to using log-linear and linear logistic models is the ready availability of computer programs for parameter estimation and hypothesis testing. We will be discussing the use of these methods in the analysis of epidemiologic data.

Fitting a log-linear or linear logistic model to data generally requires a computer, which is appropriate for a large amount of data. However, sometimes one only has access to a hand calculator, in which case the calculations are often formidable. A number of procedures for making statistical inferences will be discussed that can readily be carried out with a hand calculator alone. We sometimes provide a variety of tests for the same hypothesis, one of which can be carried out without the aid of a computer. These methods do have limitations with regard to the type of information that can be obtained but are valid so long as the appropriate assumptions are realized.

STUDY DESIGN AND ANALYSIS

To some extent, the strategy for analyzing any set of data is determined by the study design. Two considerations in an epidemiologic study are (1) the time frame in which a condition manifests itself and (2) whether special sampling procedures have been used in an attempt to make the study more efficient. The former consideration will affect the interpretation of results, and the latter will influence the assumptions used in estimating parameters and testing hypotheses.

Many studies in perinatal epidemiology consider the outcome of a pregnancy, such as whether the infant exhibits a certain congenital abnormality. Such a condition may be observed immediately, so that for all practical purposes there is no period of follow-up for the infant. The outcome in this case becomes the proportion of infants in a particular risk group who have the anomaly. Other conditions develop over a period of time; thus it is more natural to consider the incidence rate as the basic quantity being measured.

When estimating the effect of two levels of risk on the disease condition of interest, we will use the odds ratio (*OR*). If we represent two risk groups by r_1 and r_2, then in a cohort study we determine the proportion (*P*) of infants with an anomaly d in each group: $Pr(d|r_1)$ and $Pr(d|r_2)$. The odds ratio is given by

$$OR(r_1, r_2) = \frac{Pr(d|r_1)\, Pr(\bar{d}|r_2)}{Pr(\bar{d}|r_1)\, Pr(d|r_2)}$$

where d and $\bar{d}$ indicate that the anomaly is present and absent, respectively. The odds ratio is often used instead of the relative risk:

$$RR(r_1 r_2) - \frac{Pr(d|r_1)}{Pr(d|r_2)}$$

When the proportion of subjects with the condition in each group is small, then *OR* and *RR* agree well. Table 16-1 indicates the percentage difference between the two quantities for various proportions diseased, and relative risks.

In a case-referent study, subjects are sampled from the group with the condition and from a reference group without it. The risk group for a particular subject is then determined, and the proportion exposed is compared for the case and referent group [i.e., $Pr(r|d)$

Table 16-1. Percentage Difference in Odds Ratio and Relative Risk by Probability of Disease in Unexposed and Relative Risk

Probability of disease in unexposed (%)	Relative risk (RR)				
	1.5	2.0	3.0	4.0	5.0
0.1	0.1	0.1	0.2	0.3	0.4
0.5	0.3	0.5	1.0	1.5	2.1
1.0	0.5	1.0	2.1	3.1	4.2
5.0	2.7	5.6	11.8	18.8	26.7
10.0	5.9	12.5	28.6	50.0	80.0

and $Pr(r|\bar{d})$. The odds ratio from such a study is given by

$$OR(r_1,r_2) = \frac{Pr(r_1|d)\,Pr(r_2|\bar{d})}{Pr(r_1|\bar{d})\,Pr(r_2|d)}$$

A cohort study is easier to conceptualize but often more difficult to conduct. The fact that the odds ratio from a case-referent study is equivalent to the cohort odds ratio (Cornfield, 1951) makes it a useful measure of association.

For a disease condition that develops over a period of time, the incidence intensity or the hazard (h) is given by $h(r_1)$ and $h(r_2)$ for the two risk groups. In this case the association of risk status with disease can be measured by the incidence intensity ratio:

$$IR(r_1,r_2) = h(r_1)/h(r_2)$$

A case-referent study of such a disease would sample new cases of the disease that occur during a study period in which the probability of any one subject developing the disease is small. Similarly, a reference group would be chosen among those without the disease. The odds ratio from such a study would yield the incidence intensity ratio (Miettinen, 1976; Breslow, 1977; Prentice and Breslow, 1978). Hence we interpret the odds ratio from a case-referent study as the ratio of odds for disease if we study a disease that is apparent after essentially no follow-up and an incidence intensity ratio if the disease develops over time.

A second aspect of study design that must be in the analysis is the method of selecting subjects. In some studies, subjects in the reference group are selected because they match subjects in the group of cases. If this is the design used, then it is only appropriate that the analytic method reflect this. When one or more referents are matched to each case, there are methods of analysis that are directly related to the methods discussed here (see Liddell et al., 1977; Breslow et al.,

1978; Breslow and Day, 1980; Holford, 1978, 1982; Holford et al., 1978; Prentice and Breslow, 1978). However, these will not be discussed in this chapter.

RATIO OF ODDS FOR DISEASE

Exposure to a putative risk factor may be recorded as simply yes or no. However, this is generally overly simplistic, and a more realistic representation will give information on the level of exposure to the factor. As a first step in the analysis of data we might compare two groups, but eventually we should describe the dose–response relationship. Log-linear models provide a framework for carrying out the analysis. Many statistical methods in epidemiology have a theoretic basis in the log-linear model that includes the special case of the linear logistic model. We will investigate the use of log-linear models in the analysis of a putative risk factor.

Estimate of the Odds Ratio

First let us consider the problem of estimating the odds ratio when only two risk groups are to be compared. For the purpose of illustration, let us consider a case-control study described by Kelsey et al. (1978) in which the effect of mother's smoking on subsequent congenital anomalies in the child was investigated. Data may be summarized as in Table 16-2. The estimate of the odds ratio is given by

$$OR = \frac{n_{11} n_{22}}{n_{21} n_{12}}$$

$$= \frac{(1988)(480)}{(980)(889)}$$

$$= 1.095 \tag{1}$$

Table 16-2. Distribution of Cases and Controls by Whether the Mother Smoked in the Third Month of Pregnancy

Mother smoked (r)	Disease status (d)	
	1. Control	2. Case
1. No	$n_{11} = 1988$	$n_{12} = 889$
2. Yes	$n_{21} = 980$	$n_{22} = 480$

where n_{ij} represents the observed frequency in the ith row and jth column of a two-way table like Table 16-2. Often we are also interested in the logarithm:

$$\ln OR = 0.0910 \tag{2}$$

The standard error of the log odds ratio can be found by

$$se(\ln OR) = \sqrt{\frac{1}{n_{11}} + \frac{1}{n_{12}} + \frac{1}{n_{21}} + \frac{1}{n_{22}}}$$

$$= \sqrt{\frac{1}{1988} + \frac{1}{889} + \frac{1}{980} + \frac{1}{480}}$$

$$= 0.0688$$

A test of the null hypothesis that $OR = 1$ is equivalent to testing $\ln OR = 0$. One such test uses the ratio:

$$W = \frac{\ln OR}{se(\ln OR)}$$

$$= \frac{0.0910}{0.0688}$$

$$= 1.32 \tag{3}$$

which can be compared to a standard normal deviate. Such a test, which makes use of a parameter estimate and its standard error, is called a Wald test (Rao, 1973, p. 417). It is common to express a Wald test as the square of the expression in eq. (3), or

$$W^2 = \frac{(\ln OR)^2}{[se(\ln OR)]^2}$$

$$= 1.75 \tag{4}$$

and compare it to a chi-square distribution on 1 df.

Log-Linear Model

An alternative method for describing a set of data is to use the log-linear model (Bishop et al., 1975; Fienberg, 1977; Haberman, 1978). One advantage of the log-linear model is that it can easily be generalized to the case where one wishes to adjust for potential confounding factors. We now describe this model for the case of one risk factor, and in the next main section (p. 386) we consider the more general case. The log-linear model is similar to an analysis of variance model on the log frequencies, but its chief advantage for our purpose is the fact that we can pick out parameters that yield the log of the odds ratio. For disease group d ($1 =$ control, $2 =$ case) and risk group r ($= 1, \ldots, R$), we have the expected frequency N_{rd} for which we observe n_{rd}. If $L_{rd} = \ln N_{rd}$, then a log-linear model gives

$$L_{rd} = \mu + \rho_r + \delta_d + (\rho\delta)_{rd} \tag{5}$$

This expression has more parameters than can be uniquely determined, so we let $\sum_r \rho_r = \sum_d \delta_d = \sum_r (\rho\delta)_{rd} = \sum_\delta (\rho\delta)_{rd} = 0$. Observed log frequencies are l_{dr}, which for our example gives:

	d	
r	1	2
1	7.5949	6.7901
2	6.8876	6.1738

The parameter μ is described as the grand mean of the log frequencies and is given by

$$\mu = \frac{1}{2R} \sum_d \sum_r L_{dr}$$

which we estimate by

$$\hat{\mu} = \frac{1}{(2)(2)} (7.5949 + 6.7901 + 6.8876 + 6.1738)$$
$$= 6.8616$$

The main effect for disease is δ_d, and because $\delta_1 + \delta_2 = 0$, we have $\delta_2 = -\delta_1$. This parameter gives the deviation of the column mean of log frequencies from the grand mean:

$$\delta_d = \frac{1}{R} \sum_r L_{rd} - \mu$$

estimated by

$$\hat{\delta}_1 = \tfrac{1}{2}(7.5949 + 6.8876) - 6.8616$$
$$= 0.3797$$

and

$$\hat{\delta}_2 = -\hat{\delta}_1 = -0.3797$$

Similarly, the main effect for risk group r is

$$\rho_r = \tfrac{1}{2} \sum_d L_{rd} - \mu$$

estimated by

$$\hat{\rho}_1 = \tfrac{1}{2}(7.5949 + 6.7901) - 6.8616$$
$$= 0.3309$$

and

$$\hat{p}_2 = -\hat{p}_1 = -0.3309$$

In the present context the main effects are not of special interest, but, as we shall see, the interactions $(\rho\delta)_{rd}$ give us the log odds ratio. In terms of the log expected frequencies, we have the deviation from a simple additive effect due to risk group and disease.

$$(\rho\delta)_{rd} = L_{rd} - (\mu + \rho_r + \delta_d)$$

estimated by

$$\widehat{(\rho\delta)}_{11} = 7.5949 - (6.8616 + 0.3797 + 0.3309)$$
$$= 0.0227$$
$$= \widehat{(\rho\delta)}_{22}$$

and

$$\widehat{(\rho\delta)}_{12} = \widehat{(\rho\delta)}_{21} = -\widehat{(\rho\delta)}_{11} = -0.0227$$

The log odds ratio is given by

$$\log \frac{n_{11}n_{22}}{n_{21}n_{12}} = l_{11} - l_{21} - l_{12} + l_{22}$$
$$= \widehat{(\rho\delta)}_{11} - \widehat{(\rho\delta)}_{21} - \widehat{(\rho\delta)}_{12} + \widehat{(\rho\delta)}_{22}$$
$$= 4(0.0227)$$
$$= 0.0908$$

which is algebraically equivalent to the value in eq. (2), the slight difference being due to rounding error. A test of the null hypothesis that the odds ratio is 1 is equivalent to testing the null hypothesis that $(\delta\rho)_{dr}$ is 0 for all d and r.

To test whether $(\delta\rho) = 0$ we can compare the fit of a model where all parameters are estimated, to the fit of a model in which the $(\delta\rho)_{rd}$ are set to 0, and the other parameters, are estimated subject to that restriction. If $(\delta\rho)_{rd} = 0$, then the expected frequency is estimated by

$$\hat{N}_{rd} = \frac{n_{r+}n_{+d}}{n_{++}} \tag{6}$$

where $n_{r+} = \sum_d n_{rd}$, $n_{+d} = \sum_r n_{rd}$ and $n_{++} = \sum_r \sum_d n_{rd}$. Using our present example, the expected cell frequencies under our null model are as follows:

	d	
r	1	2
1	1968.86	908.14
2	999.14	460.86

The Pearson chi-square statistic is one that may be used as a test of the null hypothesis,

$$\chi^2 = \sum_r \sum_d \frac{(n_{rd} - \hat{N}_{rd})^2}{\hat{N}_{rd}}$$

$$= \frac{(1988 - 1968.86)^2}{1968.86} + \frac{(889 - 908.14)^2}{908.14}$$

$$+ \frac{(980 - 999.14)^2}{999.14} + \frac{(480 - 460.86)^2}{460.86}$$

$$= 1.75$$

This would be compared to a chi-square distribution with $(R - 1) = 1$. When we have only two risk groups $(R = 2)$, we have the simplified expression for the chi-square statistic:

$$\chi^2 = \frac{(n_{11}n_{22} - n_{12}n_{21})^2 n_{++}}{n_{1+}n_{2+}n_{+1}n_{+2}} \tag{7}$$

Another statistic that is often computed is the likelihood ratio statistic given by

$$G^2 = 2 \sum_r \sum_d n_{rd} \ln(n_{rd}/\hat{N}_{rd})$$

$$= 2\left[1988 \ln\left(\frac{1988}{1968.86}\right) + 889 \ln\left(\frac{889}{908.14}\right) \right.$$

$$\left. + 980 \ln\left(\frac{980}{999.14}\right) + 480 \ln\left(\frac{480}{460.86}\right) \right]$$

$$= 1.74$$

This statistic would also be compared to chi-square on $(R - 1) = 1 \, df$.

We have so far given three chi-square tests for the null hypothesis that the odds ratio is 1: the Wald test, W^2; the Pearson chi-square, χ^2; and, the likelihood ratio statistic, G^2. They all gave very similar values, although they are not algebraically equivalent. In large samples all three of these become equivalent, and on this basis there is little to choose among them. These tests are useful when the expected frequencies are at least five, but for smaller frequencies it is preferable to use Fisher's exact test (see Armitage, 1971, pp. 135–138).

Dose–Response Relationships

DISPLAYING A TREND

In our discussion thus far we have just considered the effect of any smoking during the third month of pregnancy on congenital mal-formations. This analysis has suggested very little in the way of an

Table 16-3. Distribution of Mothers of Cases and Controls According to Average Number of Cigarettes Smoked per Day During the Third Month of Pregnancy

Number of cigarettes mothers smoked/day (r)	Disease status (d)	
	1. Controls	2. Cases
1.　0	1988	889
2.　1–10	426	182
3. 11–20	420	203
4. 21–30	86	55
5.　$\geqslant$31	48	40

Source: Modified from Kelsey et al. (1978).

effect due to smoking, but the measurement of exposure in just two categories is very crude. A better indication of exposure can be determined by the average number of cigarettes smoked per day. In Table 16-3 we have a more detailed breakdown of cigarette consumption. The parameters from the log-linear model are shown in Fig. 16-1. Once again we focus on the (disease × smoking) interaction to measure the association of smoking with disease. If we choose the risk group r_0 as a reference, then the log odds ratio comparing group r to r_0 is estimated by

$$\ln OR(r,r_0) = (\rho\delta)_{r_0 1} - (\rho\delta)_{r_0 2} - (\rho\delta)_{r1} + (\rho\delta)_{r2}$$

Fig. 16-1. Log-linear model parameters for data in Table 16-3.

Grand mean:
　5.3019

Disease (δ):
Control	Case
-0.3012	0.3012

Smoking (ρ):
Number of cigarettes

0	1–	11–	21–	31–
1.8906	0.3273	0.3749	-1.0711	-1.5218

Disease × smoking ($\rho\delta$):
	0–	1–	11–	21–	31–
Control	0.1012	0.1240	0.0624	-0.0777	-0.2101
Case	-0.1012	-0.1240	-0.0624	0.0777	0.2101

For example, to compare the ⩾31 cigarette group with nonsmokers, we obtain

$$\ln OR(⩾31,0) = 0.1012 - (-0.1012) - (-0.2101) + 0.2101$$
$$= 0.6226$$

and

$$OR = e^{0.6226}$$
$$= 1.86$$

To investigate the trend in the log odds ratio with average number of cigarettes smoked, we can carry out a similar calculation for each smoking category. Alternatively, we may compute the quantity.

$$\ln(P_{r2}/P_{r1}) = L_{2r} - L_{1r}$$
$$= (\delta_2 - \delta_1) + [(\delta\rho)_{2r} - (\delta\rho)_{1r}] \tag{8}$$

The term $(\delta_2 - \delta_1)$ is constant, independent of risk group r; hence the trend can be observed by only considering $(\delta\rho)_{2r} - (\delta\rho)_{1r}$. Another reason for ignoring $(\delta_2 - \delta_1)$ is that it depends on the proportion of subjects who develop the disease in question, which is not possible, generally, from a case-referent study. A plot of $(\rho\delta)_{r2} - (\rho\delta)_{r1}$ (Fig. 16-2) indicates the trend in log odds for disease with cigarette

Fig. 16-2. Trend in odds ratio for congenital malformations by average number of cigarettes. Solid line, linear trend for all groups; dashed line, linear trend among smokers only.

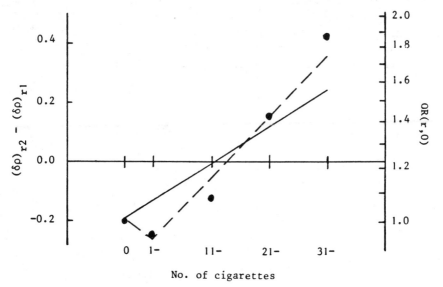

consumption. The right vertical shows the corresponding odds ratio relative to nonsmokers giving the corresponding antilog for the left vertical. It is useful to give both axes, the left giving the actual quantity being plotted. The right axis is useful for reference purposes, as most investigators are more familiar with the odds ratio. Choosing a reference group for the odds ratio is necessarily arbitrary, but a different choice would only shift the right axis leaving the pattern unchanged.

To test for an association between cigarette smoking by the mother and a congenital malformation in the child, we can use either the Pearson chi-square or the likelihood ratio statistics. For the data in Table 16-3 we obtain a Pearson chi-square:

$$\chi^2 = 13.11$$

($df = 4$, $p = 0.011$). In contrast to the earlier results, the more precise measurement of exposure does suggest an association between congenital malformations and smoking in the third month of pregnancy by the mother. Figure 16-2 suggests a dose–response relationship, but up to this point we have not made use of the natural ordering of risk groups in our significance test.

LINEAR LOGISTIC MODEL

For a systematic trend such as that observed in Fig. 16-2, one should try to describe it further. Taking the analysis further can give greater power to a significance test by considering a more specific null hypothesis. In addition, it has the advantage of giving a parsimonious summary of the results in terms of a model or equation. One method of model fitting is the use of a linear logistic model. To describe the association between a risk factor and disease, the linear logistic model assumes

$$\ln(P_{2r}/P_{1r}) = \alpha + X_1\beta_1 + X_2\beta_2 + \cdots + X_p\beta_p \tag{9}$$

where X_1, X_2, ..., X_p are regressor variables and α, β_1, β_2, ..., β_p parameters to be estimated. This expression can generate the log odds of eq. (8) by defining

$$
\begin{aligned}
X_1 &= 1 && \text{if } r = 1 \\
&= -1 && \text{if } r = 5 \\
&= 0 && \text{otherwise} \\
X_2 &= 1 && \text{if } r = 2 \\
&= -1 && \text{if } r = 5 \\
&= 0 && \text{otherwise}
\end{aligned}
$$

380

$$X_3 = \quad 1 \qquad \text{if } r = 3$$
$$= -1 \qquad \text{if } r = 5$$
$$= \quad 0 \qquad \text{otherwise}$$
$$X_4 = \quad 1 \qquad \text{if } r = 4$$
$$= -1 \qquad \text{if } r = 5$$
$$= \quad 0 \qquad \text{otherwise}$$

The correspondences among parameters are

$$\delta_2 - \delta_1 = \alpha$$
$$(\delta\rho)_{21} - (\delta\rho)_{11} = \beta_1$$
$$(\delta\rho)_{22} - (\delta\rho)_{12} = \beta_2$$
$$(\delta\rho)_{23} - (\delta\rho)_{13} = \beta_3$$
$$(\delta\rho)_{24} - (\delta\rho)_{14} = \beta_4$$
$$(\delta\rho)_{25} - (\delta\rho)_{15} = -(\beta_1 + \beta_2 + \beta_3 + \beta_4)$$

An advantage of using the linear logistic representation of eq. (9) is that we can also consider a linear trend with dose:

$$\ln(P_{2r}/P_{1r}) = \alpha \mid X_r\beta$$

where X_r gives the dose. For the present data we might use midpoints for the smoking categories, for example:

$$X_r = \quad 0 \qquad \text{for nonsmokers}$$
$$= \quad 5 \qquad \text{for } 1\text{–}10 \text{ cigarettes/day}$$
$$= 15 \qquad \text{for } 11\text{–}20 \text{ cigarettes/day}$$
$$= 25 \qquad \text{for } 21\text{–}30 \text{ cigarettes/day}$$
$$= 35 \qquad \text{for } \geqslant 31 \quad \text{cigarettes/day} \qquad (10)$$

A test of the null hypothesis that the slope $\beta = 0$ indicates whether there is significant linear trend in the log odds ratio.

SIMPLE TEST FOR TREND

One method of fitting a model is by the method of maximum likelihood. This method yields estimates that have optimal statistical properties; however, the amount of calculation required to fit a model by this method may be large. The reason for this is that for some models one cannot obtain a simple expression for the parameter. Instead one uses an iterative technique whereby one guesses a value for the parameter and subsequently modifies it until one is sufficiently near the optimal value. Other models can be fitted directly, because one can give an equation for the parameters. One such model is the null model when $\beta = 0$. In this case the expected frequencies are given by eq. (6). A statistical test that only requires fitting a null model is the score test (Rao, 1973, pp. 417, 418), and for linear trend in the log odds for disease this is given by

$$S^2 = \frac{\left[\sum_r X_r(n_{r2} - \hat{N}_{r2})\right]^2}{V\left(\sum_r X_r n_{r2}\right)}$$

where $\hat{N}_{r2}$ is given by eq. (6) and

$$V\left(\sum_r X_r n_{r2}\right) = \frac{n_{+1}n_{+2}}{n_{++}^2}\left[\sum_r n_{r+}(X_r - \bar{X})^2\right]$$

where $\bar{X} = \sum_r n_{r+}X_r/n_{++}$ is the mean observed dose. When using a calculator it is convenient to note that

$$\sum_r n_{r+}(X_r - \bar{X})^2 = \sum_r n_{r+}X_r^2 - \frac{\left(\sum_r n_{r+}X_r\right)^2}{n_{++}}$$

This test was proposed by Armitage (1955) as a test of linear trend for proportions, but it is also a test of linear trend for the log odds ratio (see Cox, 1970, pp. 61–65). Intermediate calculations for the data in Table 16-3 are shown in Table 16-4. This gives

$$V\left(\sum_r X_r n_{r2}\right) = \frac{(2968)(1369)}{(4337)^2}\left[351,300 - \frac{(18,990)^2}{4337}\right]$$

$$= 57,925.11$$

and

$$S^2 = \frac{(6730 - 5994.40)^2}{57,925.11}$$

$$= 9.34$$

which is compared to a chi-square distribution ($df = 1$, $p = 0.0022$).

Table 16-4. Intermediate Calculations for Score Test of Linear Trend for Data in Table 16-3

X_r	n_{2r}	N_{2r}	n_{+r}	$X_r n_{2r}$	$X_r N_{2r}$	$X_r n_{+r}$	$X_r^2 n_{+r}$
0	889	908.14	2877	0	0	0	0
5	182	191.92	608	910	959.60	3040	15,200
15	203	196.65	623	3045	2949.75	9345	140,175
25	55	44.51	141	1375	1112.75	3525	88,125
35	40	27.78	88	1400	972.30	3080	107,800
Totals				6730	5994.40	18,990	351,300

MODEL FITTING

Although the chief advantage of the score test is ease of computation, a disadvantage is that parameter estimates are not obtained and the assumptions regarding trend are not investigated. To fit this model we use a computer program for the linear logistic model. The response is the number of cases out of the total number of subjects in a particular response group. Equation (10) can be used as the independent variable, although there is some advantage to using

$$X_r^* = X_r - \tilde{X}$$

where $\tilde{X}$ is a simple mean of X over the 5 risk groups. The slope β is unaffected by this coding scheme, and $X_r^*\beta$ gives fitted log odds values standardized so that $\sum_r X_r^*\beta = 0$. Hence these may be plotted in Fig. 16-2 to investigate the adequacy of the model. The result of fitting gives parameter estimates and their standard errors

		Estimate	Standard error
Intercept (α)		0.6324	0.05635
X^*	(β)	0.01231	0.00404

A Wald test of the null hypothesis that the slope is 0, uses the parameter estimate and its standard error:

$$W^2 = \left(\frac{0.01231}{0.00404}\right)^2$$

$$= 9.28$$

($df = 1$, $p = 0.0023$), which is analogous to S^2 of the score test in the previous subsection. The fitted trend line ($X_r^*\beta$) is shown by the solid line in Fig. 16-2. This suggests a systematic departure of the trend from the smoothed line. The points in the graph suggest that instead of a smooth increase in risk, there may be a threshold, in that there appears to be very little effect for mothers who smoke one to ten cigarettes per day. A test of fit for the model can be obtained by comparing observed and fitted values using either Pearson chi-square ($\chi^2 = 3.37$) or the likelihood ratio statistic ($G^2 = 3.38$), both with 3 df. Neither of these tests of fit is statistically significant, and they could not attain significance at the nominal 0.05 level even if a single parameter (i.e., 1 df) could account for the lack of fit.

Comparing the likelihood ratio statistics G^2 with and without the variable X^* included gives the contribution to fit by the independent variable X^*. The change that results in the goodness of fit statistic is

$$\nabla G^2 = G^2(0) - G^2(\hat{\beta})$$

where $G^2(0)$ is the likelihood ratio statistic when X^* is not included (i.e., $\beta = 0$) and $G^2(\hat{\beta})$ when it is (i.e., β is estimated). In our present example we have

$$\Delta G^2 = 12.52 - 3.38$$
$$= 9.14$$

($df = 1$, $p = 0.0025$), which is yet another test of the null hypothesis, $\beta = 0$. We have given three tests of significance for β: the score test, the Wald test, and now the likelihood ratio test. All three are equivalent in large samples (Rao, 1973, p. 418), and any one of them may be used. The advantage of either the likelihood ratio or Wald tests is that the slope parameter has been estimated in the process. However, the score test can be very easily computed using a hand calculator.

When fitting a model to data one must be prepared to consider alternatives when an initial idea seems inappropriate. We have already indicated a systematic departure from a simple linear relationship shown in Fig. 16-1. Another model might exclude the contribution of nonsmokers to the trend line by introducing an indicator variable for nonsmokers. This gives two independent variables for our model: X_1 as defined in eq. (10) and

$$X_2 = 1 \qquad \text{if nonsmoker}$$
$$= 0 \qquad \text{otherwise}$$

Now we have the contribution for nonsmokers, $\alpha + \beta_2$ and smokers $\alpha + X_1\beta_1$. Such a model may be the result of a fundamental difference between smoking and nonsmoking mothers. Alternatively, a threshold below which there is no effect of smoking would also be consistent with the present data.

Normalizing values of the independent variables by subtracting the mean over all groups gives

X_1^*	X_2^*	Average number of cigarettes/day
−16	0.8	0
−11	−0.2	1–10
−1	−0.2	11–20
9	−0.2	21–30
19	−0.2	≥31

Parameter estimates resulting from the fit using X_1^* and X_2^* as independent variables are

Source	Estimate	Standard error
Intercept	−0.6201	0.0567
β_1	0.0207	0.0065
β_2	0.1831	0.1112

A Wald test of $\hat{\beta}_2$,

$$W^2 = \left(\frac{0.1831}{0.1112}\right)^2$$
$$= 2.71$$

$(df = 1, p = 0.10)$, indicates whether nonsmokers are significantly off the line for a simple linear relationship. The likelihood ratio statistic for goodness of fit is now $G^2 = 0.65$ $(df = 2, p = 0.72)$, and the change from the model with only X_1^* included gives a likelihood ratio test of the null hypothesis $\beta_2 = 0$

$$\Delta G^2 = 3.38 - 0.65$$
$$= 2.73$$

which corresponds to the Wald statistic. The fit of this model is shown by a plot of $X_1^*\hat{\beta}_1 + X_2^*\hat{\beta}_2$ given by the broken line in Fig. 16-2. No systematic departure is now apparent, but neither is there a significant improvement in fit.

When searching for an equation that adequately describes the relationship between a potential risk factor and disease, it is important to display the results so that one can see how well the model does. Systematic departures from fit and a significant lack of fit indicate that the equation is not appropriate for the data. An exploration of the data to find an appropriate model will sometimes involve consideration of additional variables such as the present example. In other situations one may wish to consider different functions of dose (e.g., log dose is often appropriate) in order to linearize the relationship. Such an exploration of the data will provide clues on an empirical basis of the relationship between risk factor and disease. The analysis of our example suggests a threshold for the effect of cigarette smoking, but there were not sufficient data to yield a statistically significant result. In any case, validation from other studies would be important when a model is arrived at using an exploratory approach such as that described above.

ADJUSTMENT FOR OTHER FACTORS

The previous section described the effect of smoking on congenital malformations. This factor was considered by itself, and no other factor was simultaneously considered as a risk factor for congenital malformations. Another potential risk factor that might be considered is tranquilizer use by the mother during pregnancy (Bracken and Holford, 1981). In Table 16-5 we see the distribution of cases

Table 16-5. Distribution of Cases with Congenital Malformations and Controls by Exposure to Tranquilizers and Cigarettes in Pregnancy

Average number of cigarettes/ day (c)	1. Control		2. Cases		(d)
	1. No	2. Yes	1. No	2. Yes	(r)
1. 0	1916	47	848	30	
2. 1–20	826	13	361	21	
3. ≥21	122	8	75	18	
Total	2864	68	1284	69	

Source: Modified from Bracken and Holford (1981).

and controls by smoking. At this point in our analysis we are only considering three smoking categories (0, 1–20, and ≥21 cigarettes/day). The frequencies in each smoking category are slightly less than those indicated in Table 16-3 because of a lack of information on tranquilizer use for some women.

If we ignore cigarette smoking and just consider the effect due to tranquilizer use alone, we obtain the odds ratio:

$$OR = \frac{(69)(2864)}{(68)(1284)}$$
$$= 2.26$$

and a Pearson chi-square test of association

$$\chi^2 = 23.13$$

($df = 1$, $p < 0.001$). However, an examination of the distribution of tranquilizer use by cigarette smoking suggests that heavy smokers are more likely to use tranquilizers than nonsmokers. At this point we might ask whether the tranquilizer effect may be due to its association with smoking. Hence we now consider the effect of tranquilizer use, adjusting for cigarette smoking as a covariate.

Model for Two Factors

The log-linear model that we now consider for disease group d (= 1,2), risk or tranquilizer group r (= 1, ..., R), and covariate or cigarette category c (= 1, ..., C) is

$$L_{rdc} = \mu + \rho_r + \gamma_c + \delta_d + (\rho\gamma)_{rc} + (\rho\delta)_{rd} + (\gamma\delta)_{cd} + (\rho\gamma\delta)_{rcd} \quad (11)$$

where $L_{rdc} = \ln N_{rdc}$, the log of the expected frequency. The usual parameterization for the log linear model requires that

$$\sum_r \rho_r = \sum_c \gamma_c = \sum_d \delta_d = \sum_r (\rho\gamma)_{rc}$$
$$= \sum_c (\rho\gamma)_{rc} = \sum_r (\rho\delta)_{rd} = \sum_d (\rho\delta)_{rd} = \sum_c (\gamma\delta)_{cd}$$
$$= \sum_d (\gamma\delta)_{cd} = \sum_r (\rho\gamma\delta)_{rcd} = \sum_c (\rho\gamma\delta)_{rcd} = \sum_d (\rho\gamma\delta)_{rcd} = 0$$

Parameters of special interest are the interaction terms that include δ or disease, as these determine the log odds ratio for disease. The log odds ratio comparing levels r to r_0 of the risk factor at level c of the covariate is

$$\ln OR(r,r_0|c) = \ln \frac{N_{r_0 1c} N_{r2c}}{N_{r_0 2c} N_{r1c}}$$
$$= L_{r_0 1c} - L_{r_0 2c} - L_{r1c} + L_{r2c}$$
$$= [(\rho\delta)_{r_0 1} - (\rho\delta)_{r_0 2} - (\rho\delta)_{r1} + (\rho\delta)_{r2}]$$
$$\quad + [(\rho\gamma\delta)_{r_0 c1} - (\rho\gamma\delta)_{r_0 c2} - (\rho\gamma\delta)_{rc1} + (\rho\gamma\delta)_{rc2}]$$

If the three-way interaction terms $(\rho\gamma\delta)$ are all zero, then the log odds ratio and the odds ratio are constant over the level of the covariate. In this case the association between risk factor and disease is given by the parameters $(\rho\delta)$. In a similar way $(\gamma\delta)$ gives the association between the covariate and disease.

Mantel–Haenszel Procedures

When the odds ratio is constant over levels of the covariate, it is reasonable to summarize the results with a single quantity that is an average value. A score test of the null hypothesis that the constant odds ratio is zero (Cox, 1970, pp. 58–61) is given by the Mantel–Haenszel (1959) statistic:

$$S^2 = \frac{\left[\sum_c (n_{11c} - \hat{N}_{11c}) \right]^2}{\sum_c V(n_{11c})} \tag{12}$$

where $\hat{N}_{11c}$ is the estimated expected frequency under the null hypothesis:

$$\hat{N}_{11c} = \frac{n_{1+c} n_{+1c}}{n_{++c}}$$

and

$$V(n_{11c}) = \frac{n_{1+c} n_{2+c} n_{+1c} n_{+2c}}{n_{++c}^2 (n_{++c} - 1)}$$

Table 16-6. Calculation of the
Mantel–Haenszel Statistic for the
Data in Table 16-5

n_{11c}	N_{11c}	$V(n_{11c})$	$\dfrac{n_{11c}n_{22c}}{n_{++c}}$	$\dfrac{n_{12c}n_{21c}}{n_{++c}}$
1916	1909.80	16.002	20.232	14.029
826	815.64	7.112	14.206	3.844
122	144.84	5.609	9.848	2.691
2864	2840.28	28.723	44.286	20.564

For our example, the intermediate calculations are shown in Table 16-6, giving

$$S^2 = \frac{(2864 - 2840.28)^2}{28.723}$$

$$= 19.59$$

which has a chi-square distribution ($df = 1$, $p < 0.001$). Mantel and Haenszel (1959) recommended a continuity correction, giving a slight modification to eq. (12):

$$S_c^2 = \frac{\left[\left|\sum_c (n_{11c} - N_{11c})\right| - \tfrac{1}{2}\right]^2}{\sum_c V(n_{11c})}$$

$$= \frac{(|2864 - 2840.28| - \tfrac{1}{2})^2}{28.723}$$

$$= 18.77$$

One estimator of the common odds ratio is given by

$$OR_{MH} = \frac{\sum_c n_{11c}n_{22c}/n_{++c}}{\sum_c n_{12c}n_{21c}/n_{++c}}$$

(Mantel and Haenszel, 1959). The fourth and fifth columns of Table 16-6 give intermediate results for our example, and our estimate of the odds ratio is

$$OR_{MH} = \frac{44.286}{20.564}$$

$$= 2.15$$

However, this is not a maximum likelihood estimate, and we must use an iterative technique to find one.

Model Fitting for Two Factors

We can find a maximum likelihood estimate of the common log odds ratio by fitting this model in eq. (11) without the parameters ($\rho\gamma\delta$). The parameter estimates and expected frequencies resulting from this are shown in Fig. 16-3. Maximum likelihood estimates of the odds ratio can be obtained using either the expected frequencies or the parameter estimates. Using the expected values for the nonsmoking group, we obtain

$$OR = \frac{(1923.24)(37.24)}{(39.76)(840.76)}$$

$$= 2.14$$

Identical values are obtained by using either of the other two smoking categories. Alternatively we can use the fact that the common log odds ratio is

$$\ln OR = (\rho\delta)_{11} - (\rho\delta)_{12} - (\rho\delta)_{21} + (\rho\delta)_{22}$$

Fig. 16-3. Log-linear model parameters and expected frequencies for the data in Table 16-5.

Grand mean:
  4.509

Disease main effect (δ):
  0.153   −0.153

Tranquilizer main effect (ρ):
  1.498   −1.498

Cigarette main effect (γ):
  0.890   0.060   −0.950

Disease–tranquilizer interaction ($\rho\delta$):
  0.191   −0.191
  −0.191   0.191

Disease–cigarette interaction ($\gamma\delta$):
  0.070   0.061   −0.131
  −0.070   −0.061   0.131

Tranquilizer–cigarette interaction ($\rho\gamma$):
  0.251   0.239   −0.490
  −0.251   −0.239   0.490

Expected values:

Cigarette	Control		Case	
	No	Yes	No	Yes
0	1923.24	39.76	840.76	37.24
1–20	821.59	17.41	365.41	16.59
≥21	119.17	10.83	77.83	15.17

Using the estimates of the $(\delta\rho)$ parameters (i.e., the disease–tranquilizer interaction), we obtain

$$\ln OR = 0.191 - (-0.191) - (-0.191) + 0.191$$
$$= 0.764$$

and the antilog gives

$$OR = 2.15$$

The slight differences in the numerical results are due to rounding and not to mathematical differences in the method. These estimates are not algebraically equivalent to the Mantel–Haenszel estimate, although they agree very well in this example.

An alternative to the Mantel–Haenszel test of the common odds ratio is the likelihood ratio test, which compares the goodness of fit including and excluding the disease–risk factor interactions. The test statistic is

$$\Delta G^2 = G^2(0) - G^2(\delta\rho)$$

where $G^2(0)$ is the goodness of fit under the null hypothesis [i.e., $(\rho\gamma\delta) = 0$ and $(\rho\delta) = 0$] and $G^2(\delta\rho)$ when the disease–risk factor association is estimated. For our example we have

$$\Delta G^2 = 25.16 - 6.71$$
$$= 18.45$$

$(df = 3 - 2 = 1, p < 0.001)$. There is also an equivalent Wald test, but most log-linear model programs do not give the appropriate variance estimate. This can be obtained by fitting a linear logistic model, if it were appropriate. However, we now have evidence that our constant odds ratio model is inappropriate. This is suggested by the likelihood ratio statistic, $G^2 = 6.71$ $(df = 2, p = 0.035)$ and the Pearson chi-square, $\chi^2 = 6.62$ $(df = 2, p = 0.037)$.

Variable Odds Ratio

To investigate the assumption of constant odds ratio further, we compute the odds ratio for each cigarette category as well as the Pearson chi-square test of association $(df = 1)$:

Number of cigarettes/day	OR	χ^2	p
0	1.44	2.41	0.121
1–20	3.70	15.11	<0.001
≥ 21	3.66	9.17	0.002

It is apparent that the association is strong among smokers but not nonsmokers. In fact, the association is not significant for nonsmokers.

The estimate of the odds ratio is nearly identical for the two smoking categories; hence, to obtain a final summary, we shall investigate whether the association is significantly different among the smoking groups.

In order to choose our own parameterization, we use the linear logistic model, where the log odds for disease is

$$\ln(P_{r2c}/P_{r1c}) = \alpha + X_{1rc}\beta_1 + X_{2rc}\beta_2 + \cdots + X_{prc}\beta_p \qquad (13)$$

For the log-linear model of eq. (11) we have the log odds for disease

$$\begin{aligned}
\ln(N_{rc2}/N_{rc1}) &= L_{rc2} - L_{rc1} \\
&= (\delta_2 - \delta_1) + [(\rho\delta)_{r2} - (\rho\delta)_{r1}] \\
&\quad + [(\gamma\delta)_{c2} - (\gamma\delta)_{c1}] + [(\rho\gamma\delta)_{rc2} - (\rho\gamma\delta)_{rc1}]
\end{aligned}$$

An equivalent parameterization for our example can be obtained by defining a linear logistic model where

$$\begin{aligned}
X_1 &= 1 &&\text{if } r = 1 \\
&= -1 &&\text{if } r = 2 \\
X_2 &= 1 &&\text{if } c = 1 \\
&= -1 &&\text{if } c = 3 \\
&= 0 &&\text{otherwise} \\
X_3 &= 1 &&\text{if } c = 2 \\
&= -1 &&\text{if } c = 3 \\
&= 0 &&\text{otherwise} \\
X_4 &= X_1 X_2 \\
X_5 &= X_1 X_3
\end{aligned}$$

Parameters are given by

$$\begin{aligned}
(\rho\delta)_{12} - (\rho\delta)_{11} &= -[(\rho\delta)_{22} - (\rho\delta)_{21}] = \beta_1 \\
(\gamma\delta)_{12} - (\gamma\delta)_{11} &= \beta_2 \\
(\gamma\delta)_{22} - (\gamma\delta)_{21} &= \beta_3 \\
(\gamma\delta)_{32} - (\gamma\delta)_{31} &= -\beta_2 - \beta_3 \\
(\rho\gamma\delta)_{112} - (\rho\gamma\delta)_{111} &= -[(\rho\gamma\delta)_{122} - (\rho\gamma\delta)_{211}] = \beta_4 \\
(\rho\gamma\delta)_{122} - (\rho\gamma\delta)_{121} &= -[(\rho\gamma\delta)_{222} - (\rho\gamma\delta)_{221}] = \beta_5 \\
(\rho\gamma\delta)_{132} - (\rho\gamma\delta)_{131} &= -[(\rho\gamma\delta)_{232} - (\rho\gamma\delta)_{231}] = -\beta_4 - \beta_5
\end{aligned}$$

The comparison of interest here is between the two smoking groups; hence we adopt a different parameterization. For the comparison of nonsmokers with the average of the two smoking groups, let

$$\begin{aligned}
X_2 &= 2 &&\text{if } c = 1 \\
&= -1 &&\text{if } c = 2, 3
\end{aligned}$$

and define X_1 and X_3 as above. Ignoring the interaction variables, X_4

and X_5, for the moment, and holding constant the tranquilizer variable X_1, we have the log odds

$$\alpha + X_1\beta_1 + 2\beta_2 \qquad \text{for nonsmokers}$$
$$\alpha + X_1\beta_1 - \beta_2 + \beta_2 \qquad \text{for smokers of 1 to 20 cigarettes}$$
$$\alpha + X_1\beta_1 - \beta_2 - \beta_3 \qquad \text{for smokers of} \geq 21 \text{ cigarettes}$$

The difference between the two smoking categories is given by

$$(\alpha + X_1\beta_1 - \beta_2 + \beta_3) - (\alpha + X_1\beta_1 - \beta_2 - \beta_3) = 2\beta_3$$

To test whether the log odds is equivalent for the two smoking categories, we consider the null hypothesis that $\beta_3 = 0$. In a similar way, the interactions $X_4 = X_1X_2$ and $X_5 = X_1X_3$ indicate the consistency of the log odds ratio. The log odds ratio for tranquilizer use is given by the difference in the log odds. Under the present parameterization we have the log odds ratio for each level of the covariate:

$$(\alpha-\beta_1+2\beta_2-2\beta_4)-(\alpha+\beta_1+2\beta_2+2\beta_4) \qquad\qquad\quad =-2\beta_1-4\beta_4 \qquad \text{if } c=1$$
$$(\alpha-\beta_1-\beta_2+\beta_3+\beta_4-\beta_5)-(\alpha+\beta_1-\beta_2+\beta_3-\beta_4+\beta_5)=-2\beta_1+2\beta_4-2\beta_5 \qquad \text{if } c=2$$
$$(\alpha-\beta_1-\beta_2-\beta_3+\beta_4+\beta_5)-(\alpha+\beta_1-\beta_2-\beta_3-\beta_4-\beta_5)=-2\beta_1+2\beta_4+2\beta_5 \qquad \text{if } c=3$$

The difference in the log odds ratio for the two smoking categories is given by

$$(-2\beta_1 + 2\beta_4 + 2\beta_5) - (2\beta_1 + 2\beta_4 - 2\beta_5) = 4\beta_5$$

Hence, a test of the null hypothesis that $\beta_5 = 0$ is a test of equivalence of log odds ratio for the two smoking categories.

For our example we have the estimated coefficients and their standard errors:

	Coefficient	Standard error
Intercept	-0.2146	0.1036
X_1	-0.4952	0.1036
X_2	-0.2087	0.0621
X_3	-0.1681	0.1437
X_4	0.1560	0.0621
X_5	-0.0025	0.1437

A Wald test of no difference in odds ratio between the two groups is

$$W^2 = \left(\frac{-0.0025}{0.1437}\right)^2$$
$$= 0.0003$$

which is obviously not significant. Similarly, the likelihood ratio test of the model that only excludes the independent variable X_5 is

$$G^2 = 0.0003$$

($df = 1$). To compare the odds ratio for nonsmokers with an average of the two smoking groups, we compare the likelihood ratio statistic when neither interaction variable is included,

$$\Delta G^2 = 6.71 - 0.0003$$
$$= 6.71$$

($df = 1$, $p = 0.010$).

The conclusion we reach from this analysis is that the association between tranquilizer use and congenital malformations depends on whether the mother is also a smoker. If the mother smokes during pregnancy, then there is an estimated 3.7-fold increase in the odds for a congenitally malformed child by using tranquilizers. The estimate of the odds ratio for a mother who does not smoke is 1.44, but this is not statistically significant at the nominal 0.05 level.

More Than Two Factors

The methods we have used in this section can be extended to the problems of adjusting for more than one covariate. One approach is to stratify by the additional covariates and compute the Mantel–Haenszel statistic as shown above. It is implicit in such a summary that the odds ratio is constant over all the strata and it does not depend on any of the covariates. As long as this is true, the method gives a valid summary of the data. The method does break down rather quickly as the number of covariates becomes large, however. Very detailed stratifications result in many instances of zero marginal frequencies in the 2×2 tables. These strata contribute no information on the disease–risk factor association, and the test statistic goes to zero.

One way to think of this problem with the Mantel–Haenszel statistic is to consider the corresponding model that would have been fitted. In this case one is effectively adjusting not only for the association between the covariate and disease, but also for all the possible interactions. This results in a very large number of parameters that are being controlled. For a large number of strata one can overfit the data, resulting in no information to test the association of interest.

An alternative to the stratification procedure is model fitting using either log-linear or linear logistic programs. This allows one considerable flexibility in the way in which covariates are controlled. When using such an approach it is important to keep in mind the fit of the data. This can be done by considering interactions and polynomial terms in the model. Another useful method is to categorize continuous variables like blood pressure in much the same way as our treatment of numbers of cigarettes smoked. This enables one to plot the log odds for disease so that the form of the relationship can be investigated. Sometimes a change of scale for a factor (e.g., the use of log dose) can result in a linear trend in the log odds for disease. In addition, one might consider a function other than the log odds for disease. The computer package GLIM (Baker and Nelder, 1978) gives one considerable flexibility in the type of model that can be considered.

CONCLUSION

The purpose of data analysis is to obtain a summary of the data. There is no formula that can always be used to give a valid summary. An analyst should explore the data and give it every opportunity to discredit one's preconceptions of the relationship between a putative risk factor and disease. We have discussed some ways of displaying the results and observing the fit of the model in order to see how well the model agrees with the data.

An important feature of all statistical methods is that some assumption must be made in order to carry out a significance test or describe the quantity to be estimated. Many of the commonly used methods in epidemiology, such as the Mantel–Haenszel test and tests for trend, can be derived as score tests of log-linear or linear logistic models. The advantage of fitting a model is that it provides a mechanism whereby one can consider more general representations of the data. However, a powerful method such as this should not be used without considerable care. It is not enough to simply run data through a computer program and report the estimated coefficients. Effort also should be expended in investigating the form of a trend and the adequacy of the fit.

Cohort studies can present special problems when the condition develops over time and one is investigating length of time until the disease occurs. The literature in this area is covered in texts by Elandt-Johnson and Johnson (1980), Kalbfleisch and Prentice (1980), and Lee (1980). Log-linear models also can be used to analyze data in this form (Holford, 1980; Laird and Olivier, 1981). The overall strategy remains one of exploring the data to find useful summaries of the results.

REFERENCES

Armitage, P. (1955). Tests for linear trends in proportions and frequencies. *Biometrics 11*, 375–386.

———— (1971). *Statistical methods in medical research.* Oxford: Blackwell.

Baker, R.J. and Nelder, J.A. (1978). *The GLIM system, release 3, generalized linear interactive modelling.* Harpenden, Herts, England: Rothamsted Experimental Station.

Bishop, Y.M.M., Fienberg, S.E., and Holland, P.W. (1975). *Discrete multivariate analysis.* Cambridge, Mass.: MIT Press.

Bracken, M.B. and Holford, T.R. (1981). Exposure to prescribed drugs in pregnancy and association with congenital malformations. *Am. J. Obstet. Gynecol. 58,* 336–344.

Breslow, N.E. (1977). Some statistical methods useful in the study of occupational mortality. In *Environmental health: Quantitative methods,* edited by A. Whittemore. Philadelphia: Society for Industrial and Applied Mathematics, pp. 88–103.

———— and Day, N.E. (1980). *Statistical methods in cancer research.* Vol. 1, *The analysis of case control studies.* Lyons, France: International Agency for Research on Cancer.

————, ————, Halvorsen, K.T., Prentice, R.L., and Sabia, C. (1978). Estimation of multiple relative risk functions in matched case-control studies. *Am. J. Epidemiol. 108,* 299–307.

Cornfield, J. (1951). A method of estimating comparative rates from clinical data. Applications to cancer of the lung, breast and cervix. *J. Ntl. Cancer Inst. 11,* 1269–1275.

Cox, D.R. (1970). *The analysis of binary data.* London: Methuen & Co.

Elandt-Johnson, R.C. and Johnson, N.L. (1980). *Survival models and data analysis.* New York: Wiley.

Fienberg, S.E. (1977). *The analysis of cross-classified categorical data.* Cambridge, Mass.: MIT Press.

Haberman, S.J. (1978). *Analysis of qualitative data.* Vol. 1, *Introductory topics.* New York: Academic Press.

Holford, T.R. (1978). The analysis of pair-matched case-control studies, a multivariate approach. *Biometrics 34,* 665–672.

———— (1980). The analysis of rates and of survivorship using log-linear models. *Biometrics 36,* 299–305.

———— (1982). Covariance analysis for case-control studies with small blocks. *Biometrics 38,* 673–683.

————, White, C., and Kelsey, J.L. (1978). Multivariate analysis of matched case-control studies. *Am. J. Epidemiol. 107,* 245–256.

Kalbfleisch, J.D. and Prentice, R.L. (1980). *The statistical analysis of failure time data.* New York: Wiley.

Kelsey, J.L., Dwyer, T., Holford, T.R., and Bracken, M.B. (1978). Maternal smoking and congenital malformations: An epidemiological study. *J. Epidemiol. Community Health 32,* 102–107.

Laird, N. and Olivier, D. (1981). Covariance analysis of censored survival data using log-linear analysis techniques. *J. Am. Stat. Assoc. 76,* 231–240.

Lee, E.T. (1980). *Statistical methods for survival data analysis.* Belmont, Calif.: Lifetime Learning Publications.

Liddell, F.D.K., McDonald, J.C., and Thomas, D.C. (1977). Methods of cohort analysis: Appraisal by application to asbestos mining. *J. R. Stat. Soc. (A) 140,* 469–491.

Mantel, N. and Haenszel, W. (1959). Statistical aspects of the analysis of data from retrospective studies of disease. *J. Ntl. Cancer Inst.* 22, 719–748.

Miettinen, O.S. (1976). Estimability and estimation in case-referent studies. *Am. J. Epidemiol.* 103, 226–235.

Prentice, R.L. and Breslow, N.E. (1978). Retrospective studies and failure time models. *Biometrika* 65, 153–158.

Rao, C.R. (1973). *Linear statistical inference and its applications*, 2nd Ed. New York: Wiley.

17

Design and Conduct of Randomized Clinical Trials in Perinatal Research

Michael B. Bracken

Randomized clinical trials (RCTs) are defined as studies in which the efficacy of one or more experimental diagnostic or therapeutic procedures is compared with that of a control procedure by randomly assigning patients to experimental or control groups and later comparing the groups for differences in outcome after follow-up for a specific time period. Such studies are increasingly being used to assess the efficacy of treatment methods in obstetrics (Bracken, 1983), perinatology, and neonatology. Their results play a prominent role in policy discussions of the risks and benefits of medical procedures; witness the importance of RCTs in the debate on electronic fetal monitoring in the United States, (Banta and Thacker, 1978; Hobbins et al., 1979; Council on Scientific Affairs, 1981). The science of designing, conducting, and analyzing RCTs is itself expanding rapidly, highlighted by the recent establishment of the Society for Clinical Trials with its own journal. Particular attention is being paid to the special problems of conducting cooperative multicenter RCTs that are necessitated by the increasing study of diseases with too small an incidence, or very rare outcomes, for investigation at a single hospital (Ederer, 1975; Sylvester et al., 1981). This chapter reviews the principles involved in designing and conducting perinatal RCTs, draws examples from some major trials in the literature, and considers the compromises that must be made when performing rigorously designed RCTs in acute-care perinatal settings.

Acknowledgment. The author is grateful to Richard A. Ehrenkrantz M.D., John C. Hobbins M.D., and Ralph I. Horowitz M.D. for their suggestions during the preparation of this chapter. Financial support was partly provided by a grant (NS 15078) from the National Institute of Neurological and Communicative Disorders and Stroke.

Investigators must pay a high price for the benefits of an RCT. They are expensive and difficult to design, and they pose significant management problems. Fredrickson's (1968) description of RCTs as "the indispensable ordeal" is appreciated by the clinical trial manager who invariably considers Murphy (of "what can go wrong, will" fame) a sublime optimist. Although RCTs are important, the question of when they are appropriate is itself a complex issue. Chalmers (1975) has argued that the first time any patient is given a new treatment he or she should be assigned by random allocation either to the new or to a standard treatment. Because deciding whether to embark on an RCT is difficult and involves questions of ethics and study design, we review these issues in detail below.

Randomized trials tend to be conducted at three distinct points when a new procedure is introduced. First, new drugs or devices are tested to evaluate their safety and efficacy prior to marketing. In the United States such studies are often conducted to meet Federal Drug Administration (FDA) requirements. Second, randomized trials are used when a drug approved and in use for one purpose is tried for another. The early trials of corticosteroids for the prevention of respiratory distress (RDS) in premature newborns exemplify this (Liggins and Howie, 1972). The third point is when a treatment procedure has entered widespread practice, but doubt arises as to its efficacy or safety. The electronic fetal monitoring (EFM) trials reflect the third point (Haverkamp et al., 1976, 1979; Renou et al., 1976; Kelso et al., 1978). The EFM trials were, as Fredrickson suggests, "a relatively late expression of uncertainty" and entered "a terrain already littered with preconceived opinion" (Fredrickson, 1968, p. 988).

The ethical dilemma underlying the debate as to when an RCT should be conducted concerns the balancing of unnecessary risks to patients currently under treatment, and who may receive what is eventually found to be the less efficacious treatment, with the possible benefits of the RCT to future patients (Calabresi, 1970). Weinstein (1974) described this as "making a transfer of welfare from the experimental subject to the future patient" (p. 1284). Stated another way, the dilemma concerns the potential conflict of the physician's role as clinician and as scientist.

PILOT STUDIES

The case for random assignment of the first patient ever to receive a new drug or medical procedure is made on the grounds that a nonrandomized pilot study makes it difficult to organize the more definitive RCT subsequently. Three reasons are given. First, the nonrandomized pilot study may so convince investigators of the benefits of the new therapy that they feel ethically unable to randomize later patients to what they consider to be the less effective treatment. Second, the new treatment is not considered beneficial, and clinicians refuse to assign future patients into that treatment group. Third, the results are equivocal, and the investigator loses interest in the new treatment and searches for other more promising innovations (Chalmers et al., 1972; Chalmers, 1975).

Because the great majority of pilot projects utilize small numbers of patients, these studies have low statistical efficiency and the chance of incorrectly proving or disproving the null hypothesis (also, respectively, called Type 1 and Type 2 errors) is high. Not only do poorly controlled pilot studies lead to premature rejection of what might be beneficial new therapies, they also lead to the premature acceptance of nonbeneficial therapies into general medical practice. The inclination of investigators to write up and of editors to publish the results of positive rather than negative pilot studies augments this phenomenon. The publication records of many new therapies show a larger proportion of positive results in the early reports with later published studies apt to refute the earlier claims of benefit. Because the results of small, uncontrolled pilot studies can be so misleading, their lack of certainty should be made obvious.

Gehan and Freireich (1974) and Weinstein (1974) argue that uncontrolled pilot studies are necessary to develop more precise estimates of dose schedules, refine surgical procedures, and obtain "preliminary estimates" of efficacy and complications. Because it is precisely the effect of such preliminary estimates on the investigator's subsequent practice that concerns Chalmers, these are irreconcilable positions. Gehan and Freireich (1974) state that "if a patient suffers severe toxicity from a new therapy in a randomized Phase 1 study, it is difficult to undertand how a clinician could derive any ethical comfort from the fact that the patient had an equal chance of receiving the conventional therapy" (p. 198). Chalmers (1975) argues that there is considerable ethical relief in randomizing patients who are at risk of complications.

Our own experience has been that pilot studies are essential before large multicenter RCTs can be set up. In addition to the reasons cited above, they are essential to refine data collection protocols and instruments, validate methods for measuring the outcome variable, identify problems in overall study management, develop intercenter contractual agreements, and establish appropriate human consent procedures. Sample size estimation also requires some preliminary knowledge of the effect of the study treatment (see Chapter 15, p. 360).

ALTERNATIVES TO RANDOMIZATION

Several alternatives to early randomization have been proposed:

1. Historical controls taken either from previously treated patients or from reports in the literature can be used.
2. Concurrent patients who *elect* to be managed by standard rather than innovative treatment can be enrolled. These patients may in some situations be "match-paired" with patients in the experimental group.
3. Patients may be enrolled who have served as controls, cases, or both in previous studies. This approach is appropriate if the investigators are engaged in a series of studies of variations in a management protocol, for example, different doses of the same drug. However, selection criteria, response measures, and other therapies must remain unchanged from one study to the next.
4. The allocation of patients to alternative treatments may be based on a decision-making strategy in which the latest evidence from the trial influences the allocation. One example, is Zelen's "play the winner rule" (Zelen, 1969). Each patient is allocated to a treatment on the basis of the success or failure of the treatment given to the previous patient in the study. If, for example, the preceding patient did well on treatment A, the next patient receives treatment A. If the first patient did poorly on treatment A, the subsequent patient is given B. It is argued that fewer patients will be given the less effective treatment than when random allocation is used.

However, in a multicenter trial, where outcomes may be assessed many months after treatment, it is hardly feasible to allocate patients to treatments on the basis of knowledge already produced by the trial. For, example, the national collaborative study on antenatal dexamethasone therapy to prevent RDS included 9-, 18-, and 36-month detailed neurologic examinations to detect any possible long-term sequelae to the steroid (Collaborative Group on Antenatal Steroid Therapy, 1981). Such a variety of long-term outcome measures precludes the use of an adaptive allocation design. Other aspects of adaptive allocation are discussed below.

ADVANTAGES OF RANDOMIZATION

Although there is much to be said for considering alternative strategies to random allocation in designing clinical trials, the double-blind randomized trial remains the optimal design. Five considerations favor randomization.

1. Many authors in the medical trial literature discuss the design of studies as if they were investigating differences in the effect of *treatments*. Actually, the great majority of RCTs evaluate differences in *managing* patients with or without inclusion of the allocated treatment (Sackett and Gent, 1979). This is not a subtle distinction. It has implications for many design issues, some of which are discussed below. Random allocation is important because it increases the probability of achieving comparable distributions of both known and unknown *confounding variables* in both treatment groups. Nonrandom allocation schemes may achieve equality in known major confounders, such as other treatment procedures, but obviously cannot do so for unidentified confounders.

2. Both known and unknown *prognostic indicators* that are characteristic of the patient or her condition need to be considered. Thus, in studies of antenatal steroids, gestational age, rupture of membranes, cervical dilation, and presence or absence of uterine contractions might all be controlled. Even within these major prognostic categories for RDS, however, great variability in prognosis could still exist. Only randomization adequately controls for these "unknown" sources of variance.

3. It is difficult to persuade reviewers, editors, and colleagues that the results of a study are valid unless random allocation is used. This is not a trivial reason for randomizing if the clinical trial is performed to influence future medical practice as it should be.

4. The proposed alternatives to randomized trials are not necessarily more ethical procedures. Byar et al. (1976) have pointed out that permitting physicians to treat their patients in the manner they consider best implies that the poorly informed physician is ethically as secure as the well-informed one who may treat patients quite differently. "It is not sufficient to practice what one believe is best; one must do what is in accord with sound scientific evidence. Ethical behavior alone is not sufficient to determine best treatment" (p. 78).

WHAT QUESTIONS SHOULD RCTs ADDRESS?

Because RCTs are expensive and complex undertakings, they should investigate only the most significant clinical questions (Peto et al., 1976). In drug trials it is almost always preferable to have a placebo against which to contrast the experimental drug. However, when a widely used therapy already exists, it is necessary to compare the new treatment to a standard therapy. Failure to use a placebo poses problems in interpreting the results of those RCTs that find no difference in the efficacy of either drug (if two drugs are being compared) or dose (if a low dose is compared with a high dose of the same drug). The investigator cannot tell whether neither of the treatments are efficacious or whether both are equally beneficial. This difficulty is intensified when the control treatment itself has not been appropriately evaluated in an RCT.

In drug trials it is advantageous to make the treatment doses as disparate as is ethically possible or, in a placebo trial, make the treatment dose as large as good clinical practice permits. Here too the investigator wishes to reduce the possibility, in the event of a null result, that the experimental dose was too low to obtain an effect. Drug trials investigate the drug regimen as well as studying drug dose. Thus it is important that the drug regimen follow accepted clinical practice. Studies with negative results are more useful if the investigator feels confident that this is not due to an inadequate drug regimen. The importance of these aspects of study design for interpreting negative RCT results is stressed, because the majority of RCTs fail to show any significant difference between treatments.

The difficulty in interpretation that can follow from inappropriate choice of study drug, comparison treatment, and drug regimen is exemplified by the RCTs of antenatal steroid therapy (Table 17-1). There is considerable variation in the amount and type of steroid used, the frequency with which the steroid was given, and the protocol for avoiding premature delivery until completion of the full course of treatment. Thus, even though all of the RCTs show a positive effect of steroids, it is not possible to decide what an optimal treatment protocol should be. This problem is further compounded by differences in patient eligibility for the study, which are reviewed later. The Collaborative Group on Antenatal Steroid Therapy (1981) results would have been much more definitive if betamethasone had been studied (to replicate the earlier work) and at higher doses (to see if further reductions in the incidence of RDS could be achieved).

Evaluation of surgical techniques (Bonchek, 1979) and adjusted dose schedules by RCTs is fraught with considerably more difficulty than are fixed dose schedule drug studies. The effectiveness of a drug is not influenced by physician skill when given in a fixed regimen, and the results of drug studies in an RCT—methodological issues not-with-standing—are usually generalizable to other medical centers. The success or failure of surgery and of drug schedules adjusted to the patient's condition depends much more on the skill of the operator and on nuances in technique that are virtually impossible to control. Additionally, surgical techniques and drug regimens are being constantly changed in subtle but critical ways. Early surgical and pharmacologic innovators may have success rates that are difficult for others to replicate. Special skills possessed by early practitioners may

Table 17-1. Comparative Treatments and Treatment Regimen for RCTs of Antenatal Steroid Therapy

Reference	Study treatments	Treatment regimen	Tocolytic protocol
Liggins and Howie (1972)	6 mg betamethasone acetate + 6 mg betamethasone phosphate vs. 6 mg cortisone acetate	On admission and 24 hours later if undelivered	Intravenous ethanol or salbutamol for 48–72 hours
Block et al. (1976)	12 mg betamethasone or 125 mg methylprednisolone vs. saline	On admission and 24 hours later if undelivered	Alcohol drip for 48 hours minimum
Taeusch et al. (1979)	4 mg dexamethasone phosphate vs. saline	On admission and every eight hours for six doses or until delivery	Tocolytics not given
Papageorgiou et al. (1979)	6 mg betamethasone acetate + 6 mg betamethasone phosphate vs. vehicle of steroid preparation (not specified)	On admission, 24 hours later, and weekly until delivery or 34 weeks gestation	Isoxsuprine hydrochloride
Doran et al. (1980)	3 mg betamethasone acetate + 3 mg betamethasone phosphate vs. vehicle of steroid preparation (not specified)	On admission and every 12 hours for four doses or until delivery	Alcohol or isoxsuprine at obstetrician's discretion
Collaborative Group on Antenatal Steroid Therapy (1981)	5 mg dexamethasone phosphate vs. placebo	On admission and every 12 hours for four doses	Ethanol or isoxsuprine hydrochloride for 48 hours minimum

make innovative surgery and drug therapy more successful than achieved by later physicians; alternatively, because techniques are still being developed, early efforts might be less successful and complication rates higher.

Similarly, much of the instrumentation used in perinatology is constantly being developed. For example, ultrasound equipment provides either static or dynamic images and offers a wide range of methods for image enhancement (Deter, 1979; Kremkau, 1980). Any trial of an instrument per se is likely to be of only historical interest by the time the data are analyzed. Moreover, any trial that required the use of ultrasound—for example, trials of fetal surgery—would need to ensure that use of a specific advanced machine is a standard part of the study protocol.

Electronic fetal monitors are also under constant development, and it is of interest that whereas two of the EFM RCTs used the same monitor (Haverkamp et al., 1976, 1979), another trial used one of two different instruments (Kelso et al., 1978) but failed to consider the type of machine used in the statistical analysis. The instrumentation for analyzing blood and the scalp electrodes also varied between these RCTs. The fourth RCT of EFM (Renou et al., 1975) did not report which monitor(s) were studied or any of the other instrumentation used. Because the decision whether or not to perform cesarean section depends to a large extent on interpreting data produced by the monitor (Murphy et al., 1981; Cohen et al., 1982), the choice of instrument is a critical consideration.

MANAGEMENT VERSUS EXPLANATORY TRIALS

Most RCTs evaluate the effect of innovations in the overall management of patients, not the efficacy of a particular treatment. This is a distinction that confuses much of the clinical trial research literature (Sackett and Gent, 1979). The steroid RCTs would only analyze those patients completing the full treatment schedule prior to delivery if they were studying the effect of the steroids themselves. Because they were, in fact, examining the possible benefit of steroid treatment in the management of threatened premature labor, all randomized patients should have been analyzed. This was only done, however, in the two most recent studies (Table 17-1).

Scheduling difficulties in emergency clinical settings are inevitable. Some patients will die before being started on treatment protocols; others will not complete all of a prescribed regimen, or some aspect of care will not be given optimally. For example, a drug might not be administered on schedule. To withdraw all of these patients from an

RCT would not simulate the role of the innovative therapy in normal clinical management. Moreover, the rate of protocol deviations may vary between treatment groups for important reasons. There may be some delay in giving one treatment over another, hence more patients may have chance to die before receiving that treatment. This crucial piece of knowledge about the impact of managing patients with the new treatment would be lost if deaths were excluded from analysis. Even if death is not caused by treatment delay, one would be reluctant to exclude the randomized dead patients' data from analysis. The first event after randomization (first administration of the drug, or death) is likely to be accidental. Thus to include both groups of patients in the trial's analysis does not lead to bias and may provide important information. In general, therefore, in clinical trials of therapeutic management all *randomized* patients enter data analysis (Peto et al., 1976, 1977). The only possible exception would be to exclude patients who were ineligible for the trial but had been incorrectly randomized.

It is important to note that multicenter trials do not demand that general management of patients be equivalent in participating centers. In a multicenter study of the effects of antenatal steroids on the newborn, it would *not* be necessary to standardize neonatal care at the participating centers. It can be assumed that if antenatal steroids were truly beneficial in reducing risk for RDS, this would occur at all centers irrespective of their neonatal management. This statement does not preclude the fact that nonsignificant, or even reverse, observations may be observed at a center because of chance. Each center must be a major stratification variable in the analysis. The possible interaction of antenatal steroid with other management procedures is an analyzable question (Armitage, 1981).

WHO SHOULD BE BLINDED IN CLINICAL TRIALS?

Blinding of Physicians

Although the question of "blinding" is often linked with randomization, it is a quite distinct design issue. Surgical trials, for example, may be randomized but not blinded. If many of the previously discussed ethical dilemmas are to be optimally resolved, physicians involved in patient care in a trial must be unaware of the ongoing results of the study; furthermore, they should preferably not know which arm of the study protocol a particular patient is in. The second important reason for blinding is to protect physicians from their own often subconscious biases toward one of the study treatments. For example,

405

because the diagnosis of RDS is frequently equivocal, it is not difficult to see how a systematic tendency to "diagnose" RDS in patients in one arm of the study could lead to a biased result.

Blinding for drug studies requires careful thought in packaging the treatments. They must look identical and have the same properties for dilution and administration. If one drug can be distinguished from another, even in a subtle way, and is thought to be the preferred dose, then serious bias can be introduced into the study even if the clinician guessed incorrectly. Clinicians may be asked to report which drug they thought their patient received as a check of whether treatment bias may have occurred. The risk of biasing the study not only stems from subconscious bias in evaluating the results of treatment but also from the way a clinician's expectations about the outcome of a particular treatment influence his or her overall management of the patient. This may include a tendency to overcompensate in other clinical maneuvers for the patient believed to be receiving the less effective treatment. The only way to protect against this type of bias is to blind the treating physicians. Where this is not possible, as in surgical trials, it is important that clinicians not involved in the patient's surgery perform the study evaluations. If this cannot be done blind because of scars or emplaced devices, objective data from X-ray films, laboratory tests, or other standardized measures should be used. A detailed report of all procedures performed on each study patient will allow for analysis of possible differences in the general treatment of the study groups.

Blinding of Patients

Patients are blinded in clinical trials for two major reasons. First, if blind, they are unlikely to withdraw from an RCT after being randomized into what they believe to be the less effective treatment. Such selective withdrawal would be extremely serious for the success of a trial. Second, blinding the patient avoids placebo effects. Ballintine (1975) reminds us that "history of medical treatment was the history of the placebo effect since until recently almost all medications were 'placebos' " (p. 763). When the outcome of a trial is a subjective response, such as a psychologic test, it is particularly important that patients not know which treatment schedule they received. A study of the efficacy of vitamin C showed that patients on placebo who thought they had vitamin C reported fewer colds than patients on vitamin C who believed they received placebo (Ederer, 1975). One simple technique for estimating whether a placebo effect has occurred is to ask patients which treatment they think they received and to anlayze the data by their response.

Blinding of Other Personnel

In addition to blinding clinical personnel it is also important to blind the coordinating managerial staff, computing personnel, and statisticians. None of these people are free of their own preconceived notions about the outcome of the trial. Whether a decision is being made to follow up a patient more intensively, to count a piece of data or to consider it missing, or to accept a statistical table as being the "final analysis," there is always room for bias.

WHICH METHOD SHOULD BE USED FOR RANDOMIZATION?

The literature is replete with accounts of major RCTs that failed to achieve a reliable result because randomization was inappropriate. Typically, patients were assigned to treatments on odd or even days, by having surnames with a certain letter, or by simple alternation. The fundamental problem with these methods of randomization is the physician's control in placing patients into treatment groups. For example, they can delay or speed up a patient's admission into hospital for the "preferred" treatment (Wright et al., 1954). Even the use of sealed envelopes does not guarantee full randomization, because the envelopes could be used other than consecutively or could be transilluminated to reveal treatment allocation (Carleton et al., 1960).

Ideally, patient randomization is performed outside the clinical setting. Physicians wishing to enter a patient into an RCT may be asked to call a central 24-hour telephone operator who will instruct them which treatment package to give the patient. The treatment packages for each patient should be uniquely numbered, so that a broken code for one patient does not jeopardize the entire RCT code. In a multicenter study each hospital's pharmacy can reconstitute drug preparations (sometimes also in a "blind" fashion) and deliver them to the treating physician.

Because the analysis of a multicenter RCT must be stratified by center, it is important that randomization ensure equivalence in treatment groups within each center. The simplest approach is to contain the randomization in a paired fashion (e.g., ABABAB) within each center. Simple pairing, however, makes it difficult to keep the study "blind," because clinic personnel can readily look for differences in treatment effects in alternating patients. It is preferable to constrain (or "block") randomization, so that within each block of six patients at any center the treatment regimen is always evenly divided (e.g., ABAABB/BAABABB). In studies with frequent patient intake, larger blocks of eight or ten might be chosen. Blocks greater than about ten, however, increase the risk of random imbalance between treatments within a participating center with a consequent loss of statistical efficiency in the study. Table 17-2 shows the randomization procedures for the antenatal steroid RCTs. For many of them the precise methods used could not be ascertained from the report, a frequent problem for many RCT publications (Der Simonian et al., 1982).

PATIENT ALLOCATION

The allocation of patients between treatment groups is an important design issue, involving three basic considerations: (1) Should assignment to treatment be balanced or unbalanced? (2) Should assignment be fixed for the entire length of the trial or adapted in some manner according to the trial's own experience? (3) Should potential confounding variables be controlled by stratification during randomization or in the analysis? These issues, more than all others, exemplify the compromises that must be made between the optimally designed study and the actual successful completion of an RCT in a clinical setting.

Fixed Balanced Allocation

Most RCTs allocate patients to study treatments using a simple balanced 1:1 (innovative treatment:control) ratio. This was used in all the antenatal steroid studies (Table 17-2). In some RCTs, unbalanced treatment allocation may be considered. For every one case given the experimental treatment, two receive a placebo or standard treatment. This may be considered if the new drug or surgical device is rare, difficult to obtain, or very expensive. Designing an unbalanced randomization algorithm is a relatively trivial problem, but it should not be undertaken lightly. Unbalanced allocation increases the risk of breaking the trial's blinding; it is also more difficult to manage and offers marginal improvement in terms of statistical efficiency, in that it requires almost as many patients as simple 1:1 allocation. Moreover, patients have more difficulty understanding unbalanced allocation when signing consent forms. If an unbalanced allocation is chosen it almost certainly should not exceed a 2:1 (control:experimental treatment) ratio. Having *fewer* controls than experimental cases is never justified.

Table 17-2. Eligibility, Allocation, Stratification, Randomization, and Blinding Aspects of the Design of the Antenatal Steroid RCTs

Reference	Eligibility criteria	Treatment allocation	Pre- or post-randomization stratification	Randomization procedures	Blinding
Liggins and Howie (1972)	Premature labor at 24–36 weeks gestation	1:1 Fixed	Post	Random order	Double
Block et al. (1976)	Premature labor, or premature with ruptured membranes, weeks unspecified	1:1 and later 1:1:1 Fixed	Post	Consecutively numbered	Double
Taeusch et al. (1979)	Premature labor ≤33 weeks, or premature with ruptured membranes, or cervical dilatation <5 cm, or >33 weeks with L/S ratio <2.0, or had infant with RDS	1:1 Fixed	Pre by gestational age	Random order	Double
Papageorgiou et al. (1979)	Premature labor at 25–34 weeks gestation, or premature with ruptured membranes	1:1 Fixed	Post	Numbered randomly	Double
Doran et al. (1980)	Premature labor or ruptured membranes at 24–34 weeks gestation	1:1 Fixed	Pre by gestational age	Randomly assigned	Double
Collaborative Group on Antenatal Steroid Therapy (1981)	High risk for premature delivery at 26–37 weeks gestation, cervical dilatation <5 cm, delivery anticipated 24 hours to seven days; if uncertain, L/S ratio <2.0	1:1 Fixed	Post	Blocked every ten patients within each center	Double

Adaptive Allocation

Much attention has been given in recent years to the issues of adaptive allocation in RCTs (Zelen, 1969; Weinstein, 1974; Hoel et al., 1975; Bailar, 1976; Simon, 1977; Healy, 1978). These include allocation designs with such fascinating titles as "Play the Winner," "One Step-Ahead," "Vector at a Time," and "Two-Arm Bandit." The essential common feature of these approaches is that they feed information from the ongoing RCT back into the allocation procedure so as to increase the proportion of patients receiving the most beneficial treatment. It is important not to confuse adaptive allocation with those rules established for sequential statistical analysis in order to *stop* the trial because one treatment has proved more successful than another. Although both treatment allocation and "stopping" procedures seek to reduce the number of patients that might be given the less efficacious treatment, they are distinct design aspects of a clinical trial and need to be considered separately.

Adaptive allocation has two advantages:

1. It allows the attending physician to treat the patient on the basis of the most recently available information.
2. It addresses the ethical argument that it is always wrong to subject a current patient to increased risks for the possible benefit to some future patient.

However, adaptive allocation schemes, although statistically quite elegant, have a number of significant problems that frequently make them unworkable in clinical settings.

1. Because treatment effects in the RCT must be known in order to adapt allocation, it increases the chance of the trial being unblinded.
2. Many trials examine outcomes that occur too late after treatment to be of use in influencing the allocation of new patients entering the trial.
3. It is exceedingly difficult to change allocation procedures on an ongoing basis, especially in a multicenter study. Clinicians, quite justifiably, would object to delays in treating their patients while some complicated allocation formula was followed.
4. The statistical analysis of RCTs with adaptive allocation is controversial. The results of such a trial could come under heavy assault from many quarters, thereby causing sufficient concern to discredit or negate any beneficial influence the trial might have on future medical practice.
5. Patients are unlikely to understand (and less likely to agree to) consent forms that describe how they will be adaptively allocated to a particular treatment.

410

6. Many response variables are *not* dichotomous (improved vs. not improved) measures but rather complex estimates of a patient's well-being. Selecting any one outcome for adaptive allocation precludes the examination of the effect of treatment on other outcomes, because distribution of the two treatment groups would no longer be unbiased.

7. Adaptive allocation precludes the study of other clinical factors that may confound or modify the effect of the particular treatment being studied. Many such clinical factors, moreover, cannot be predicted before the trial is analyzed.

8. Most clinical trials assess the relative effectiveness of one treatment against another while accounting for a comparison of risks for each treatment. At present there is no satisfactory statistical technique for analyzing this type of cost–benefit ratio on multiple variables in a manner appropriate for influencing allocation into an ongoing RCT.

Crossover Designs

One of the most elegant designs for an RCT is the crossover design in which patients act as their own control group. Each patient is assigned to one of the trial's treatments on a random basis and then followed to obtain a response. The patient is next switched to the other treatment and followed to obtain a second response. However, only chronic conditions (such as intractable pain) or recurring episodic illnesses (typically colds and flu) are generally amenable to this type of study design.

Crossover designs are appealing to the statistician because they eliminate variation among patients. This variation, if uncontrolled, can be more troublesome than the variance found between treatment groups. However, crossover designs introduce at least three serious difficulties (Brown, 1978). First, the effects of the two treatments may not be independent—that is, the *sequence* in which two treatments are given may itself influence response because of the interactions between the two treatments. This is particularly true if long biologic half-lives of compounds cause them to intrude on the second treatment stage. Second, the "disease" may be altered by the first treatment, so that the second treatment is actually for a different disease state. Third, the patient's own subjective response to treatment—for example, a "pain response" to the analgesic effects of a drug—may be conditioned by the effects of the first treatment.

Even if crossover designs were practically feasible, one would not wish to use them from one pregnancy to the next because of the importance of parity in many outcomes. Thus they are likely to play a limited role in perinatal research.

ENTRANCE ELIGIBILITY AND WITHDRAWAL CRITERIA

Several authors have reviewed design aspects of the entrance criteria for RCTs (Truelove, 1964; Weinstein, 1974; Ederer, 1975; Bailar, 1976; Peto et al., 1976). Several issues are discussed elsewhere in this chapter. A summary of generally accepted guidelines follows.

Eligibility

Only patients who meet specified diagnostic criteria for the disease should be eligible for study. It is unethical (and inefficient) to study patients who are not genuine candidates for the study treatment. This point is not as obvious as it seems when one thinks of the different prognoses for various stages and severities of any one disease entity. When the disease under study is highly specified, then the study will have more statistical power and will have less ambiguous results. Patients presenting likely follow-up difficulties, or those who have not given consent, must be considered ineligible. It is extremely important that all randomized patients can be eligible to receive all treatments. Any question about some patients being too ill, or not ill enough, to receive a treatment should be handled by modifying the eligibility criteria, preferably during the pilot study. It is critical that all decisions about eligibility be made *before* randomization. The loss of patients before randomization reduces the generalizability of the study but does not introduce bias. Reduced generalizability is not necessarily a problem, although there would be little point to doing an RCT that could not be generalized at all. Bias, however, is always a danger and can be sufficient to invalidate the entire RCT.

The major eligibility criteria for the antenatal steroid studies are shown in Table 17-2. Whereas these are generally comparable, some RCTs were much more specific than others, particularly in only including women in later pregnancy whose baby was at higher risk of developing RDS, by additional specification of low Lecithin/ Sphingomyelin (L/S) ratios.

Because withdrawal of patients after randomization can introduce serious bias into a study, it is preferable to postpone randomization until immediately before administration of the study treatments. This principle is based on practical rather than theoretical grounds. In theory, if patient randomization were entirely unbiased it would not matter what time it occurs before treatment. In practice, knowing (or guessing) the randomized treatment of a patient puts strong unconscious pressure on the physician to manage patients differentially or even to withdraw them prior to actual treatment. This leads to a breakdown in the comparability of treatment groups. In general, then, eligibility criteria should be developed to reduce subsequent patient withdrawals.

Patient Withdrawal

Once patients have been randomized into a study they can never be withdrawn. This is not to say that treatment cannot be discontinued, or a patient not followed up, but rather that in some manner or other all randomized patients must be accounted for in the analysis. Patients who withdraw their consent to continue in a clinical trial, or who are withdrawn by their physicians because of medical complications, can still provide informative data if they can be followed up, even if only to ascertain whether, say, they miscarried or had a livebirth. There is considerable debate among ethicists, however, as to how much information should be used from patients who refuse or withdraw consent (Jonas, 1970; Fried, 1974; Veatch, 1975).

In collaborative RCTs it is useful to insist that a detailed written report be provided of the reasons for withdrawal. This provides important documentation and reduces withdrawal for trivial reasons. Withdrawal from the study through loss to follow-up is another source of potentially serious bias. Every attempt should be made to obtain some information for every patient so that, at least, the reasons for loss to follow up can be compared for any possible associations with treatment.

When a protocol violation occurs, a decision must be made about the patient's status. If a scheduled drug dose is missed, it may be possible to give the drug immediately on discovering the error and so maintain the schedule. If too long a time has elapsed, the drug regimen will have to be discontinued. The ground rules for these decisions must be worked out in the pilot study, must be unambiguous, and should make pharmacologic sense (thus, protocol violations may depend on the time it takes for drug blood levels to fall). In all circumstances, however, the data obtained on an incomplete treatment regimen can still provide useful information and should be analyzed.

Failure to follow eligibility criteria will cause other withdrawals. There can be no rule of thumb here except that the study protocol should try to anticipate the causes of withdrawal and spell out the procedures to be followed. When it is found that certain patients have not given consent or were initially misdiagnosed, for example, these patients should be immediately put on appropriate standard therapy. Patients who were randomized in error and who violate criteria established for methodologic rather than ethical or clinical reasons may, under some circumstances, be continued in the experimental treatment. It becomes inefficient to exclude these patients once they have been started on treatment, and they may provide useful data although it would not be used in testing the major study hypothesis.

Even though randomization may be delayed until the moment prior to treatment, there will still be patients who die or who do not receive treatment after being randomized for some other reason. Should these patients be withdrawn from the analysis? This question was reviewed earlier within the context of whether the RCT is a study of overall patient management or a pharmacologic study of the drug per se. If the former is the case, the patient must be retained in the analysis, because it is important to know whether some feature of the drug administration itself influences the patient's outcome. All withdrawals from the study must be carefully monitored and documented to ensure they are occurring equally in each treatment group. If they are not, then some error in randomization, break in treatment blinding, or other serious protocol violation must be suspected.

PRE- OR POSTRANDOMIZATION STRATIFICATION

The manner in which confounding or effect-modifying variables should be controlled presents one of the most challenging decisions in designing RCTs. First, one must decide whether they should be controlled by stratification before randomization or by post hoc adjustment during analysis. In the present context, confounding risk factors are those that distort the true relative risk of the study treatment on the disease outcome, because the risk factor is itself associated with both exposure and disease outcome. An effect modifier interacts with study treatment and outcome to increase the precision of the estimate of true relative risk. Effect modifiers may be part of the causal pathway between treatment and disease outcome (Kleinbaum et al., 1982).

One method of prerandomization stratification is to limit the study to specific medical conditions, excluding patients with conditions known to confound the association of treatment with outcome. This can be a useful technique for a multicenter trial. Effect modifiers, however, cannot be used to exclude patients because they are of clinical and theoretical importance, and a decision to stratify before randomization or in the analysis must be made (Armitage, 1981).

Prerandomization stratification has two major advantages. First, it leaves less to chance in the randomization procedures; the number of cases and controls across each stratum of the effect modifiers is more likely to be balanced. Except in extremely large trials, randomization

414

cannot guarantee equal numbers of patients across all strata of all effect modifiers. In the Collaborative Group on Antenatal Steroid Therapy (1981) RCT for example, women in the steroid treatment arm were treated later in gestation than the placebo group. This imbalance could only be corrected in the analysis and resulted in considerable loss of statistical power. If the randomization had been blocked within gestational age categories this problem would have been avoided. Second, prerandomization stratification is conceptually easier to understand than is post hoc adjustment by multivariate analysis. Hence the results of the RCT are more likely to be accepted by the medical community.

Two considerations weigh against prerandomization stratification. First, statistical analysis is committed to methods that must account for the strata. This is particularly problematic when confounding factors, which were not prestratified, must be additionally controlled for in analysis (Peto et al., 1977). Second, patient entry into a prestratified study can be extremely complicated. It is possible to develop algorithms, based on knowledge of the patient's risk status, for assigning patients to treatment in a stratified fashion. However, these procedures can be quite complex, are prone to error, and can delay entry of the patient into treatment (Meier, 1981).

SAMPLE SIZE

The number of patients required by a clinical trial is a function of (1) the treatment effect that it is deemed clinically important for the trial to demonstrate, (2) the significance levels chosen to demonstrate that any observed treatment difference is not due to chance (called the α level and typically set at a 95% chance of an observed difference being correct), and (3) the probability of no observed difference between the treatments being a correct result (called the β level and usually ranges from an 80 to 95% probability). An erroneous treatment difference found in an RCT is called a Type 1 error. If no treatment differences are observed in an RCT when they actually exist, this is called a Type 2 error. See Chapter 18 for a more detailed discussion of this point.

Enormous numbers of patients are required for RCTs that set both α and β levels at 95%. In practice it is the β level that is relaxed in order to reduce the number of patients required for a study. This rests on the assumption that it is preferable to increase the chance of making a Type 2 error in a study than Type 1. The trial that fails to show a treatment effect when one actually exists has less serious consequences than one that mistakenly shows a new treatment to be an improvement over the standard treatment. The effect of a Type 1 error on (1) the welfare of future patients and (2) the progress of scientific research can be disastrous. The clinician should remember, however, that there is nothing sacrosanct about an α value of 0.05. In very rare medical conditions or where drugs are expensive, an RCT might be designed with α set at 0.1. This is preferable to not running an RCT at all because of a shortage of resources, although it is certainly not an optimal design.

In any RCT the number of patients needed increases when greater statistical power is demanded, smaller differences between treatments need to be detected, or the α level is lowered. A strong argument can be made in multicenter trials for calculating sample sizes at $\alpha = 0.01$ and $\beta = 0.95$ because of the need to stratify the analysis by center, to account for sample blocking, and to maintain the power of any necessary additional multivariate analyses (Brown, 1978).

Should one- or two-tailed statistical tests be used? The former will permit a smaller sample size. The one-tailed test is principally for when the RCT is testing only one hypothesis, for example: Drug A is more efficacious than placebo. In many clinical trials, however, the investigator is ethically committed also to determine whether the drug is significantly *worse* than placebo. In these studies a two-tailed statistical test is essential.

In reporting the results of an RCT, it is important to provide both the statistical power used to plan the study and also the power calculations for the data used in the final analyses. This will inform the reader of the actual probabilities of Types 1 and 2 errors for the study. This information was not provided for any of the four EFM trials and in only two of the five antenatal steroid trials. In general, study power appears to be the most underreported piece of information in published accounts of RCTs (Der Simonian et al., 1982).

SOME METHODS FOR INCREASING THE POWER OF AN RCT

A major epidemiologic problem in conducting RCTs of relatively rare conditions, or of more common conditions having rare outcomes, is the need to increase the statistical power of these studies. Multicenter studies are one method of increasing the number of available cases. Modification of the traditional α and β levels or use of one-tailed significance tests are other, albeit less satisfactory, approaches. There are at least six other general methods for increasing statistical power without requiring larger numbers of patients.

First, if studying a rare drug or a particularly expensive surgical intervention, the innovation to control allocation can be changed from the typical 1:1 to 1:2. Increasing the number of controls for each case reduces the number of cases in the experimental regimen that must be studied at any given level for α and β. The increase in efficiency is not great and, as described earlier, unbalanced allocation may cause other difficulties in the trial that preclude its use. Second, a study that uses survival time (e.g., how *long* patients survive, rather than the number of survivors) will gain additional power. Life table methods of analysis are used in this type of study. These techniques are straightforward and amenable to presentation in an understandable format (Peto et al., 1977). Third, the study outcome might be brought forward in time, for example, by using a prognostic rather than diagnostic indicator as an outcome measure, or by measuring morbidity rather than mortality. Fourth, more complete follow-up is essential to increase study efficiency. Brown (1978) has observed that six years follow-up on 2000 angina patients provides the same information as three years follow-up on 4000. In many RCTs, especially those of rare conditions, recruitment costs are expensive, and it is clearly preferable to ensure very complete case follow-up. For this reason, patients who are known to be difficult to follow-up (e.g., illegal aliens or patients transferred long distances from home) should not be randomized. Fifth, patient eligibility can be restricted to those patients with conditions thought to be most responsive to the experimental treatment. Sixth, the outcomes may be limited to those thought to be most influenced by treatment.

CONCLUSION

This chapter has reviewed only selected issues in the design and conduct of perinatal RCTs. We have not, for example, examined the design of questionnaires and other data collection instruments (Oppenheim, 1966; Gorden, 1969), methods of sequential (Armitage, 1975) and other statistical analyses (Peto et al., 1977), or the management aspects of an RCT, which range from daily staffing to the establishment of national monitoring committees (Klimt, 1981; Meinert, 1981).

The present chapter suggests that a tension often exists between the optimal design and conduct of an RCT, and clinical practice. To reduce this tension, an RCT should mimic as closely as possible normal medical practice and should interfere with routine patient care as little as possible. Sophisticated and complex RCT designs should be avoided unless they are essential. When essential they should be insisted on. Most perinatal RCTs in the foreseeable future are unlikely to require unbalanced and crossover or adaptive allocation. It is essential, however, that perinatal RCTs be blind, randomized, and have appropriate statistical power.

The principle of simplicity should guide the design of all aspects of the RCT. For example, data collection instruments should be specific to the study at hand and avoid at all costs the "since we're collecting data anyway, why not look at ..." philosophy. Sample sizes will usually be fixed in advance and the study hypothesis analyzed at the end of the study. Ongoing analysis will usually be limited to study of treatment complications. When an elegantly designed study founders on the hard realities of clinical practice it has served both investigators and patients badly. Moreover, launching the next trial is made even more difficult.

Obstetricians, pediatricians, and, more recently, neonatologists and perinatologists have constantly sought to improve their clinical practice, although the use of RCTs has not been a dominant methodology (Chalmers and Richards, 1977). Perinatal trials are often more complex than those of other disciplines and frequently require very long follow-up periods to ascertain the safety to both the mother and offspring of a treatment given to the mother for the benefit of her fetus. We should recall that significant numbers of young women with clear cell adenocarcinoma of the vagina and cervix were the subjects of RCTs to assess the value of diethylstilbestrol in reducing their mother's risk of spontaneous abortion (Herbst et al., 1979). In spite of these difficulties the number of perinatal RCTs reported in the literature have increased dramatically in recent years (Chalmers, 1980), as have useful reviews of specific RCTs including those of routine iron and vitamin use in pregnancy (Hemminki and Starfield, 1978), tocolytic drugs (Hemminki and Starfield, 1978a), and EFM (Chalmers, 1979).

If ongoing laboratory or clinical study is fortunate enough to discover an innovative approach that will impact dramatically on the management of the pregnant mother or her fetus, it will not be tested in an RCT. Penicillin, quite correctly, was never put into an RCT because its obvious efficacy was beyond dispute. The present reality for perinatal research, however, is that new therapies are likely to make only modest gains. When the increased benefits of new treatments are small they are correspondingly more difficult to evaluate. It is therefore crucial that each incremental improvement in perinatal patient management be secure in the knowledge that the improvement is real. The RCT is an essential tool for ensuring that each small but unequivocal gain in patient management provides a firm base on which to evaluate the next potentially advantageous maneuver.

Randomized clinical trials are essential for identifying the red herrings and blind avenues that plague perinatal, and indeed all clinical research, so that new investigation can focus on potentially even more beneficial treatment innovations.

REFERENCES

Armitage, P. (1975). *Sequential medical trials*, 2nd Ed. New York: Wiley.
—— (1981). Importance of prognostic factors in the analysis of data from clinical trials. *Controlled Clinical Trials 1*, 347–353.
Bailar, J.C. (1976). Patient assignment algorithms—An overview. In *Proceedings of the 9th International Biometric Conference*, Vol. 1. Raleigh, N.C.: Biometric Society, pp. 189–209.
Ballintine, E.J. (1975). Objective measurements and the double-masked procedure. *Am. J. Ophthalmol. 79*, 763–767.
Banta, H.D. and Thacker, S.B. (1978). *Costs and benefits of electronic fetal monitoring*. National Center for Health Services Research, U.S. Dept of Health, Education and Welfare.
Block, M.F., Kling, O.R., and Crosby, W.M. (1976). Antenatal glucocorticoid therapy for the prevention of respiratory distress syndrome in the premature infant. *Obstet. Gynecol. 50*, 186–190.
Bonchek, L.I. (1979). Are randomized trials appropriate for evaluating new operations? *N. Engl. J. Med. 301*, 44–45.
Bracken, M.B. (1983). Epidemiologic approaches to the evaluation of obstetrical innovations. *Mead Johnson Symp. Perinat. Dev. Med. 30*, 3–11.
Brown, B.W. (1978). *Statistical controversies in the design of clinical trials*, Technical Report No. 37, Division of Biostatistics, Stanford University, Stanford, Calif.
Byar, D.P., Simon, R.M., Friedewald, W.T., Schlesselman, J.J., DeMets, D.L., Ellenberg, J.H., Gail, M.H., and Ware, J.H. (1976). Randomized clinical trials: Perspectives on some recent ideas. *N. Engl. J. Med. 295*, 74–80.
Calabresi, G. (1970). Reflections on medical experimentation in humans. In *Experimentation with human subjects*, edited by P.A. Freund. New York: Braziller, pp. 178–196.
Carleton, R.A., Sanders, C.A., and Burack, W.R. (1960). Heparin administration after acute myocardial infarction. *N. Engl. J. Med. 263*, 1002–1005.
Chalmers, I. (1979). Randomized controlled trials of fetal monitoring 1973–1977. In *Perinatal medicine*, edited by O. Thalhammer, K. Baumgarten, and A. Pollack. Stuttgart: George Thieme.
—— (1980). *Clinical trials in perinatal medicine*. Paper presented at the Symposium on the Application of the Randomized Controlled Trial to Perinatal Medicine and Pediatrics, Faculty of Health Sciences, McMaster University, Hamilton, Ontario, October 27–28.
—— and Richards, M. (1977). Intervention and causal inference in obstetric practice. In *Benefits and hazards of the new obstetrics*, edited by T. Chard and M. Richards. Philadelphia: J.B. Lippincott.

Chalmers, T.C. (1975). Randomization of the first patient. *Med. Clin. North Am. 59*, 1035–1038.

———, Block, J.B., and Lee, S. (1972). Controlled studies in clinical cancer research. *N. Engl. J. Med. 287*, 75–78.

Cohen, A.B., Klapholz, H., and Thompson, M.S. (1982). Electronic fetal monitoring and clinical practice. A survey of obstetric opinion. *Med. Decision Making 2*, 79–95.

Collaborative Group on Antenatal Steroid Therapy (1981). Effect of antenatal dexamethasone administration on the prevention of respiratory distress syndrome. *Am. J. Obstet. Gynecol. 141*, 276–286.

Council on Scientific Affairs (1981). Electronic fetal monitoring. *J.A.M.A. 246*, 2370–2373.

Der Simonian, R., Charette, J., McPeek, B., and Mosteller, F. (1982). Reporting on methods in clinical trials. *N. Engl. J. Med. 306*, 1332–1337.

Deter, R.L. (1979). Advances in imaging. In *Diagnostic ultrasound in obstetrics*, edited by J.C. Hobbins. New York: Churchill Livingstone.

Doran, T.A., Swyer, P., MacMurray, A., Mahon, W., Enhorning, G., Bernstein, A., Falk, M., and Wood, M.M. (1980). Results of a double-blind controlled study on the use of betamethasone in the prevention of respiratory distress syndrome. *Am. J. Obstet. Gynecol. 136*, 313–320.

Ederer, F. (1975). Practical problems in collaborative clinical trials. *Am. J. Epidemiol. 102*, 111–118.

Fredrickson, D.S. (1968). The field trial: Some thoughts on the indispensable ordeal. *Bull. N.Y. Acad. Med. 44*, 985–993.

Fried, C. (1974). *Medical experimentation: Personal integrity and social choice*. In *Clinical Studies*, Vol. 5, edited by A.G. Bearn, D.A.K. Black, and H.H. Hiatt. New York: American Elsevier.

Gehan, E.A. and Freireich, E.J. (1974). Non-randomized controls in cancer clinical trials. *N. Engl. J. Med. 290*, 198–203.

Gorden, R.L. (1969). *Interviewing: Strategy, techniques and tactics*. Homewood, Ill.: Dorsey Press.

Haverkamp, A.D., Orleans, M., Langendoerfer, S., McFee, J., Murphy, J., and Thompson, H.E. (1979). A controlled trial of the differential effects of intrapartum fetal monitoring. *Am. J. Obstet. Gynecol. 134*, 399–412.

———, Thompson, H.E., McFee, J.G., and Cetrulo, C. (1976). The evaluation of continuous fetal heart rate monitoring in high risk pregnancy. *Am. J. Obstet. Gynecol. 125*, 310–320.

Healy, M.J.R. (1978). New methodology in clinical trials. *Biometrics 34*, 709–712.

Hemminki, E. and Starfield, B. (1978). Routine administration of iron and vitamins during pregnancy: Review of controlled clinical trials. *Br. J. Obstet. Gynaecol. 85*, 404–410.

——— and ——— (1978a). Prevention and treatment of premature labour by drugs: Review of controlled clinical trials. *Br. J. Obstet. Gynaecol. 85*, 411–417.

Herbst, A.L., Scully, R.E., and Robboy, S.J. (1979). Prenatal diethylstilbestrol exposure and human genital tract abnormalities. In *Perinatal carci-*

420

nogenesis, edited by J.M. Rice. National Cancer Institute Monograph 51. U.S. Dept. of Health, Education and Welfare Publ. No. (NIH) 79-1633. Washington, D.C.: National Institutes of Health.

Hobbins, J.C., Freeman, R., and Queenan, J.T. (1979). The fetal monitoring debate. *Pediatrics 63*, 942–951.

Hoel, D.G., Sobel, M., and Weiss, G.H. (1975). A survey of adaptive sampling for clinical trials. *Perspect. Biometrics 1*, 29–61.

Jonas, H. (1970). Philosophical reflections on experimenting with human subjects. In *Experimentation with human subjects*, edited by P.A. Freund. New York: Braziller, pp. 1–29.

Kelso, I.M., Parsons, R.J., Lawrence, G.F., Shyam, S.A., Edmonds, D.K., and Cooke, I.D. (1978). An assessment of continuous fetal heart rate monitoring in labor. *Am. J. Obstet. Gynecol. 131*, 526–532.

Kleinbaum, D.G., Kupper, L.L., and Morgenstern, H. (1982). *Epidemiologic research*. Belmont, Calif.: Lifetime Learning Publications.

Klimt, C.R. (1981). The conduct and principles of randomized clinical trials. *Controlled Clinical Trials 1*, 283–293.

Kremkau, F.W. (1980). *Diagnostic ultrasound: Physical principles and exercises*. New York: Grune & Stratton.

Liggins, G.C. and Howie, R.N. (1972). A controlled trial of antepartum glucocorticoid treatment for prevention of the respiratory distress syndrome in premature infants. *Pediatrics 50*, 515–525.

Meier, P. (1981). Stratification in the design of a clinical trial. *Controlled Clinical Trials 1*, 355–361.

Meinert, C.L. (1981). Organization of multicenter clinical trials. *Controlled Clinical Trials 1*, 305–312.

Murphy, J.R., Haverkamp, A.D., Langendoerfer, S., and Orleans, M. (1981). The relation of electronic fetal monitoring patterns to infant outcome measures in a random sample of term size infants born to high risk mothers. *Am. J. Epidemiol. 114*, 539–547.

Oppenheim, A.N. (1966). *Questionnaire design and attitude measurement*. New York: Basic Books.

Papageorgiou, A.N., Desgranges, M.F., Masson, M., Colle, E., Shatz, R., and Gelfand, M.M. (1979). The antenatal use of betamethasone in the prevention of respiratory distress syndrome: A controlled double-blind study. *Pediatrics 63*, 73–79.

Peto, R., Pike, M.C., Armitage, P., Breslow, N.E., Cox, D.R., Howard, S.V., Mantel, N., McPherson, K., Peto, J., and Smith, P.G. (1976). Design and analysis of randomized clinical trials requiring prolonged observation of each patient. I. Introduction and design. *Br. J. Cancer 34*, 585–612.

Peto, R., Pike, M.C., Armitage, P., Breslow, N.E., Cox, D.R., Howard, S.V., Mantel, N., McPherson, K., Peto, J., and Smith, P.G. (1977). Design and analysis of randomized clinical trials requiring prolonged observation of each patient. II. Analysis and examples. *Br. J. Cancer 35*, 1–39.

Renou, P., Chang, A., Anderson, I., and Wood, C. (1976). Controlled trial of fetal intensive care. *Am. J. Obstet. Gynecol. 126*, 470–476.

Sackett, D.L. and Gent, M. (1979). Controversy in counting and attributing events in clinical trials. *N. Engl. J. Med. 301*, 1410–1412.

Simon, R. (1977). Adaptive treatment assignment methods and clinical trials. *Biometrics 33*, 743–749.

Sylvester, R.J., Pinedo, H.M., De Pauw, M., Staquet, M.J., Buyse, M.E., Renard, J., and Bonadonna, G. (1981). Quality of institutional participation in multicenter clinical trials. *N. Engl. J. Med. 305*, 852–855.

Taeusch, H.W., Frigoletto, F., Kitzmiller, J., Avery, M.E., Hehre, A., Fromm, B., Lawson, E., and Neff, R.K. (1979). Risk of respiratory distress syndrome after prenatal dexamethasone treatment. *Pediatrics 63*, 64–72.

Truelove, S.C. (1964). Therapeutic trials. In *Medical surveys and clinical trials: Some methods and applications of group research in medicine*, edited by L.J. Witts. London: Oxford University Press, pp. 148–164.

Veatch, R.M. (1975). Ethical principles in medical experimentation. In *Ethical and legal issues of social experimentation*, edited by A.M. Rivlin and P.M. Timpane. Washington, D.C.: Brookings Institution.

Weinstein, M.C. (1974). Allocation of subjects in medical experiments. *N. Engl. J. Med. 291*, 1278–1285.

Wright, I.S., Marple, C.D., and Beck, D.F. (1954). *Myocardial infarction*. New York: Grune & Stratton, p. 9.

Zelen, M. (1969). Play-the-winner rule and the controlled clinical trial. *J. Am. Stat. Assoc. 64*, 134–146.

18

Methodologic Issues in the Epidemiologic Investigation of Drug-induced Congenital Malformations

Michael B. Bracken

Perinatal epidemiologists face a unique set of problems when they seek to investigate the etiology of congenital malformations. Since the early 1940s, when the first observations were made that exposure to an environmental agent, rubella, during pregnancy could lead to malformations in offspring (Gregg, 1941), over 1500 compounds have been studied for their teratogenic potential (Schardein, 1976; Shepard, 1980). The Collaborative Perinatal Project observed over 225 discrete congenital anomalies (Heinonen et al., 1977), and new defects such as the fetal alcohol syndrome (see Chapter 9) and the fragile X chromosome (Chapter 1) continue to be identified. This chapter reviews five issues perinatal epidemiologists should consider when undertaking studies of drug etiologies for congenital malformations. First, congenital malformations are difficult to classify, a problem that reflects their complex etiology; this complexity must be recognized if the findings of epidemiologic studies are to correlate with our knowledge of embryologic development. Second, specific congenital anomalies are rare, so that the design and statistical efficiency of epidemiologic studies become a crucial concern. Third, assessment of the time and degree of exposure to potential teratogens is important. Fourth, various approaches to the choice of control subjects can be taken. Fifth, new insights into placental metabolism of drugs have pointed the way to potentially rewarding new epidemiologic studies of the drug etiology of congenital malformations.

Acknowledgment. The author is grateful to Carol Bryce-Buchanan M.A. and Daniel H. Freeman Jr. Ph.D. for their suggestions during preparation of this chapter. Financial support was partly provided by a grant (HD 11357) from the National Institute of Child Health and Human Development.

PROBLEMS IN CLASSIFYING CONGENITAL MALFORMATIONS

Deformational Malformations

These may be defined as those malformations that are the result of normal tissue being modified, restructured, or destroyed because of external forces. Examples of these malformations include congenital dislocation of the hip, talipes (clubfoot), and limb reduction deformities. Although an understanding of the cause of these malformations dates from Hippocrates, they have most recently been described in detail by Dunn (1976). The principal source of pressure on the developing fetus comes from reduced intrauterine volume. This is itself associated with primigravidity and breech presentation, as well as less common factors such as the presence of large fibroids, a bicornuate uterus, and oligohydramnios. Ectopic and abdominal pregnancies can also exert unusually great pressure on the fetus, as can the presence of a twin (Dunn, 1976). Evidence for the origin of deformational malformations relatively late in pregnancy comes, at least in part, from their relative rarity in abortuses (Nishimura, 1970). Clinically, however, it is often difficult to diagnose a malformation as having a deformational versus developmental etiology. For example, a limb reduction deformity may be due to a genetic defect, an environmental agent (such as thalidomide) affecting growth of the limb buds, or positional pressure leading to necrosis of a previously normally developed limb (Wolpert, 1976). Only detailed examination of each individual case is likely to differentiate the specific etiology. Epidemiologic studies should attempt to diagnose their subjects with this level of detail if etiologic hypotheses are to be tested with greater precision.

Developmental Malformations

These are malformations that result from errors occurring in the gene or chromosome, or during primary morphogenesis. Gene and chromosome anomalies are the subject of detailed review elsewhere in this volume (Chapter 1). A large number of congenital malformations appear to be caused by either inherited or *de novo* genetic defects, or by environmental teratogens that themselves may be mutagenic or may disrupt morphogenetic development. For example, pyloric stenosis appears to have a genetic component to its etiology (Spence and Gladstein, 1978) but has also been associated with exposure to Bendectin in the first trimester of pregnancy (Eskenazi and Bracken, 1982). Because a family history of a malformation can bias a subject's exposure to a potential teratogen, it is important that epidemiologic studies incorporate family histories of congenital malformations into their data collection.

The Analysis of Syndromes

It is often unclear, in analyzing a series of congenital malformations, how complex syndromes should be classified. For example, the most frequent syndrome encountered is Down syndrome, which may or may not include cardiac anomalies in any single case. Generally, although not always, the Down syndrome will be correctly coded as the primary diagnosis. Analyses that have used only the primary diagnosis should therefore have appropriately classified all Down syndrome cases. More problematic is whether the analysis of newborns with congenital heart malformations should include or exclude the Down syndrome babies who also have cardiac defects. Because the cause of most cardiovascular anomalies is unknown, we cannot draw on a knowledge of their etiology for guidance in answering this question. At least two general etiologic hypotheses exist: (1) Some cardiac anomalies may be due to genetic errors that are linked to the trisomy associated with Down syndrome, and (2) some cardiac anomalies are due to environmental agents that act with increased effect on a trisomic fetus. The greater association of specific cardiac anomalies, such as endocardial cushion defects (Rudolph, 1974), with Down syndrome lends some support to the first hypothesis, but only detailed epidemiologic study using a variety of classification schemes can being to address the problem.

Even the classification of malformations that are not generally considered to be syndromes requires considerable care. Elwood and Elwood (1979) review in detail the classification of anencephalus and spina bifida. They indicate how detailed subclassification is necessary if the investigator is to understand the role of environmental fators on the etiology of these malformations, particularly on such crucial issues as whether some cases of spina bifida are due to reopening of a closed neural tube rather than initial failure of the tube to close.

STUDY DESIGN AND STATISTICAL POWER

Study design and power pose particular problems in the epidemiologic investigation of congenital malformations. Although reported total malformations range in incidence from 3 to 5% of livebirths, as described above, very little can be learned from studies grouping all malformations together. Thus, analysis of specific defects or natural groupings of them based on their embryologic development become necessary. Study of specific diagnostic groups further reduces the incidence rates to, at most, 6 to 8 per 1000 livebirths (e.g., for ventricular septal defects) and more usually to 1 or 2 per 1000 livebirths (Bracken, 1983). A number of strategies have been developed to increase the statistical power of studies, including using case-control study designs, modifying the α and β levels for which the study is designed to accept or reject the null hypothesis, and using one-tailed statistical tests.

Case-Control Studies

One of the most important advances in the epidemiologic study of rare diseases has been the development and refinement of case-control (also called case-referent) studies. In these studies a group of cases are defined, which may be newborns with a particular congenital malformation. A reference group of newborns without the malformation is also identified, and the frequency of exposure of the newborns in both groups to a putative risk factor is compared.

There is some confusion in the perinatal epidemiologic literature as to whether the newborn or the newborn's mother should be considered as the "case". Two issues need to be considered:

1. Mothers may enter long-lasting studies more than once for different pregnancies. However, because the exposures for each pregnancy are likely to be highly correlated, investigators must identify such women, and preferably, only consider one (often the first) pregnancy in the analysis.
2. Women with twin or other multiple pregnancies may deliver one newborn with a malformation and another without. Multiple pregnancies with mixed outcomes contribute nothing to the statistical analysis of the role of an environmental risk factor in case-control studies and may bias the exposure estimate if both fetuses are equally affected or unaffected. Thus, multiple pregnancies should be examined separately in etiologic analyses.

If the above precautions are taken, it is immaterial whether mother, or her offspring is defined as a case. There is some virtue, however, in using teminology consistent with epidemiologic studies in other disciplines and thus to defining the "diseased" newborn as the case.

Case-control studies permit a calculation of the odds ratio, which estimates the probability of exposure to a putative risk factor in cases

compared to the probability of exposure in the reference group. Holford has shown (Chapter 16) that where the incidence of disease is low the odds ratio provides a very good estimate of the relative risk. The relative risk is calculated from prospective studies and compares the proportion of mothers exposed to a risk factor who deliver a malformed child, with the proportion of unexposed mothers delivering a malformed child. The incidence of all congenital malformations is sufficiently low so that the odds ratio closely estimates relative risk.

The effect of a case-control study in gaining statistical power is shown by the following example. Let us assume we are designing a case-control study to detect with 90% power and an α level (two-tailed) of 5% of the relative risk of 3.0 for Down syndrome among women using spermicides at conception compared to nonusers. We further assume that 5% of mothers of healthy newborns use spermicides at conception and that three referent subjects will be studied for every case. Using a formula of Miettinen (1969), as programmed by Rothman and Boice (1979), we can calculate that this study would require 156 cases of Down syndrome and 469 controls for a total of 625 subjects.

To design a prospective study using the same parameters, we would require an estimate of the incidence of Down syndrome in women not using spermicides. This is assumed to be 1.5 per 1000 livebirths. A cohort of 35,000 pregnancies is required to identify a threefold risk of Down syndrome in the 5% of women using spermicides at conception.

Although it is more efficient to conduct case-control studies for many investigations of specific congenital malformations, and whereas these will provide odds ratios that accurately estimate relative risk, the design of case-referent studies raises many problematic issues. A number of these have been reviewed previously (Ibrahim, 1979; Breslow and Day, 1980; Schlesselman, 1982). Later in this chapter (p. 435), the choice of control groups in studies of congenital malformations is discussed more extensively. Other problems reviewed in the chapter pertain equally to case-control and to cohort studies.

Study Power

The choice of power in studies of the etiology of congenital malformations poses a major paradox. Typically, in performing epidemiologic studies, we test the null hypothesis (H_0), that no association exists between a putative risk factor and a disease. We design the study so as to accept a 5% risk (defined as α) that H_0 will be *incorrectly rejected*; that is, an association between the risk factor and disease will be reported when none actually exists (also called a Type 1 error). Additionally, we accept another level of risk (defined as β), that H_0 will be *incorrectly accepted*; that is, no association will be found where one truly exists (called Type 2 error). This level of risk is usually set within a range of 5 to 20%. The β level is relaxed in order to reduce the number of subjects necessary for a study. We elect to reduce the β rather than the α level because in science the burden of proof is always placed on an investigator to demonstrate that associations exist. The incorrect reporting of a risk factor–disease association in the epidemiology literature can result in wasting scarce epidemiologic resources because of the effort to replicate and eventually refute the original report. Moreover, epidemiologic studies often have a major influence on a public policy, societal behavior, and legislation. Thus, epidemiologic studies flawed with a Type 1 error will set in motion public actions based on erroneous results. However, studies that incorrectly fail to report an association are more likely to remain unpublished or, if published, are less likely to come to the attention of policy makers.

There are two particular considerations for the epidemiologist. First, the credibility of an investigation will be threatened if it departs too radically from traditional scientific criteria. Any such deviation should be clearly justified in all reports emanating from the study. Second, the benefits as well as the risks of an investigatory drug need to be evaluated. For example, investigators studying the association of oral contraceptives with congenital malformations might adopt a fairly stringent α level for rejecting the null hypothesis, because the benefits of oral contraception for family planning will for most women far outweigh any possible risks to the few who use the pill inadvertently in pregnancy (World Health Organization, 1981). In contrast, investigators studying Bendectin as a possible risk factor for congenital malformations face a different situation. Bendectin has not been well documented as being efficacious in preventing nausea in pregnancy, although it is widely used for this purpose (Kolata, 1982). Should the investigator therefore elect to adopt a less stringent α level because the potential risks of Bendectin to many of its users early in pregnancy could pose a considerable public health problem without any concomitant benefit? The use of many products in pregnancy— including alcohol, caffeine, cigarettes, and most prescription drugs— fall into a similar category.

The dilemma investigators face can be described simply: Should epidemiologic studies be conducted conservatively but at the risk of failing to challenge potentially dangerous medical and public health practices? If epidemiologists follow the traditional scientific dictum and design studies that increase the risk of Type 1 error in preference to Type 2, the evaluation of many investigatory drugs as risk factors for congenital malformations will incorrectly suggest that they are safe. However, we currently do not have guidelines that permit investigators to make decisions concerning the power of their studies based on a general risk–benefit analysis of the drug under investigation. Until criteria are developed for making such decisions, it is almost certainly preferable for investigators to use traditional power estimates.

Several investigators have used one-tailed statistical tests rather than the traditional two-tailed test in designing epidemiologic studies of the role of drugs in the etiology of congenital malformations. For any particular level of α, a one-tailed test has the advantage of reducing β. Stated another way, and undoubtedly reflecting why one-tailed tests are used, a one-tailed statistical test can be performed on fewer subjects than a two-tailed test for any given level of α or β.

The rationale for using one-tailed tests relies on the notion that the investigator is testing a unidirectional hypothesis, namely that exposure to a risk factor is associated with an *increased* risk for malformations and is unlikely to reduce risk. Thus, it is argued, one can ignore the need to look for a "protective" effect of exposure to the drug. However, care must be taken in evaluating the effect of a drug on congenital malformations observed at term delivery. It is possible that some drug exposures (e.g., alcohol or cigarette smoking) increase the rate of spontaneous abortion of fetuses with a defect. If, as is likely, this occurs for some drug exposures (Chapter 2), then a reduction in exposed fetuses seen at birth with the defect is theoretically possible. This possibility should be amenable to statistical analysis through the use of two-tailed tests.

Furthermore, reporting one-tailed tests is problematic because of the difficulty in comparing study results. It may be possible for another investigator to reconstruct published tables so that two-tailed significance tests can be recalculated. General readers, including some reviewers and editors, are less likely to be sensitive to the nuances of one- versus two-tailed tests. Thus, findings that are "positive" using a one-tailed test may be published in preference to a study obtaining essentially the same result but reporting it as a "negative" finding when using a two-tailed test. Some standardization of reporting is desirable to assist the public in evaluating the results of perinatal epidemiologic studies. It should be noted that studies designed to test their results using one-tailed test offer only a small increase in study power. For example, if a prospective study was designed to examine the risk of spermicide use at conception on the risk for a congenital malformation, we might assume that 17% of women used spermicides and 1.5% of unexposed pregnancies resulted in a congenitally malformed newborn; and we wished to detect a relative risk of 2.0. Setting α equal to 0.05 and the sample size to 10,000, we can calculate the study power of $(1-\beta)$ to be 0.954 for two-tailed, and 0.974 for one-tailed significance testing.

Multiple Observations

For many of the reasons cited above, it is usually inefficient to design studies of the possible relationship of a single drug to a specific congenital malformation. Thus, investigators frequently analyze the effect of several drugs, used over a number of different time exposures (before pregnancy, first trimester, second trimester, etc.), on many kinds of congenital malformations. In any one study, therefore, a great many associations are being examined. Such complexity can result in the finding of several relationships that are statistically significant merely by chance—for example, 1 in 20 at the $p < 0.05$ level. How can researchers protect themselves against this problem?

First, investigators may consider that they are actually performing several studies in one (i.e., separate investigations of each exposure) malformation relationship and reject entirely the notion that they should account for multiple observations.

Second, a number of adjustments during data analysis may be made. For example, the Bonferoni procedure simply divides the usual p value by the number of observations being made (Miller, 1966). Thus, if one were studying 20 congenital malformations over five exposure periods a p value of 0.0005 would be considered as being equivalent to the usual 0.05 p value. Given the difficulties of low statistical power in congenital malformation studies to begin with, the additional Bonferoni adjustment further increases the likelihood that these studies will fail to detect true risks. In other situations the investigator may be contrasting the mean drug exposures associated with different congenital malformations and a control group. In this situation the methods of adjustment for multiple comparisons described by Scheffé (1953) and Dunn (1958) may be appropriate.

Another solution to this problem, admittedly not entirely satisfactory, is to report the findings unadjusted for multiple comparisons and then to report further those continuing to be significant after adjustment. This reports a calculation that careful readers would wish to know and lets them decide how to evaluate the "true" significance of the reported association.

EXPOSURE ASSESSMENT IN STUDIES OF CONGENITAL MALFORMATIONS

Time of Exposure

In order to evaluate fully the teratogenic risk of exposure to a drug, it is necessary to know with some precision the time of drug exposure with reference to embryologic development. For example, transposition of the great vessels would occur as a result of exposure to a teratogen between 23 and 32 days gestation, whereas ventricular septal defects require exposure later in pregnancy (37–42 days).

Two factors lead to difficulty in the assessment of such precise exposure during pregnancy:

1. In the majority of pregnancies neither the respondent nor her physician can precisely estimate what the gestational age is. The usual method of calculating the estimated date of delivery uses the last menstrual period, leaving an average two-week margin of error. Gestational dating by ultrasonography provides only marginal improvement in accuracy.
2. Few respondents are able to recall exactly when they used a particular drug. This is especially true in case-control studies when women who have delivered are asked to remember drug use in the early part of pregnancy. Recall is particularly imprecise if a substance was used only once or twice, as occurs with a large number of compounds. Women who chronically used a drug throughout their pregnancy are more likely to recall its use accurately, but their exposure covers such a long period of embryologic development that it is of minimal benefit in testing specific etiologic hypotheses.

In a few instances, such as the use of hormones for pregnancy testing and diethylstilbestrol (DES) to reduce the risk of miscarriage, exact dates of exposure may be known. It is also important to identify exposures that cannot be related to the defect. For example, exposure to a drug after Day 32 of pregnancy cannot be responsible for transposition of the great vessels. Thus, when evaluating the risk for this defect, subjects using potential teratogens in most of the second and all of the third months of pregnancy should be considered unexposed. Exposure prior to some embryologic period is more difficult to evaluate in that the drug or its metabolites may remain in the body. Thus the biologic half-life of the drug and its metabolites needs to be considered.

Finally it is important to recognize that many behavioral teratogens (Chapter 9) may exert their influence at any time in pregnancy but especially in the third trimester.

Extent of Exposure

The frequency of drug use in early pregnancy can be observed from a study of 3208 women interviewed during pregnancy by the Yale Perinatal Epidemiology Unit in Connecticut between May 1980 and April 1982. All the women obtained their antenatal care with private obstetricians in the New Haven area. A total of 4973 separate drug usages were reported, and 69.1% of the respondents reported having used at least one drug at the time of interview. Among the drugs used, 68.8% were nonprescription, the remainder being prescribed products. The 20 most frequently used products are ranked by order of use in Table 18-1. Tylenol is by far the most commonly used product, followed by Bendectin. Of the nonprescription drugs, 61.4% were analgesics taken orally, followed by antacids and cold or allergy preparations (10.5 and 8.7% of nonprescription products, respectively). Among prescription drugs, those most frequently used were the autonomic and central nervous system agents including analgesics and tranquilizers (27.6 and 17.0% of prescribed drugs, respectively).

Table 18-1. The 20 Most Frequently Reported Drugs Used in Pregnancy

Drug	N (%)[a]	Prescription status[b]	Classification[c]
Tylenol Tablets	1091 (21.9)	N	Analgesic
Bendectin	391 (7.9)	P	Autonomic
Tylenol Extra Strength	378 (7.6)	N	Analgesic
A.S.A. Enseals	286 (5.8)	N	Analgesic
Penicillins	153 (3.1)	P	Antiinfective
Analgesics and antipyretics	123 (2.5)	P	Analgesic
Maalox	98 (2.0)	N	Antacid
Bayer Aspirin	89 (1.8)	N	Analgesic
Bufferin	77 (1.5)	N	Analgesic
Robitussin	68 (1.4)	N	Antitussive
Mylanta	65 (1.3)	N	Antacid
Excedrin	64 (1.3)	N	Analgesic
Antihistamines	61 (1.2)	P	Antihistamine
Sudafed	60 (1.2)	N	Cold and allergy
Tranquilizers	58 (1.2)	P	Tranquilizer
Thyroid and antithyroid	57 (1.1)	P	Hormones
Anacin	56 (1.1)	N	Analgesic
Pepto-Bismol	51 (1.0)	N	Antidiarrheal
Metamucil	45 (0.9)	N	Weight control
Diuretics	44 (0.9)	P	Electrolytic

[a] A total of 4973 drug usages were reported by respondents.
[b] P, Prescription; N, Nonprescription.
[c] According to American Society of Hospital Pharmacists (1980) and National Professional Society of Pharmacists (1979).

In the same study, 31.9% of women used one drug, 20.8% two drugs, and 16.4% three or more. Table 18-1 also shows that even the most frequently used drugs are generally taken by fewer than 5% of pregnant women.

It may be possible to estimate the extent of a specific drug exposure from recommended treatment doses. However, these may not have been followed, especially with nonprescription drugs. Exposure information can also be improved by asking women to recall the brand names of drugs used. These can be reclassified into generic compounds using standard reference works such as those of the American Society of Hospital Pharmacists (1980) for prescribed medications, and the National Professional Society of Pharmacists (1979) for nonprescription drugs.

The importance of using brand names to ascertain drug exposures is exemplified in a study of some 300 mothers who were asked about their "aspirin" use just prior to delivery. There were no positive responses, although 10% of infants had cord serum salicylate. The discrepancy was found to result from respondents not realizing that the products they had consumed contained aspirin (Palmisano and Cassady, 1969). Recall of the use of drugs can be aided by probes that ask respondents if they have taken medications for any of a list of reasons, such as (1) to help control nausea, (2) for fluid retention (swelling and/or bloating), (3) for diet or weight loss, (4) to help them sleep. It is realistic to ask about drug use for each week of pregnancy, although often recall may be limited to a particular month.

In studies where specific groups of drugs are the subject of inquiry (e.g., oral contraceptives), many investigators have found it useful to provide interviewers with "pill books." These are either colored photographs or actual samples of each pill dispenser and package ever marketed. This permits more accurate identification of the exact product used. Additionally, the interviewers should be blind to the study hypothesis and should not know if they are interviewing a case or a control.

In evaluating the risk of a particular drug it is important to recognize that many drugs contain multiple components. For example, Bendectin, a widely used drug for treating nausea in early pregnancy and the subject of several epidemiologic studies, contains an antihistamine, doxylamine succinate, and vitamin B_6. In many countries the product also contains a muscle relaxant, dicyclomine, which was removed from the U.S. product in 1976. The component drugs in Bendectin are also found in other products. In order to avoid the unknown but potentially confounding effects of other drugs, therefore, women exposed to the drug of interest should be contrasted with women who did not use any drugs in pregnancy.

433

Moreover, to isolate the independent effect of exposure to a specific drug, analysis of its effect should be examined among women who used only that drug and no other.

Understanding for what condition a drug was prescribed is important in order to determine whether the drug or the condition itself might be associated with congenital malformations. Particularly troublesome in this respect is the use of Dilantin (diphenylhydantoin) for seizures (Monson et al., 1973), insulin for diabetes (Landauer, 1972), and antiemetics for nausea and vomiting (Eskenazi and Bracken, 1982). If patients can be identified who had symptoms of equal severity but did not use the drug, then the independent effects of the drug can be evaluated.

Recall Bias

Because the great majority of epidemiologic studies of congenital malformations use the case-control design, recall bias is an issue of particular importance. Recall bias may be defined as the *differential likelihood* that subjects with a disease or other condition leading to their definition as a "case," will recall prior exposures to potential risk factors for the disease, as compared with subjects without the disease and defined as "controls." Case subjects are generally thought to be more likely to recall prior exposures, because their disease prompts a more careful review of their past experience. It may be, however, that cases are less likely to recall a past exposure because they deny or repress behaviors about which they feel guilty, such as heavy smoking or illicit drug use. Although recall bias has been the source of considerable discussion in the literature (e.g., see Sackett, 1979), it has received mixed empirical support. Klemetti and Sáxen (1967) found that neither being a mother of a dead or malformed newborn nor being interviewed long after delivery (as long as 15 months) differentially influenced the recall of drug use.

More recent studies, which compared responses at interview with medical and pharmacy records, found fairly accurate recall of drug histories ranging from a low of 69% for barbiturates to 87% for anti-hypertensives with no evidence for differential recall in cases (women with breast cancer) and (community) controls (Paganini-Hill and Ross, 1982). Stolley et al. (1978) also report equal agreement (89%) by cases (thromboembolic patients) and controls (women hospitalized for another condition) on the recall of the name of the most recently used oral contraceptive, and on the date usage stopped, when interview responses were compared with prescriber's records. The cases showed better agreement for the starting date of drug use and, for all women, the dates and names of less recently used drugs were less well remembered. A greater mismatch of similar-sounding brand names (e.g., Ovral and Ovulen) was also noticed. Glass et al. (1968) also found good agreement of recent oral contraceptive use with prescription records. The age when oral contraception was first used was accurately remembered by only 55.4% of women, and 87.7% remembered within 1 year over an average recall of 9.1 years (Bean et al., 1979).

Much research needs to be done on the phenomenon of recall bias, not only on a psychological level so as to understand what disease states and other events may prompt differential recall, but also empirically in order to assess the extent of any bias. There is not yet any overwhelming evidence that recall bias poses a major problem in studies of drug exposure and congenital malformations.

One would not expect, in the types of comparative studies described above, to find complete agreement between interview responses and prescription records. Some women may fill prescriptions and not use them, or they may obtain drugs from other sources. Nonetheless, the underreporting of drug exposure, even if it occurs equally by case and control subjects, will reduce the chance of finding a positive association between drug use and congenital malformations if one truly exists (Bross, 1954; Barron, 1977). A dose–response relationship between a drug exposure and birth outcome should still be evident, however, despite random misclassification (Marshall et al., 1981; Schlesselman, 1982).

CHOICE OF CONTROL SUBJECTS

It was shown earlier that case-control studies are statistically the most efficient study design for many investigations of congenital malformations. This is because of the relative rarity of both specific congenital malformation diagnostic groups and, in many instances, the drug exposures of interest. This section focuses on the considerations involved in choosing control groups in case-control studies.

Number and Choice of Controls

For many case-control studies it is desirable to use two or more control groups (Jick and Vessey, 1978; Janerich et al., 1979). For example, an investigator may elect to utilize a community-based control group and a second control group from patients admitted to hospital with a diagnosis unrelated to that under investigation. In perinatal studies, however, this is rarely necessary. A single control group of newborns not manifesting any evidence of being congenitally malformed is the most appropriate comparison group. In some studies the investigator may wish to observe the infants for up to a year before finally classifying them as cases or controls, because only about 50% of congenital malformations are observed at delivery (World Health Organization, 1981). In this way a number of defects not always evident at birth, such as ventricular septal defects and pyloric stenosis, can be more completely ascertained. A study will be more useful if the control group is a proportionate random sample of all nonmalformed newborns being delivered in the same hospital(s) from which the cases were obtained and over the same period of time. This control group permits the exact calculation of the incidence of congenital malformations occurring in the study population (a useful check on the completeness of case ascertainment) and also allows estimation of the prevalence of drug exposures (providing a means of comparing rates in different study populations). A random sample of controls also permits a calculation of the attributable risk, an estimate of the proportion of cases that may be due to use of the drug (Walter, 1978).

It is often preferable to design case-control studies using a ratio of controls to cases of 2:1 or 3:1. This provides the study with an increase in statistical power, particularly when the subjects are stratified according to other possible risk factors. However, an increase in the control:case ratio beyond 3:1 provides less incremental benefit for the additional cost of studying the extra controls (for discussion see Schlesselman, 1982, p. 150). The perinatal epidemiologist has an advantage in sampling healthy newborns as controls, because they are readily available in large numbers. This availability usually precludes the need to consider using matched control groups, which are the focus of much attention in other epidemiologic disciplines (Schlesselman, 1982, p. 105).

Using Other Cases as "Controls"

In recent years a few investigators have chosen to use newborns with "other" malformations as "controls" for the diagnostic malformation groups of interest, the cases. The risks of exposures to caffeine (Rosenberg et al., 1982) and Bendectin (Cordero et al., 1981; Mitchell et al., 1981) for subsequent congenital malformations have been studied using this method. The development of this approach results from concern over recall bias but is also a matter of convenience, because studies are less expensive if healthy controls do not need to be interviewed.

However, it is not evident that using other cases as "controls" will avoid recall bias, because often the cases have more serious and life-threatening malformations than do the "controls." Thus, if exposure recall bias were a function of the severity of the congenital lesion, recall bias could still exist in these studies.

The case against using "case controls" rests on three points: (1) etiologic heterogeneity, (2) statistical indeterminacy, and (3) impossible generalizability.

ETIOLOGIC HETEROGENEITY

The rationale for using "case controls" rests on the assumption that a particular drug exposure is unlikely to cause more than one birth defect. Thus we are told, for example: "No human teratogen has yet been identified that causes defects uniformly across the broad spectrum of malformations" (Rosenberg et al., 1982, p. 1432).

In fact, we do not yet know whether most drugs are only teratogenic for a single defect. Case-control studies of specific malformations cannot determine whether other defects (not studied) are also associated with the same drug. Conversely, prospective studies of a particular drug exposure cannot determine whether other drugs (not studied) might cause the same birth defect. However, evidence from the laboratory (Schardein, 1976) and from studies of several congenital malformations and drug exposures (Bracken and Holford, 1981; Heinonen et al., 1977) indicates that exposure to a single drug may be associated with defects in several organ systems and, conversely, development of a particular organ system may be influenced by several drugs. It appears likely that the point in *time* that a specific teratogenic insult occurs during embryologic development is as important as the nature of the teratogen itself. Even if specific drugs were only associated with a single malformation, the lack of precision in determining the time of drug exposures described earlier indicates that exposure to a drug for the case malformation is likely to be also correlated with the "control" malformations.

It is important to note that thalidomide, which is often considered the prime example of a drug causing specific defects, was associated with other than upper limb defects in some 30% of affected cases (Mellin and Katzenstein, 1962). These included malformations of the lower limbs, esophagus, duodenum, heart (tetralogy of Fallot), and kidney (renal agenesis).

There seems to be little rationale, at least with respect to embryologic development, in selecting which malformations are to be considered cases and which controls. In one study (Rosenberg et al., 1982), for example, the cases of interest were simply the six defects for which the investigators had more than 100 cases. The diagnostic groups so selected were inguinal hernia, cleft lip with and without cleft palate, cardiac defects, isolated cleft palate, and neural tube defects, none of which have much in common. All other malformed infants were considered controls. Thus, congenital malformations that might be expected to share their developmental etiology are divided between the cases and the "case controls."

STATISTICAL INDETERMINACY

If there is no true relationship between a drug exposure and a particular fetus becoming a case, in a study using other malformations as controls the observed relationship will only accurately predict the true situation if the cases being used as controls are also unrelated to the exposure. If the controls themselves have a positive relationship with the exposure, the observed relationship between cases and exposure will always be less than the true relationship.

The earlier discussion of heterogeneous etiology suggests that if a drug is teratogenic for the case of interest, there is a reasonably high likelihood that it may also be associated in the data set with some of the "control" malformations. In this situation a true positive relative risk will be spuriously reduced.

A converse bias will occur if the drug exposure has a "protective" relationship with the "control" malformation. The prevalence of congenital malformations at delivery is, in part, a function of the true incidence of the malformation minus the number of affected fetuses miscarried (Hook, 1982). Thus, a teratogen may cause embryonic malformation but may also induce early miscarriage in malformed fetuses that would otherwise have been delivered. Consequently, drug exposure may result in a reduced prevalence of some malformations at delivery. If this occurs, studies using "case controls" will observe relative risks greater than unity.

Without any a priori reason to expect that a teratogen will affect a particular organ system, we must assume that all organs are at equal risk of being developmentally malformed. Studies that define one or two birth defects as cases, using all other birth defects as controls, have a very low probability of including affected organ systems in their cases of interest and a very high probability of including affected organ systems among the "controls."

IMPOSSIBLE GENERALIZABILITY

A series of studies using case-control (with healthy controls) or cohort designs should provide relatively similar estimates of the strength of association of a particular congenital malformation with specified exposure. Because of the methodologic difficulties described in this chapter, the extant literature does not provide an example of this point from studies of congenital malformations. However, case-control and cohort studies of oral contraceptive use prior to pregnancy and the associated possible increased risk of a multiple pregnancy show notable similarity in their findings (Table 18-2). Relative risk is used as the measure of association and shows no significant difference from unity in any of the studies. The close similarity in the results of these studies, which were performed in several countries, is due partially to the similar assessment of oral contraceptive exposure and partially to the ease and agreement in diagnosing the study outcome, a "multiple pregnancy."

The relative risks for the same drug exposure in studies using "case controls", however, will vary depending on which malformations were selected as "controls." The difficulty in generalizing from one study to another is enhanced by the case of interest in one study being used as a "control" in another. For example, Cordero et al. (1981) found an association between esophageal atresia, encephalocele, and Bendectin, whereas in the Bendectin study of Mitchell et al. (1981), esophageal atresia and encephalocele cases were part of the control group.

Whenever future investigation implicates an exposure as causing a congenital malformation, all preceding studies that used that malformation as a "control" are invalidated. Mitchell et al. (1981) used as controls in their Bendectin study a large number (50%) of patients with gastrointestinal defects, a proportion of which would include pyloric stenosis. A more recent study (Eskenazi and Bracken, 1982), however, has implicated Bendectin as a possible risk factor for pyloric

Table 18-2. Studies of Multiple Births to Women Who did or Did Not Use Oral Contraceptives Prior to Conception

	Oral contraceptive users		Nonusers		
Reference	Number of women	Multiple births per 1000	Number of women	Multiple births per 1000	Relative risk
Royal College of General Practitioners (1976)	4477	10.1	9511	10.9	0.9
Rothman (1977)	6002	10.1	2616	11.0	0.9
Harlap and Davies (1978)	2953	13.6	13,630	14.5	0.9
Bracken (1979)	1341	17.9	2269	15.0	1.2
Vessey et al. (1979)	1798	9.5	2214	14.5	0.7

Source: Modified from World Health Organization (1981), Table 12.

stenosis, thereby casting doubt on the validity of the earlier study. This is a particular problem in epidemiology, where we generally seek to replicate an association in several studies before feeling confident that the association is a true one.

Studies using "case controls" cannot estimate the attributable risk due to a particular exposure. Attributable risk permits an estimate of the excess burden of disease that might be attributed to the exposure and depends on knowing the proportion of the population that is at risk of disease, that is exposed to the drug, and the relative risk of exposure (Walter, 1978). It is an important index in considering the public health importance of a potential teratogen. Neither the proportion of mothers in the normal population exposed to a potential teratogen nor an unbiased estimate of the relative risk can be derived from the studies that do not use healthy infants as controls.

PLACENTAL METABOLISM OF MULTIPLE DRUGS AND RISK FOR CONGENITAL MALFORMATION: A HYPOTHESIS

Two recent findings from an epidemiologic study of maternal drug exposures as possible risk factors for congenital malformations in offspring, conducted in Connecticut from 1974 to 1977, prompted examination of the pharmacology literature and the development of a hypothesis for explaining the possible role of placental metabolism of ingested maternal drugs to explain an apparent synergistic relationship of multiple drug exposures on the risk for congenital malformations. The hypothesis is testable in future epidemiological studies both of congenital malformations and various other perinatal problems.

The first finding concerned oral contraceptive use in pregnancy (Bracken et al., 1978). Maternal oral contraceptive use was unrelated to malformations in offspring when exposure occurred most recently in the year before conception (odds ratio, $OR = 0.9$, $p = 0.25$) or during pregnancy, actually the first month of pregnancy for almost all respondents ($OR = 1.3$, $p = 0.30$). Women who smoked more than 20 cigarettes daily, in the same study, had a significantly increased risk for malformation in offspring (relative risk = 1.6; Kelsey et al., 1978). For both risk factors, adjustment for other confounding maternal variables did not change the risk ratios in any substantial manner. Of particular interest was the finding of a significant interaction for the effect of combined exposure to both oral contraception and cigarette smoking in early pregnancy (Bracken et al., 1978). Women so exposed were more than 13 times as likely to deliver a malformed infant as

440

women exposed to neither (OR = 13.2, lower 95% Confidence Limit (CL) = 1.6).

The second finding of interest involved use of prescribed tranquilizers in pregnancy. Tranquilizer use was more common among mothers of infants with a congenital malformation (OR = 2.3, lower 95% CL = 1.5), and the effect of tranquilizer use significantly increased ($p < 0.01$) among women who also smoked in pregnancy. Among tranquilizer users, women who smoked one pack or fewer cigarettes daily and women who smoked more than 20 cigarettes daily had the same risk (OR = 3.7, p = 0.0002) as compared to women who smoked but did not use tranquilizers. Among nonsmokers, tranquilizer use increased the risk of being a case by 44% (Bracken and Holford, 1981; see also Chapter 16, p. 385).

In recent years it has become established that the placenta is able to synthesize drugs so that their potential teratogenic effects are modified. Tuchmann-Duplessis (1975) has suggested that various drugs may be teratogenic in some animals but not others because of interspecies differences in the metabolic pathways used to synthesize drugs. In humans the placenta has been shown to contain many enzyme systems responsible for drug biotransformations, particularly by hydrolysis and reduction (Juchau, 1976). Placental metabolism, moreover, is significantly influenced by environmental agents (Yaffe and Stern, 1976).

In a series of important studies, Welch and colleagues (1968, 1968a, 1969) reported that the placentas of women who smoke will hydrolyze benzo[a]pyrene, a reaction that protects the fetus from its potentially teratogenic and carcinogenic effects. Other polycyclic hydrocarbons found in cigarette smoke were also found to initiate benzo[a]pyrene hydroxylation in rats. Benzpyrene hydroxylase formation has, moreover, been reported to occur less frequently in early pregnancy (Juchau et al., 1968; Juchau, 1971; Pelkonen et al., 1972) and to be inhibited in the presence of estrogens and progesterones (Juchau, 1976). Correspondingly, it has been shown that carbon monoxide inhibits the metabolism of 19-norsteroids to estrogens in human placental tissue (Meigs and Ryan, 1971). These observations have led Juchau (1976) to suggest that drugs and steroids may utilize the same enzymes for some metabolic reactions, although human placental hydroxylation of benzo[a]pyrene does not itself appear to be catalyzed by the same enzyme system as that by which steroids are synthesized.

Existing pharmacologic research suggests two basic mechanisms by which concurrent maternal exposure to cigarettes and another drug have a synergistic effect on increasing risk for congenital malformations in offspring. First, transformation of tranquilizers and estrogens

441

or progesterones into less teratogenic metabolites may be inhibited in the placentas of mothers who smoke. Second, hydroxylation of benzo[a]pyrene may be inhibited by tranquilizers or oral contraceptives or their metabolized products, when the mother uses these concurrently. These hypotheses are not necessarily competing because, at least theoretically, either might operate depending on which combination of exposures is considered and on other modifying maternal factors such as gestational age.

The existing literature on the risk for human congenital malformations after maternal exposure to cigarette smoking and to prescription drugs is complex and frequently conflicting. Schardein (1976) has reviewed exposure to over 1500 compounds, and one is hard pressed to find even one drug for which exposure, in human studies, consistently results in a specific congenital malformation. The literature generally suggests that a single compound may produce several kinds of defects or that a specific organ malformation may be caused by any one of several compounds. In either case many reported associations are quite modest (e.g., Heinonen et al., 1977). Our failure to predict more accurately which drug exposures increase teratogenic risks is partially due to methodological difficulties in epidemiologic studies, some of which were discussed above. Another reason for this failure, however, may be the rarity with which we estimate concurrent risk exposures, such as smoking, when looking at drug exposures. To what can we attribute this shortcoming in available studies? There are at least seven issues.

1. Interaction effects have not been routinely sought, either because the necessary statistical tools were not available or because the study design did not permit collection of required data. Some aspects to this issue are as follows:

    a. In regression analyses interaction terms are not frequently used.

    b. Computer programs for log-linear analyses that permit searches for interactions are only now becoming more widely available.

    c. The relevant theoretical work has only recently appeared in the epidemiologic literature (Rothman, 1974, 1976; Kupper and Hogan, 1978; Walter and Holford, 1978; Rothman et al., 1980).

    d. Epidemiologists do not read the pharmacologic journals, and pharmacologists do not read the epidemiologic journals.

    e. Most studies of maternal drug use have not collected reliably detailed smoking data, and past studies of smoking in pregnancy have not estimated reliable detailed drug usage.

    f. One of the tenets of epidemiologic analysis has been that a variable must be associated with both the major risk factor of interest and the disease before it is controlled. If smoking is not found to have an effect on the outcome, it is not considered further as an effect modifier in terms of the drug exposure and malformations.

g. In samples where 30% of mothers smoked and only 15% of smokers used more than 20 cigarettes daily, the simple classification of the variable into smokers versus nonsmokers could mask a heavy smoking effect and also remove smoking as a variable from consideration as an effect modifier.

h. When a variable is identified as a confounder it is often simply controlled in the analysis and not analyzed in detail for potential synergistic relationships.

2. The incidence of most malformations is low (<1%; Bracken, 1983), and the frequency of exposure to specific drugs in pregnancy (except smoking, which is about 30%; Kelsey et al., 1978) is also very low (1 to 2%; Bracken, 1983 and Table 18-1); thus studies of many thousands of women are required to detect concurrent drug effects. The use of spontaneous abortions as a screening device for malformations may reduce the number of cases required (Kline et al., 1977).

3. Exposure to drugs must occur at very specific points in embryologic development for a specific malformation to occur. Such detailed information is difficult for women to remember and for epidemiologists to measure. Many investigators assess, at best, exposure by each month of pregnancy (see earlier discussion on p. 431).

4. The effect of environmental agents may be dose related either linearly or in a threshhold type of relationship. Exact dose amounts are also difficult for respondents to remember.

5. Mothers who expose themselves to one risk factor, such as smoking, are also more likely to have used prescription drugs and alcohol, and to be exposed to other risk factors. This intercorrelation of risk factors further weakens the power of statistical studies, because control of confounding and examination of effect modifiers only utilizes a subset of the study sample.

6. Maternal exposure to drug risk factors is only one possible cause of malformations; others include genetic mutations, inherited characteristics, and other ambient environmental effects. The contribution of a specific maternal risk factor (the attributable risk) to the overall incidence of the malformation is therefore quite small. In the Connecticut study, smoking had a population attributable risk of between 6 and 9% (Kelsey et al., 1978).

7. Two drugs having no independent effect on the fetus but that might be teratogenic in combination would not be detected in most studies, because the first stage of analysis, the search for main effects, would routinely eliminate them from later analysis of interactive effects.

443

The above list includes some methodologic reasons for possible failure to detect synergistic effects of multiple drug exposures. One would not, however, expect that *all* concurrent exposures increase risk.Biosynthesis of some drugs in the placenta might occur without interfering with the simultaneous biosynthesis of others. In the Connecticut study (Bracken and Holford, 1981), no interaction was found between cigarettes smoked daily in pregnancy and concurrent use of narcotic analgesics. This may be because of some of the methodologic issues raised above or because narcotic analgesics, unlike tranquilizers, are not metabolized by enzyme systems that compete with the metabolism of compounds present in cigarettes. Nor, in the same study, did concurrent use of tranquilizers and narcotic analgesics show any interactive effects. Harlap and Shiono (1980) did not find any interaction between cigarettes smoked in pregnancy and concurrent use of alcohol as risk factors for second-trimester spontaneous abortion, alcohol having a stronger independent effect than smoking. An interaction was found, however, between maternal weight and alcohol use, the effect of alcohol on mid-trimester miscarriage being much greater in the lighter women.

Although the synergistic impact of multiple drug usage as a risk factor for perinatal problems has not been widely examined, there are other examples in the epidemiology literature where concurrent exposures enhance risk. Combined exposure to cigarettes and oral contraceptives has a synergistic relationship to increased risk of myocardial infarction (Mann and Inman, 1975) as well as related cerebro vascular events (Jain, 1977; Royal College of General Practitioners, 1977; Vessey et al., 1977). People exposed to both cigarettes and asbestos incur much higher risks of lung cancer than those exposed to either risk factor alone (Saracci, 1977).

Although the foregoing discussion has focused on congenital malformations, concurrent maternal exposures to multiple drugs might further explain the etiology of other perinatal outcomes as well. Fetal alcohol syndrome, for example, does not occur universally in women who drink heavily. The effect of alcohol might be modified by concurrent use of cigarettes or other drugs. Placental alcohol dehydrogenase may be inhibited in the presence of other compounds. Such a phenomenon could explain why the effect of maternal alcohol use on spontaneous abortion (Harlap and Shiono, 1980), intrauterine growth retardation (Ouellette et al., 1977), and low birthweight (Little, 1977) was not observed earlier. If some concurrent maternal drug use interferes with the biosynthesis of benzo[a]pyrene, we might hypothesize that offspring exposed to both drugs and cigarettes *in utero* have increased risks of cancer later in life. This is a hypothesis deserving urgent examination. Similarly, not all women who were exposed to DES as fetuses because of maternal use develop vaginal carcinomas. The effect of DES could be enhanced in mothers who concurrently smoked or used other drugs in pregnancy.

The hypothesis for a synergistic effect of multiple drug exposures on increasing teratogenic risk does not conflict with recent work on the genetic control of drug metabolism and congenital malformations. These studies suggest that individual differences in the teratogenic susceptibility of fetuses to a drug are due to genetically determined variation in the rates of forming and detoxifying drug metabolites (Spielberg, 1982). For example, mouse studies have shown that fetuses with the genotype for high genetic cytochrome *P*-450 activity, which mediates the oxidation of benzo[*a*]pyrene, have more congenital malformations when exposed to benzo[*a*]pyrene than fetuses with less cytochrome *P*-450 activity (Shum et al., 1979). Moreover, the mother's own genetically determined rate of drug metabolism may further determine the susceptibility of her fetus to a particular drug exposure. Genotypic variations in drug metabolism would explain why one twin of a dizygous pair may be affected by the mother's use of a drug while the other twin is not affected (Phelan et al., 1982).

Fortunately, the statistical tools, epidemiologic theory, and clinical knowledge have advanced to a point where perinatal epidemiologists can look for the interactive effect of concurrent risk exposures. However, this search must be accompanied by an understanding of the pharmacologic and biologic processes that might be involved, because examination of a large number of interaction effects in a complex data set will assuredly reveal many spurious associations. If careful attention is paid to developing a priori hypotheses, such studies may provide considerable new knowledge on the etiology of perinatal disorders and permit more sensitive and insightful counsel to pregnant patients and their physicians.

REFERENCES

American Society of Hospital Pharmacists (1980). *American hospital formulary service.* Washington, D.C.: American Society of Hospital Pharmacists.

Barron, B.A. (1977). The effects of misclassification on the estimation of relative risk. *Biometrics 33*, 414–418.

Bean, J.A., Leeper, J.D., Wallace, R.B., Sherman, B.M., and Jagger, H. (1979). Variations in the reporting of menstrual histories. *Am. J. Epidemiol. 109*, 181–185.

Bracken, M.B. (1979). Oral contraception and twinning: An epidemiologic study. *Am. J. Obstet. Gynecol. 133*, 432–434.

—— (1983). The epidemiology of perinatal disorders. In *Principles and practice of perinatal medicine maternal–fetal and newborn care*, edited by J.B. Warshaw and J.C. Hobbins. Menlo Park, Calif.: Addison-Wesley.

—— and Holford, T.R. (1981). Exposure to prescribed drugs in pregnancy and association with congenital malformations. *Obstet. Gynecol. 58*, 336–344.

——, ——, White, C., and Kelsey, J.L. (1978). Role of oral contraception in congenital malformations of offspring. *Int. J. Epidemiol. 7*, 309–317.

Breslow, N.E. and Day, N.E. (1980). *Statistical methods in cancer research.* Vol. 1, *The analysis of case-control studies.* Lyons, France: International Agency for Research on Cancer.

Bross, I.D.J. (1954). Misclassification in 2 × 2 tables. *Biometrics 10*, 478–486.

Cordero, J.G., Oakley, G.P., Greenberg, F., and James, L.M. (1981). Is Bendectin a teratogen? *J.A.M.A. 245*, 2307–2310.

Dunn, O.J. (1958). Estimation of the means of dependent variables. *J. Am. Stat. Assoc. 29*, 1095–1111.

Dunn, P.M. (1976). Congenital postural deformities. *Br. Med. Bull. 32*, 71–76.

Elwood, J.M. and Elwood, J.H. (1979). *Epidemiology of anencephalus and spina bifida.* Oxford: Oxford University Press, p. 15.

Eskenazi, B. and Bracken, M.B. (1982). Bendectin (Debendox) as a risk factor for pyloric stenosis. *Am. J. Obstet. Gynecol. 144*, 919–924.

Glass, R., Johnson, B., and Vessey, M.P. (1968). Accuracy of recall of histories of oral contraceptive use. *Br. J. Prev. Soc. Med. 28*, 273–275.

Gregg, N.M. (1941). Congenital cataract following German measles in the mother. *Trans. Ophthalmol. Soc. Aust. 3*, 35–41.

Harlap, S. and Davies, A.M. (1978). *The pill and births: The Jerusalem Study.* Bethesda, Md.: Center for Population Research, National Institute of Child Health and Human Development.

—— and Shiono, P. (1980). Alcohol, smoking, and incidence of spontaneous abortions in the first and second trimester. *Lancet 2*, 173–176.

Heinonen, O.P., Slone, D., and Shapiro, S. (1977). *Birth defects and drugs in pregnancy.* Littleton, Mass.: Publishing Sciences Group.

Hook, E.B. (1982). Incidence and prevalence as measures of the frequency of birth defects. *Am. J. Epidemiol. 116*, 743–747.

Ibrahim, M. (1979). The case-control study: Consensus and controversy. *J. Chron. Dis. 32*, 1–144.

Jain, A.K. (1977). Mortality risk associated with the use of oral contraceptives. *Stud. Fam. Plann. 8*, 50–54.

Janerich, D.T., Glebatis, D., Flink, E., and Hoff, M.B. (1979). Case-control studies on the effect of sex steroids on women and their offspring. *J. Chron. Dis. 32*, 83–88.

Jick, H. and Vessey, M.P. (1978). Case-control studies in the evaluation of drug-induced illness. *Am. J. Epidemiol. 107*, 1–7.

Juchau, M.R. (1971). Human placental hydroxylation of 3,4-benzpyrene during early gestation and at term. *Toxicol. Appl. Pharmacol. 18*, 665–675.

—— (1976). Drug biotransformation reactions in the placenta. In *Perinatal pharmacology and therapeutics*, edited by B.L. Mirkin. New York: Academic Press.

————, Niswander, K.B., and Yaffe, S.J. (1968). Drug metabolizing systems in homogenates of human immature placentas. *Am. J. Obstet. Gynecol.* *100*, 348–356.

Kelsey, J.L., Dwyer, T., Holford, T.R., and Bracken, M.B. (1978). Maternal smoking and congenital malformations: An epidemiological study. *J. Epidemiol. Community Health 32*, 102–107.

Klemetti, A. and Sáxen, L. (1967). Prospective versus retrospective approach in the search for environmental causes of malformation. *Am. J. Public Health 57*, 2071–2075.

Kline, J., Stein, Z.A., Strobino, B., Susser, M., and Warburton, D. (1977). Surveillance of spontaneous abortions. Power in environmental monitoring. *Am. J. Epidemiol. 106*, 345–350.

Kolata, G. (1982). FDA to reexamine Bendectin data. *Science 217*, 335.

Kupper, L.L. and Hogan, M.D. (1978). Interaction in epidemiologic studies. *Am. J. Epidemiol. 108*, 447–453.

Landauer, W. (1972). Is insulin a teratogen? *Teratology 5*, 129–135.

Little, R.E. (1977). Moderate alcohol use during pregnancy and decreased infant birthweight. *Am. J. Public Health 67*, 1154–1156.

Mann, J.I. and Inman, W.H. (1975). Oral contraceptives and death from myocardial infarction. *Br. Med. J. 2* (5965): 245–248.

Marshall, J.R., Priore, R., Graham, S., and Brasure, J. (1981). On the distortion of risk estimates in multiple exposure level case-control studies. *Am. J. Epidemiol. 113*, 464–473.

Meigs, R.A. and Ryan, K.J. (1971). Enzymatic aromatization of steroids. 1. Effects of oxygen and carbon monoxide on the intermediate steps of estrogen biosynthesis. *J. Biol. Chem. 246*, 83–87.

Mellin, G.W. and Katzenstein, M. (1962). The saga of thalidomide. Neuropathy to embryopathy, with case reports of congenital anomalies. *N. Engl. J. Med. 267*, 1184–1193, 1238–1244.

Miettinen, O.S. (1969). Individual matching with multiple controls in the case of all or none responses. *Biometrics 25*, 339–354.

Miller, R.G. (1966). *Simultaneous statistical inference.* New York: McGraw-Hill, p. 8.

Mitchell, A.A., Rosenberg, L., Shapiro, S., and Slone, D. (1981). Birth defects related to Bendectin use in pregnancy. 1. Oral clefts and cardiac defects. *J.A.M.A. 245*, 2311–2314.

Monson, R.R., Rosenberg, L., Hartz, S.C., Shapiro, S., Heinonen, O.P., and Slone, D. (1973). Diphenylhydantoin and selected malformations. *N. Engl. J. Med. 289*, 1049–1052.

National Professional Society of Pharmacists (1979). *Handbook of nonprescription drugs*, 6th Ed. Washington, D.C.: American Pharmaceutical Association.

Nishimura, H. (1970). Incidence of malformations in abortions. In *Congenital malformations*, edited by F.C. Fraser and V.A. McKusick. Amsterdam and London: Excerpta Medica (International Congress Series, No. 204), pp. 275–283.

Ouellette, E.M., Rosett, H.L., Rosman, N.P., and Weiner, L. (1977). Adverse effects on offspring of maternal alcohol abuse during pregnancy. *N. Engl. J. Med. 297*, 528–530.

Paganini-Hill, A. and Ross, R.K. (1982). Reliability of recall of drug usage and other health-related information. *Am. J. Epidemiol. 116*, 114–122.

Palmisano, P.A. and Cassady, G. (1969). Salicylate exposure in the perinate. *J.A.M.A. 209*, 556–560.

Pelkonen, O., Jouppila, P., and Karki, N.T. (1972). Effect of maternal cigarette smoking on 3,4-benzpyrene and N-methylaniline metabolism in human fetal liver and placenta. *Toxicol. Appl. Pharmacol. 23*, 399–407.

Phelan, M.C., Pellock, J.M., and Nance, W.E. (1982). Discordant expression of fetal hydantoin syndrome in heteropaternal dizygotic twins. *N. Engl. J. Med. 307*, 99–101.

Rosenberg, L., Mitchell, A.A., Shapiro, S., and Slone, D. (1982). Selected birth defects in relation to caffeine-containing beverages. *J.A.M.A. 247*, 1429–1432.

Rothman, K.J. (1974). Synergy and antagonism in cause-effect relationships. *Am. J. Epidemiol. 99*, 385–388.

——— (1976). The estimation of synergy or antagonism. *Am. J. Epidemiol. 103*, 506–511.

——— (1977). Fetal loss, twinning, and birthweight after oral contraceptive use. *N. Engl. J. Med. 297*, 468–471.

——— and Boice, J.D., Jr. (1979). *Epidemiologic analysis with a programmable calculator.* Washington, D.C.: U.S. Department of Health, Education and Welfare, Public Health Service, National Institutes of Health, National Cancer Institute, Environmental Epidemiology Branch.

———, Greenland, S., and Walker, A.M. (1980). Concepts of interaction. *Am. J. Epidemiol. 112*, 467–470.

Royal College of General Practitioners (1976). The outcome of pregnancy in former oral contraceptive users. *Br. J. Obstet. Gynaecol. 83*, 608–616.

——— Oral Contraception Study (1977). Mortality among oral-contraceptive users. *Lancet 2* (8041), 727–731.

Rudolph, A.M. (1974). *Congenital diseases of the heart.* Chicago: Year Book Medical Publishers, p. 265.

Sackett, D.L. (1979). Bias in analytic research. *J. Chron. Dis. 32*, 51–63.

Saracci, R. (1977). Asbestos and lung cancer: An analysis of the epidemiological evidence on the asbestos-smoking interaction. *Int. J. Cancer 20*, 323–331.

Schardein, J.L. (1976). *Drugs as teratogens.* Cleveland, Ohio: CRC Press.

Scheffé, H. (1953). A method of judging all contrasts in the analysis of variance. *Biometrics 40*, 87–104.

Schlesselman, J.J. (1982). *Case-control studies.* New York: Oxford University Press.

Shepard, T.H. (1980). *Catalog of teratogenic agents*, 3rd Ed. Baltimore: The Johns Hopkins University Press.

Shum, S., Jensen, N.M., and Nebert, D.W. (1979). The murine *Ah* locus: In utero toxicity and teratogenesis associated with genetic differences in benzo[a]pyrene metabolism. *Teratology 20*, 365–376.

Spence, M.A. and Gladstein, K. (1978). Pyloric stenosis and the simulation of mendelism. In *Genetic epidemiology*, edited by N.E. Morton and C.S. Chung. New York: Academic Press, pp. 331–351.

Spielberg, S.P. (1982). Pharmacogenetics and the fetus. *N. Engl. J. Med. 307*, 115–116.

Stolley, P.D., Tonascia, J.A., Sartwell, P.E., Tockman, M.S., Tonascia, S., Rutledge, A., and Schinnar, R. (1978). Agreement rates between oral contraceptive users and prescribers in relation to drug use histories. *Am. J. Epidemiol. 107*, 226–235.

Tuchmann-Duplessis, H. (1975). *Drug effects on the fetus.* Sydney, Australia: ADIS Press.

Vessey, M.P., McPherson, K., and Johnson, B. (1977). Mortality among women participating in the Oxford/Family Planning Association Contraceptive Study. *Lancet 2* (8041), 731–733.

———, Meisler, L., Flavel, R., and Yeates, D. (1979). Outcome of pregnancy in women using different methods of contraception. *Br. J. Obstet. Gynaecol. 86*, 548–556.

Walter, S.D. (1978). Calculation of attributable risks from epidemiological data. *Int. J. Epidemiol. 7*, 175–182.

——— and Holford, T.R. (1978). Additive, multiplicative and other models for disease risks. *Am. J. Epidemiol. 108*, 341–346.

Welch, R.M., Harrison, Y.E., Conney, A.H., Poppers, P.J., and Finster, J. (1968). Cigarette smoking: Stimulatory effect on metabolism of 3,4-benzpyrene. *Science 160*, 541–542.

———, ———, Gomni, B.W., Poppers, P.J., Finster, M., and Conney, A.H. (1969). Stimulatory effect of cigarette smoking on the hydroxylation of 3,4-benzpyrene and the N-demethylation of 3-methyl-4-monomethyl-aminoazobenzene by enzymes in human placenta. *Clin. Pharmacol. Ther. 10*, 100.

———, Poppers, P.J., Harrison, Y.E., and Conney, A.H. (1968a). Stimulatory effect of cigarette smoking on the metabolism of 3,4-benzpyrene (BP) by enzymes in human placenta. *Proc. Am. Soc. Exp. Biol. 27*, 301.

Wolpert, L. (1976). Mechanisms of limb development and malformation. *Br. Med. Bull. 32*, 65–70.

World Health Organization (1981). *The effect of female sex hormones on fetal development and infant health.* Technical Report Series 657. Geneva: WHO.

Yaffe, S.S. and Stern, L. (1976). Clinical implications of perinatal pharmacology. In *Perinatal pharmacology and therapeutics*, edited by B.L. Mirkin. New York: Academic Press, pp. 355–428.

19

Assessment of Occupational and Environmental Exposures

Jane E. Gordon

In the search for causes of reproductive failure, investigators have focused their efforts on a spectrum of reproductive outcomes in each parent, the developing fetus, and the newborn. The range of outcomes includes sexual dysfunction, germ cell and semen abnormalities, subfertility, fetal loss, chromosomal and congenital abnormalities, prematurity, childhood developmental disability, morbidity, and mortality. This list of end points is neither exhaustive nor necessarily mutually exclusive. Each outcome mentioned is subject to errors of its own in terms of diagnosis, self-report, biologic significance, and interpretation (Bloom, 1981). In planning and conducting perinatal research, the difficulty of defining outcome events complicates the search for etiologic agents and for biologic mechanisms, as well as the identification of populations at greatest risk.

Scientific research has always placed a high priority on the determination of cause–effect relationships. In that vein, a wide variety of exposures have been studied as possible causes for diagnosed perinatal disease or less than optimum perinatal health. Although we will focus on identifying types of exposure, it may be useful to distinguish first between intrinsic and extrinsic factors.

Intrinsic factors relate to the characteristics or conditions of an individual. Such factors can be considered elements of exposure because they exert a direct effect on the diesase process or on an individual's susceptibility to disease, and therefore impact on the exposure–disease relationship. Sociodemographic factors such as age, ethnicity, social class (education/occupation), and marital status are often used as the most basic descriptors of a population's exposure or risk status.

450

Standardized schemes have been devised for coding occupational and industrial classifications: The *Alphabetical Index of Industries and Occupations* (U.S. Dept. of Commerce, 1982), the *Dictionary of Occupational Titles* (U.S. Dept. of Labor, 1977), and the *Standard Industrial Codes* (Office of Management and Budget, 1972) have all been widely used. Newer schemes that link known or presumed exposures to specific occupations have also been developed and are undergoing testing and revision (Hoar, 1980; U.S. Dept. of Health and Human Services, 1982).

Personal and family history of disease can indicate genetic diseases or traits that may influence the health of an individual or relate to the chance of his or her offspring being affected. Other traditional risk factors that help to define exposure or susceptibility come from an individual's medical history of specific, acute, and chronic diseases. This may extend to the reproductive history of a couple or of each partner.

Sometimes in perinatal research, what may be an outcome of interest in one study may be used in another study to define exposure status. For example, studies of the effectiveness of diethylstilbestrol (DES) in preventing miscarriage led to later investigation of the effects of the drug in possibly limiting the reproductive potential of the offspring (Gill et al., 1978; Barnes et al., 1980; Herbst et al., 1980).

Extrinsic factors refer to the variety of agents introduced into our environment voluntarily or otherwise. Among these are drug usage (further classified as prescription, over the counter, and illicit), consumption of caffeine, alcohol, and tobacco, and nutritional factors. The remaining category of extrinsic exposure factors is the primary focus of this chapter, namely exposures in the occupational and ambient (indoor and outdoor) environments.

Three major issues predominate in assessing environmental and occupational exposures: (1) their measurement, (2) where, when, and to whom they occur, and (3) consequences of determining measurements and occurrence.

EXPOSURE MEASUREMENT

The technology of environmental sampling and laboratory evaluations is beyond the scope of this discussion (U.S. Dept. of Health and Human Services, 1973; Patty, 1977). However, consideration of the possible problems in collecting samples in the field, and interpreting the results, are critical elements to an epidemiologist attempting to quantify exposures. The list of parameters to be considered when undertaking field sampling in both the occupational and ambient environments also indicates the numerous opportunities that exist for introducing measurement error. Lippmann and Schlesinger (1979) have carefully reviewed the elements of environmental measurement. Although theirs is not an epidemiologic perspective, the following points are relevant nonetheless.

Choosing which agents are to be measured requires extensive technical and professional experience, particularly when many agents coexist in the workplace or surrounding environment, and their association with the outcome of interest is not established or may not even be suspected.

The selection of which materials are to be sampled and analyzed for levels of a specific agent can clearly affect the ultimate classification of exposure status. For example, if occupational exposure to chemicals were measured only in terms of inhalable vapors, exposure status could be subject to error if dermal and oral sources of exposure were not also considered. In environmental settings, the appropriateness of sampling air, water, soil, food, biota, or biologicals may be clear, as in an outbreak of gastrointestinal illness after the annual picnic, but less so when exposure is presumed to be toxic waste materials and the effect is adverse reproductive outcomes among area residents, as was the case in the Love Canal area of New York State (Paigen, 1982).

The type of sample examined can provide a range of information but is subject to misinterpretation in terms of assessing whether the correct type of sample was taken for the association in question. Thus, source samples (e.g., effluents from smokestacks or discharge pipes) provide quantitative information about the elements measured at the source, but little about actual external exposures to population groups, and nothing about an individual's internal dose.

Outdoor ambient samples measure representative air and watershed locations within designated areas, often to monitor environmental standards. Such measurements would be of limited usefulness in determining an individual's dose or the source of the potential (specific) exposure. This would also be true, but to a lesser degree, of samples collected in indoor environments, particularly in the home.

Personal samples measure elements (usually in the air) in the individual's immediate environment (e.g., inhalation exposures of workers) and are often collected with pieces of equipment worn by the subject. The value of measures made on samples of this sort depends on cooperation on the part of the subjects. Anecdotal reports abound of individuals being studied who have covered, removed, or overexposed the sampling equipment to influence study results for motives of their own.

Finally, process samples are collected within equipment used for a specific industrial process or transfer line, to describe rates of flow or composition of materials. This type of measure may show the highest concentration of many elements, but reflects very little about environmental or personal exposure.

The timing of sampling (from fractions of a minute to seasons of the year), whether continuous or point measures are taken, as well as the precise locations in a workplace or geographic area, can clearly affect the concentration of measured substances. For example, particulate airborne lead in the workplace is measured as a function of weight per cubic meter. This does not account for size of the particle. Therefore, if samples were taken close to the emission source, the amount of lead in the air would be high, but this would include a large proportion of nonrespirable particles that would not be of importance in the assessment of a worker's dose.

Similarly, for environmental measurement of pesticidal chemicals, seasonality is an important factor. Measures taken during planting or harvesting seasons would give different impressions of potential human exposure than would be generated from samples taken during the winter or even during the growing periods. Within the peak application periods, the time between chemical treatment of land or crops and collection of the environmental samples will provide a wide range of exposure data. Use of measurements at any point within this range can be justified, but careful interpretation and qualification of results of ensuing studies would be essential.

In general, the timing of sampling includes parameters such as distance from the source of the agent, air currents in the measurement area, temperature and other atmospheric conditions, the representativeness of the sample in terms of its presence in a particular process at any chosen time, and the chemical and physical properties of the agent being collected. These and other sources of potential bias must be carefully evaluated prior to field work and incorporated into the design of a specific study.

Temporal and spatial sampling parameters relate closely to the number of samples of each type that must be drawn at each location in order to approximate "true" exposure to people. If continuous measures are not feasible, samples collected at various times throughout a typical set of workdays would be a reasonable alternative. Determinations of the sampling intervals and of how the collected samples must be stored and shipped must be made in order to avoid introducing systematic error into the laboratory analyses.

Sound principles of measurement are predicated on the use of appropriate, accurate, and uniformly calibrated equipment. Calibration of equipment involves comparing each device in use to a reference instrument and to a standard sample of the substance being measured. The underlying purpose is to ensure the validity of the measure (the ability to measure what the instrument claims to measure) and its reliability (i.e., precision, repeatability), which refers to the replicability of the measure. The degree of replicability depends on the variability of the instrument, the observer, and the subject (particularly in cases where biologic, physiologic, or behavioral measures are involved). Calibrating equipment and standardizing the techniques for drawing, processing, and analyzing samples must include the training of responsible personnel. Such training should include strategies relevant to the particular study that will minimize both within-observer and between-observer variability. Part of the training program should include work with standard samples or subjects and be followed up by field testing under actual conditions.

The purpose of attending to the components of measurement variation is to minimize the chance of introducing biased (systematic) error into the study from either the observers, the subjects, or both. Systematic error cannot be reduced by increasing sample size; it is hard to quantify, it can often go unrecognized, and conclusions or comparisons made on such data are distorted. Random error, in contrast, can often be adjusted for if sample size is increased and if the magnitude of the measurement variation is known. However, the true association being examined may be obscured or inaccurately estimated (Rose et al., 1982).

Even presuming cooperation on the part of the people being sampled, and the skill and impartiality of the observers, the process of obtaining quality measurements on any single agent is complex. Moreover, the integration of the elements of each of the measurement parameters described is a multifaceted task that remains complex in its interpretation on the technical (instrumentation), statistical, and biologic levels.

Strobino, Kline, and Stein (1978) have compiled an extensive list of individual agents and their effect on human reproduction. Other listings also exist that aim at identifying chemical hazards to human reproduction (Clement Associates, 1981). These lists are very useful, but they do not address the increasing degree of complexity that exists when one considers that people are simultaneously exposed to multiple agents within their workplace, and concurrently, to multiple agents from their outdoor and indoor environments (Sever, 1981). Consideration of exposures—including environmental pollutants found in air, water, soil, and food, hobbies, fumes from home heating fuels, and use of some home cleaning products—might well be made to construct an overall exposure score that would represent more closely an individual's total exposure to the main elements in their personal environment.

Personal habits such as cigarette smoking and alcohol use may modify the effects of occupational and environmental exposures. Perhaps the best known example of this comes from the research done on smoking and asbestos. Asbestos workers had a risk of dying from lung cancer that was five times that of controls in both smoker and nonsmoker groups. However, the combined effect of smoking and asbestos exposure appeared to fit a multiplicative rather than additive model; that is, the mortality ratio for the group with both exposures was close to 55 times that of controls with neither exposure, whereas smoking alone increased the death rate about 11 times and asbestos alone increased it 5 times (Hammond, et al., 1979; U.S. Dept. of Health and Human Services, (1980).

If personal habits promote behavior that removes the person from the exposure source (e.g., they were too intoxicated to work or succumbed quickly to dust or fumes because of reduced lung function from smoking), their absolute exposure might actually be low and result in an apparent net protection from the exposure agent. Alternatively, subjects may be more susceptible to even minimal exposures, and therefore be at greater risk of ill effects, because of the nature of their impaired physical state, as in the smoking–asbestos example above. The risk factors of smoking and drinking are particularly important in relation to their potential effects on occupational and environmental exposures in perinatal research because of their demonstrated independent associations with pregnancy outcome (Landesman-Dwyer and Emanuel, 1979; Streissguth et al., 1980).

EXPOSURE OCCURRENCE

Although any single type of exposure may be relatively constant, the situations in which each is found and measured may be unique. If occupational and environmental exposures are simplistically assumed to be chemical, biologic, or physical (e.g., noise, heat, radiation), measurements of a specific agent in a factory setting, when contrasted with the same substance in the environment, could require different technical measurement strategies. The resulting measures could lead to different interpretations regarding the levels of exposure to people in each environment.

Lead exposure provides an example of this problem. The examination of worker exposure to lead might take the form of measurements of airborne particulates in the workplace supplemented by blood lead levels to assess systemic evidence of the exposure. Concentrations of lead in effluent discharged by a plant into a river could be a measure of potential community lead exposure, whereas the measurement of lead content in drinking water delivered to homes via lead pipes can be used to quantify personal exposure. Children's exposure to particulate lead brought home on the clothing, skin, or hair of their occupationally exposed parents constitute yet another level of exposure. This set of illustrations demonstrating how lead exposure can reach individuals in and around an industrial setting can also serve to highlight the fact that it may be the individual's cumulative exposure from *all* sources that is the most accurate measure of actual external exposure to any single agent.

Difficult though it is to define an individual's level of exposure to one or more agents from occupational sources, it is even more difficult to define the additional effect of indirect exposure to the same agents the worker faces at home, and to which the worker's family may also be subjected (possibly stemming from materials that are inadvertently brought home on clothing, skin, or hair, or are in drinking water, as in the example with lead) (Ratcliffe, 1981). The source of exposure may affect the hypothesized mechanism of biologic effects manifest in these individuals. For example, X-radiation, which may be potentially carcinogenic to the person with primary exposure in the workplace or elsewhere, may also damage germ cells and sperm, and thereby future development of a fetus. Thus an agent may be simultaneously classified as a mutagen and a teratogen. The biologic effect being studied often reflects the researcher's hypothesis as to whether teratogenesis, mutagenesis, carcinogenesis, or developmental toxicity is presumed to be in operation in relation to exposure to a specific agent (Hunt, 1979). Furthermore, multiple exposures may exist for the developing fetus. Exposures that may have preconceptionally affected the germ cells of one or both parents in occupational or environmental settings may do so again postconceptionally through continued direct (e.g., on the job) or indirect (e.g., from contaminated clothing or water) maternal exposure (Selevan, 1981).

The determination of who is actually exposed must accommodate the biologic question of whether an environmental sample (an external measure of exposure) is an adequate surrogate for what the human body absorbs, metabolizes, stores, and excretes (the internal evidence of exposure). External measurement of exposure includes (1) the concentration of the specific agent, per unit of a relevant medium (e.g., air, water), that can reach an individual, and (2) the rate of intake of the exposure medium per unit time. This is not the same as an individual's internal exposure or dose. Dose refers to the amount of the specific agent (via its medium) that can reach an organ or other site of effect. Because the site of effect is not always known or directly measurable, biologic specimens (e.g., blood, tissue, urine, feces) are often used as surrogates. Even biologic specimens may give only a partial indication of "true" exposure. Ratcliffe (1981) discusses the exposure and dose concepts in conjunction with a metabolic model that evaluates quantitative and qualitative aspects of absorption, distribution, deposition, accumulation, and excretion of lead. The kinetics of these processes in any given part of the body will affect both our measurement and our assessment of whether or not exposure has occurred or affected an individual. Furthermore, biologic samples used for evidence of the effect of a presumed toxicant depend not only on the kinetics of its metabolism but on the initial rates of its intake. For instance, an individual's rate and depth of breathing would influence the dose of respirable material, as would the contents of a person's gut affect the dose of ingested matter (related to the absorption rate). Parameters such as these, in addition to age, sex, body size, health status, and so forth, must be considered in the assessment of evidence of apparent dose–effect relationships (the gradation of a biologic effect with increasing dose) and dose–response relationships (the frequency of each level of a biologic effect in the population studied relative to increasing dosage).

Regardless of how highly specific the biologic index of lead exposure may be, the biologic significance of a given dose will be different in childhood and in the fetal stages of life from that of adults as a result of differences in body weight, metabolic rate, and rate of tissue growth. Ratcliffe (1981) cites animal and human evidence relating to the particular physiologic vulnerability or dose-specific susceptibility of the young to lead. She also describes epidemiologic studies of lead neurotoxicity, mental retardation, and hyperactivity in children. Although the study findings are inconsistent and often limited by a lack of comparability among the study populations in measurements of dose and in the definition of an effect, there is clear evidence for a positive correlation between lead in cord and in maternal blood, with the suggestion that the placental transfer begins at approximately the third month of gestation and increases throughout the pregnancy. This evidence provides the necessary link between maternal, prenatal, and postnatal lead exposure, and its potential contribution to neurologic effects in children (see also Chapter 9).

One might suspect that male or female fetuses may be differentially susceptible to toxicants if hormones or storage in fat cells play a part in the manifestation of effects of certain exposures, such as those to pesticides. Chlorinated hydrocarbon pesticides (e.g., DDT and its derivatives DDD and DDE; BHC, dieldrin, heptachlor epoxide) are stored in body fat and blood (Hayes, 1975). Because females generally have more body fat than males, and blood volume and metabolic rate increases during pregnancy, it is not surprising to find that cord blood and many fetal tissues are laden with these chemicals (Curley et al.,

1969). Animal studies further document female excesses in the storage of this class of chemicals in all tissues (Hayes, 1975). Selective survival of fetuses exposed to such toxins could also be a function of their sex. Perhaps this could explain a portion of the deviation from the normal livebirth sex ratio of infants born with anencephaly, spina bifida, or trisomy 18 (Stein et al., 1975; Elwood and Elwood, 1980).

It is not sufficient in epidemiology to consider only who is at risk of exposure or who is actually exposed. One must also consider who is *classified* as being exposed and the effect that classification has on measures of association. The potential for misclassifying "exposed" individuals as "unexposed," or vice versa, is an important research issue whether the exposures come from occupational or from environmental settings. The effect of such misclassification reduces the chance of detecting a true association when one exists between exposure and outcome, or will tend to conceal the true strength of the association (Kleinbaum et al., 1982).

How exposure agents have their impact may vary by the timing of each insult. From a research perspective, one should consider the issues of acute, possibly one-time exposure, chronic exposure at uniform or variable dosage levels, and the importance of summarizing these types of exposure for a cumulative dose while taking into consideration possible synergistic or antagonistic effects. Gordon and Shy (1981) developed an exposure-scoring system that evaluated the simultaneous exposure to several types of agricultural chemicals in relation to congenital cleft lip or palate. It was only when the summary exposure score was used that a pattern of positive, statistically significant, results was suggested. Expanding the strategies for composite indices of risk is challenging and difficult. Applying such indices would require different assumptions and techniques in prospective, cross-sectional, and historical study time frames. Although not linked to a specific study strategy, the National Institute for Occupational Safety and Health (NIOSH) is in the process of developing a risk algorithm that ranks occupations as potentially hazardous on the basis of literature reports of known toxic chemical agents that exist in the various occupational settings (U.S. Dept. of Health and Human Services, 1982).

Modeling exposure with a view to several temporal issues could refine the dose parameter of the crucial dose–effect and dose–response relationships. There are several issues involved, the first of which is the age at first exposure, including in utero exposure. This focuses on the susceptibility of rapidly growing tissues to potentially toxic agents, as previously mentioned for the effects of lead on the fetus and in children.

The second concern is the timing (i.e., age) at peak exposure. This too relates to susceptibility, in that the youngest or oldest individuals

458

may be at increased risk because of factors such as immature or weakened immune responses to biologic insults. From another perspective, the identical dose (80 μg/dl of lead) to a healthy adult may not result in any overt symptoms, whereas a child may develop acute symptoms (lead poisoning or encephalopathy) (Ratcliffe, 1981).

The third related issue is cumulative lifetime exposure. Except where resistance to an agent is possible, it would be reasonable to presume that as the duration of exposure increases, so will the likelihood that the dose will increase (particularly if the toxicant is stored in the body); thereby the threshold for a biologic effect will be reached, potentially increasing the severity of an effect with increasing dose (over time).

It is not clear whether the sequence in which exposures are encountered has any effect on outcomes observed. If more were known about the biologic interactions of the agents, including their absorption, distribution, and excretion, then single or combined metabolic processes might be identified that could mediate or possibly prevent adverse biologic effects. Research on how nutritional status might affect disease processes is being developed. This has been rapidly expanding in the field of cancer research (National Research Council, 1981). Nutritional deficiencies or excesses, and their relation to teratology, are outside the scope of this chapter. However, Hurley (1977) has summarized the influence of nutritional elements during the prenatal period. Work relating susceptibility to lead toxicity and various nutritional factors (calcium, phosphorous, iron, copper, zinc, protein, fat, and vitamin D) have been summarized by Ratcliffe (1981), with particular attention paid to the effects on children. She concludes that a diet low in protein, minerals, and certain vitamins may very likely increase a growing child's vulnerability to a systemic dose of lead and actually enhance the effect of that dose.

CONSEQUENCES OF DETERMINING MEASUREMENTS AND OCCURRENCES OF EXPOSURE

Health professionals carry much of the responsibility for researching the associations between exposure factors and health outcomes and for implementation of the research findings. We have already seen examples of this in disease prevention or health education (e.g., genetic counseling) (Stein et al, 1975) and antismoking campaigns (Doll and Hill, 1950, 1964; Doll and Peto, 1976), medical therapies for cancer, or a commitment to routine screening, surveillance, and monitoring programs (e.g., alphafetoprotein) (Goldberg and Oakley, 1979), birth defects (U.S. Dept. of Health and Human Services, 1974), chromosomal and cytogenetic monitoring of specific occupational groups at high risk (Bloom, 1981), and well-established cancer registries like that in Connecticut.

The clinically oriented health professional also has the opportunity to help in collecting and recording medical information from patients in a comprehensive, uniform manner that will be of considerable value in direct patient care as well as in research. Some examples of relevant areas for such data gathering include the diagnosis and classification of congenital malformations for entry onto hospital and birth records, and the need for information about occupational history on hospital, birth (parental occupations), and death records. The extensiveness of the occupational history will vary with the capacity of the recording system, and also the nature of the agents and outcomes under study. Key occupational parameters in perinatal research should focus on (1) each parent's occupation(s) and place of employment pre-, post-, and at conception, (2) the duration of each, (3) a checklist of known or suspected hazardous agents, and (4) a description of materials handled and duties on the job.

The greatest psychosocial impact of scientific research on the public is through the variety of media that are reporting ever more stories about both exposures and disease. Jargon that is commonplace in scientific circles may not be clear or have the same meaning for lay readers. The danger of misinterpretation, overacceptance, disbelief, or fear among the lay public may affect their attidues and behavior on health and safety issues. Scientists should consider the ethical ramifications of how their data can be used, particularly by the public. For example, some women have had themselves sterilized in order to obtain or to keep high-paying jobs working with agents labeled as teratogenic (Hunt, 1979).

The level of the public's misinterpretation of scientific findings, or belief about a potential hazard, may result in biases that might complicate the process of conducting future research. A current example of this potential bias surrounds the increasing reports of clusters of adverse pregnancy outcomes among female users of video display terminals (VDTs) (Microwave News, 1981). A few women have presumed that they are exposed to X-radiation from the terminals in spite of reports to the contrary (U.S. Dept. of Health and Human Services, 1981) and have taken to wearing lead aprons at work. Another aspect of the bias could be differential recall of information related to exposure or outcome among the groups being compared. The problems created for researchers would be compounded if all female VDT operators believed they would spontaneously abort their pregnancies if they did not leave their jobs, thereby effectively eliminating the exposed study group before their true risk could be evaluated. Alternatively, if the exposed group decided to report exposures or adverse reproductive outcomes to confirm their own ideas about the cause–effect relationship, the data would be systematically biased, and the study results would be distorted.

There are legal and political ramifications of much research on the health effects of industrial exposures in the workplace and emissions into the general environment. The establishment of federal exposure standards, their evaluation, enforcement, and revision are often challenged by industrial and labor officials, and by scientists. The strengths and weaknesses of data supporting environmental standards, or a set of research findings, are frequently being aired in courtrooms, where workers or exposed persons are suing for compensation for their ill health (e.g., asbestos workers suing their former employer). Longo (1980) raises some interesting questions as to where this type of litigation may lead if in fact the fetus, born damaged but alive, sues its mother for "wrongful birth or life," for exposing it to harmful agents, or the manufacturer of that agent, or the medical practitioner who failed to test for or warn against such exposure. It is almost certain that the legal arguments in any case like this would rely heavily on the parameters discussed in this chapter pertaining to the measurement and occurrence of exposures in the occupational and ambient environments.

Beyond research and health education, technology must be used to advantage in order to enhance environmental exposure measurement capability and interpretability. Environmental safety must be built into newly constructed and created industries, for the protection of the workforce and the community, and to provide for the safe, permanent disposal of hazardous wastes. Tackling the complexities of creating a safe environment, innovatively assessing the substances that will remain to be monitored, and providing the epidemiologic research that will identify true perinatal risks can improve our chance of benefiting from, and of meeting, the new environmental challenges that accompany technology.

REFERENCES

Barnes, A.B., Colton, T., Gunderson, J., Noller, K.L., Tilley, B.C., Strama, T., Townsend, D.E., Hatab, P., and O'Brien, P.C. (1980). Fertility and pregnancy outcomes in women exposed *in utero* to diethylstilbestrol: Preliminary findings from the DESAD project. *N. Engl. J. Med. 302*, 609–613.

Bloom, A.D., editor (1981). *Guidelines for studies of human populations exposed to mutagenic and reproductive hazards.* White Plains, N.Y.: March of Dimes Birth Defects Foundation.

Clement Associates, Inc. (1981). *Chemical hazards to human reproduction.* Report prepared for the Council on Environmental Quality. Washington, D.C.: U.S. Government Printing Office.

Curley, A., Copeland, M.F., and Kimbrough, R.D. (1969). Chlorinated hydrocarbon insecticides in organs of stillborn and blood of newborn babies. *Arch. Environ. Health 19*, 628–632.

Doll, R. and Hill, A.B. (1950). Smoking and carcinoma of the lung. *Br. Med. J. 2*, 739–748.

———— and ———— (1964). Mortality in relation to smoking: Ten years' observation of British doctors. *Br. Med. J. 1*, 1399–1410, 1460–1467.

———— and Peto, R. (1976). Mortality in relation to smoking: 20 years' observations on male British doctors. *Br. Med. J. 2*, 1525–1536.

Elwood, J.M. and Elwood, J.H. (1980). *Epidemiology of Anencephalus and spina bifida.* New York: Oxford University Press.

Gill, W.B., Schumacker, G.F., and Bibbo, M. (1978). Genital and semen abnormalities in adult males two and one half decades after *in utero* exposure to diethylstilbestrol. In *American College of Obstetrics and Gynecology DES Symposium Proceedings*, edited by A.L. Herbst. Chicago: American College of Obstetrics and Gynecology, pp. 53–57.

Goldberg, M.F. and Oakley, G.P. (1979). Prenatal screening of anencephaly and spina bifida: Some epidemiological projections for a national program. In *Service and education in medical genetics*, edited by I.H. Porter and E.B. Hook. New York: Academic Press.

Gordon, J.E. and Shy, C.M. (1981). Agricultural chemical use and congenital cleft lip and/or palate. *Arch. Environ. Health 36*, 213–220.

Hammond, E.C., Selikoff, I.J., and Seidman, H. (1979). Asbestos exposure, cigarette smoking, and death rates. *Ann. N.Y. Acad. Sci. 330*, 473–490.

Hayes, W.J. (1975). *Toxicology of pesticides.* Baltimore: Williams and Wilkins.

Herbst, A.C., Hubby, H.M., Plough, R.R., and Azizzi, F. (1980). A comparison of pregnancy experience in DES exposed and DES unexposed daughters. *J. Reprod. Med. 24*, 62–69.

Hoar, S. (1980). Computerized occupation–exposure crosslinkage system. Personal communication.

Hunt. V.R. (1979). *Work and the health of women.* Boca Raton, Fla.: CRC Press.

Hurley, L.S. (1977). In *Handbook of teratology: General principles and etiology*, edited by J.G. Wilson and F.C. Fraser. New York: Plenum Press.

Kleinbaum, D.G., Kupper, L.L., and Morgenstern, H. (1982). *Epidemiologic research: Principles and quantitative methods.* Belmont, Calif.: Lifetime Learning Publications.

Landesman-Dwyer, S. and Emanuel, I. (1979). Smoking during pregnancy. *Teratology 19*, 119–125.

Lippmann, M. and Schlesinger, R.B (1979). *Chemical contaminants in the human environment.* New York: Oxford University Press.

Longo, L.D. (1980). Environmental pollution and pregnancy: Risks and uncertainties for the fetus and infants. *Am. J. Obstet. Gynecol. 137*, 162–173.

462

Microwave News (1981). Birth defect and miscarriage clusters stir up more fears over VDTs. October 1981, pp. 1–3.

National Research Council (1981). *Diet, nutrition and cancer.* Washington, D.C.: National Academic Press.

Office of Management and Budget (1972). *Standard industrial classification manual.* Washington, D.C.: U.S. Government Printing Office.

Paigen, B. (1982). Controversy at Love Canal. *Hastings Center Report 12*, 29–37.

Patty, F., Clayton, G., and Clayton, F. (1977). *Industrial hygiene and toxicology*, 3rd Ed., Vol 1. New York: Wiley.

Ratcliffe, J.M. (1981). *Lead in man and the environment.* New York: Wiley.

Rose, G.A., Blackburn, H., Gillum, R.F., and Prineas, R.J. (1982). *Cardiovascular survey methods*, 2nd Ed. Geneva: World Health Organization Monographs No. 56.

Selevan, S.G. (1981). Design considerations in pregnancy outcome studies of occupational populations. *Scand. J. Work, Environ. Health 7* (Suppl. 4), 76–82.

Sever, L.E. (1981). Reproductive hazards of the workplace. *J. Occup. Med. 23*, 685–689.

Stein, Z., Susser, M., Warburton, D., Wittes, J., and Kline, J. (1975). Spontaneous abortion as a screening device. *Am. J. Epidemiol. 102*, 275–290.

Streissguth, A.P., Landesman-Dwyer, S., Martin, J.C., and Smith, D.W. (1980). Teratogenic effects of alcohol in humans and laboratory animals. *Science 209*, 353–361.

Strobino, B.R., Kline, J., and Stein, Z. (1978). Chemical and physical exposures of parents: Effects on human reproduction and offspring. *Early Hum. Dev. 1*, 371–399.

U.S. Department of Commerce, Bureau of the Census (1982). *1980 Census of population alphabetical index of industries and occupations.* Washington, D.C.: U.S. Government Printing Office.

U.S. Department of Health and Human Services (Centers for Disease Control) (1974). *Birth defects monitoring program*, Congenital Malformations Surveillane Bimonthly Reports.

U.S. Department of Health and Human Services (NIOSH) (1973). *The industrial environment—its evaluation and control.* Washington, D.C.: U.S. Government Printing Office.

U.S. Department of Health and Human Services (NIOSH) (1980). *Workplace exposure to asbestos—review and recommendations.* Washington, D.C.: U.S. Government Printing Office.

U.S. Department of Health and Human Services (NIOSH) (1982). *NIOSH risk identification model—preliminary report.* Personal communication.

U.S. Department of Health and Human Services, Public Health Services, Food and Drug Administration, Bureau of Radiologic Health (1981). *An evaluation of radiation emission from video display terminals.* Washington, D.C.: U.S. Government Printing Office.

U.S. Department of Labor (1977). *Dictionary of occupational titles*; 4th Ed. Washington, D.C.: U.S. Government Printing Office.

20

Detection of Neurobehavioral Dysfunction in Infancy: Current Methods, Problems, and Prospects

David T. Scott

Adults caring for an infant often wonder about the child's future life. This is all the more true when the child is in some sense medically exceptional or at risk. Some infants are placed at risk by forces at work before their conception; some experience chronic stresses during gestation or more acute insults during labor and delivery; still others encounter problems during the newborn period. But whenever there is a suspicion of damage to the central nervous system, urgent questions are asked: What exactly has happened and how serious is it? What is the prognosis? What can be done to facilitate recovery? At present these questions are often difficult, if not impossible, to answer.

This chapter reviews some of the work that has been done in the detection of neurobehavioral dysfunction since the Second World War. An effort is made to identify some areas of special promise for future investigations.

ASSESSMENTS OF GESTATIONAL AGE

There is little disagreement with the assertion that comprehensive neurologic and behavioral assessments of infants must be conducted with reference to a set of expectations or norms based on the infant's degree of maturity. For example, infants born after a gestation of only 26 to 28 weeks commonly exhibit a degree of hypotonia or "floppiness" that would be quite pathologic in a full-term infant. Likewise, in the term neonate, the absence of a well-formed Moro reflex (see below) may be regarded as a sign of neurologic dysfunction, whereas the *presence* of a well-formed Moro reflex after six to nine months of age is often a sign of dysfunction (Peiper, 1963; Fiorentino, 1972).

Thus, in order to evaluate the significance of the infant's neurobe-havioral attributes, we must determine whether there are any exten-uating circumstances (e.g., maternal anesthesia) that might alter the infant's neurobehavioral functioning, and we must compare our clinical findings with expectations based on the infant's level of maturity.

In the case of preterm infants, one uses the gestational age up until term; thereafter, the "corrected age," the age computed from the maternal due date, is employed (Drillien, 1964; Saint-Anne Dargassies, 1972). Maturational assessments thus play a special role in the care of preterm infants, in that they determine both the maturational expec-tations in the neonatal period and the corrected age thereafter. Furthermore, many neonatologists prefer maturational assessments based on a clinical examination of the neonate (Lubchenco, 1975). Gestational assessments based on the date of the last menstrual period (LMP) are subject to a variety of systematic biases. The LMP may be altered by contraceptive medication or by breast-feeding in a recent pregnancy, and vaginal spotting or bleeding after a new pregnancy has begun may often be mistaken for a menstrual phe-nomenon.

For well over a century, experienced individuals have possessed the means to determine the approximate length of gestation of a fetus by examining the fetal morphology (e.g., His, 1882). However, it was not until much more recently that investigators codified this informa-tion into more formal scales that could be used in a clinical setting to establish the approximate length of gestation, usually within one or two weeks of the putative actual value.

The Amiel-Tison Method

A group of investigators in Paris developed a collection of matura-tional items involving primarily developmental changes in muscle tone and reflexes (Thomas and Saint-Anne Dargassies, 1952; Saint-Anne Dargassies, 1955, 1966; Minkowski et al., 1966). Subsequently, Amiel-Tison (1968) organized these techniques into an inventory that she proposed for practical clinical application. She included five tests of "passive tone," that is, the resistance an examiner encounters in attempting to move the infant's extremities while the infant is at rest. First, the infant's overall body *posture* is observed. The preterm infant at 28 weeks gestation typically lies with all four extremities fully extended and, like a rag doll, offers little or no resistance to exoge-nous movement. In the second test, the examiner flexes the infant's legs at the hips, taking care that the pelvis remains on the examining surface. In infants of 28 weeks gestation, there is so little passive tone that flexion continues until the heels are brought right to the ears, or very nearly so. With infants nearer and nearer term, this *heel-to-ear maneuver* encounters more and more resistance, and the heels stop short of the ears at a greater and greater distance as flexor tone increases.

At this point the *popliteal angle* may also be measured. Amiel-Tison recommends flexion and partial abduction at the hip to achieve a knee-on-chest position. Then an attempt is made to raise the lower leg away from the thigh. The popliteal angle is the angle formed when the lower leg is maximally extended in this position. At 28 weeks gestation, it is commonly measured at about 150°, but it becomes progressively more acute as the infant matures, and by term the maximum extension yields a popliteal angle of only about 80°. The fourth test involves *dorsiflexion of the foot* against the lower leg. Even though in general more passive tone is observed in infants close to term than in infants born very prematurely, the range of motion observed in pedal dorsiflexion is greatest in the full-term neonate, in whom the foot can often be fully dorsiflexed until it is virtually parallel to the lower leg. Only partial dorsiflexion (forming an angle of 40 to 50°) is observed prior to term, in preterm infants come to term, and in older infants.

The two remaining passive-tone assessments advocated by Amiel-Tison are the *scarf sign* and the *return to flexion of the forearm*. In the "scarf" maneuver, the examiner grasps one of the infant's hands and attempts to move the infant's arm across the midline and then across the contralateral shoulder. In the 28-week premature, very little resistance is encountered, and the arm may be wrapped over the contralateral shoulder almost like scarf. Nearer to term, progressively more resistance is encountered, largely because of the increasing flexion of the upper extremities. By 40 weeks from the LMP, the infant's elbow often will not cross the midline. *Return to flexion of the forearm* involves the recoil observed in an infant near term after the arms have been fully extended for half a minute and then quickly released. This recoil, or return to flexion, is weak or entirely absent before about 32 to 34 weeks gestation.

Amiel-Tison's approach to the assessment of active tone takes advantage of the caudocephalic progression in the development of tone up to term. At 30 to 32 weeks, one looks for an extensor tone in the lower extremities that is sufficient to bear at least some body weight when the infant is held in a vertical suspension. At about 36 weeks, the caudocephalic progression of tone should enable the infant to achieve reasonably full extension of the trunk, especially when the soles of the feet are stimulated by weight-bearing. Finally, at about term there should be sufficient active tone in the neck muscles to permit transient head righting. If this does not occur spontaneously in the seated infant while the head is flexed forward, the infant's trunk may be gradually tilted backward in order to facilitate lifting up the head with the nuchal extensor muscles. Alternatively, the supine infant may be pulled to sit by his hands or forearms; during this traction maneuver, the examiner determines the amount of head lag, or, obversely, the ability of the infant to use the neck flexor muscles to lift the head up from a hyperextended position.

Finally, Amiel-Tison recommended six "primary reactions" or reflexes. *Sucking* is commonly weak and poorly organized in the very premature infant of 28 to 30 weeks but is adequate for oral feedings by about 34 to 36 weeks. *Rooting* comprises movement of the face and head in response to perioral stimulation such that the infant's mouth is brought closer to the source of stimulation. This reflex, which clearly facilitates feeding in the more adaptive full-term neonate, is also sluggish and unreliable in the very premature infant. The *grasp reflex* refers to the infant's tendency to flex the fingers when the palms are rubbed by a small object. The toes can also be made to flex in a plantar grasp when the soles of the feet are stimulated in a similar manner. [Indeed, Peiper (1963) displayed photographs of infants suspended from a taut horizontal cord by the strength of their grasp reflexes.] Amiel-Tison used the extent to which the infant can bear weight by means of the palmar grasp as an index of maturity, with greater weight-bearing in the more mature infants.

The *Moro reflex* is also employed by Amiel-Tison in assessing maturation. Moro (1918) originally elicited this reflex by suddenly striking with both hands the surface on which the infant lay resting in supine position. It is now more commonly elicited by letting the infant's head drop backward a few centimeters in the sagittal plane. Alternatively, the examiner may hold the infant in supine position and then allow the infant's entire body to "drop" suddenly for a few centimeters. The full Moro response in a mature infant consists of abduction and partial extension of the arms, fanning of the fingers, and crying. Before 32 weeks, Amiel-Tison found the Moro reflex to be weak or incomplete and easily exhausted during repeated trials.

The crossed *extension* reflex is elicited by stimulation of the sole of one foot while that leg is held in extension. The response is observed in the contralateral leg and in full form comprised extension of the contralateral leg, adduction, and fanning of the toes. Amiel-Tison describes this response as largely random before about 30 weeks but fully formed by about 36 weeks.

The final test in the Amiel-Tison battery is *automatic walking* or *stepping*. When the infant is held in vertical suspension with the soles of the feet resting lightly on a horizontal surface, automatic stepping movements will be observed in many infants. The full-term infant, with better foot dorsiflexion, will appear to walk down on the soles of the feet, whereas the preterm infant will walk in a less organized manner (often on tiptoes) or not at all.

One of the drawbacks of the method set forth by Amiel-Tison is the absence of clearly delineated procedures for interpreting the information derived from each of the above tests. Others have objected that most of the individual items in the Amiel-Tison battery show considerable variation from infant to infant in the precise gestational ages at which they can be elicited (e.g., Dubowitz et al., 1970). The *return to flexion* or elbow-recoil maneuver, for example, has been shown to be rather poorly correlated with gestational age. On the one hand, partial elbow recoil may be observed in some infants as early as 28 weeks of gestation; on the other, there are isolated full-term infants in whom this response is totally absent.

The Dubowitz Scale

In order to address these problems, Dubowitz and her colleagues (Dubowitz et al., 1970) accumulated a number of additional items, many of which were "external" or morphologic in nature and derived from the work of Farr and others (Farr et al., 1966, 1966a). Dubowitz and her colleagues then attempted to select from this collection of items those with the highest interrater reliability that were minimally affected by the infant's state of arousal or neurologic condition. (The authors did not specify how these determinations were made.) In addition, each item was graded on an ordinal scale on which the number of ordinal scores was set equal to the number of distinctions that the several raters could reliably make.

On the Dubowitz subscale containing neurologic items, as in the Amiel-Tison method, the first item is *posture*, which, again, rates the degree of caudocephalic progression of flexion. The second item is called *square window*, which is the minimum angle formed by the hand when it is flexed toward the ventral surface of the forearm. Next are *dorsiflexion of the foot* and *arm recoil*, which are much the same as in Amiel-Tison's battery. *Leg recoil* is also measured by holding the supine infant's lower extremities fully flexed against the trunk for five seconds, then pulling the legs into total extension briefly before releasing them; in the full-term infant the legs usually snap back rapidly into flexion, whereas they may remain in extension in the very premature infant. The next four Dubowitz neurologic items—*popliteal angle, heel to ear, scarf sign,* and *head lag*—involve procedures similar to those described by Amiel-Tison. The final item on the

Dubowitz neurologic subscale is called *ventral suspension*. In this maneuver, the examiner evaluates the posture of the prone infant who is suspended at the chest with his weight supported by the examiner's hand. With increasing maturation, infants are able to mount more and more of an extensor response in an effort to overcome the pull of gravity.

In addition to the 10 neurologic signs just described, the Dubowitz system also employs 11 evaluations of the degree of physical maturity of the infant's body. The amount of *edema* (which is said to diminish with increasing maturation) is evaluated on a three-point scale. Five-point scales are used to evaluate the *skin texture, skin color,* and *skin opacity*. Skin texture generally exhibits increasing thickness with increasing maturation, while the color changes from dark red to a pink or paler color, and the skin opacity increases, making it harder to see the underlying vascular structures as the infant matures. The soft fine hair on the infant's back, known as *lanugo*, is also rated: Lanugo first increases and then decreases with increasing maturation. A five-point scale is also used to assess the development of *plantar creases* on the soles of the infant's feet.

Four-point scales are used to assess the maturity of the infant's *nipple formation* and the amount of *breast tissue*, as well as *ear form* (ranging from shapeless to mature incurvation) and *ear firmness* (the degree of recoil reflecting the progression of cartilaginous tissue). Finally the *genitalia* are assessed: In the male one notes the degree of testicular descent into the scrotum, and in the female, the size and development of the labia majora.

The Dubowitz scale is scored by summing the scores of the 10 neurologic items and the 11 "external" morphologic items. Dubowitz et al. examined 167 infants born to mothers with well-established LMPs. The subtotal from the 10 neurologic items and the subtotal from the 11 external morphologic items were each correlated with the putative gestational age by dates. A linear regression model proved to be most suitable. There was a slight tendency for the external morphologic items to be more highly correlated ($r = .91$) than the neurologic items ($r = .89$). However, the sum of all 21 items was an even better predictor of gestational age ($r = .93$) than either of the subtotals. The 95% confidence limits of an individual examination was ± 2 weeks; the 95% confidence limits could be reduced to 1.4 weeks by performing two independent examinations of the same infant. The authors presented evidence from a subseries of 70 infants who had been examined repeatedly, suggesting that the infant's state of arousal and age (up to five days) made relatively little difference on the results obtained.

The Shortened Ballard Scale

Ballard and her co-workers have developed a streamlined version of the Dubowitz scale in order to (a) reduce the time required for assessing gestational age and (b) reduce further the extent to which the assessment is contaminated by nonmaturational factors such as neurologic dysfunction (Klaus and Fanaroff, 1973; Ballard et al., 1977). Ballard and her colleagues retained 6 of the 10 Dubowitz neurologic items: posture, square window, arm recoil, popliteal angle, heel to ear, and scarf sign. From the 11 external morphologic items on the Dubowitz scale, Ballard derived 6 items: skin texture, color, and opacity are combined into one composite item; nipple formation and breast size are likewise combined into a single item, as are ear form and ear firmness. The other items are all retained, with the exception of the edema item, which was discarded. The Ballard scale is scored using the same sort of arithmetic sum as employed by the Dubowitz scale. The Ballard and Dubowitz scores, not surprisingly, were found to be highly correlated ($r = .975$) in a series of 284 infants. In a series of 86 infants with reliable dates, the external morphologic characteristics were again more highly correlated with gestational age by dates than were the neurologic characteristics. However, again the total score from all 12 items was more highly correlated ($r = .952$) with gestational age than either of the two subtotals alone. The Ballard exam has subsequently gained wide acceptance in American newborn units, largely, no doubt, because it takes only about five minutes to administer and it does not include some Dubowitz items (e.g., ventral suspension) that may be contraindicated in infants who are very immature or acutely ill.

ASSESSMENTS OF NEONATAL NEUROLOGIC STATUS

The modern neurologic examination is derived in large measure from work in clinical neurology during the last decades of the nineteenth century, together with work in experimental neurology during the late nineteenth and early twentieth centuries (McHenry, 1969; Spillane, 1981). The clinicians included Jean Martin Charcot and his student Joseph Babinski in France, Sir William Gowers in England, and Carl Westphal, William Heinrich Erb, and Herman Oppenheim in Germany. The experimental work of Rudolf Magnus at Utrecht and of Sir Charles Scott Sherrington at Oxford also influenced the development of the clinical neurologic examination, as well as the inferences drawn from clinical findings.

Whereas neurologists prior to 1870 restricted themselves largely to detached observations of the patient, there followed a period of rapid change during which various forms of manipulation of the patient assumed increasing importance. Thus, the *patellar* or *knee-jerk reflex* was introduced by Erb and Westphal in 1875, quickly followed by many other deep-tendon stretch reflexes. Likewise, a number of putative pathologic or pathognomonic "signs" were also advanced. One of the best known of these was introduced by Joseph Babinski (1896) in a one-page report. Babinski's pathologic sign consisted of the extension and fanning of the toes in response to a longitudinal scratch along the lateral plantar surface of the patient's foot; this stimulus ordinarily elicits flexion of the toes in mature normal patients. As Peiper (1963) has demonstrated, the use of Babinski's sign has a fascinating history, and its significance in infancy has been the subject of protracted controversy. No fewer than 117 contradictory papers were published on this subject between Babinski's 1896 report and a thorough review published 39 years later by Richards and Irwin (1935). These reviewers differentiated a number of distinguishably different responses to the recommended stimulus. Not surprisingly, therefore, Richards and Irwin themselves achieved an interrater reliability of only 77%.

Inasmuch as many of these reflexes and signs were named after the investigator who discovered them, there was a rapid influx of such "discoveries" into the neurologic literature (McHenry, 1969). Although it is certainly true that many of these signs and abnormal reflexes may often be observed in disease states, it is equally clear that some of these indicators are occasionally either present in the absence of detectable disease or absent in the presence of disease. Thus, even with adult patients, there is still some variation in the techniques employed in routine clinical neurologic examination—and in the methods used to draw inferences from the findings. There is still some art to neurologic inference.

These difficulties are compounded when the patient in question is an infant. Some infant reflexes (e.g., automatic walking) are commonly absent in the very premature infant and present in the infant born at term or come to term, only to disappear again thereafter in the normal infant (though sometimes not in the infant with neurologic sequelae). Thus, again, the results of the neurologic examination of the infant must be evaluated with respect to the infant's level of maturity. However, as Prechtl (1977) has pointed out, to the extent that the maturity determination is based on neurologic tests such as those included by Amiel-Tison, Dubowitz, and Ballard, there is an obvious potential for a dangerous circularity of reasoning.

During the postwar years, there was in Europe a quickening of interest in the neurologic examination of the infant. Albrecht Peiper published his encyclopedic review *Die Eigenart der kindlichen*

Hirntätigkeit in Leipzig in 1949. Peiper was consciously influenced by Pavlov, Magnus, and von Uexküll, and his prodigious review of neonatal reflexes gives ample witness to his indebtedness. Despite the comprehensiveness of Peiper's review, however, there are no clearly demarcated boundaries around a set of procedures that Peiper could be said to recommend for routine use.

The Paris school included André-Thomas, Saint-Anne Dargassies, and Amiel-Tison, as well as a number of others. The Paris school showed a greater interest in developing rather more standardized procedures that could provide comparative data from a variety of clinical situations (Thomas and Saint-Anne Dargassies, 1952, 1960, 1972; Minkowski et al., 1966). Many of their procedures designed for assessments of neonatal maturation have been discussed above.

Finally, the third European center of special activity in this area has been the University of Groningen, where Prechtl and his colleagues (Prechtl and Beintema, 1968; Prechtl, 1977) have developed a still more standardized neurologic examination that, however, is intended for use mainly with full-term infants.

Prechtl's Method

Like his predecessors before 1870, Prechtl does not forget, first of all, to *observe the patient*. At the outset of Prechtl's examination, the infant's state of arousal (ranging from coma to vigorous crying) is noted; the arousal state is monitored constantly throughout the examination, inasmuch as many of the procedures are intended to be conducted only when the infant is in the state appropriate to that procedure. During the observation period, the examiner also notes any spontaneous "startles"—described by Peiper (1963) as sudden flexor spasms that are therefore the opposite of the sudden extensor reaction seen in the Moro reflex. As in Amiel-Tison's examination, the infant's resting *posture* is noted, with flexion or semiflexion of the extremities being the normal expectation in mature neonates. *Spontaneous motor activity* is rated as to type and intensity. Of special interest are any so-called *athetoid postures* or *movements*, which are most often seen following birth asphyxia and related insults. The frequency and amplitude of any *tremor* or *clonus* are noted; a clonic type of tremor observed (apart from crying) in an infant several days old is a worrisome sign according to both Prechtl (1979) and Saint-Anne Dargassies (1972). During this initial observation period, Prechtl also recommends watching for other suspicious or abnormal movements (marked overshooting of limb movements, muscle twitchings, tonic or clonic convulsions, etc.), and assessing skin color and the rate and regularity of the infant's respirations.

472

The initial observation period completed, the infant is then lifted onto the examination table for an examination of the head. The shape and circumference of the head are noted, along with the size and condition of the fontanelles and the sutures. In examining the face, special attention is paid to any asymmetries (which may suggest a facial palsy) and to any structural irregularities or malformations (which may be associated with structural malformations of the nervous system). Prechtl recommends testing for *Chvostek's reflex* (Chvostek, 1876), which is a spasm of the facial muscles in response to a finger tap on the facial nerve. This reflex is normally absent, but is seen occasionally in tetany. Other facial reflexes that Prechtl includes are the *lip reflex* (a pursing of the lips in response to a finger tap just above or just below the mouth), the *jaw jerk* or *masseter reflex* (an upward jerk of the jaw in response to a tap on the chin), and the *glabella reflex* (a momentary blinking of the eyes in response to a tap on the forehead just above the nose). The lip, jaw, and glabella reflexes are all normally present and, perhaps more important, symmetrical. Their absence may indicate a general neurologic depression, which characterizes what Prechtl calls the "apathetic" infant, or a more focal impairment, e.g., of a cranial nerve.

After undressing the infant and placing him in a supine position, Prechtl reevaluates *posture, spontaneous motor activity, respirations,* and the *skin.* Then three "skin reflexes" are tested. First, the *abdominal reflex* is tested by scratching the abdomen in each quadrant, horizontally from the flank toward the midline. An asymmetric response may suggest a lesion proximal to the area being tested. Evaluation of this reflex is complicated, however, by the fact that habituation often occurs with repeated stimulation, and a complete absence (as opposed to an asymmetry) of the abdominal reflex response is occasionally observed in normal infants. The second Prechtl skin reflex, the *cremaster reflex,* is tested in male infants by scratching the medial aspect of the thigh with a sharp object; in normal male infants the response consists of a rostral elevation of the ipsilateral testis or of both testes. The third skin reflex, the *anal reflex,* is tested by pricking or scratching the perianal skin with a pin. In normal infants, this results in a contraction of the external anal sphincter, commonly termed an "anal wink." This reflex is often absent in spina bifida or in other lesions of the lower spinal cord.

Prechtl then observes the eyes in order to detect limitations or asymmetries of the extraocular movements; occasional dysconjugate eye movements may be observed in some normal neonates, however. Chronic downward deviation of both eyes may suggest an upward-gaze palsy secondary to increased intracranial pressure. Sustained nystagmus is regarded by Prechtl to be frankly abnormal. Deviation of the eyes in a single direction may signify an otherwise subclinical seizure. Weak or absent *pupillary responses* to light (in all but the most premature infants, in whom they are quite difficult to evaluate in any case) suggest coma or other significant dysfunction, as do asymmetric pupillary reflexes. Blinking in response to a sudden noise (*acoustic blink reflex*) or to a bright light (*optical blink reflex*) is normally found in the full-term infant in an alert state. The fifth cranial nerve is tested in eliciting the *corneal reflex* by touching the cornea with a few strands of cotton. The *doll's-eye test* (Bartels, 1910) entails watching the infant's eyes while the head is passively rotated from side to side. In normal full-term newborns and many preterm infants, the eyes move in a direction opposite to the movement of the head; according to Prechtl, this response normally changes during the first ten days of life, as visual fixation develops.

In the *asymmetric tonic neck reflex* (ATNR), which is normally absent, the infant assumes a "fencing" position when the head is rotated laterally, with the arm nearest the face extended and the arm nearest the occiput flexed. A similar though less well-developed response may occasionally be observed in the lower extremities. Peiper (1963) attributed a positive ATNR to "the elimination of higher, usually inhibitory, centers," that is, an instance of motoric disinhibition.

At this point in the examination, Prechtl evaluates the infant's passive tone and active tone (although he avoids these words on the grounds that they have proved confusing in their application). In gauging passive tone, one assesses the resistance to passive movement offered by the musculature of the resting infant. Normal full-term infants are neither limp (hypotonic) nor stiff (hypertonic). In assessing active tone, one rates the *power* with which active movements are conducted: Active movements with little force are easily resisted by the examiner and thus have little power, and so on. Again, the active movements of normal full-term infants are neither too weak nor too forceful, but intermediate in degree or perhaps nearer the forceful end of the continuum. Generalized weakness may be seen in neurologic depression or in neuromuscular disease. Unilateral weakness would, in contrast, suggest a more focal condition such as hemiparesis. Prechtl also checks the *forearm recoil at the elbow* and feels the *consistency of the muscles*, with the expectation of finding intermediate or moderately high values for both tests in normal infants.

Prechtl also tests many of the same reflexes that have been reviewed previously. The *biceps reflex* is a deep-tendon reflex comprising a quick contraction of the biceps muscle that can normally be elicited by tapping the distal tendon of the biceps just above the elbow. As with the *knee jerk*, which is tested along with the biceps reflex, one looks for responses that are unusually sluggish or unusually brisk (relative to the infant's gestational age), or for bilateral asymmetry. Quickly pushing the normal infant's foot into dorsiflexion does not ordinarily elicit *ankle clonus*, a rapid flexion–extension alternation measured in "beats" of clonus. Prechtl regards sustained ankle clonus in the full-term neonate as evidence for neurologic impairment. The *palmar* and *plantar grasps* are also evaluated for their strength and bilateral symmetry. They may all be diminished in marked neurologic depression. The plantar grasps may also be absent in spinal cord lesions. Interrelationships among several reflexes may also be observed: Sucking often strengthens the palmar grasp, but the elicitation of the palmar grasp may inhibit the Moro reflex (Peiper, 1963).

Prechtl also includes checking for *Babinski's sign*, which he considers normally present in normal full-term newborns, even though its presence in older patients would be considered pathognomonic of a corticospinal lesion. Prechtl recommends noting the vigor with which the toes fan upward. Prechtl also describes a *magnet response*, by which he means extension of the lower extremity in response to light pressure on the soles. Contrarily, there is flexion of the lower extremity, or a *withdrawal response*, in response to scratching the sole of the foot. In both cases, the examiner assesses the vigor and symmetry of the responses to plantar stimulation.

The tests performed next, which have all been discussed above, are *rooting*, *sucking*, the *pull-to-sit* or *traction test* (in which both arm flexion and head control are assessed), and the Moro reflex. Prechtl regards the absence of a Moro response in a full-term neonate as a sign of serious dysfunction.

With the infant in the prone position, Prechtl examines the spinal *vertebrae* and assesses the infant's ability to maneuver the head for *spontaneous head movements*. He watches as well for *spontaneous crawling* movements, and if none occur, attempts to facilitate them with light pressure on the soles of the feet (Bauer's response). Another deep-tendon reflex, the *ankle jerk*, is also elicited. *Trunk incurvation*, or *Galant's response*, is tested by slowly scratching alongside the infant's spine with a pin: Many older infants and some newborns will respond to this stimulus with a lateral flexion of the pelvis toward the source of stimulation. An asymmetric response, as usual, is cause for concern, as is a response that consistently stops at the same vertebral level. The last procedure performed in the prone position is a *prone suspension*, described above as Dubowitz's *ventral suspension*.

Finally, three procedures are performed with the infant held in an upright (standing) position. *Placing* is tested by allowing the upper (dorsal) surface of the infant's foot to brush against the lower surface of a table edge; the full-term neonate typically responds by lifting the lower extremity and stepping up onto the table top. Once there, the examiner watches for *stepping movements*, also known as *automatic walking*. Finally, while holding the infant vertically, facing the examiner, and at arm's length, the examiner rotates 90° to the left and to the right. Normal infants ordinarily turn eyes and head toward the direction in which they are being turned, as if to see where they are going.

Prechtl ends his examination with the infant in supine position once more. *Spontaneous motor activity* is assessed for a third time. If the Moro response was previously weak or incomplete, the test is repeated at this time, thus affording another opportunity for an assessment of the quality and vigor of the infant's cry.

The examiner who has completed the administration of Prechtl's examination will have generated a sizeable quantity of clinical data. It is natural at this point to ask how one should go about drawing inferences from these data. Regrettably, although Prechtl does hint at the kinds of procedures he favors, a great deal is left unsaid, quite possibly because a great deal is still unknown. Some findings suggest a specific diagnosis; others are of equivocal significance.

There have been two major styles of approaching clinical data derived from observation and examination of the patient: the *pathognomonic sign* approach and the *level of performance* approach. The standard approach of clinical neurology has been the pathognomonic sign approach, in which the detection of a sign (or a set of signs) is perhaps sufficient to warrant at least a preliminary diagnosis. Thus, a febrile child with nuchal rigidity, Kernig's sign (inability to extend the legs at the knees while sitting but not while supine; Kernig, 1882), and Brudzinski's neck sign (involuntary flexion of the lower extremities coincident with exogenous flexion of the neck; Brudzinski, 1909) will certainly suggest to most clinicians a diagnosis of meningitis. However, the recurring difficulty with this approach in neonatal neurology is that the pathognomonic signs that work quite reliably in older patients are often absent or misleading in the newborn. For example, many neonates with documented meningitis have not exhibited any of the classic pathognomonic signs noted above. Furthermore, there is still controversy regarding the age until which an infant may safely have the upturning toes of Babinski's sign.

Because the standard pathognomonic sign approach has not proved wholly satisfactory in application to infants, Prechtl offers modifications to this approach. In one instance the modification is semiquantitative: Before diagnosing a hemisyndrome in an infant, Prechtl requires, not a single asymmetric finding, but rather three or more asymmetric findings. Another recommended approach is to group a number of clinical findings together into "syndromes" that appear to be similar to what other investigators have termed a priori "clusters" (e.g., Als, 1978). Thus, Prechtl has so far defined three syndromes or clusters. The hyperexcitable infant has tremors, possibly brisk reflexes, easily elicited Moro responses, and sometimes an increased activity level and increased passive tone. The apathetic infant responds weakly and only after relatively vigorous stimulation, and may be hypoactive and hypotonic. The comatose infant, a more familiar entity in clinical neurology, shows little or no arousal even to nociceptive stimuli and may have abnormal respirations. Unfortunately, Prechtl did not offer much in the way of follow-up data with which to evaluate the efficacy of either the semi-quantitative approach or the syndromic approach. Thus, the usefulness of these classifications remains to be further evaluated.

However, Prechtl also advocates an "optimality concept" that breaks away from the pathognomonic sign tradition in incorporating some features of the level-of-performance tradition. The "optimality score" that Prechtl recommends is simply a count of the number of items on which an infant received the "optimal" or best possible score. Because many non-optimal scores are still within normal limits, this is a stricter standard that will presumably stretch the distribution of scores across a broader range, making fine discriminations along the scale more feasible. Again, however, Prechtl did not present follow-up data with which to evaluate the predictive validity of this assessment method.

Current American Methods: Volpe's Approach

If the recent clinical work in Leipzig, Paris, and Groningen can be traced back to Charcot, Gowers, and Sherrington, perhaps it is not too irreverent to suggest that the current clinical practice in America must be derived in part from Thomas Edison. Even though the clinical neurologic examination of the infant may remain the "cornerstone" of neonatal neurology (Volpe, 1981), that cornerstone is surely heavily buttressed by an impressive array of technically sophisticated instrumentation. Electron microscopy is now often employed to study the ultrastructure of fetal and neonatal tissues. The development in Britain of computerized tomographic (CT) scanning introduced fundamental changes into the practice of newborn neurology by making it possible to visualize the gross structures of the central nervous system in the living infant without resorting to surgical procedures.

477

More recently, echoencephalography has made possible serial visualizations without risk from radiation exposure. Many centers are now equipped to measure cerebral blood flow in newborns, either with a Doppler ultrasound technique or with a radioisotope of xenon, which can be monitored by gamma cameras. In addition, currently under development are applications of positron-emission tomography (PET scanning), which will provide new kinds of information about the metabolic status of living human nervous systems.

Perhaps it is partly because of these new technical developments that recent investigators have felt more free to discard some of the accumulation of reflexes and signs that had been incorporated over the years into the neurologic examination of the infant. Thus, one leading American neonatal neurologist, Joseph Volpe, employs an examination that is rather more concise than that of Prechtl (Volpe, 1981).

Volpe begins, as expected, with an assessment of gestational age. Only four indicators are ordinarily employed: ear cartilage, breast tissue, maturity of the genitalia, and proliferation of the plantar creases.

Volpe places primary importance on the infant's level of alertness relative to gestational age. Periods of alertness appear more readily and more spontaneously as the infant gains maturity.

Next the functioning of the cranial nerves is examined, using many of the standard procedures. The examiner determines whether the infant blinks to light, fixes, and follows; the optic fundi are visualized. The pupillary reflexes are evaluated in relation to gestational age. Extraocular movements are noted, using the doll's head maneuver if necessary. The face is observed, with attention to movements of the facial muscles both at rest and during various activities, such as sucking and crying. Auditory competence is assessed by means of the acoustic reflex and by noting whether there are changes in the infant's activity level, respirations, or facial expressions in response to noise. The sucking, swallowing, and gagging reflexes are checked.

Volpe's motor examination is ideally performed in an alert infant who has had at least 24 hours to recover from delivery. Tone, posture, movement, and power are assessed. Three tendon reflexes—biceps, knee, and ankle—are evaluated. The amount of ankle clonus is recorded, although Volpe regards as many as five to ten beats of clonus as within normal limits for the neonate. Volpe uses a fingernail to elicit the Babinski reflex—and he reports that he ordinarily obtains downward (plantar) flexion in normal newborns.

Only three "primary neonatal reflexes" are tested: the Moro, the palmar grasp, and the tonic neck response, previously termed the asymmetric tonic neck response (ATNR). Volpe had discarded many

478

of the tests from previous examinations (e.g., heel-to-ear, scarf sign, popliteal angle) because he has not found them to be clinically useful in his own practice.

Volpe's approach to the clinical neurologic examination, somewhat like Ballard's approach to the maturity assessment, seems to be a distillation of previous experience, in that unnecessary and possibly unreliable tests have been discarded. Perhaps future investigators will be able to conduct a more formal and more quantitative item analysis in order to verify the currently favored batteries of tests for maturational assessment and neurologic evaluation.

BEHAVIORAL ASSESSMENTS

It will become apparent that the distinction between neonatal neurologic assessments and behavioral assessments is sometimes an uncertain one. There is a great deal of overlap in the item content of the assessment instruments. However, the neurologic approaches have tended to favor evaluating the patient for the presence of punctate signs of pathology in an attempt to make binary or dichotomous judgments about the presence or absence of disease. The behavioral approaches, in contrast, have tended toward the evaluation of relatively continuous levels of performance. Because the boundaries of behavioral dysfunction may be said to be less sharply demarcated than the boundaries of neurologic dysfunction, perhaps the behavioral approaches have made a virtue of necessity. Nevertheless, each approach has distinctive features that make it better suited for some applications.

Graham's Scale

In the early 1950s, a behavioral scale for newborn infants was developed by Frances Graham, along with Ruth Matarazzo and Bettye Caldwell (Graham et al., 1956). It had previously been noted that ostensibly comparable episodes of perinatal asphyxia had widely discrepant infant outcomes. This scale was designed to determine which infants had sustained brain damage as a consequence of antenatal or perinatal insult. Although the problem that Graham addressed was considered largely neurologic in nature, the approach she took was rather more psychometric. In fact, she acknowledged her indebtedness to Psyche Cattell (1940), Arnold Gesell (1941), and Ruth Griffiths (1954), all of whom had developed scales of infant development.

Graham's scale comprised five subscales. The first subscale was a measure of *pain threshold* and as such seems today rather more psychophysical than psychometric. The pain was generated by electric shock; although the current delivered was no doubt very small (the exact amount was not specified), the voltage ranged up to 530 V. The minimum voltage to elicit a reliable response (leg movement) was taken as the threshold measure.

The second subscale was termed a *maturation scale*, and there were nine items. The *prone head reaction* comprised placing the infant in a prone position with the head in the midline, thus threatening the airway; the infant's efforts to turn or lift the head were then noted. Also noted were any alternating thrusting movements of the legs simulating *crawling*. With the infant still prone, an item designated *pushes feet* (Prechtl's magnet response) was performed. The infant's *auditory reaction* was assessed by repeated trials of graded sounds from a rattle and a bell; any systematic changes in the infant's behavior coincident with these auditory stimuli were taken as a response.

Two other items involved the infant's defensive reactions to a threatened obstruction of the airway. In the first of these, a piece of cotton was held across the nostrils for 20 seconds; in the second item a rectangle of paper (cellophane) was held across both the nose and the mouth. In both instances the examiners watched for defensive reactions such as head turning or head retraction. The *persistence* and *vigor* of any such defensive responses were assessed. Finally the strength of the infant's palmar *grasp* was assessed by means of a small spring-balance device.

The third subscale assessed *vision* in the infant. The infant's ability to fix on and follow common objects was rated.

Irritability, the fourth subscale, was evaluated by determining the intensity of stimulation required to elicit crying, by noting the quality of the cry, and by noting the ease with which the infant could be consoled. These determinations were then used to characterize the infant as "normal," "fussy," or "irritable."

The fifth subscale comprised bipolar ratings of *muscle tension*. The infant was scored on a five-point scale, ranging from "flaccid" to "marked tension," by assessing posture, passive tone, postural response to the pull-to-sit maneuver, spontaneous activity, and "trembling." The "trembling" in question was not further described, but this term probably referred to tremors or possibly jitteriness.

The concurrent validity of Graham's scale was addressed in a standardization study of 81 insulted infants (who had survived episodes of perinatal hypoxia) and of 265 normal controls. Significant differences were detected on all five subscales. The insulted infants had higher pain thresholds, lower scores on the maturation scale and the vision scale, and higher incidences of abnormal irritability and

480

muscle tension. Graham's scale was better at identifying infants who had experienced relatively severe insults, as opposed to infants who had experienced milder insults, as determined by independent pediatric reviewers.

Regrettably, Graham's scale generated relatively little data on predictive validity. A follow-up of Graham's samples of normal and asphyxiated patients at three years of age found little relationship between the scores on Graham's scale and subsequent functioning on a variety of other instruments including the Stanford–Binet Intelligence Scale (Graham, 1962).

The Graham–Rosenblith Behavioral Examination of the Neonate

Rosenblith (1979) revised Graham's original scale in light of her own experience with it. Rosenblith reorganized Graham's scale, subdividing Graham's maturity scale, for instance, into two subscales: a *motor scale* and a *tactile–adaptive scale*. The motor scale retains four of Graham's nine maturity scale items: prone head reaction, crawling, grasp, and vigor of response to cotton and cellophane. The pushes feet (magnet response) item was moved to the muscle tone assessment, and the auditory reactions to rattle and bell were moved to a separate sensory evaluation. The primary response to cotton and paper (cellophane), together with the persistence of that response, were collected onto the tactile–adaptive scale. The pain threshold determinations, mercifully, were dropped altogether. The scoring of many items was revised, often by stretching the scale to permit finer graduations.

Rosenblith was able to conduct follow-up assessments at eight months and at four years of age on over 1000 infants who had been evaluated neonatally with the Graham–Rosenblith scale. The motor scale was found to be significantly correlated with all of the seven types of assessment that were performed at age eight months; there were fewer significant correlations between the tactile–adaptive scale and the eight-month follow-up test scores. At four years of age, however, quite the opposite pattern obtained: The neonatal tactile–adaptive scale was the better predictor, although, not surprisingly, with the passage of time there had been some erosion of the predictive validity of the neonatal assessment.

Brazelton's Neonatal Behavioral Assessment Scale

T. Berry Brazelton's well-known scale (Brazelton, 1973) is in part an offshoot that includes among its forebears both Prechtl's neurologic examination and Graham's behavioral scale. Brazelton's method includes 20 elicited responses from Prechtl's examination: plantar grasp, hand (palmar) grasp, ankle clonus, Babinski's reflex, standing, automatic walking (stepping), placing, incurvation (Galant's response), crawling, glabella reflex, tonic deviation of head and eyes, nystagmus, tonic neck reflex, Moro reflex, rooting, sucking, and resistance to passive movement in each of the four extremities.

The behavioral examination has two parts. The infant's response to 11 standardized procedures is reflected in 11 scores; an additional 16 scores assess more global aspects of the infant's behavior during the administration of the scale. Most of these 27 items are scored along nine a priori ordinal scales.

Among the 11 items in the first category, there are four assessments of habituation, or of the diminution of the infant's responses to repeated stimulation with four test objects: a flashlight, a rattle, a bell, and a pin. Graham's scale had also included repeated stimulation, but Brazelton's scale directs the scoring to the rate at which the infant shuts down his responses to repeated stimulation. As Volpe (1981) observed, habituation requires temporal integration of the incoming stimulation, which in many instances is thought to involve at least some cortical mediation. Thus, these four habituation items may have some potential for providing information about the functioning of the neonatal cortex. Likewise, the temporal juxtaposition of the rattle and bell items offers some opportunities to examine auditory discrimination, which may also involve cortical mediation.

The next four specific behavioral scores reflect the infant's responses to animate and inanimate stimuli presented in the visual and auditory channels—for example, a ball, a rattle or bell, a face, and a voice. In the ninth test, face and voice are presented simultaneously.

The last two tests are *pull-to-sit* (as in Prechtl's traction test) and *defensive movements* (similar to Graham's cotton and paper items). Pull-to-sit is scored with reference to head control and changes in muscle tone. The defensive movements item is scored in much the same way as on Graham's test, although Brazelton offers finer graduations on his nine-point scale.

The 16 global scores entail assessing the degree of alertness, as well as the overall impression of motor tone and of motor maturity. A number of items address the changes in the infant's state of arousal throughout the examination. One rates the overall level of irritability, the peak of irritability, the volatility of state changes, the degree of difficulty encountered in consoling the infant, and the extent to which the infant can quiet himself. Tremors, startles, and smiles are noted. Finally, records are made of the examiner's impressions of the infant's overall activity level and of the degree to which the infant cuddles.

Assessments of Infant Temperament

A rather different approach to infant assessment was begun in New York City in 1956. In that year, Alexander Thomas, Stella Chess, and Herbert Birch founded the New York Longitudinal Study. A total of 141 children from 85 (mostly middle-class) families were enrolled over a six-year period. Several additional samples from other social backgrounds were subsequently collected and studied (Thomas et al., 1963, 1968; Thomas and Chess, 1977).

The *modus operandi* of the New York Longitudinal Study was to gather extensive information about children from their parents via a series of intensive interviews by specially trained interviewers. The interview records from the first 22 infants entered into the project were examined in order to identify temperament categories by "inductive content analysis." This method led to the induction of nine categories of temperament, which were then each fitted to three-point scales with which to perform content analysis of subsequent interview protocols.

The first category, *activity level*, was used to assess the degree of motor activity that characterized the child's daily behavior cycle. Each child was rated as high, medium, or low in this area.

The temporal predictability of daily activities was designated *rhythmicity* or *regularity*. Biologic functions such as feeding, sleeping, and toileting were included. The scale values were regular, variable, and irregular.

The *approach or withdrawal* scale assessed the child's reaction to new situations. The descriptive terms were adaptive, variable, and nonadaptive.

The child's ability to adjust to changes in his environment or routine was assessed with the *adaptability* scale. The scale values were adaptive, variable, and nonadaptive.

The *threshold of responsiveness* scale sought to measure the intensity of stimulation ordinarily required to elicit a response from the child. The intensity was described as high, medium, or low.

In contrast, the intensity of the child's responses was scored with the *intensity of reaction* scale. Reactions were rated as positive, variable, or negative.

The *quality of mood* in the child was described as positive, variable, or negative.

The *distractibility* scale was used to gauge the ease with which extraneous stimulation could capture the child's attention. The ratings were distractible, variable, and nondistractible.

The final category was a composite of *attention span* and *persistence*. The duration of the child's attention, as well as the effort required to divert his attention, were rated simultaneously. The scale values were persistent, variable, and nonpersistent.

The New York Longitudinal study team employed both factor analysis and nonquantitative methods to arrive at three temperamental types. Most children fit one of these three types.

The first type was designated the *easy child*. This term was applied to the 40% of the study sample who were characterized mostly by the desirable scale values described above—that is they were regular, adaptable, and had mostly positive moods. By contrast, the 10% of the study sample who fell into the *difficult child* classification were irregular, unable to adapt to change, and negative in mood. The third type, the *slow-to-warm-up child*, was characterized by initial withdrawal from new situations, followed eventually by adjustment.

The New York Longitudinal Study investigators rejected some of the demands of predictive validity by denying that their infant temperament data could be used to predict the future course of development for individual children. To the contrary, they stressed the interaction of the child and his environment and argued that the infant's temperament was only a place from which the child–environment transactions got under way. Nevertheless, there were significant patterns of association between infant temperament ratings and outcomes such as behavior disorders several years later.

In view of the labor-intensive nature of the interview method employed by the New York group, it was difficult to transplant their methods into other settings. A pediatrician in Philadelphia set out to devise a procedure that could be used, for example, by pediatricians in community practice. Dr. William B. Carey compiled a series of 70 multiple-choice questions with which to capture the same infant attributes measured by the more elaborate interview procedures (Carey, 1970, 1973). These 70 questions were assembled into a questionnaire that could be completed by the infant's mother in about 20 minutes.

Application of this questionnaire to Carey's own clinical practice yielded distributions that were similar to those that had been obtained in New York by the interview method. Carey's questionnaire has subsequently been employed by a number of investigators. Carey used the instrument himself, for example, to investigate the temperamental attributes of infants with sleep disturbances (Carey, 1974). Moreover, Sostek and Anders (1977) found significant intercorrelations among temperament measurements, certain scoring dimensions from the Brazelton scale, and subsequent performance on the Bayley Scales of Infant Development.

Emerging Clinical Applications of Behavioral Research

As Lipsitt (1977) has suggested, until recently the reader of the literature on neonatal assessment might well assume that the infant is a decorticate preparation. The last 30 years of experimental research have made it quite clear that infants are capable fairly early of rather complex perceptual discriminations. More interesting still, there is a growing literature suggesting that considerable cortical mediation may be involved in some of the habituation and discrimination phenomena that have been described in the experimental literature.

Engen and Lipsitt (Engen et al., 1963; Engen and Lipsitt, 1965), for example, studied habituation of activity level and respiratory responses to repeated presentations of olfactory stimuli. In a counterbalanced design, one group was exposed to odorant A repeatedly, followed by repeated exposures to odorant B; the other group had corresponding exposures to B first, followed by A. Both groups showed vigorous responses to the initial odorant presentations, followed by a gradual erosion or habituation of the responses. The response rates demonstrated a quick, if partial, recovery once the second odorant was introduced, thus implying temporal integration of the stimuli at some level in the infant nervous system. Moreover, further trials with combinations of odorants lent support to the hypothesis that the temporal integration or mediation occurred at a cortical, rather than a peripheral, level. Recovery from habituation (dishabituation) could be obtained by presenting in pure form an odorant that had been a major constituent of a mixture of odorants to which habituation had been obtained. Because pure odorant had been present in the initial mixture, the dishabituation phenomenon could not be explained away as a peripheral fatigue artifact. Thus, central structures are implicated.

A different kind of evidence for sophisticated, probably cortical, processing of complex stimuli comes from research on speech perception in infancy. Eimas and his collaborators at Brown University studied the infant's perception of a feature of speech that has been termed "voice onset time" (Eimas et al., 1971). Voice onset time is the temporal relationship between oral articulatory activity and laryngeal activity or "voicing." Voice onset time is involved in the distinctions between certain pairs of stop-consonants, such as /b/ and /p/. A remarkable feature of the perception of voice onset time in adults is that it appears to be "categorical." In other words, adults are exquisitely sensitive to acoustic variations near the boundaries between phonemes (speech sounds such as /b/ and /p/) but remarkably *insensitive* to comparable variations occurring within phonemes, which therefore have no linguistic significance. Thus, it appears that

485

the adult's speech perception apparatus is in some sense specially "tuned" to focus on variations that are meaningful in all (or nearly all) human languages.

More remarkable still, Eimas, using the habituation paradigm, assembled persuasive evidence that infants in the second month of life are *already* perceiving voice onset time categorically. Because speech sounds are very complex, and because such invariances as have been detected across speakers may involve higher order relationships, it seems exceedingly unlikely that phonomena such as categorical perception could be mediated at a peripheral level, and thus central, perhaps cortical, structures are again implicated. However, whether the structures eventually prove to be cortical or subcortical may be of secondary importance. The lesson to be learned here is that these heretofore experimental techniques may open the way to new avenues in the evaluation of the functional status of the infant nervous system. Evaluations of "higher" functions may be of more significance in determining long-term prognosis than many of the classic motor-based procedures have been.

CONCLUSION

In his remarks at the end of a monograph on the Brazelton Neonatal Behavioral Assessment Scale, Sameroff (1978) reviewed the findings on the scale's predictive validity and concluded that "a way of tapping the essence of the newborn still eludes us." He continued by wondering "whether the resolution of this problem lies in the construction of better tests or in a better understanding of the infant."

It does seem clear that the assortment of neurologic examinations and behavioral assessments have perhaps left many with a sense of disappointment. Nevertheless, it seems premature to abandon further work in the areas of prediction and prognosis. Just as there are limits to the explanatory power of the simple cause–effect models of development that Sameroff had denounced (Sameroff and Chandler, 1975), so there may be limits or at least qualifications to the transactional model that has been offered as a replacement. Although it is probably futile to try to account for all of child development with factors endogenous to the neonate, it may be equally wrong to shift the focus too far away. The work of Eimas and others strongly suggests that there are some biologic facts that need to be included in any prognostic equation.

Sameroff has attributed relatively little importance to perinatal insults such as birth asphyxia (Sameroff and Chandler, 1975). This conclusion has typically been drawn from studies in which infants who were presumed to have been asphyxiated were compared with normal controls. In many such studies, group differences diminished over time and in some cases even failed to achieve statistical significance in samples of moderate size. Yet most perinatal clinicians know of all too many cases in which insulted infants became children with severe static impairments. Group means may show evidence for recovery; however, that is unfortunately not the prospect enjoyed by all the individuals. The shortcomings of neonatal prognostication to date may arise not so much from the inherent mutability of the child as from our ignorance in determining the answer to the questions that we raised at the outset: What exactly has happened to this insulted infant and how serious is it? We have until recently been remarkably poorly equipped to distinguish between the low-Apgar neonate who has experienced only a transient stress during the final stages of delivery, and the low-Apgar infant who has been irreversibly compromised as a result of a long-standing insult.

Fortunately, this state of affairs allows us to end on a note of cautious optimism. We anticipate major technological advances in our understanding of the biologic substrate of neonatal neurobehavioral assessment. These advances may introduce an era in which there will be equally important contributions in the area of brain–behavior correlations. A recent article (Lou, 1979) has reported a significant relationship between a measure of neonatal cerebral blood flow and a measure of developmental outcome many months later. Further progress of this sort may greatly augment our abilities to detect precursors of dysfunction in time to apply efficacious therapies.

REFERENCES

Als, H. (1978). Assessing an assessment: Conceptual considerations, methodological issues, and a perspective on the future of the Neonatal Behavioral Assessment Scale. In *Organization and stability of newborn behavior: A commentary on the Brazelton Neonatal Behavior Assessment Scale,* edited by A.J. Sameroff. *Monographs of the Society for Research in Child Development 43* (Serial No. 177), 14–28.

Amiel-Tison, C. (1968). Neurological evaluation of the maturity of newborn infants. *Arch. Dis. Child. 43*, 89–93.

Babinski, J.F.F. (1896). Sur le réflexe cutané plantaire dans certains affections organiques du système nerveux central. *C.R. Soc. Biol. (Paris) 3* (Ser. 9), 207.

Ballard, J.L., Kazmaier, K., and Driver, M. (1977). A simplified assessment of gestational age. *Pediatr. Res. 11*, 374.

Bartels, M. (1910). Über Regulierung der Augenstellung durch den Ohrapparat. *Arch. Ophthalmol. 76*, 1–97.

Brazelton, T.B. (1973). *Neonatal behavioral assessment scale.* London: Heinemann.

Brudzinski, J. (1909). Un signe nouveau sur les membiers inférieurs dans les méningites chez les enfants. *Arch. Med. Enf. 12,* 745–752.

Carey, W.B. (1970). A simplified method for measuring infant temperament. *J. Pediatr. 77,* 188–194.

—— (1973). Measurement of infant temperament in pediatric practice. In *Individual differences in children,* edited by J.C. Westman. New York: Wiley, pp. 293–306.

—— (1974). Night waking and temperament in infancy. *J. Pediatr. 84,* 756–758.

Cattell, P. (1940). *The measurement of intelligence in infants and young children.* New York: Psychological Corporation.

Chvostek, F. (1876). Beitrag zur Tetanie. *Wien Med. Presse 17,* 1201.

Drillien, C.M. (1964). *The growth and development of the prematurely born infant.* Edinburgh: E. & S. Livingstone.

Dubowitz, L.M.S., Dubowitz, V., and Goldberg, C. (1970). Clinical assessment of gestational age in the newborn infant. *J. Pediatr. 77,* 1–10.

Eimas, P.D., Siqueland, E.R., Jusczyk, P., and Vigorito, J. (1971). Speech perception in infants. *Science 171,* 303–306.

Engen, T. and Lipsitt, L.P. (1965). Decrement and recovery of responses to olfactory stimuli in the human neonate. *J. Comp. Physiol. Psychol. 59,* 312–316.

——, ——, and Kaye, H. (1963). Olfactory responses and adaptation in the human neonate. *J. Comp. Physiol. Psychol. 56,* 73–77.

Farr, V., Kerridge, D.F., and Mitchell, R.G. (1966). The value of some external characteristics in the assessment of gestational age at birth. *Dev. Med. Child Neurol. 8,* 657–660.

——, Mitchell, R.G., Neligan, G.A., and Parkin, J.M. (1966a). The definition of some external characteristics used in the assessment of gestational age in the newborn infant. *Dev. Med. Child Neurol. 8,* 507–511.

Fiorentino, M.R. (1972). Normal and abnormal development. Springfield, Ill.: Charles C Thomas.

Gesell, A.L. and Amatruda, C. (1941). *Developmental diagnosis.* New York: Hoeber.

Graham, F.K., Ernhart, C., Thurston, D., and Craft, M. (1962). Development three years after perinatal anoxia and other potentially damaging newborn experiences. *Psychol. Monogr. 76(3),* 1–53.

——, Matarazzo, R.G., and Caldwell, B.M. (1956). Behavioral differences between normal and traumatized newborns. *Psychol. Monogr. Vol 70(20),* 1–33.

Griffiths, R. (1954). *The abilities of babies.* New York: McGraw-Hill Book Co.

His, W. (1882). Anatomie menschlicher Embryonen. II. Gestalt- und Grossenentwicklung bis zum Schluss des 2 Monats. Leipzig: F.C.W. Vogel.

Kernig, V.M. (1882) Ein Krankheitssymptom der acuten Meningitis. *St. Petersburg Med. Wochenschr. 7,* 398.

Klaus, M.H. and Fanaroff, A.A. (1973). *Care of the high-risk neonate.* Philadelphia: W.B. Saunders.

Lipsitt, L.P. (1977). The study of sensory and learning processes of the newborn. *Clin. Perinatol.* 4, 163–186.

Lou, H.C., Skov, H., and Pedersen, H. (1979). Low cerebral blood flow: A risk factor in the neonate. *J. Pediatr.* 95, 606–609.

Lubchenco, L.O. (1975). Assessment of weight and gestational age. In *Neonatology: Pathophysiology and management of the newborn*, edited by G.B. Avery. Philadelphia: J.B. Lippincott, pp. 127–149.

McHenry, L.C. (1969). *Garrison's history of neurology.* Springfield, Ill.: Charles C Thomas.

Minkowski, A., Larroche, J.C., Vignaud, J., Dreyfus-Brisac, C., and Saint-Anne Dargassies, S. (1966). Development of the nervous system in early life. In *Human development*, edited by F. Falkner. Philadelphia: W.B. Saunders, pp. 254–325.

Moro, E. (1918). Das erste Trimenon. *München Med. Wochenschr.* 65, 1147–1150.

Peiper, A. (1963). *Cerebral function in infancy and childhood.* New York: Consultants Bureau.

Prechtl, H.F.R. (1977). *The neurological examination of the full term newborn infant.* London: Heinemann.

—— and Beintema, D. (1964). *The neurological examination of the full-term newborn infant.* London: Heinemann.

Richards, T.W. and Irwin, O.C. (1935). Studies in infant behavior II. *Univ. of Iowa Studies: Studies in Child Welfare 11*, 1–146.

Rosenblith, J.F. (1979). The Graham/Rosenblith behavioral examination for newborns: Prognostic value and procedural issues. In *Handbook of infant development*, edited by J.D. Osofsky. New York: Wiley, pp. 216–249.

Saint-Anne Dargassies, S. (1955). La maturation neurologique du prématuré. *Études néo-natales 4*, 71–116.

—— (1966). Neurological maturation of the premature infant of 28–41 weeks' gestational age. In *Human development*, edited by F. Falkner. Philadelphia: W.B. Saunders, pp. 306–325.

—— (1972). Neurodevelopmental symptons during the first year of life. *Dev. Med. Child Neurol. 14*, 235–264.

Sameroff, A.J. (1978). Summary and conclusions: The future of newborn assessment. In *Organization and stability of newborn behavior: A commentary on the Brazelton Neonatal Behavior Assessment Scale*, edited by A.J. Sameroff. *Monographs of the Society for Research in Child Development 43* (Serial No. 177), pp. 102–117.

—— and Chandler, M.J. (1975). Reproductive risk and the continuum of caretaking casualty. In *Review of child development research 4*, edited by F.D. Horowitz. Chicago: University of Chicago Press, pp. 187–244.

Sostek, A.M. and Anders, T.F. (1977). Relationships among the Brazelton Neonatal Scale, Bayley Infant Scales, and early temperament. *Child Dev. 48*, 320–323.

Spillane, J.D. (1981). *The doctrine of the nerves: Chapters in the history of neurology.* Oxford: Oxford University Press.

Thomas, A., Chesni, Y., and Saint-Anne Dargassies, S. (1960). *The neurological examination of the infant.* London: National Spastics Society.

——— and Saint-Anne Dargassies, S. (1952). *Études neurologique sur le nouveau-né et le jeune nourrisson.* Paris: Masson.

Thomas, A. and Chess, S. (1977). *Temperament and development.* New York: Brunner/Mazel.

———, ———, and Birch, H.G. (1968). *Temperament and behavior disorders in children.* New York: New York University Press.

———, ———, ———, Hertzig, M.E., and Korn, S. (1963). *Behavioral individuality in early childhood.* New York: New York University Press.

Volpe, J. (1981). *Neurology of the newborn.* Philadelphia: W.B. Saunders.

21

Methodological Considerations in the Analysis of Perinatal Mortality Rates

Howard J. Hoffman, Olav Meirik, Leiv S. Bakketeig

The perinatal mortality rate has been used as an indicator for the quality and utilization of medical care services within and between populations (Falk and Wranne, 1973; Karlberg and Priolisi, 1977; Bakketeig et al., 1978; Ericson et al., 1979; Bowes, 1981; Paneth et al., 1982; Williams and Chen, 1982; Meirik, 1983). The advantage of the perinatal mortality rate is its sensitivity to changes over relatively short time periods. Also, the perinatal mortality rate is a robust measurement because it deals with dichotomized events which are easily recognized.

In recent years, the perinatal mortality rate in several countries has declined to very low levels. These reductions have been attributed both to improvements in social conditions and advances in medical and health care (Baird et al., 1953; Baumgartner and Erhardt, 1953; Illsley, 1955; Gruenwald, 1968; Rantakallio, 1969; MacMahon et al., 1972; Chase, 1974; Baird, 1975; Alberman, 1977, 1980; Dowding, 1981). In the subsequent analyses of data, the two components of the perinatal mortality rate, late fetal and early neonatal deaths, were considered to represent two different types of mortality risk from a health care services viewpoint. At present, the prevention of fetal deaths requires either a primary preventive approach to ameliorate risk factors in pregnant mothers (i.e., reduction of smoking and alcohol consumption), or secondary prevention strategies to monitor intrauterine conditions which may require

The authors wish to thank and acknowledge the assistance of Professor Tor Bjerkedal and his staff at the Medical Birth Registry of Norway for providing birthweight-specific perinatal mortality data, 1967–80, for inclusion in this chapter. Also, we want to thank Director Anders Ericson of the Swedish Medical Birth Registry, National Board of Health and Welfare of Sweden, for providing the Swedish birth and mortality data used in the tables and figures. In addition, we wish to thank Ms. Dorothy Day for her outstanding assistance in typing the numerous drafts of this chapter.

therapy in high-risk pregnancies. However, the prevention of early neonatal mortality, and the continued maintenance of the current low levels which prevail in most developed countries, is a matter of mostly medical care based on complex and costly technology for intervention and treatment of very high-risk infants (Phibbs et al., 1981; Paneth et al., 1982).

This chapter will address a number of interrelated methodological issues that frequently arise in research on perinatal epidemiology. A number of editorials, letters to the editor, and full-length articles have appeared in the medical and public health literature during the past five years debating these methodological issues (North and MacDonald, 1977; Lee et al., 1976, 1980; Bakketeig and Hoffman, 1979, 1980; Philip et al., 1981; Terrin and Meyer, 1981; Erickson and Bjerkedal, 1982; Guyer et al., 1982; Paneth, 1982; Wallace et al., 1982; Williams and Chen, 1982; Shapiro, 1982). Our purpose here is to consolidate this methodological discussion in light of a growing amount of substantive information scattered in the published literature.

Since birthweight and other indices of fetal maturity such as gestational age invariably have the major impact on perinatal mortality rates, it is not surprising that most methodological issues hinge upon the interpretation of birthweight-specific (and joint birthweight and gestational age-specific) perinatal mortality rates. When these rates have not been available for study, similar methodological issues have arisen based on the low birthweight rate as the surrogate measure of perinatal outcome (Chase, 1977; Lee, et al., 1980; Rooth, 1980).

The crown–heel length of the newborn is an additional indicator of fetal well-being. Earlier publications by Clifford et al. (1953), Gruenwald (1969), Miller and Hassanein (1971), Fryer et al. (1977), Hoffman et al. (1978), Daikoku et al. (1979), and Bakketeig and Hoffman (1984) have suggested the importance of this additional measure for predicting perinatal survival. The Medical Birth Registries of Norway and Sweden are both exceptionally good sources (due to the standard recording of this information) for elucidating the importance of the crown–heel length of the newborn to further refine and classify perinatal mortality risks.

MATERIALS AND METHODS

The accumulated records for 14 years of Norwegian births, 1967–80 were used as the basis for the tables and graphs in this chapter. During this time period, there were 825,913 births, which included livebirths and fetal deaths with a gestational age of 16 weeks or more recorded in the Norwegian Medical Birth Registry. Of these births, 10,170 were fetal deaths and 5238 of the liveborn infants died within the first week of life (Bjerkedal, 1983). The completeness of recording of critical measurements for judging the maturity of the infant is very high in this registry. For example, the birthweight was not available in less than 0.5% of deliveries and gestational age at birth was missing in less than 3% of infants (Bjerkedal and Bakketeig, 1975; Hoffman et al., 1977; Bakketeig et al., 1979).

Records encompassing eight years of Swedish births, 1973–80, were also available for the analysis. These data were collected by the Swedish Medical Birth Registry, which includes all livebirths plus fetal deaths of 28 weeks or more gestational age (Karlberg and Ericson, 1979; Karlberg, 1980). The completeness of information in this registry is comparable to that of the Norwegian Medical Birth Registry (National Central Bureau of Statistics, 1983).

Data from the United States were provided by the National Center for Health Statistics and through state centers for health statistics in, Minnesota, Missouri, and North Carolina. In addition, crown–heel length data for U.S. births were examined using the Collaborative Perinatal Study of the National Institute of Neurological Diseases and Stroke (Niswander and Gordon, 1972).

Historical data are based on the *Historical Statistics of Norway* published by the Norwegian Central Bureau of Statistics. International comparisons of perinatal mortality data have been obtained from selected volumes of the United Nations *Demographic Yearbook* or, when necessary, through direct contacts with the central statistical bureaus of various countries.

Terminology

Comprehensive discussions of the definitions relating to the perinatal period have been published elsewhere (World Health Organization, 1977; Dunn, 1979). Definitions of the following three terms are included here to clarify their meaning in this chapter.

Fetal mortality rate. The number of fetal deaths occurring at 20 weeks or more of gestational age per 1000 total births. The "late" fetal mortality rate refers to the number of deaths occurring in fetuses of gestational age 28 weeks or more per 1000 total births. Birthweight greater than or equal to 1000 g was used in the definition of late fetal mortality if gestational age was missing.

Neonatal mortality rate. The number of deaths in the first 28 days of life per 1000 livebirths. The "early" neonatal mortality rate refers to the number of deaths occurring 0–6 days after birth per 1000 live-births. Both of these rates are occasionally defined per 1000 *total* births, rather than per 1000 livebirths, which is the case in Table 21-1 of this chapter.

Perinatal mortality rate. The number of late fetal deaths plus early neonatal deaths per 1000 total births. Occasionally, this term is used in a broader sense to include all deaths in fetuses of gestational age 20 weeks or more. In this chapter, it is not used to include neonatal deaths occurring past the first week of life.

Statistical Methods

We have used simple smoothing techniques and linear regression to display time trends more clearly. Standardization of rates is men-tioned with several references provided to assist the interested reader.

The only sophisticated methodology employed is that of contour estimation for bivariate distributions of birthweight and crown–heel length. Similar contour plots are also derived for perinatal mortality rates as a joint function of birthweight and crown–heel length. The methodology is the same as that described earlier for bivariate plots of birthweight and gestational age in Hoffman et al. (1974, 1977). Gold-stein and Peckham (1976) and Wilcox (1981) provide additional in-formation on contour diagrams.

RESULTS OF METHODOLOGICAL INVESTIGATIONS

The analysis of time trends and geographical differences in perina-tal mortality not only provides epidemiologic insights but also has significance for underlying methodological issues. Although any en-deavor in descriptive epidemiology is circumscribed by time and place, these limitations require frequent reevaluation when plan-ning and conducting research studies. In the following section, data for very long-term trends in perinatal mortality rates have been abstracted from published historical statistics in Norway. Although much has been written concerning the origins and instructions for registration of these data, it is impossible to know the quality through-out such a long period of time (Backer, 1947, 1948; Gille, 1949; Ofstad, 1949). Setting aside the issue of data precision, these mortality rates are shown since they are practically unique in providing information over such a considerable time period. The overall perspective afforded by these data is worthwhile, even if individual features in the graph may be better explained in terms of changes in methods of registration, patterns of emigration, or other external events.

Long-Term Time Trends

In examining time trends in perinatal mortality rates, it is important to be aware not only of the trend in recent decades but also of trends over a much longer span of years. The magnitude of recent improvements can then be easily appreciated in the context of the time required to achieve similar relative gains in preceding years. Perinatal mortality rates in the United States are not available before 1922 (U.S. Bureau of the Census, 1960), and there have been reliable data only since 1945 (Burnham, 1982). However, data do exist, or have been reconstructed, over a much longer period of time in some European countries (Gille, 1949; Backer and Aagenaes, 1967; Mitchell, 1975; Hofsten and Lundstrøm, 1976; Tomasson, 1977; Lithell, 1981). For example, in Fig. 21-1, perinatal mortality rates are shown over an entire century in Norway, starting with 1876. Fetal mortality rates are available from the same source (Central Bureau of Statistics of Norway, 1979) beginning in 1801, and infant mortality rates are published from 1836 on.

Figure 21-1 illustrates the long-term pattern of general decline in perinatal mortality rates. During this century, there were only two periods when successive five-year perinatal mortality rates did not decline: the five years from 1891–95, and the years surrounding the Great Depression, 1926–40. From 1876 until 1925, there was a gradual improvement in the perinatal mortality rate, from a rate of 50 to approximately 35 perinatal deaths per 1000 births. During 1930s the perinatal mortality rates increased again to the level prevailing at the turn of the 20th century: 40 deaths per 1000 births. Since the beginning of the Second World War, the perinatal mortality rates have been improving at a rate three times higher than that accomplished in the preceding half-century. However, a word of caution is needed before accepting these data at face value. The apparent increase in perinatal mortality rates that began in the late 1920s may be attributable in part to the improvement of procedures for registration of vital events as a result of the increasing number of deliveries taking place in hospitals (Backer and Aagenaes, 1967; National Board of Health and Welfare, 1973).

The fetal mortality rates extending back to 1801 suggest an earlier period of increased mortality. There is a slight increase in the fetal mortality rate from 1871–75, which is also part of a much broader increase in this rate that began after 1815 and reached a maximum in the 1850s. An understanding of this pattern requires more knowledge

495

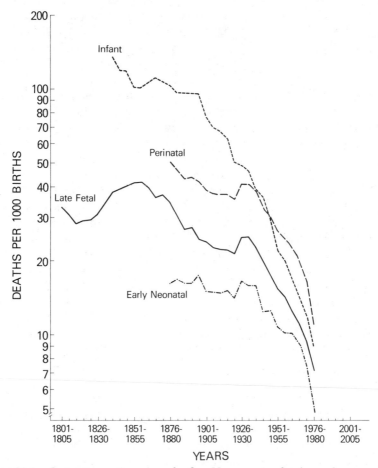

Fig. 21-1. Long-term time trends for Norway in fetal, early neonatal, perinatal, and infant mortality rates. Data are presented as five year averages and were abstracted from the *Historical Statistics* volumes published by the Central Bureau of Statistics of Norway.

of the social and economic climate within Norway during the first half of the 19th century than is possible to sketch here (Amneus, 1900; Derry, 1957; Drake, 1969, 1972). What is striking is the similarity between the fetal and perinatal mortality rates throughout the 100 years where both rates are available. In contrast, the early neonatal mortality rates were relatively constant until after the Second World War when they began to fall sharply.

The infant mortality rates, also shown in Fig. 21-1, are not closely related to either the fetal or perinatal mortality rates. The infant mortality rate has fallen at a continued rapid pace since 1900. Before 1900, the infant mortality rate also was declining but at a slower pace.

After the Second World War, the infant mortality rates in Norway, and in several other developed countries, declined to a level below that of the perinatal mortality rate, a condition which had never existed previously. For instance, in 1880 in Norway the infant mortality rate was twice the perinatal mortality rate.

The remaining analyses in this chapter are based on data from more recent time periods. Nevertheless, before interpreting recent time trends, it is intriguing to consider that the current status is the extrapolation of a pattern that has prevailed for almost a 100 years. The assumption here is, of course, that the mortality rates in Norway reflect those of other industrialized populations. A number of publications suggest that this is true in recent time periods (Chase, 1967; Weatherall, 1975; Bakketeig et al., 1984). For trends covering a longer span of years, Rooth (1979) has published infant and perinatal mortality rates in Sweden from 1915 through 1976. These data provide evidence for very similar historical patterns in Sweden compared to Norway during these 60 years. Even more extensive data are available for Sweden than for Norway on stillbirth and infant mortality rates, and the time trends are similar when rates are known for both countries (Gille, 1949; National Central Bureau of Statistics, 1969; Hofsten and Lundstrøm, 1976).

Geographic Variations and Short-Term Declines

Within the last two decades, reductions in perinatal mortality have become a widespread phenomenon in the industrialized countries (Weatherall, 1975; Manciaux, 1976; Nordic Council, 1981; United Nations, 1981). In Table 21-1, perinatal mortality, and its individual components of late fetal and early neonatal mortality, is presented for the United States and 22 other countries at two points in time, 1973 and 1978. The latter year, 1978, is the most recent year for which data are readily available from a variety of developed countries. In most of these countries, the perinatal mortality rate has declined between 30 and 45% in this span of only five years. Evaluation of the decline in late fetal and early neonatal mortality rates separately suggests that both of these components were substantial contributors to the general decline in most countries.

Particular attention should be focused on the countries that in 1978 had achieved a perinatal mortality rate of less than 12 per 1000 births. In the six countries identified in the table—Finland, Sweden, Switzerland, Denmark, Japan, and Norway—with the lowest perinatal mortality rates, there was practically no variation in the rates of early neonatal mortality. The average early neonatal mortality rate for these six countries was 4.6 per 1000 births. In contrast, these six

Table 21-1. Number of Births (live plus stillborn) and Rates of Late Fetal Mortality (LFM), Early Neonatal Mortality (ENM), and Perinatal Mortality (PM) per 1000 Births[a]

	1973				1978			
	Births	LFM	ENM	PM	Births	LFM	ENM	PM
Finland	57,143	6.2	7.4	13.6	64,297	4.9	4.4	9.3
Sweden	110,451	7.1	6.8	14.0	93,703	4.9	4.6	9.5
Switzerland	88,183	7.5	7.8	15.4	71,810	6.1	4.6	10.7
Denmark	72,418	7.2	7.3	14.5	62,400	5.8	5.0	10.8
Japan	2,111,412	9.2	5.8	15.0	1,720,005	6.6	4.5	11.1
Norway	61,783	9.3	7.3	16.6	52,095	6.6	4.5	11.1
Netherlands	196,775	9.1	7.2	16.3	176,809	7.1	5.3	12.4
New Zealand	61,285	9.1	8.3	17.4	51,393	7.1	5.8	12.9
Canada	346,239	8.3	9.3	17.6	361,088	6.2	6.7	12.9
U.S. white	2,571,417	7.9	10.4	18.3	2,697,417	6.0	7.0	13.0
West Germany	641,319	8.9	13.3	22.2	580,119	6.3	7.4	13.7
Australia	250,592	11.7	10.5	22.1	225,915	6.7	7.1	13.8
U.S. Total	3,164,560	8.7	11.3	20.1	3,355,567	6.6	7.9	14.6
France	868,170	12.1	8.5	20.6	744,182	9.6	5.2	14.7
Austria	98,918	8.9	15.8	24.6	85,964	6.5	8.4	14.9
Scotland	75,265	11.6	10.9	22.5	64,819	8.1	7.3	15.4
England & Wales	683,889	11.6	9.4	21.0	601,526	8.5	7.1	15.5
Israel	89,368	9.2	11.8	21.0	93,433	8.9	8.3	17.2
Poland	603,725	8.6	12.5	21.1	671,131	7.1	11.3	18.4
Italy	888,265	13.3	15.2	28.5	719,312	8.8	11.2	20.0
Yugoslavia	382,075	7.9	14.7	22.6	384,284	7.5	13.0	20.6
U.S. nonwhite	593,143	12.2	15.4	27.6	658,119	9.1	11.8	20.9
Greece	139,223	12.2	13.9	26.1	148,091	10.1	11.5	21.6
Hungary	157,623	8.9	24.4	33.3	169,524	8.0	16.7	24.8
Portugal	175,640	18.9	14.2	33.1	169,757	13.5	13.0	26.5

[a] Based in part on data contained in the 1980 United Nations Demographic Yearbook (special subject—mortality statistics).

countries do show some variation in their rates of late fetal mortality. The average rate is 5.8 per 1000 births, but with a range from 4.9 to 6.6 per 1000 births.

This situation contrasts with that obtaining for the five countries in Table 21-1, who in 1978 experienced perinatal mortality rates ranging from 15 to 20 per 1000 births. For these five countries, late fetal mortality rates were practically identical at 8.3 per 1000 births. However, the early neonatal mortality rates ranged from a low of 7.3 to a high of 11.3 per 1000 births. Hence, the explanation for variations among countries may depend both on the separate components of the perinatal mortality rate and the actual level of perinatal mortality reflected by the relative rankings of countries. These rankings depend ultimately on the whole complex association between technological development and the delivery of health care services within individual countries. Countries at different stages of development should be expected to have different trends in the declining rates of fetal and neonatal mortality.

A more detailed examination of geographical and time variations in perinatal mortality is possible for selected industrial countries. In the following discussion, the focus will be primarily on comparing data from various Scandinavian countries with data from the United States. The completeness of recorded data and the extent of information available make it feasible to explore both time trends and information pertaining to fetal maturity at birth, such as weight, gestational age, and in some instances, crown–heel length.

In Table 21-2, perinatal mortality rates covering the 15-year period 1966–80 are provided for Denmark, Norway, Sweden, and the United States (white and nonwhite rates shown separately). In each national or ethnic group the perinatal mortality rates were reduced in half

Table 21-2. Comparison of Time Trends in Perinatal Mortality Rates (PMR) in the United States and Three Scandinavian Countries

Year	Denmark	Norway	Sweden	United States White	United States Nonwhite
1966	21.6	20.8	18.8	24.3	39.2
1967	19.2	20.5	18.7	23.7	38.2
1968	18.9	19.7	18.3	23.5	37.0
1969	18.7	20.2	16.2	21.8	34.3
1970	17.9	19.1	16.4	21.0	32.7
1971	17.4	17.7	15.7	19.8	30.2
1972	16.1	17.5	14.3	19.3	29.6
1973	14.5	16.6	14.0	18.3	27.6
1974	13.9	15.4	13.2	17.3	26.0
1975	13.3	14.1	11.3	16.0	25.0
1976	12.6	13.2	10.7	15.1	23.8
1977	10.6	13.1	10.1	13.8	21.7
1978	10.8	11.1	9.5	13.0	20.9
1979	9.9	11.6	9.1	12.5	19.3
1980[a]	9.0	10.8	8.5	12.0	18.0
Average PMR (15 years)	15.0	16.1	13.6	18.1	28.2

[a] Provisional data.

499

over the 15-year time span. During this period, Denmark averaged perinatal mortality rates approximately 10% higher than Sweden, and the Norwegian rates were approximately 20% higher than Sweden. Also, the United States white perinatal mortality rates were 33% higher than Sweden, and the nonwhite perinatal mortality rates were more than 100% higher, on average, than the rates prevailing in Sweden. It is remarkable that these different countries or ethnic groups remained in such a relatively stable configuration throughout the 15-year period. In general, one would not expect to find such a statistical result among five different population groups. This situation affords an unique opportunity to examine the two separate components of perinatal mortality, late fetal and early neonatal mortality, and to study the available data for birthweight-specific time trends.

Birthweight-Specific Mortality Rates

A number of authors have recently stressed the need for a more detailed birthweight-specific analysis of perinatal mortality rates (Chalmers, 1979; Macfarlane and Chalmers, 1981). In addition, a number of studies from different countries have already been carried out to examine trends through time in these rates (Erkkola et al., 1982; Forbes et al., 1982; Williams and Chen, 1982; Meirik, 1983). All of these studies have shown dramatic improvements in birthweight-specific perinatal mortality rates during the 1970s. Such comparisons are generally unavailable prior to 1970, although two reports, Alberman (1974) and Pharoah and Alberman (1981), have extended birthweight-specific perinatal mortality comparisons as far back as 1953 based on births in England and Wales. Their results will be discussed below in reference to data recently made available from Norway (Bjerkedal, 1983).

A comparison of birthweight-specific fetal mortality rates for the United States, Norway, and Sweden in 1972–73 is provided in Table 21-3. The U.S. data for this table were derived from three states (Minnesota, Missouri, and North Carolina) representing approximately 7% of the total United States. These three states were selected from a number of states which had linked infant death and live-birth certificate data for these years. They were selected in part because they were among the first states to adopt the revised 1968 United States certificate of birth which, for the first time, requested the date of the last normal menstrual period (LMP) prior to pregnancy. In addition, each of these states reports annually about the same number of births as do Norway and Sweden (between 50,000 and 100,000 births annually). Morever, during this time period these three states were typical of the U.S. average if judged by the infant

Table 21-3. Birthweight-Specific Fetal Mortality Rates, 1972–73

Birthweight (g)	United States[a]		Sweden[b]	Norway
	Nonwhite	*White*		
–999	389.4	425.6	269.8	710.6
1000–1499	183.0	193.1	266.6	316.0
1500–1999	86.8	91.3	111.5	159.6
2000–2499	30.3	25.3	34.2	44.5
2500–2999	6.2	7.1	10.8	12.6
3000–3499	4.8	2.8	3.1	3.9
3500–3999	5.7	2.4	2.1	2.2
4000–4499	9.6	2.9	2.3	2.0
4500+	49.3	8.3		6.3
Not stated	702.7	605.8	183.2	215.3
Total	19.4	10.2	7.8	12.6

[a] Data from three states with approximately 7% of total births.
[b] Swedish data for 1973 only.

mortality rate for the country as a whole: Missouri was frequently the median state while Minnesota and North Carolina were only slightly above or below the average for the country, respectively (Wegman, 1974).

Fetal deaths for Norway and the United States shown in Table 21-3 are based on the broadest definition possible, including births registered as early as 16 weeks gestation in Norway and from 20 weeks gestation in the United States. In Sweden, only data using the narrow definition, from 28 weeks of gestation on, are recorded and available. This limitation in the Swedish data primarily affects the fetal mortality rate below 1000 g. The Swedish and Norwegian rates are higher than the United States rates for birthweight categories less than 3000 g. Above 3500 g, the Swedish and Norwegian fetal mortality rates are less than the United States rates. The most striking differences between the United States, Norway, and Sweden occur in the fetal mortality rates of infants weighing between 1000 and 2000 g (differences in excess of 40%). One possible explanation for these discrepancies is that "fetal" and "early neonatal" deaths are labeled differently in the United States and Scandinavia (Hoffman et al., 1978, 1984).

To circumvent this possibility, it is necessary to compare perinatal mortality rates using the same data sets (Table 21-4). The perinatal mortality rates for infants born weighing less than 2000 g are much more similar than the fetal mortality rates shown in the Table 21-3. In spite of attempts by the World Health Organization to standardize international conventions, there are still these detectable differences

Table 21-4. Birthweight-Specific Perinatal Mortality Rates, 1972–73

Birthweight (g)	United States[a]		Sweden[b]	Norway
	Nonwhite	White		
–999	868.5	905.3	818.6	948.9
1000–1499	437.2	519.5	529.8	592.8
1500–1999	159.1	222.3	211.5	285.8
2000–2499	46.7	54.4	61.6	72.0
2500–2999	9.9	12.9	15.4	20.4
3000–3499	6.9	4.9	5.0	5.7
3500–3999	8.1	4.2	3.3	3.2
4000–4499	12.7	4.6	3.7	3.3
4500+	74.0	12.1		7.2
Not stated	858.1	735.3	480.9	340.3
Total	35.9	20.0	14.2	19.4

[a] Data from three states with approximately 7% of toal U.S. births.
[b] Swedish data for 1973 only.

in what is labeled a "fetal" as opposed to an "early neonatal" death (Hoffman et al., 1978; World Health Organization, 1978; Davies, 1980).

Although the use of perinatal mortality eliminated the effect of labeling fetal deaths or early neonatal deaths differently in various countries, there is still a marked difference in birthweight-specific perinatal mortality rates in the United States, Norway, and Sweden which needs to be accounted for. The United States apparently has a lower birthweight-specific perinatal mortality rate than either Norway or Sweden for babies weighing less than 3000 g. Also, from Table 21-4 it is clear that the same finding is true for U.S. nonwhites in comparison to U.S. whites. That is, for babies born weighing between 1500 and 1999 g, the perinatal mortality rate for Nonwhites is almost 30% less than it is for whites, 159.1 versus 222.3 per 1000 births. Similar differences in New York City data from 1958 to 1961, led Erhardt et al. (1964) to carefully examine their information on fetal maturity as reflected by gestational age data based on the last normal menstrual period measurement. They concluded that the improved survival for nonwhites at lower birth weights was not due to the known and observed differences in gestational age between white and black races. Furthermore, there are only very slight differences between the gestational age distributions of births for U.S. whites compared to Scandinavia (Hoffman et al., 1983).

Therefore, it is necessary to look for a different explanation in order to account for the observed ethnic differences. One significant factor is the consistent difference for the U.S. nonwhite versus white

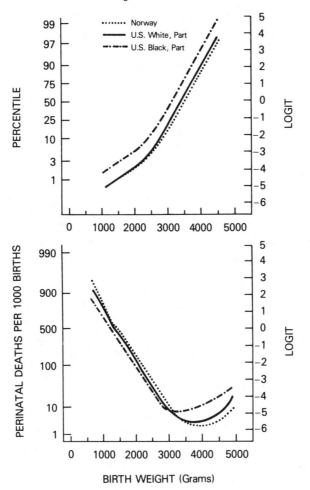

Fig. 21-2. Cumulative birth weight distributions and birth weight-specific perinatal mortality rates in singleton deliveries for Norway and United States white and black samples in 1972 and 1973 combined.

populations, and for Scandinavian versus the U.S. populations, in the relative frequency of low birthweight deliveries. For example, 14% of the nonwhite births in these U.S. data were low birthweight (less than 2500 g), but only 7% of the U.S. white births were low birthweight. In Norway and Sweden these low birthweight percentages were only 5 and 4% of births, respectively. It appears, then, that the distribution of birthweights within different populations influence the birthweight-specific perinatal mortality rates. This effect is displayed graphically in Fig. 21-2 where the cumulative birthweight distributions and the birthweight-specific perinatal mortality rates for Norway and the U.S. white and nonwhite populations are plotted, based on the data in Table 21-4.

An enhanced comparison between ethnic or national groups can be developed by further adjusting the birthweight-specific perinatal mortality rates for the differing percentiles of the cumulative birthweight distributions in the underlying populations. In an analogous fashion, Rooth (1980) has proposed an adjustment to standardize the comparison of low birthweight rates between countries. Additional efforts could be directed toward establishing some "standard" population birthweight and gestational age distributions. Then, data pertaining to different ethnic or national groups could be adjusted to a universal standard for more detailed evaluation. Of course, the standard would be specific for a particular time period. Such a standard could also be used to clarify changes which occur as medical care practices and socioeconomic conditions change through time. A number of common approaches for calculating a set of standardized rates may be employed (Fleiss, 1973), or other adjustment procedures based on regression techniques may be used (Feldstein, 1966; Mosteller and Tukey, 1977).

Birthweight-specific perinatal mortality data for the United States are extremely difficult to obtain. Although individual states may have linked infant mortality and birth certificate data, there are no multistate data sets available for epidemiologic research since 1974. The National Center for Health Statistics (NCHS) has coordinated the preparation of a multistate linked perinatal data set in cooperation with the World Health Organization report (1978), and these data have since been used to make comparisons with a complete U.S. linked data set constructed by NCHS for 1960 (Armstrong, 1972; Chase, 1972; Kleinman et al., 1978). Fetal mortality rates for the United States are the only data generally available for comparison to other countries. These data are routinely published in the *Vital Statistics of the United States* volumes, the most recent year being 1977 (U.S. Department of Health and Human Services, 1981). In Table 21-5, comparisons in fetal mortality rates for the year 1977 are shown for the United States and Norway. Comparing the data in this table with that shown earlier for 1972–73 (Table 21-3) makes it obvious that the birthweight-specific fetal mortality rates have improved considerably: 30% improvement for U.S. blacks, 20% for U.S. whites, and 10% for Norway. In births of infants weighing 3500–3999 g, this improvement is even more striking: 50% for U.S. whites and Norwegians and over 100% for U.S. blacks during this five-year interval. These trends suggest that routine records of fetal (and early neonatal) mortality within the United States could be extremely

Table 21-5. Birthweight-Specific Fetal
Mortality Rates, 1977

| Birthweight (g) | United States | | Norway |
	Nonwhite	White	
−499	494.7	533.8	990.9
500–999	298.9	322.7	668.5
1000–1499	132.1	151.3	320.0
1500–1999	59.7	67.9	122.5
2000–2499	17.3	20.0	49.8
2500–2999	4.4	5.2	12.3
3000–3499	2.5	2.2	3.1
3500–3999	2.4	1.6	1.5
4000–4499	5.3	2.1	.9
4500–4999	16.6	4.4	.7
5000+	66.0	20.2	.0
Not stated	468.1	437.1	127.1
Total	14.6	8.7	11.4

helpful in health care planning, and in furthering our understanding of perinatal epidemiology.

Time Trends in Birthweight-Specific Mortality Rates

Time trends in birthweight-specific perinatal mortality rates have recently become available for several countries. The data presented here for Norway cover 14 years, beginning with 1967 when the Medical Birth Registry in Norway was first introduced. In Table 21-6, the improvement in perinatal mortality rates within each birthweight category is shown through time. In order to increase the stability of rates, the annual data have been combined into three-year averages. The overall reduction in the perinatal mortality rate has been approximately 45% during these 14 years. Apart from the two lowest-weight groups, and the highest-weight group, the reduction in mortality has been of the same order in each weight group.

This finding is also illustrated in the right-hand panel of Fig. 21-3 where the mortality curves are parallel. The other two panels demonstrate the importance of separating the two components of perinatal mortality when studying time trends. There has been essentially no change in fetal mortality for the extremely low-weight births. However, the reduction in mortality is substantial for average sized and heavy births, particularly for those infants weighing more than 4500 grams. For the early neonatal mortality rates in the middle panel

505

Table 21-6. Time Trends in Birthweight-Specific Perinatal Mortality Rates in Norway

Birthweight (g)	1967–68	1969–71	1972–74	1975–77	1978–80
–499	1000.0	1000.0	1000.0	1000.0	997.3
500–999	949.6	950.5	933.8	904.7	833.9
1000–1499	660.7	659.5	585.6	514.8	412.5
1500–1999	295.5	295.4	278.7	214.6	171.4
2000–2499	102.4	98.2	76.4	65.4	58.6
2500–2999	22.4	18.9	19.7	14.7	14.2
3000–3499	8.0	6.9	5.7	5.0	4.5
3500–3999	4.3	4.3	3.2	2.7	2.7
4000–4499	3.6	4.3	3.5	2.5	2.5
4500–4999	4.5	6.4	5.4	3.3	3.3
5000+	26.9	12.5	11.5	7.6	5.6
Not stated	290.9	290.7	358.9	257.7	226.5
Total	22.4	21.2	18.8	16.4	14.4

of Fig. 21-3, however, it is apparent that the greatest improvements have occurred among the lowest-weight births. As an example, neonatal mortality dropped 64% for births weighing 1500–1999 g compared to a drop of 15% among births weighing 4000–4499 g.

It is important to reiterate that the separate components of perinatal mortality (fetal versus neonatal mortality) have developed differently as a function of birthweight over time. The sharp fall in neonatal mortality (especially for low-weight births during the 1970s) is probably attributable to the rapid development and dissemination of modern obstetric and neonatal intensive care. However, the opposite association with weight shown for the fetal mortality trends is most likely due to the improved quality and more extensive use of modern antenatal surveillance and obstetric care.

The next two illustrations show the time trends in birthweight-specific fetal mortality rates (Fig. 21-4) and early neonatal mortality rates (Fig. 21-5) in a more detailed fashion. Due to the fluctuations from year to year in these rates, a fitted linear regression line is drawn through the actual data for each of the birthweight categories. These figures can be contrasted with published data from England and Wales (Alberman, 1974; Pharoah and Alberman, 1981), from Sweden (Meirik, 1983), and a few from other countries (Erkkola et al., 1982; Forbes et al., 1982).

The data in Fig. 21-4 confirm that in Norway the same tendency holds as noted for England and Wales by Alberman and colleagues. Fetal mortality rates have improved at a relatively more rapid pace

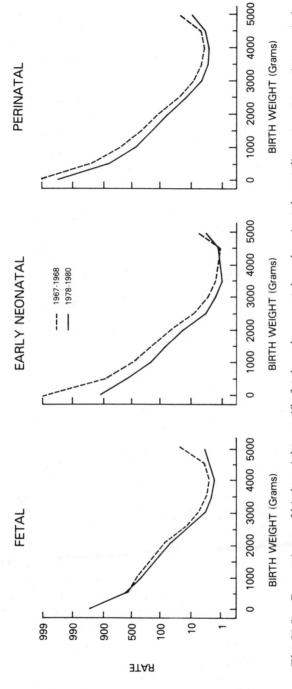

Fig. 21-3. Comparisons of birth weight-specific fetal, early neonatal, and perinatal mortality rates at two time periods, 1967–68 and 1978–80, in Norway. *Source:* Professor Tor Bjerkedal, personal communication.

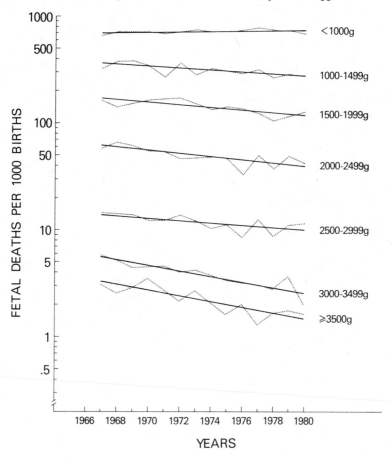

Fig. 21-4. Time trends for recent years in Norway showing the decline in birth weight-specific fetal mortality rates. The solid lines represent linear, least-squares regression fits to the annual fetal mortality rates (dotted lines) within each birth weight category. The steepest fall in fetal mortality rates occurred for births weighing 3,000 grams or more. *Source:* Professor Tor Bjerkedal, personal communication.

for the larger birthweight infants. The rates in Fig. 21-4 are plotted on a logarithmic scale so that the slope of the fitted regression line indicates the rate of improvement for each birthweight group. The data in Fig. 21-5 also support the findings of Alberman and colleagues. The early neonatal mortality rates have improved more rapidly for births weighing less than 2500 g. The only slight exception is for births weighing less than 1000 g. However, unlike the fetal mortality rates at these extremely low birthweights, there is a detectable trend in the direction of improved neonatal survival if these infants are born alive.

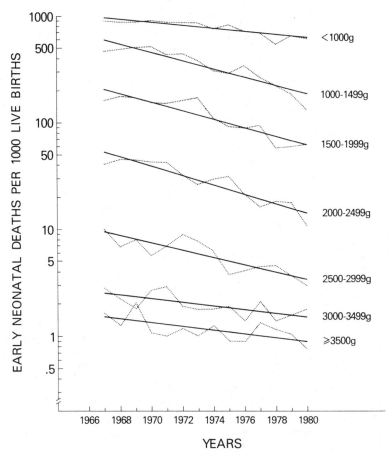

Fig. 21-5. Time trends for recent years in Norway showing the decline in birth weight-specific early neonatal mortality rates. The solid lines represent linear, least-squares regression fits to the annual early neonatal mortality rates (dotted lines) within each birth weight category. The steepest fall in early neonatal mortality rates occurred for births weighing between 2,000 and 2,499 grams. *Source:* Professor Tor Bjerkedal, personal communication.

Mortality Risks as a Joint Function of Birthweight and Gestational Age

The need to consider other indices of maturity at birth besides weight in assessing perinatal mortality risks has long been recognized (Lubchenco et al., 1963; Erhardt et al., 1964; Yerushalmy et al., 1965, 1967; Gruenwald, 1966; Van Den Berg and Yerushalmy, 1966; Battaglia and Lubchenco, 1967; Ghosh and Daga, 1967; Lubchenco et al., 1972).

Gestational age is the most direct and obvious indicator of fetal maturity to use in refining the mortality risks established with birthweight alone. Unfortunately, gestational age as measured by the mother's recall of the first day of her last normal menstrual period (LMP), is "unknown" or "uncertain" in a rather high proportion of cases, often between 20 and 30% of mothers in the United States (Hoffman et al., 1977). Even when the LMP date is known, the variable length of the menstrual cycle may further reduce the usefulness of this measure, but this does not seem to be a major problem (Treloar et al., 1967; Hammes and Treloar, 1970). Nevertheless, when gestational age is available from medical or vital records, it has been used profitably to classify further fetal, neonatal, and perinatal mortality risks (Hoffman et al., 1974; Goldstein and Peckham, 1976; Bakketeig et al., 1979, 1983; McIlwaine et al., 1979; Philip et al., 1981; Williams et al., 1982).

Much of the impetus for employing gestational age as an additional indicator of fetal maturity has come from the recognition that small preterm infants are subjects to quite different morbidity and mortality risks as compared to small term or posterm infants. These latter babies are called small-for-dates (SFD), intrauterine growth retarded (IUGR), or small-for-gestational-age (SGA). It has been customary to define the growth-retarded infants as those below the 10th percentile (occasionally, the 5th or 3rd percentile) of birthweight for given gestational age (Lubchenco et al., 1963; Bjerkedal et al., 1973; Hoffman et al., 1974). However, some investigators, notably Usher and McLean (1969) and Ounsted (1965, 1969), prefer to define limits above and below the average fetal growth curve based on one or two standard deviations of birthweight for given gestational age.

Several research workers have refined these fetal growth percentiles to take into account a number of additional factors such as maternal age, parity, race, height, or weight, etc. (Tanner and Thomson, 1970; Chamberlain et al., 1975). However, a recent study at the University of Kansas Medical Center in Kansas City conducted by Miller (1981) has greatly exceeded these earlier attempts to allow for a few maternal or fetal variables when calculating intrauterine growth curves. After searching the literature for factors known or thought to reduce the fetal growth potential, this study was designed and carried out prospectively to identify all such maternal–fetal pairs. For example, maternal smoking, medical complications in pregnancy or delivery, congenital malformations, and a host of other factors were used to exclude maternal–fetal pairs. These mothers and infants were then excluded from the baseline population for purposes of calculating norms, in particular birthweight percentiles at given gestational ages. The limitation of sample size to approximately 2500 mothers has made

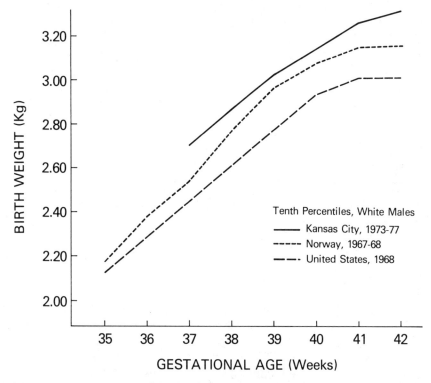

Fig. 21-6. Comparison of the tenth percentiles of birth weight for gestational age from three different populations. The solid line is based on a selected cohort of births born at the University of Kansas Medical Center in Kansas City from 1973 through 1977. This cohort was selected to represent "normal" births, excluding all those births which had any influence from factors known to restrict the fetal growth potential (Miller and Merritt, 1979). The dashed and dotted line represents the tenth percentile based on all births in Norway for two years, 1967 and 1968 (Bjerkedal et al., 1973). The dashed line represents the tenth percentile in the United States (36 states plus the District of Columbia) using gestational age information from the revised live birth certificate in 1968 (Hoffman et al., 1974).

it necessary to compute percentiles only at gestations ranging from 37 to 42 weeks (Miller and Merritt, 1979).

Figure 21-6 illustrates the 10th percentile line for white male infants based on Miller's "normal" maternal–fetal pairs. For contrast, the 10th percentiles of birthweight for gestational age are shown from the two earlier, less discriminating studies of Bjerkedal et al. (1973) and Hoffman et al. (1974). The Norwegian birthweight 10th percentile line is above that of the United States as expected, but falls

Table 21-7. Selected Percentiles of Birth Weights (kg) for Gestational Age for White Male Births Derived From Different Fetal Growth Standards

Gestational Age (weeks)	Kansas City[1] 5th Centile	Norway[2] 10th Centile	United States[3] 15th Centile
35	–	2.17	2.26
36	–	2.38	2.41
37	2.63	2.54	2.61
38	2.77	2.77	2.76
39	2.91	2.97	2.88
40	3.04	3.08	3.01
41	3.16	3.15	3.10
42	3.27	3.16	3.11

[1] Data from Miller and Merritt (1979).
[2] Data from Bjerkedal et al. (1973).
[3] Data interpolated from Hoffman et al. (1974).

considerably short of Miller's refined standard. In Table 21-7, it is shown that Miller's 5th percentile of birthweight for gestational age agrees quite closely with the 10th percentile of Norwegian births, and the 15th percentile for U.S. births. It seems reasonable that if mothers and infants at risk are excluded before birthweight percentiles, are calculated, as was done in Miller' study, then a standard based on the 5th percentile would be more generally useful for clinical practice or epidemiologic studies. In this light, the 10th or 15th percentile based on unselected birth populations is useful as well as for future research studies on small-for-gestational-age births. This conclusion is possible as a result of Miller's careful and painstaking research study.

Preterm Births

Since preterm labor, and the resulting preterm birth, poses an increased risk of perinatal mortality, this is a major clinical and public health problem (Fedrick and Anderson, 1976; Rush et al., 1976; Eisner et al., 1978; Bakketeig and Hoffman, 1981). In Table 21-8, perinatal mortality rates are shown as a function of broad gestational age categories for single and multiple births in the United States and Norway. The data used here are the same as described earlier for birthweight and perinatal mortality (Table 21-4). However, only data from one state, Minnesota, was used in calculating these rates. In Minnesota for 1972–73, only 1% of either fetal deaths (with 20 or more

Table 21-8. Gestational Age-Specific Perinatal Mortality Rates, 1972–73

	Single births		Multiple births	
Gestational age (wks)	U.S. white[a]	Norway	U.S. white[a]	Norway
≤26	862.5	868.9	1000.0	978.9
27–32	323.3	428.1	338.9	427.7
33–38	22.2	36.0	39.1	51.9
39–44	5.2	5.8	31.7	21.2
44+	8.9	10.8	–	–
Not stated	262.3	22.0	500.0	157.1
Number of births	107,044	124,677	1900	2388
Perinatal mortality rate	18.4	19.4	104.7	106.4

[a] Based on data from Minnesota.

weeks of gestation) or livebirths had missing gestational age information. The other two states in this linked data set had a much higher proportion of missing LMP dates and therefore have been excluded from this comparison.

The differences in perinatal mortality rates for the United States and Norway shown in this table are not very large in the very preterm infants (less than 26 weeks gestation) and in the term births (39 or more weeks gestation). However, the perinatal mortality rates for infants born between 27 and 38 weeks are strikingly lower for the United States as compared to Norway. The frequency of infants born in the United States at this gestational age range is about 25% higher than in Norway. The issue of the need to standardize comparisons based on cumulative gestational age distributions is similar to the argument used earlier in regard to cumulative birthweight distributions.

The perinatal mortality comparisons between single and multiple births are consistent for both the United States and Norway. Multiple births do not show much increased risks of perinatal deaths until after 32 weeks of gestation. This finding suggests that growth retardation as a result of multiple fetuses plays an increasing role as gestation advances beyond 32 weeks. At term gestational ages, multiple births are between four and five times more likely to die in the perinatal period compared to single deliveries. It should be pointed out, however, that if one member of a twin set dies *in utero*, birth does not usually occur until the surviving twin reaches full-term gestation. This effect will naturally tend to bias the perinatal mortality rates upward at term for multiple births.

Ante- and Intrapartum Fetal Deaths

A recent perinatal mortality survey in Scotland conducted by McIlwaine and colleagues (1979) has been able to distinguish the relative contributions made to perinatal mortality by preterm low-birthweight infants from that made by small-for-gestational-age births. As expected, when both of these categories are combined they contribute a substantial amount of all perinatal deaths. Out of 1012 single perinatal deaths occurring in Scotland during 1977, 265 were due to fetal abnormalities (140 cases with central nervous system malformations). Of the 747 normally formed infants, the largest single cause of death was classified as low birthweight for mothers who had no complications of pregnancy, a total of 302 cases (40%). Of these low-birthweight infants, 127 were preterm (42%) and 103 were small for gestational age (34%). When these preterm and growth-retarded infants were examined in relation to time of death (antepartum, intrapartum, or postpartum), a very significant finding emerged. Almost three-quarters of the preterm infants were born alive and died after birth. Conversely, approximately three-quarters of the growth-retarded infants died before the onset of labor (McIlwaine et al., 1979).

As infant and neonatal mortality rates have progressively declined over the past several decades, the contribution of low-birthweight infants to perinatal and infant mortality risk has correspondingly risen (Backer and Aagenaes, 1967; Alberman, 1974, 1977; Davies, 1980; Forbes et al., 1982). As a result, there is a need to repeat population-based research studies similar to that undertaken by McIlwaine and colleagues at frequent time intervals in order to elucidate these trends. Geographical studies (among states in developed countries, and between developed and developing countries) rely on the rates of very low birthweight deliveries and the relative proportions of preterm and growth-retarded infants as monitored through time for interpretation of results (Lee et al., 1980; Villar and Belizan, 1982). Trends in cause-specific perinatal mortality rates also contribute greatly to our understanding of declining perinatal mortality, but as a result of the limitations in the quality of such data, there are very few illustrative studies (Edouard and Alberman, 1980; Forbes et al., 1982).

In addition to the usual definition of fetal growth retardation which relies on the 10th percentile of birthweight for gestational age, a number of researchers have pointed out a group of high-risk infants who are in the normal weight range, above 2500 g, at birth (Clifford et al., 1953; Gruenwald, 1969; Miller and Hassanein, 1971; Daikoku et al., 1979; Bakketeig and Hoffman, 1984). The interest of these authors has been in collecting and analyzing the infants ponderal index, or crown–heel length, in relation to birthweight.

514

Table 21-9. Birthweight-Specific Fetal Deaths in Norway, 1967–73

Birthweight (g)	Deaths during labor	Total fetal deaths	Percent occurring during labor
–999	165	1800	9.2
1000–1499	57	792	7.2
1500–1999	84	676	12.4
2000–2499	88	637	13.8
2500–2999	134	696	19.3
3000–3499	156	655	23.8
3500–3999	119	405	29.4
4000–4499	54	144	37.5
4500+	22	73	30.1
Not stated	12	192	62.5
Total	891	6070	14.7

Data from Bakketeig et at. (1977).

An analysis of birthweight-specific intrapartum fetal deaths is given in Table 21-9. The data of McIlwaine et al. on low birthweight and perinatal deaths did not emphasize findings with regard to fetal deaths occurring during labor. From this table, it is clear that intrapartum fetal deaths are more common among heavier births. Although the overall proportion of intrapartum fetal deaths in Norway during these seven years was 15%, the proportion corresponding to births weighing in excess of 3500 g was 31%. In contrast, the proportion of intrapartum fetal deaths of births weighing less than 2500 g was only 10%. Further analyses of these data indicate that much of the excess intrapartum risk among the heavy births is attributable to those infants who are "light-for-length," i.e. their birthweights were relatively small in comparison to their length (Hoffman and Bakketeig, 1984).

Crown–Heel Length of the Newborn

The increased perinatal mortality rates for U.S. blacks compared to U.S. whites, and also for U.S. whites compared to Norwegians, for births weighing in excess of 3500 g may be attributable to a diminished capacity for support of continued fetal growth *in utero* during the last trimester of pregnancy. Gruenwald (1969) has summarized the issue succinctly:

It is apparent that about the time that the human neonate ceases to be in danger by prematurity, its liability to damage from abnormally low growth support *in utero* increases. While the mortality rate declines at this time, the *number* of infants born late in gestation is so much larger that the number of deaths is greater...This is less obvious but needs investigation just as badly as do the causes of pre-term birth.

Unlike the fetal weight, which increases very rapidly during the third trimester of pregnancy, the crown–heel length increases at a relatively more rapid pace during the first and second trimesters. Thus, at 20 weeks gestational age, the fetus already has attained approximately 50% of the expected length at term, but the weight of the fetus is only about 12% of that expected at term (Villar and Belizan, 1982). The ponderal index of the newborn, defined by Rhorer's Index = [birthweight $\{g\}$/(crown–heel length $\{cm\})^3$] $\times$ 100, is a good indicator of the infant's nutritional status at birth (Burke et al., 1943; Naeye, 1965; Miller and Hassanein, 1971; Daikoku et al., 1979; Walther and Raemaekers, 1982).

Although a number of articles have shown norms for crown–heel length at given gestational ages (Lubchenco et al., 1966; Usher and McLean, 1969; Bjerkedal and Skjaerven, 1980), there has been very little information available for the joint bivariate distribution of crown–heel length and birthweight. In Fig. 21-7, three different bivariate distributions are shown using contour diagrams. Each of these bivariate distributions is ellipsoidal, particularly for the two innermost contour levels. These ellipsoids indicate that the data are well represented by a bivariate Gaussian, or "normal," distribution. The U.S. data were collected through the Collaborative Perinatal Study (Niswander and Gordon, 1972). The Norwegian data have been routinely available since 1967 as a result of the Medical Birth Registry. The fact that the innermost contour level for U.S. black births is inscribed inside that for U.S. white births, which in turn is inscribed inside that of the Norwegian births, fits well with the hypothesis of fetal constraint *in utero* (Ounsted, 1965; Gruenwald, 1969; Kaltreider and Johnson, 1976; Bakketeig et al., 1979, 1983; Tejani, 1982).

The contours for crown-heel length and birthweight distributions differ in an important respect from those published earlier for bivariate gestational age and birthweight distributions. In the latter instance, two bulges were present in the contour diagrams beyond 39 weeks of gestation. One bulge corresponded to infants who were heavy but born at term, whereas the other bulge corresponded to infants born past term but with average birthweights. The validity of reported LMP dates used to calculate gestational age has been questioned recently by obstetricians who have used ultrasound

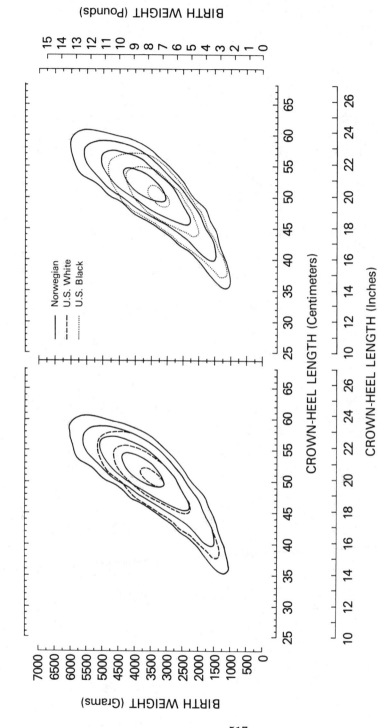

Fig. 21-7. Contour levels of the joint birth weight and crown–heel length bivariate distributions for Norwegian (solid lines) and United States White singleton births (dashed lines) in the left-hand panel, and also for Norwegian and United States Black singleton births (dotted lines) in the right-hand panel. The Norwegian data represent all births from the Medical Birth Registry for the years 1967 through 1973 (Bakketeig and Hoffman, 1979), and the United States data represent information collected through the National Collaborative Perinatal Study (Niswander and Gordon, 1972).

517

determinations to date the progress of pregnancy (Eik-Nes et al., 1983). This issue will be debated for some time as more extensive ultrasound data become available for study. It suffices here to note that the joint distribution of crown–heel length and birthweight does not have any similarly irregular features. There is only a slight curvature in the structural "ridge" regression which is accounted for by the tendency of crown–heel length to increase more rapidly than birthweight in the second trimester, and the reverse during the third trimester of pregnancy.

Perinatal mortality rates in relation to the joint bivariate crown–heel length and birthweight distribution are shown in Table 21-10. These rates have been calculated from records on seven years of Norwegian births, 1967–73. Below 2000 g the influence of birthweight appears to dominate that of crown–heel length in altering these rates. However, infants who have appropriate crown–heel length for birth-

Table 21-10. Perinatal Mortality Rates in Norway by Crown–Heel Length and Birthweight, 1967–73

Birthweight (g)	≤30	31–36	37–40	41–44	45–46	47–48	49–50	51–52	53–54	55–56	57–58	59–60
5501–6000									0	26	42	125
5001–5500								0	0	10	37	53
4501–5000							0	2	3	5	39	211
4001–4500						62	3	2	3	11	64	
3501–4000					45	8	2	3	6	44	214	
3001–3500				286	54	3	8	8	43	252		
2501–3000			300	195	18	12	19	79	349			
2001–2500		539	630	96	60	83	235	457				
1501–2000		684	446	229	330	562	950					
1001–1500	917	755	591	646	840	750						
501–1000	984	934	922	929								
≤500	1000	1000										

Crown–Heel Length (cm)

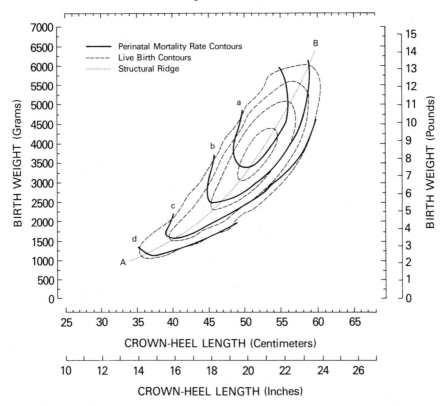

Fig. 21-8. Contour levels of perinatal mortality rates (solid lines, labeled "a" through "d") for Norwegian singleton births, 1967 through 1973. The dotted line, labeled A—B, represents the "structural" ridge regression for singleton births in relation to the joint birth weight and crown-heel length distribution (dashed lines) for singleton births. The perinatal mortality rates increase as one moves from the innermost contour level "a" to the outermost level "d." The actual perinatal mortality rates which were used in constructing the smoothed contour levels are provided in Table 21-10. For example, the outermost contour level "d" corresponds to a perinatal mortality rate of approximately 600 deaths per 1,000 singleton births, whereas the innermost level "a" is equivalent to a rate of approximately 6 perinatal deaths per 1,000 singleton births.

weight fare decidedly better if their weight is above 1000 g. In the range from 2000 to 3500 g, both birthweight and crown–heel length have a major influence on perinatal mortality, with those infants who are "appropriate" for both measurements having the best outcomes.

The ponderal index of newborns is the major determinant of perinatal mortality risk above 3500 g. Thus, an infant who weighs

4000 g and has a length of 55 or more centimeters is at a much greater risk of perinatal death in comparison to infants of similar length but weighing between 4500 and 5000 g. An examination of the two components of perinatal mortality separately reveals that the increased risk is mostly in late fetal deaths, not in early neonatal deaths. The identification of these fetuses before delivery should lead to improved obstetric management and to reductions in the perinatal mortality rates.

Figure 21-8 is a composite drawing which has superimposed contour levels for the perinatal mortality rates (solid lines) on top of contour levels for the bivariate distributions of births (dashed lines). In addition, a structural ridge regression line (labeled A–B) indicates the modal frequencies of births as a function of joint crown–heel length and birthweight. The perinatal mortality contour levels are based on the information provided in Table 21-10. The innermost contour level corresponds to the least risk of perinatal death. All births occurring on a given contour level have the same level of risk. The levels of perinatal mortality risk increase in directions orthogonal to the contour levels (or from the innermost to the outermost contour levels). This figure greatly simplifies the task of assigning the risk of perinatal mortality to any specific combination of crown–heel length and birthweight.

This figure is similar to earlier published bivariate contour diagrams for fetal mortality by Hoffman et al. (1974, 1977) and for neonatal mortality by Goldstein and Peckham (1976). These earlier contour diagrams indicated that birthweight was a much more important variable in predicting fetal and neonatal viability than was gestational age. The present contour diagrams are more informative because the value of the crown–heel length measurement is clearly indicated.

CONCLUSIONS

In 1978, Bakketeig et al. demonstrated that the association between available perinatal services and perinatal survival was stronger for births with average to above average weights than for low-weight infants. They emphasized that when monitoring the possible effects of improvements in care, one should not merely concentrate on the outcome among low-weight infants. It may well be that measures of outcome among births of normal weight are just as sensitive and important indicators of the improvement in social and medical conditions.

In a recent study in Norway (Larssen et al., 1981, 1982), a perinatal audit showed that 30% of all perinatal deaths were considered possibly avoidable. A considerable portion of these deaths occurred before the onset of labor. Many of them were of relatively low weight, but a large number were of average size or greater. It is reasonable to think that further reductions in perinatal mortality will derive from the elimination of many of these average-size intrauterine deaths. Evidence for such developments can be found in the comparison of birthweight specific perinatal mortality rates between countries such as Norway and Sweden. The perinatal mortality rate was 27% higher in Norway compared to Sweden in 1980 (10.8 versus 8.5 per 1000 births). If these mortality differences are closely examined, it becomes apparent that the perinatal mortality is more than 50% higher for average-size births (weighing 3000 g or more) in Norway. Moreover, the major difference in perinatal mortality rates between these two countries stems from differences in the fetal mortality rate for average-size births (NOMESCO, 1982). An attempt to apply the Norwegian perinatal audit classification to Swedish perinatal deaths has indicated that as the level of mortality is further reduced the average size fetal deaths tend to disappear (Bakketeig, 1983).

Some impact on declining perinatal mortality rates will continue to derive from reductions in the relative proportion of infants born prematurely. Efforts are underway to identify mothers at high risk of preterm delivery, and programs for intervention are under evaluation (Papiernik-Berkhauer et al., 1969, 1974, 1979; Creasy et al, 1980; Herron et al., 1981). Using North Carolina data from 1968 through 1977, David and Siegel (1982) have shown a 19% reduction in the low-birthweight rate. Also, consistent with the data presented in this chapter, they have demonstrated a considerable improvement in the birthweight-specific mortality rates. To determine the relative contributions made by these two factors to the decline in neonatal mortality rates during this decade, they calculated that approximately one-third of the decline was attributable to an improvement in the birthweight and gestational age characteristics of the newborn population. However, the shift toward "better babies" was more evident in the early part of the decade and among the white population.

The recently increased use of birthweight and gestational-age-specific mortality rates resulted from the availability of this information from hospital and population-based birth registries in the 1960s and 70s. Other accessible quantitative data should also be assessed and, if appropriate, utilized for the identification of fetuses and newborns at high risk. Two such indices are crown–heel length and head circumference of the newborn. Additional qualitative indicators have been suggested (Dennis and Chalmers, 1982) but their usefulness remains to be established. However, as the current low perinatal mortality rates in developed countries continue to drop, more sensitive endpoints—which will probably be more difficult to acquire—will force their way into perinatal surveillance and epidemiology.

REFERENCES

Alberman, E. (1974). Stillbirths and neonatal mortality in England and Wales by birthweight 1953–71. *Health Trends 6*, 14–17.

────── (1977). Facts and figures. In *Benefits and hazards of the new obstetrics. Clinics in Developmental Medicine, No. 64*, edited by T. Chard and M. Richards, Spastics International Medical Publications. London: Heinemann, pp. 1–33.

────── (1980). Prospects for better perinatal health. *Lancet i*, 189–192.

Amneus, G. (1900). Population. In *Norway, official publication for the Paris exhibition 1900*, edited by S. Konow and K. Fischer. Kristiania, Norway: Aktie-Bogtrykkeriet, pp. 85–126.

Armstrong, R.J. (1972). *A study of infant mortality from linked records by birthweight, period of gestation and other variables, United States, 1960 live-birth cohort*. National Center for Health Statistics, Vital and Health Statistics, Data from the National Vital Statistics System, Series 20, No. 12, U.S. DHEW Publ. No. (HSM) 72-1055, Rockville, Maryland, 90 pp.

Backer, J.E. (1947). Population statistics and population registration in Norway. Part 1. The vital statistics of Norway, an historical review. *Popul. Studies 1*, 212–226.

────── (1948). Population statistics and population registration in Norway. Part 2. Health and recruitment statistics. *Popul. Studies 2*, 318–338.

────── and Aagenaes, Ø. (1967). *Infant Mortality Problems in Norway*. National Center for Health Statistics, Vital and Health Statistics, Analytical Studies, Series 3, No. 8, U.S. DHEW Publ. No (PHS) 1000, Washington, D.C., 40 pp.

Baird, D., Thomson, A.M., and Duncan, E.H.L. (1953). The causes and prevention of stillbirths and first week deaths. *J. Obstet. Gynaecol. Br. Emp. 60*, 17–30.

────── (1975). The interplay of changes in society, reproductive habits, and obstetric practice in Scotland between 1922 and 1972. *Br. J. Prev. Soc. Med. 29*, 135–146.

Bakketeig, L.S., Hoffman, H.J., and Sternthal, P.M. (1978). Obstetric service and perinatal mortality in Norway. *Acta Obstet. Gynecol. Scand., Suppl. 77*, 1–19.

────── and ────── (1979). Perinatal mortality by birth order within cohorts based on sibship size. *Br. Med. J. ii*, 693–696.

──────, ──────, and Harley, E.E. (1979). The tendency to repeat gestational age and birth weight in successive births. *Am. J. Obstet. Gynecol. 135*, 1086–1103.

────── and ────── (1980). Interpreting survey data. In *Perinatal audit and surveillance*, edited by I. Chalmers and G. McIlwaine, Royal College of Obstetricians and Gynaecologists, London, pp. 249–262.

—— and —— (1981). Epidemiology of preterm birth: results from a longitudinal study of births in Norway. In *Preterm labor*, edited by M.G. Elder and C.H. Hendricks, Butterworths International Medical Reviews (Obstetrics and Gynecology 1), London, pp. 17–46.

—— and —— (1984). The tendency to repeat gestational age and birth weight in successive births, related to perinatal survival. *Acta Obstet. Gynecol. Scand.* (In press).

——, ——, and Oakley, A.T. (1984). The epidemiology of perinatal mortality. In *Perinatal epidemiology*, edited by M.B. Bracken. New York: Oxford University Press (this volume, Chap. 6).

——, Bjerkedal, T., and Hoffman, H.J. (1984). Small-for-gestational age births in successive pregnancy outcomes: results from a longitudinal study of births in Norway. *Early Hum. Develop.* (In press).

—— (1983). Personal communication. Department of Community Medicine, University of Trondheim, Norway.

Battaglia, F.C. and Lubchenco, L.O. (1967). A practical classification of newborn infants by weight and gestational age. *J. Pediat. 71*, 159–163.

Baumgartner, L. and Erhardt, C. (1953). Some observations on the factors in the incidence of prematurity and fetal death. In *Pregnancy wastage*, edited by E.T. Engle. Springfield, Ill.: C.C. Thomas, pp. 146–174.

Bjerkedal, T., Bakketeig, L.S., and Lehmann, E.H. (1973). Percentiles of birth weights of single, live births at different gestation periods. Bases on 125,485 births in Norway, 1967 and 1968. *Acta Paediat. Scand. 62*, 449–457.

—— and —— (1975). *Medical registration of births in Norway during the 5-year period, 1967–71.* Institute of Hygiene and Social medicine, University of Bergen, Bergen, Norway.

—— and Skjaerven, R. (1980). Percentiles of birth weight and crown–heel length in relation to gestation period for single live births. *T. Norske Laegeforen 100*, 1088–1091.

—— (1983). Personal communication. Medical Birth Registry of Norway, Oslo, Norway.

Bowes, W.A. Jr. (1981). A review of perinatal mortality in Colorado, 1971 to 1978, and its relationship to the regionalization of perinatal services. *Am. J. Obstet. Gynecol. 141*, 1045–1052.

Burke, B.S., Harding, V.V., and Stuart, H.C. (1943) Nutrition studies during pregnancy. IV. Relation of protein content of mother's diet during pregnancy to birth length, birth weight and condition of infant at birth. *J. Pediat. 23*, 506–515.

Burnham, D. (1982). Personal communication. Mortality Statistics Branch, National Center for Health Statistics, Hyattsville, Maryland.

Central Bureau of Statistics of Norway (1978). *Historical statistics, 1978.* Oslo, Norway.

Chalmers, I. (1979). Better perinatal health: the search for indices. *Lancet 2*, 1063–1065.

Chamberlain, R., Chamberlain, G., Howlett, B., and Claireaux, A. (1975). *British Births 1970. I. The First Week of Life.* London: Heinemann.

Chase, H.C. (1967). *International comparison of perinatal and infant mortality: the United States and six West European countries.* National Center for Health Statistics, Vital and Health Statistics, Analytical Studies, Series 3, No. 6, U.S. DHEW Publ. No. (PHS) 1000, Washington, D.C., 97 pp.

——— (1972). *A study of infant mortality from linked records: comparison of neonatal mortality from two cohort studies: United States, January-March 1950 and 1960*. National Center for Health Statistics, Vital and Health Statistics, Data from the National Vital Statistics System, Series 20, No. 13, U.S. DHEW Publ. No. (HSM) 72-1056, Rockville, Maryland, 99 pp.

——— (1974). Perinatal mortality, overview and current trends. *Clin. Perinatol. 1*, 3–17.

——— (1977). Time trends in low birthweight in the United States, 1950–1974. In *Epidemiology of prematurity*, edited by D.M. Reed and F.J. Stanley. Baltimore: Urban & Schwarzenberg, pp. 17–37.

Clifford, S.H., Reid, D.E., and Worchester, J. (1953). Indices of fetal maturity. In *Pregnancy wastage*, edited by E.T. Engle. Springfield, Ill.: C.C. Thomas, pp. 208–221.

Creasy, R.K., Gummer, B.A., and Liggins, G.C. (1980). System for predicting spontaneous preterm birth. *Obstet. Gynecol. 55*, 692–695.

Daikoku, N., Johnson, J., Graf, C., Kearney, K., Tyson, J.E., and King, T.M. (1979). Patterns of intrauterine growth retardation. *Obstet. Gynecol. 54*, 211–219.

David, R.J. and Siegel, E. (1983). Decline in neonatal mortality, 1968 to 1977: better babies or better care? *Pediatrics 71*, 531–540.

Davies, P.A. (1980). Perinatal mortality. *Arch. Dis. Child. 55*, 833–837.

Dennis, J. and Chalmers, I. (1982). Very early neonatal seizure rate: a possible epidemiological indicator of the quality of perinatal care. *Br. J. Obstet. Gynaecol. 89*, 418–426.

Derry, T.K. (1957). *A short history of Norway*. London: George Allen & Unwin, 281 pp.

Dowding, V. (1981). New assessment of the effects of birth order and socio-economic status on birthweight. *Br. Med. J. 281*, 683–688.

Drake, M. (1969). *Population and society in Norway 1735–1865*. The University Press, Cambridge, 255 pp.

——— (1972). Fertility controls in pre-industrial Norway. In *Population and social change*, edited by D.V. Glass and R. Revelle. London: Arnold, E. & Co., pp. 185–198.

Dunn, P.M. (1979). Perinatal terminology, definitions and statistics. In *Perinatal Medicine, Sixth European Congress, Vienna*, edited by O. Thalhammer, K. Baumgarten, and A. Pollak. Stuttgart: Georg Thieme, pp. 1–19.

Edouard, L. and Alberman, E. (1980). National trends in the certified causes of perinatal mortality, 1968 to 1978. *Brit. J. Obstet. Gynaecol. 87*, 833–838.

Eisner, V., Pratt, M.W., Hexter, A., Chabot, M.J., and Sayal, N. (1978). Improvement in infant and perinatal mortality in the United States 1965–1973. I. Priorities for intervention. *Am. J. Public Health 68*, 359–364.

Eik-Nes, S.H., Persson, P.-H., and Grøttum, P. (1983). Revaluation of standards for human fetal growth. *Br. Med. J.* (In press).

Erhardt, C.L., Joshi, G.B., Nelson, F.G., Kroll, B.H., and Weiner, L. (1964).

Influence of weight and gestation on perinatal and neonatal mortality by ethnic group. *Am. J. Public Health 54*, 1841–1855.

Erickson, J.D. and Bjerkedal, T. (1982). Fetal and infant mortality in Norway and the United States. *J.A.M.A. 247*, 987–991.

Ericson, A., Eriksson, M., and Zetterstrom, R. (1979). Analysis of perinatal mortality rate in the Stockholm area. *Acta Paediat. Scand. Suppl. 275*, 35–40.

Erkkola, R., Kero, P., Seppala, A., Gronroos, M., and Rauramo, L. (1982). Monitoring perinatal mortality by birth weight specific mortality rates. *Int. J. Gynaecol. Obstet. 20*, 231–235.

Falk, G. and Wranne, L. (1973). Perinatal mortality in Orebro County. *Lakartid. 70*, 2539–2541.

Fedrick, J. and Anderson, A.B.M. (1976). Factors associated with spontaneous pre-term birth. *Br. J. Obstet. Gynaecol. 83*, 342–350.

Feldstein, M.S. (1966). A binary variable multiple regression method of analyzing factors affecting perinatal mortality and other outcomes of pregnancy. *J. Roy. Statist. Soc., Series A 129*, 61–73.

Fleiss, J.L. (1973). *Statistical methods for rates and proportions*. New York: Wiley.

Forbes, J.F., Boddy, F.A., Pickering, R., and Wyllie, M.M (1982). Perinatal mortality in Scotland: 1970–9. *J. Epidemiol. Commun. Health 36*, 282–288.

Fryer, J.G., Harding, R.A., Ashford, J.R., and Karlberg, P. (1977). Some indicators of maturity. In *Fundamentals of mortality risks during the perinatal period and infancy. Illustrations by a comparative study between Goteborg and Palermo.* Monographs in Paediatrics, Vol. 9, edited by F. Falkner. Basel: S. Karger, Switzerland, pp. 33–65.

Ghosh, S. and Daga, S. (1967). Comparison of gestational age and weight as standards of prematurity. *J. Pediat. 71*, 173–175.

Gille, H. (1949). The demographic history of the northern European countries in the eighteenth century. *Popul. Studies 3*, 3–65.

Goldstein, H. and Peckham, C. (1976) Birthweight, gestation, neonatal mortality and child development. In *The Biology of human fetal growth*, edited by D.F. Roberts and A.M. Thomson. London: Taylor & Francis, pp. 81–102.

Gruenwald, P. (1966). Growth of the human fetus. I. Normal growth and its variation. *Am. J. Obstet. Gynecol. 94*, 1112–1119.

——— (1966). Growth of the human fetus. II. Abnormal growth in twins and infants of mothers with diabetes, hypertension, or isoimmunization. *Am. J. Obstet. Gynecol. 94*, 1120–1132.

——— (1968). Fetal growth as an indicator of socio-economic change. *Public Health Reports 83*, 867–872.

——— (1969). Growth and maturation of the foetus and its relationship to perinatal mortality. In *Perinatal problems—the second report of the 1958 British perinatal mortality survey*, edited by N.R. Butler and E.D. Alberman. Edinburgh: E. & S. Livingstone, pp. 141–162.

Guyer, B., Wallach, L.A., and Rosen, S.L (1982). Birthweight-standardized neonatal mortality rates and the prevention of low birth weight: how does Massachusetts compare with Sweden? *N. Engl. J. Med. 306*, 1230–1233.

Hammes, L.M. and Treloar, A.E. (1970). Gestational interval from vital records. *Am. J. Public Health 60*, 1496–1505.

Herron, M.A., Katz, M., and Creasy, R.K. (1982). Evaluation of a preterm birth prevention program: Preliminary report. *Obstet. Gynecol. 59*, 452–456.

Hoffman, H.J., Stark, C.R., Lundin, F.E. Jr., and Ashbook, J.D. (1974). Analysis of birth weight, gestational age, fetal viability, U.S. births, 1968. *Obstet. Gynecol. Survey 29*, 651–681.

———, Lundin, F.E. Jr., Bakketeig, L.S., and Harley, E.E. (1977). Classification of births by weight and gestational age for future studies of prematurity. In *The epidemiology of prematurity*, edited by D.M. Reed and F.J. Stanley. Baltimore: Urban & Schwarzenberg, pp. 297–333.

———, Bakketeig, L.S., and Stark, C.R. (1978). Twins and perinatal mortality: A comparison between single and twin births in Minnesota and in Norway, 1967–1973. In *Twin research (Part B): Biology and epidemiology*, edited by W.E. Nance, G. Allen and P. Parisi. New York: Alan R. Liss, pp. 133–142.

——— and ——— (1984). Fetal and perinatal mortality comparisons between the United States and Norway. *Int. J. Gynecol. Obstet.* (In press).

Hofsten, E. and Lundström, H. (1976). *Swedish Population History. Main Trends from 1750 to 1970*. National Central Bureau of Statistics, Norstedts Tryckeri, Stockholm, Sweden, 186 pp.

Illsley, R. (1955). Social class selection and class differences in relation to stillbirths and infant deaths. *Br. Med. J. 2*, 1520–1524.

Kaltreider, D.F. and Johnson, J.W.C. (1976). Patients at high risk for low-birth-weight delivery. *Am. J. Obstet. Gynecol. 124*, 251–256.

Karlberg, P. and Priolisi, A. (1977). Clinical evaluation of similarities and dissimilarities between two city surveys. In *Fundamentals of mortality risks during the perinatal period and infancy. Illustrations by a comparative study between Goteborg and Palermo*. Monographs in Paediatrics, Vol. 9, edited by F. Falkner. Basel: S. Karger, pp. 165–192.

——— and Ericson, A. (1979). Perinatal mortality in Sweden. Analyses with international aspects. *Acta Paediat. Scand. Suppl. 275*, 28–34.

——— (1980). Medical Birth Registration in Sweden. In *Perinatal Audit and Surveillance*, edited by I. Chalmers and G. McIlwaine. London: Royal College of Obstetricians and Gynaecologists, pp. 221–227.

Kleinman, J.C., Kovar, M.G., Feldman, J.J., and Young, C.A (1978). A comparison of 1960 and 1973–1974 early neonatal mortality in selected states. *Am. J. Epidemiol. 108*, 454–469.

Larssen, K.E., Bakketeig, L.S., Bergsjø, P., and Finne, P.H. (1981). *Perinatal Service in Norway During the 1970's*. Norwegian Institute for Hospital Research (Report 6/81), Trondheim, Norway.

———, ———, ———, ———, Laurini, R., Knoff, H., Holt, J., Vogt, H., and Hapnes, C. (1982). *Perinatal Audit in Norway 1980*. Norwegian Institute for Hospital Research (Report 7/82), Trondheim, Norway.

Lee, K.-S., Tseng, P.I., Eidelman, A.I., Kandall, S.R., and Gartner, L.M. (1976). Determinants of the neonatal mortality. *Am. J. Dis. Child. 130*, 842–845.

————, Paneth, N., Gartner, L.M., Pearlman, M.A., and Gruss, L. (1980). Neonatal mortality: an analysis of the recent improvement in the United States. *Am. J. Public Health 70*, 15–21.

————, ————, ————, and ———— (1980). The very low birthweight rate: principal predictor of neonatal mortality in industrialized populations. *J. Pediat. 97*, 759–764.

Lithell, U.-B. (1981). Infant mortality rate and standards of living in the past. *Scand. J. History 6*, 297–315.

Lubchenco, L.O., Hansman, C., Dressler, M., and Boyd, E. (1963). Intrauterine growth as estimated from liveborn birth-weight data at 24 to 42 weeks of gestation. *Pediatrics 32*, 793–800.

————, ————, and Boyd, E. (1966). Intrauterine growth in length and head circumference as estimated from live births at gestational ages from 26 to 42 weeks. *Pediatrics 37*, 403–408.

————, Searls, D.T., and Brazie, J.V. (1972). Neonatal mortality rate: Relationship to birth-weight and gestational age. *J. Pediat. 81*, 814–822.

Macfarlane, A.J., Chalmers, I., and Adelstein, A.M. (1980). The role of standardization in the interpretation of perinatal mortality rates. *Health Trends 12*, 45–50.

———— and ———— (1981). Problems in the interpretation of perinatal mortality statistics. In *Recent Advances in Paediatrics 6*, edited by D. Hull. Edinburgh: Churchill Livingstone.

MacMahon, B., Kovar, M.G., and Feldman, J.J. (1972). *Infant mortality rates: Socioeconomic factors.* National Center for Health Statistics, Vital and Health Statistics, Data from the National Vital Statistics System, Series 22, No. 14, U.S. DHEW Publ. No. (HSM) 72-1045, Rockville, Maryland, 68 pp.

Manciaux, M. (1976). Perinatal morbidity and mortality in Council of Europe member states and Finland. In *Fifth European Congress of Perinatal Medicine, Upsala*, edited by G. Rooth and L.-E. Bratteby. Stockholm: Almqvist & Wiksell International, pp. 18–25.

McIlwaine, G.M., Howat, R.C.L., Dunn, F., and Macnaughton, M.C. (1979). The Scottish perinatal mortality survey. *Br. Med. J. 2*, 1103–1106.

Meirik, O. (1983). Declining perinatal mortality in Sweden 1973–80. Where are the gains? *Lakartid.* (In press).

Miller, H.C. and Hassanein, K. (1971). Diagnosis of impaired fetal growth in newborn infants. *Pediatrics 48*, 511–522.

———— and Merritt, T.A. (1979). *Fetal Growth in Humans.* Chicago: Year Book Medical Publishers, 180 pp.

———— (1981). Intrauterine growth retardation—An unmet challenge. (Abraham Jacobi Lecture). *Am. J. Dis. Child. 135*, 944–948.

Mitchell, B.R. (1975). *European Historical Statistics.* London: MacMillan.

Mosteller, F. and Tukey, J.W. (1977). *Data Analysis and Regression: A Second Course in Statistics.* Reading, Mass.: Addison-Wesley.

Naeye, R.L. (1965). Malnutrition, probable cause of fetal growth retardation. *Arch. Pathol. 79*, 284–291.

National Board of Health & Welfare (1973). *Organization of Obstetric Care.* Stockholm: AB Allmanna Forlaget, 195 pp.

National Central Bureau of Statistics (1969). *Historical Statistics of Sweden. Part 1. Population, Second Edition, 1720–1967.* Stockholm: K.L. Beckmans Tryckerier AB, 144 pp.

―――― (1983). *Medical Birth Registration in 1979 and 1980.* Stockholm: Statistical Reports (HS 1983:5), Liber, 64 pp.

Niswander, K.R. and Gordon, M. (1972). *The Women and their Pregnancies. The Collaborative Perinatal Study of the National Institute of Neurological Diseases and Stroke.* Philadelphia: W.B. Saunders.

Nomesco (1982). *Births in the Nordic Countries. Registration of the Outcome of Pregnancy 1979.* Reykjavik, Iceland.

Nordic Council (1981). *Yearbook of Nordic Statistics, 1980, Vol. 19.* Stockholm: Nordic Statistical Secretariat, Norstedts Tryckeri.

North, A.F. and Macdonald, H.M. (1977). Why are neonatal mortality rates lower in small black infants than in infants in similar birthweight? *J. Pediat. 90,* 809–810.

Ofstad, K. (1949). Population statistics and population registration in Norway. Part 3. Population censuses. *Popul. Studies 3,* 66–75.

Ounsted, M. (1965). Maternal constraint of foetal growth in man. *Develop. Med. Child Neurol. 7,* 479–490.

―――― (1969). Familial factors affecting fetal growth. In *Perinatal Factors Affecting Human Development.* Pan American Health Organization, Scientific Publication 185, pp. 60–67.

Paneth, N. (1982). Infant mortality reexamined—Editorial. *J.A.M.A. 247,* 1027–1028.

――――, Kiely, J.L., Wallenstein, S., Marcus, M., Pakter, J., and Susser, M. (1982). Newborn intensive care and neonatal mortality in low-birthweight infants—A population study. *N. Engl. J. Med. 307,* 149–155.

Papiernik-Berkhauer, E. (1969). Coefficient of risk for premature labor. *Presse Méd. 77,* 793–794.

―――― and Kaminski, M. (1974). Multifactorial study of the risk of prematurity at 32 weeks of gestation. I. A study of the frequency of 30 predictive characteristics. *J. Perinat. Med. 2,* 30–36.

―――― (1979). Development of risk during pregnancy. In *Perinatal Medicine, Sixth European Congress, Vienna,* edited by O. Thalhammer, K. Baumgarten and A. Pollak. Stuttgart: Georg Thieme, pp. 118–125.

Pharoah, P.O.D. and Alberman, E.D. (1981). Mortality of low birthweight infants in England and Wales 1953 to 1979. *Arch. Dis. Child. 56,* 86–89.

Phibbs, C.S., Williams, R.L., and Phibbs, R.H. (1981). Newborn risk factors and the costs of neonatal intensive care. *Pediatrics 68,* 313–321.

Philip, A.G.S., Little, G.A., Polivy, D.R., and Lucey, J.F. (1981). Neonatal mortality risk for the eighties: the importance of birth weight/gestational age groups. *Pediatrics 68,* 122–130.

Rantakallio, P. (1969). Groups at risk in low birth weight infants and perinatal mortality. *Acta Paediatr. Scand. Suppl. 193,* 1–71.

Rooth, G. (1979). Better Perinatal Health: Sweden. *Lancet 2,* 1170–1172.

―――― (1980). Dogma disputed: Low birthweight revised. *Lancet 1,* 639–641.

Rush, R.W., Keirse, M.J.N.C., Howat, P., Baum, J.D., Anderson, A.B.M., and Turnbull, A.C. (1976). Contributions of preterm delivery to perinatal mortality. *Br. Med. J. 2*, 965–968.

Shapiro, S. (1982). Decline in perinatal mortality—letter to the editor. *N. Engl. J. Med. 306*, 62–63.

Tanner, J.M. and Thomson, A.M. (1970). Standards for birth weight at gestation periods of 32 to 42 weeks allowing for maternal height and weight. *Arch. Dis. Child. 45*, 566–569.

Tejani, N.A. (1982). Recurrence of intrauterine growth retardation. *Obstet. Gynecol. 59*, 329–331.

Terrin, M. and Meyer, M.B. (1981). Birth weight-specific rates as a bias in the effects of smoking and other perinatal hazards. *Obstet. Gynecol. 58*, 636–638.

Tomasson, R.F. (1977). A millennium of misery: the demography of the Icelanders. *Popul. Studies 31*, 405–427.

Treloar, A.E., Behn, B.G., and Cowan, D.W. (1967). Analysis of gestational interval from vital records. *Am. J. Obstet. Gynecol. 99*, 34–35.

United Nations (1981). *Demographic yearbook, 1980.* New York: Department of Economic and Social Affairs, Statistical Office.

U.S. Department of Health and Human Services (1981). *Vital statistics of the United States, 1977. Vol. I—Natality, and Vol. II—Mortality, Part A.* Washington, D.C.: U.S. Government Printing Office, DHHS Publ. Nos. (PHS) 81-1101/3.

U.S. Bureau of the Census (1960). *Historical statistics of the United States, colonial times to 1957.* Washington, D.C.: U.S. Government Printing Office.

Usher, R. and Mclean, F. (1969). Intrauterine growth of live-born Caucasian infants at sea level: standards obtained from measurements in 7 dimensions of infants born between 25 and 44 weeks of gestation. *J. Pediat. 74*, 901–910.

Van den Berg, B.J. and Yerushalmy, J. (1966). The relationship of the rate of intrauterine growth of infants of low birthweight to mortality, morbidity and congenital anomalies. *J. Pediat. 69*, 531–545.

Villar, J. and Belizan, J.M. (1982). The relative contribution of prematurity and fetal growth retardation to low birth weight in developing and developed societies. *Am. J. Obstet. Gynecol. 143*, 793–798.

—— and —— (1982). The timing factor in the pathophysiology of the intrauterine growth retardation syndrome. *Obstet. Gynecol. Survey 37*, 499–506.

Wallace, H.M., Goldstein. H., and Ericson. A (1982). Comparison of infant mortality in the United States and Sweden. *Clin. Pediat. 21*, 156–162.

Walther, F.J. and Raemaekers, L.H.J. (1982). The ponderal index as a measure of the nutritional status at birth and its relation to some aspects of neonatal morbidity. *J. Perinat. Med. 10*, 42–47.

Weatherall, J.A.C. (1975). Infant mortality: international differences. *Popul. Trends 1*, 9–12.

Wegman, M.E. (1974). Annual summary of vital statistics—1973. *Pediatrics 54*, 677–681.

Wilcox, A.J. (1981). Birth weight, gestation, and the fetal growth curve. *Am. J. Obstet. Gynecol. 139*, 863–867.

Williams, R.L. and Chen, P.M. (1982). Identifying the sources of the recent decline in perinatal mortality rates in California. *N. Engl. J. Med. 306*, 207–214.

———, Cunningham, G.C., and Norris, F.D. (1982). Fetal growth and perinatal viability in California. *Obstet. Gynecol. 59*, 624–632.

World Health Organization (1977). Recommended definitions, terminology and format for statistical tables related to the perinatal period and use of a new certificate for cause of perinatal deaths. *Acta Obstet. Gynecol. Scand. 56*, 247–253.

——— (1978). *Social and biological effects on perinatal mortality. Volumes 1 and 2. Report on an international comparative study.* Statistical Publishing House, Budapest, Hungary.

Yerushalmy, J., Van den Berg, B.J., Erhardt, C.L., and Jacobziner, H. (1965). Birth weight and gestation as indices of "immaturity." *Am. J. Dis. Child. 109*, 43–57.

——— (1967). The classification of newborn infants by birth weight and gestational age. *J. Pediat. 71*, 164–172.

Index

Page numbers in *italics* indicate illustrations.
Page numbers followed by *t* indicate tables.

531

Child mortality, definition of, 256

Childbearing, legal abortion versus, public health impact of, 308–9

Childhood, early, deaths in, from chromosome abnormalities, 15–16

Chimera, whole-body, 160–61

Chlordiazepoxide, neurobehavioral effects of, 236

Chloroprocaine, neurobehavioral effects of, 234, 235

Chorion, shared, by monozygotic twins, 160

Chromosomally normal conceptus, risk of aborting, maternal age and, 34

Chromosome abnormalities, 318
  antisocial behavior and, 17
  autoimmunity and, 18
  birth order and, 8
  congenital defects from, 16
  consanguinity and, 11
  deaths from
    embryonic, 14–15
    in early childhood, 15–16
    fetal, 14–15
    in infancy, 15–16
  environmental factors in, 11–14
  ethnic factors in, 10
  family clustering of, 8–9
  inbreeding and, 11
  infertility and, 17
  malignancy and, 18
  maternal age and, 6–7
  mental retardation from, 16
  morbidity from, 14–18
  mortality from, 14–18
  oral contraceptives and, 13
  paternal age and, 7–8
  prevalence of, at different stages of life, 4–6
  racial factors in, 10
  radiation and, 11–13
  seasonality and, 9
  sexual differentiation abnormalities and, 17
  socioeconomic factors in, 10–11
  spatial clustering of, 9
  spontaneous abortions and, 17, 28–31
  temporal clustering of, 9
  type of, 3–4
  viruses and, 13

Chvostek's reflex in Prechtl's neurologic examination, 473

Cigarette smoking, maternal. *See* Smoking, maternal

Circulatory anastomosis between placentas of DZ twins, 159–60

Classification of exposure in assessment of occupational and environmental exposures, 458

Clomiphene, neurobehavioral effects of, 233

Clonus in Prechtl's neurologic examination, 472

Clustering of multiple births, analysis of, for statistical studies of multiple births, 157

Coital frequency, twinning rate and, 171–72

Comparative studies, sample size determination in, 357–69. *See also* Sample size, determination of, in comparative studies

Conception, intendedness of, attitudes toward pregnancy and, 284–85

Conceptus
  chromosomally normal, risk of aborting, maternal age and, 34
  monosomy X, risk of aborting maternal age and, 32–33
  trisomic, risk of aborting, maternal age and, 33–34

Congenital defects
  from chromosome abnormalities, 16
  classification of, problems in, 424–25
  deformational, definition of, 424
  developmental definition of, 424–25
  drug-induced, epidemiologic investigation of
    analysis of syndromes in, 425
    case-control studies in, 426–27
    classification problems in, 424–25
    controls in: number of, 435–36; other cases as, 436–40; selection of, 435–40
    exposure assessment in, 431–35; extent of exposure in, 432–34; recall bias in, 435–35; time of exposure in, 431
    methodologic issues in, 423–45
    multiple observations in, 430
    one-versus two-tailed tests in, 429–30

544

Sexual differentiation, abnormalities of, chromosome abnormalities and, 18

Shift, minimum detectable, as continuous variable in sample size determination, 361–62

Skin
in Dubowitz scale for gestational age assessment, 469
in Prechtl's neurologic examination, 473

Sleep disturbances in fetal alcohol syndrome, 220

Slow-to-warm-up child, description of, 484

Smoking, maternal
effects of, on offspring, 221–24
and oral contraceptives, congenital malformations and, 440–42
perinatal mortality and, 123
prematurity and, 77, 78t
spontaneous abortion and, 36–37
sudden infant death syndrome and, 347
and tranquilizers, congenital malformations and, 441–42

Social class
perinatal mortality and, 111–14
twinning rate and, 167–68

Social drinker, offspring of, 220–21

Society and SIDS, 351

Sociodemographic attributes of mother, SIDS and, 348

Socioeconomic status
chromosome abnormalities and, 10–11
congenital infection incidence and, 193
hydatidiform mole and, 331
nervous system malformations and, 64
prematurity and, 78t, 80

Solvents, neurobehavioral effects of, 240

Spatial clustering of chromosome abnormalities, 9

Speech disorders, chromosome abnormalities and, 17

Spermicides
chromosome abnormalities and, 13
spontaneous abortion and, 38–39

Spina bifida, 52–66
case series of, 52–53
diagnosis of, 55

population studies of
in Charleston: comparison of, with other communities, 62–63; results of, 58–62
choosing population for, 55–58
considerations in, 53–55
medical facilities in, 57–58
population composition in, 56
population dispersion and stability in, 56
population size in, 55–56
possible risk factors for, 63–65

Spinal anesthesia, neurobehavioral effects of, 235

Spinal vertebrae in Prechtl's neurologic examination, 475

Spontaneous abortion(s), 23–44
ascertainment of, 27–28
causes of, 31–44
definitions of, 24, 26
gravidity and, 35–36
heterogeneity among, 28–31
incidence of, estimates of, 23–24, 25t
induced abortion and, 39–43
intrauterine devices in, 38–39
irradiation and, 43–44
maternal age and, 32–34
maternal alcohol drinking and, 37
maternal cigarette smoking and, 36–37
missed, hydatidiform mole and, 333
multiple, chromosome abnormalities and, 17
occupational exposures and, 42–43
oral contraceptives and, 38–39
parental age in, 32–34
paternal age and, 34
previous spontaneous abortions and, 35–36
risks of, 31–44
spermicides in, 38–39
statistics on, 27–28
twinning rate and, 172–73

Spontaneous motor activity in Prechtl's neurologic examination, 472, 473, 476

Standard error of log odds ratio, 374

Standardization of twinning rates for statistical studies of multiple births, 153–55

Startles in Prechtl's neurologic examination, 472

547

Tranquilizers
neurobehavioral effects of, 236
and smoking, congenital malformations and, 441–42
Tremor in Prechtl's neurologic examination, 472
Trend in odds ratio
displaying of, for dose-response relationship, 377–80
simple test for, in dose-response relationship, 381–82
Trimethadione, neurobehavioral effects of, 230–31
Triplets, 158–59. *See also* Multiple births
Trisomic conceptus, risk of aborting, maternal age and, 33–34
Trisomy(ies). *See also* Chromosome abnormalities
at conception maternal age and, 33
family clustering of, 8–9
maternal age and, 6–7
Trunk incurvation in Prechtl's neurologic examination, 475
Tubes, fallopian, infertility and, 276
Turner syndrome, autoimmunity and, 18
Twinning
dizygotic
genesis of, control points in, 169–70
variants of, 159–60
monozygotic, variants of, 160
rates of
body build and, 167–68
geographic variation in, 163–64
heredity and, 161–63
maternal age and, 161, *162*
nutrition and, 167–68
parity and, 161, *162*
pharmacologic agents and, 168–69
race and, 161–63
social class and, 167–68
standardization of, for statistical studies of multiple births, 153–55
temporal variation in: long-term, 165, *167*; short-term, 164–65, *166*
variables affecting, 161–69; for MZ twinning, 161
variation in: causes of, proposed, 169–76; coital frequency and, 171–72; demographic selection and, 173–74; failure of fertilization and, 171–72; failure of implantation

and, 171; gonadotropin levels and, 170–71; inbreeding and, 173; noxious environmental and, 175–76; psychoendocrine effects on, 174–75; spontaneous abortion and, 172–73
third type of, 160–61
Twins, 152–81. *See also* Multiple births
in birthweight studies, 179–81
in congenital anomalies studies, 176–79
statistics on, collection of, for statistical studies of multiple births, 153
uses of, in perinatal epidemiology, 176–81
zygosity classification of, for statistical studies, 155–56

United States, prematurity in
criteria for, 70–71
historic trends in, 75–76
Unwanted pregnancy, 283–97
concept of, 283–86
federal estimates of, 287–91
National Natality Survey in, 289–91
National Survey of Family Growth in, 287–89
implications of, for programs and policies in, 296–97
Urbanization, twinning rates and, 175
Uterus, rupture of, perinatal mortality and, 131

Vaccine
hepatitis B, in prophylaxis of hepatitis B infection in newborn, 205
rubella, use of, 208
inadvertent, during pregnancy, 208–9
Valium, neurobehavioral effects of, 236
Variables in sample size determination
continuous, 360–63. *See also* Continuous variables in sample size determination
dichotomous, 363–67. *See also* Dichotomous variables in sample size determination